Handbook of Palliative Care

HANDBOOK OF PALLIATIVE CARE

EDITED BY

Richard Kitchen
LOROS Hospice and Leicester Medical School

Christina Faull
LOROS Hospice and University of Leicester

Sarah Russell
Portsmouth Hospitals University NHS Trust

Jo Wilson
Royal Free Hospitals London NHS Foundation Trust

Fourth edition

WILEY Blackwell

Contents

List of Contributors

Gemma Allen
Palliative Care Inclusion and Community Partnerships Lead, The Mary Stevens Hospice, Chair of Palliative Care for People with Learning Disabilities Network (PCPLD) UK

Nikki Archer, MSc nursing, BSc, RGN, AdvDip Counselling
Counsellor and Doctorate student, former director of supportive care
Formerly supportive care director, St Giles Hospice, UK

Michelle Aslett, BPharm (Hons), MRPharmS, CEPIP, PgClinDip
Specialist Palliative Care Pharmacist
Marie Curie Hospice West Midlands, UK

Dr Idris Baker
Consultant in Palliative Medicine, Swansea Bay University Health Board and Honorary Senior Clinical Lecturer Swansea University Medical School
Tŷ Olwen, Morriston Hospital, Swansea, UK

Dr Rachael Barton, MA, MSc, DM, MRCP, FRCR
Consultant Clinical Oncologist
The Queen's Centre for Oncology and Haematology, Hull, UK

Dr Laura L. Calamos, PhD, MSN RN, FNP-BC, FHEA
Clinical Assistant Professor
University of Michigan School of Nursing, USA

Dr Rachel Campbell, MBChB, BSc, MRCP
Palliative Medicine Consultant
South Eastern Health and Social Care Trust, UK

Lesley Charman, RN, BN (Hons), MSc
Team Leader – Palliative Care Team
Leeds Teaching Hospitals NHS Trust, UK

Professor Andrew Chilton, MBBS, FRCP
Consultant Gastroenterologist and Endoscopist, Regional Endoscopy Lead Midlands
Kettering General Hospital Foundation Trust, UK

Monica Compton, BSc (High Honours)
Dietetic Prescribing Advisor for Northamptonshire ICB
Northamptonshire Healthcare Foundation Trust (NHFT), UK

Dr Jenny Cross, PhD, MRCP
Consultant Nephrologist
Royal Free London Hospitals NHS Foundation Trust, UK

Dr Matthew Doré, MBChB, BSc (Hons), MRCP, PGCME
Palliative Care Consultant
Northern Ireland Hospice and Belfast Trust, UK

Carolyn Doyle, RGN, DNSPQ, BSc, PGCE Soul Midwife
Visiting lecturer
City University, London, UK

Dr Alistair Duncan, MBChB, PGDip (Palliative Care and Oncology)
Consultant in Palliative Medicine
Strathcarron Hospice, UK

Professor Christina Faull, BMedSci, MBBS, MD, MRCP, PGCert Med Ed, Dip Clin Hypnosis
Consultant in Palliative Medicine
LOROS Hospice and University of Leicester, UK

Dr Amy Gadoud, MRCP, PhD
Senior Clinical Lecturer and Honorary Consultant in
Palliative Medicine
Lancaster University and Trinity Hospice, Blackpool, UK

Professor Liz Grant, MA, PhD, FRSE, FRCPE, MFPH
Assistant Principal
University of Edinburgh, UK

Professor Karen Hodson, BSc Pharm, MSc, PhD
Professor of Pharmacy Practice and Royal Pharmaceutical
Society Wales (RPS) Policy & Practice Lead
Cardiff University and RPS Wales, UK

Dr Frances Hakkak, MBBS, BSc, MSc, FRCP
Medical Director & Consultant in Palliative Medicine
Compton Care, Wolverhampton, UK

**Emeritus Professor Margaret Louise Holloway, PhD, BA
(Hons), CQSW**
Emeritus Professor
University of Hull, UK

Dr Jed Jerwood, PhD, MA Art Psych
Principal Art Psychotherapist for Community Services,
Birmingham and Solihull Mental Health Foundation Trust
Honorary Research Fellow, Institute of Clinical Sciences
University of Birmingham, UK

Dr Paul Keeley, MBChB, MSc, FRCP
Consultant in Palliative Medicine
Glasgow Royal Infirmary, UK

**Dr Richard Kitchen, BSc, MBChB, MRCP, MA
(Med Ed), PGCert (Clin Onc)**
Consultant in Palliative Medicine and Honorary Senior
Lecturer
LOROS Hospice and Leicester Medical School, UK

Dr Yifan Liang, BM, BCh, MA, DCH, FRCPCH
Consultant in Paediatric Palliative Medicine
Birmingham Women's and Children's NHS Foundation
Trust & Birmingham Community Healthcare NHS
Foundation Trust, UK

Rachel Lukwago, BSc
Health and Social Care Masters in Social work Masters in
Practice Education;

Principal Social Worker/Co-Chair Black Asian & Minority
Ethnic + A staff network
Kingston Adult Social Care, UK

Dr Linda Machin, PhD
Honorary Research Fellow
Keele University, UK

**Dr Rachael Marchant, MBChB, MRCGP, MSc in
Palliative Medicine for Healthcare Professionals**
GP, Medical Director Havens Hospices, RCGP/Marie
Curie End-of-Life Care Clinical Support Fellow
Havens Hospices, UK

Dr Catherine Millington-Sanders, MBBS, FRCGP
GP and RCGP/Marie Curie National End-of-Life Care
Clinical Champion
NHS South West, London, UK

**Dr Kerrie Noonan, BA (Psych), MPsych (Clinical), PhD
MAPS**
Director
Death Literacy Institute, Australia

Professor David Oliver, PhD, FRCP, FRCGP, FEAN
Honorary Professor / Retired Consultant in Palliative
Medicine
Tizard Centre, University of Kent, Canterbury, UK

Kerry Parker, MPharm (Hons), PgClinDip, PgCert
Macmillan Specialist Palliative Care Pharmacist
University Hospitals Coventry and Warwickshire NHS
Trust, UK

Dr Wendy Prentice, MBBS, MA, FRCP
Consultant in Palliative Medicine
Cicely Saunders Institute, King's College Hospital NHS
Foundation Trust, UK

Noura Rizk, BPharm, MPH
Research Officer
Marie Curie, UK

Dr William E. Rosa, PhD, APRN, FAANP, FPCN, FAAN
Assistant Attending Behavioral Scientist & Associate
Editor, Palliative & Supportive Care and Journal of Pain &
Symptom Management;

Department of Psychiatry and Behavioral Sciences,
Memorial Sloan Kettering Cancer Center, New York, NY,
USA

Dr John P. Rosenberg, RN BN, GDNsg (PallCare), MPallC, PhD
Senior Lecturer
University of the Sunshine Coast, Caboolture, Australia

Dr Sarah Russell, RN DHRes, MSc, PGDip, BA (Hons)
Nurse Consultant, Trust Lead Palliative and End-of-Life Care
Portsmouth Hospitals University NHS Trust, UK

Dr Nikhil Sanyal, MBChB, MRCP, BSc (Hons)
Consultant in Palliative Medicine
George Eliot Hospital, Nuneaton, UK

Tes Smith, BA, MA, Social Work NLP Master Practitioner & Coach
Director of Services (Caldicott Guardian & CQC registered manager)
Saint Francis Hospice, Romford, UK

Dr Katie Spencer, MB, BChir, MA (Hons, Cantab), FRCR, PhD
Honorary Consultant Clinical Oncologist and University of Leeds Clinical Academic Fellow
Leeds Cancer Centre and Leeds Institute of Health Sciences, University of Leeds, UK

Professor Paul Thomas, MB, ChB, DCH, MRCGP, MD, DSc (Hons)
GP and Co-Chair Community-Oriented Integration Network (COIN)
London, UK

Revd Susan van Beveren, MA, PGD Bus (Org Chge & Devt), CCPE, Cert Coaching
Head of Pastoral & Spiritual Support Services
Hospital NHS Foundation Trust with Hounslow & Richmond Community Healthcare NHS Trust, UK

Professor Derek Willis, MBChB (Hons), FRCP, MRCGP, Msc, Dip Clin Ed
Visiting Chair University of Chester and Consultant in Palliative Medicine, UK

Dr Jo Wilson, BSc (Hons), RGN, DipHSM, BA (Hons), PhD
Macmillan Consultant Nurse Palliative Care
Royal Free Hospitals London NHS Foundation Trust, UK

Dr Barbara-Anne Wren, C. Psychol CSci, AFBPsS, FFOM (Hons), RCPI
Consultant Psychologist
Wren Psychology Associates and Royal Free London NHS Foundation Trust, UK

Foreword

'I think that light and shadow have exactly the same duality that exists between life and death'. (Manuel Alvarez Bravo)

Few things in life are as certain as that we are all going to die. This means we should all have a vested interest in developing, testing and implementing services and training staff, in order to be able to deliver high quality palliative and end-of-life care for all. We now live in an ageing society where the benefits of living longer may be outweighed by the burden of multiple comorbidities. We are seeing many more patients living with dementia, which rises year on year as the possibility of developing it approximately doubles every five years after the age of sixty five. Frailty is now recognised as a condition and brings its own challenges for health and social care workers, who endeavour to promote and encourage independence, alongside living as well as possible for as long as possible. We need to truly understand dementia and older frail persons' palliative needs in order to be able to deliver the best and most appropriate care to them. We must also remember, and cast an eye over, the informal carers of these patients who must be supported and valued to ensure they have the resilience to continue in their unpaid and extremely important and necessary roles.

The conundrum of choice for patients who have life limiting conditions has boundaries which clinicians need to be mindful of, particularly prior to embarking on advance care planning conversations. We strive for seamless and coordinated care for our patients in the right place at the right time by the right people but resourcing this can be expensive and challenging and often not seen as a priority for commissioning. We cannot guarantee timely and suitable care and/or interventions out of hours, which then falls to urgent care providers who are frequently not prepared or equipped to deliver it. Ambulance services are increasingly filling gaps in community care provision and, as generalist clinicians whose focus of training is to provide life-saving and emergency interventions, recognising dying as opposed to a condition that is potentially reversible, and considering a palliative and end-of-life care approach, requires a massive paradigm shift. More emphasis is now rightly being placed on furnishing generalists with palliative and end-of-life care skills. This will go some way to improve their knowledge and confidence in this important area of care.

Alongside this is our ageing workforce. We need to refocus and reframe our attitudes to training our clinicians of the future. Work is progressing in developing competencies and a framework for nursing, and medical schools are building on their palliative care specialist training, but we need to accolade the significance of this area of care and pay attention to safeguarding our recruitment and retention strategies. A key area of that is providing education and training to hone a workforce fit for purpose and one that is able to safely care for this patient population.

As a society we welcome a public health approach to death and dying. There is a desire to move away from the medical model and work more collaboratively with communities to improve the experience of death, dying and bereavement. Working with, and sharing an understanding of people's different faiths, cultures, ethnicity and sexual orientations, will positively influence the way we care by demonstrating skill, empathy, compassion and sensitivity to their specific needs.

This book, now in its 4th edition, and edited by Professor Christina Faull, Dr Rich Kitchen, Dr Sarah Russell and Dr Jo Wilson offers contemporary information and reference material for the generalist palliative care provider, in primary and secondary care. In addition to the key chapters, there are sections related to frailty, mental health and learning disability. These new chapters indicate and highlight the novel challenges we are encountering in health care and they are warmly welcomed to help with symptom control and decision making.

It is refreshing and pleasing to see a chapter on wellbeing – both for health care professionals and the patients and carers. It is vital we pay due attention to the welfare of ourselves and colleagues. We cannot be expected to care for others if we do not care for ourselves. Sourcing appropriate avenues of support, both professionally and personally, is recognised as being of paramount importance. In addition, the patient and carers need to maintain and preserve their strength in order to receive and manage the care required and develop a robust infrastructure of support.

The book provides a pragmatic approach to care by generalists and, most importantly, in any care setting. It is practical and informative with helpful detail of what and how to do things safely and with assurance that the clinician is providing evidence based care. The variety of topics addressed aims to serve to equip the reader with sufficient knowledge and confidence in managing this cohort of patients and their carers, and enable them to die well in their place of choice.

Dying well should not necessarily be dependent on a specialist palliative care team. Many patients can be safely, effectively and compassionately cared for by the multi-disciplinary team which will include the General Practitioner/doctor, nursing/community team, social care, allied health professionals and the ambulance and urgent care providers. I believe this book will provide a necessary and valuable source of information, guidance, signposting and support for generalists delivering palliative and end-of-life care and I therefore recommend its place on your bookshelf.

Dr Diane Laverty DCP MSc BSc (Hons) RGN
Macmillan Nurse Consultant: Palliative Care
London Ambulance Service NHS Trust

Preface

We four have practiced in palliative and end-of-life care as nurses and doctors for over a 100 years between us in hospital, hospice, care home and community settings. We have a passion for education to improve palliative and end-of-life care and Faull and Kitchen have previously led e-ELCA, the UK national end-of-life care e-learning programme from e-Learning for Healthcare. We want professionals to have ready access to up-to-date and current thinking and hope that this 4th edition of the *Handbook of Palliative Care* provides that in an accessible and engaging way. The COVID-19 pandemic has shone a spotlight on the importance of compassionate palliative and end-of-life care, skilled discussions about preferences, weighing of the burdens and benefits of treatments and the vital integration of families and loved ones into care. It has also revealed the impact caring for dying patients can have on the staff, especially if circumstances mean that care is not able to be provided in the ideal of 'a good death' with human comfort, minimised distress, and with the family present.

As before, the aim of this handbook is to provide a practical and pragmatic approach to supporting patients and those around them. The book does include a good amount of detail, and could also be used as a source of reference. The text is particularly targeted towards those supporting patients with palliative care needs, in the community (General Practitioners, district nurses and others) and in the hospital (a number of members of the multi-disciplinary team). The book is also likely to be useful for those learning their trade as specialists in palliative and end-of-life care.

This 4th edition focuses on holistic care and therapeutic interventions, including several new chapters building on previous editions with content significantly updated to reflect new evidence and practice.

A new chapter 16 Palliative and end-of-life care: Frailty, dementia and multi-morbidity' looks at these increasingly important areas of practice. As global populations age, it is imperative that staff can effectively and compassionately support people with these conditions. The chapter utilises current evidence to highlight principles of optimal palliative care in these groups.

Talking to patients and those around them about their preferences for the future is an important aspect of supporting patients with palliative care needs. The chapter 9 'Recognising deterioration, preparing, and planning for dying' discusses offering and supporting discussions in a timely fashion, allowing patients to receive care that is consistent with their values, goals and preferences.

There is increased recognition of the importance of supporting professionals caring for those with palliative care needs. The chapter 23 'Creating space, clarity, and containment in order to sustain staff: managing the emotional impact of palliative care work' highlights the emotional challenges that staff face, and outlines strategies and interventions that can protect staff.

The *Handbook of Palliative Care* has previously covered 'Palliative Care in the Community', and the chapter in this edition looks at important contemporary publications such as the Daffodil Standards for GPs, reviewing how these can be used to deliver best care. The book also now contains a new complementary chapter 5 'Hospital palliative care', which focusses on how teams can effectively work together in a hospital setting to best support patients.

We hope you enjoy reading each of the chapters as much as we have.

Acknowledgements

This 4th edition has only been made possible through the great endeavour of the many chapter authors, who have contributed much of their own time towards this book. Their time was during the COVID-19 pandemic, with all its consequent increased commitments, so we are particularly appreciative. We are also grateful for the authors' commitment to building the palliative care knowledge of readers and trying to ensure that high-quality palliative care is available to all who need it.

Cover Illustration
About the cover art: This is a water-colour titled "Between Night and Day" (1995) by artist Michele Angelo Petrone, who sadly died in 2007. It is reproduced with kind permission of ONCA, an arts and environment charity which has been looking after Michele Angelo's work since 2017, when it was entrusted with the assets of the MAP Foundation. MAP was an arts in health organisation founded by Michele Angelo to promote expression, communication, and understanding for people affected by life-threatening illness.

1 The Context and Principles of Palliative Care

Christina Faull

Introduction

In my 30 years as a specialist in adult palliative care I consider myself immensely privileged to have worked with patients and their families and learnt so very much from them. As I write this chapter I find myself recalling many of them;

- the man I looked after in my first weeks as a doctor, who had taken an overdose because of his lung cancer;
- the couple with a clear advance directive of "no-intervention" for whom, in the end, it was the right thing to be admitted to intensive care;
- the man who despite multiple pathological fractures needed to travel for a trial chemotherapy as "giving-up" was beyond his ability to cope with;
- the silent lady I couldn't reach;
- the English man with Native American spiritual beliefs who was terrified of being buried alive.

Dying happens to us all and although there is some uniformity in the physical experience of this, all of us live this last part of our life and die in our own, unique way. I am profoundly humbled by the psychological, spiritual, and socio-cultural diversity of approaches that people have expressed in their living and their dying. I also recognise the challenge that this poses for health and care staff in providing effective, personalised care at the end-of-life.

Every man must do two things alone; he must do his own believing and his own dying. Martin Luther King

Dying is a wild night and a new road. Emily Dickinson

Indeed, Allah [alone] has knowledge of the Hour and sends down the rain and knows what is in the wombs. And no soul perceives what it will earn tomorrow, and no soul perceives in what land it will die. Indeed, Allah is Knowing and Acquainted. (Quran, 31:34)

Irrespective of your particular specialty or place of work, most health and care professionals will encounter people with advanced illness, and caring for people in the last months, weeks, and days of life is an important and valued part of their work [1, 2]. It is estimated that 40 million people worldwide require palliative care of whom 69% are adults over sixty years of age and 6% are children [3]. Caring for someone who is nearing the end of their life can be an extremely rewarding area of practice, and this satisfaction is enhanced by confidence in core interpersonal skills and through a basic knowledge of physical and non-physical symptom management [4, 5].

In the developed world at least, most people die from conditions that have been diagnosed for some time and they have multiple contacts with healthcare professionals, offering numerous opportunities for discussions about deterioration, dying and the "trade-offs" or personal priority setting so eloquently argued by Atul Gawande in his book *Being Mortal* [6]. However, we know that these conversations are challenging and there is an ambivalence on the part of professionals to initiate such discussions for a number of well-intended reasons. The COVID-19 pandemic exposed healthcare professionals in a new way to the needs of patients and families for open and honest conversations about prognosis and individual requirements and preferences [7]. This Handbook aims to build your confidence and diminish your ambivalence in having such discussions with people in the last stage of their lives. It will aim to equip you with knowledge and skills in assessment of the patient's needs and context, in physical symptom management and in communication, enabling your practice in empathetic, personalised, holistic care.

Palliative care offers much to patients with advanced illness and to their families. For some patients this is the main approach in their care. For many patients it can improve the quality of their life when used as shown in Figure 1 not as an alternative to other care (brink-of-death care) but as a complementary and vital part of their management, integrated alongside appropriate care to reverse illness or prolong life [8]. The challenges of the parallel approaches of trying to improve physical well-being and prolong life while also addressing the realistic probability of deterioration and death are significant, especially in those illnesses characterised by episodes of acute deterioration. Perhaps one of the biggest challenges we face in medicine and indeed in society is balancing the clinical and ethical "pros and cons" (weighing the burdens, benefits, and risks) of investigation and intervention in those with advanced illness and in the frail elderly. In the United Kingdom, the General Medical Council (GMC) has recommended that end-of-life should be an explicit discussion point when patients are considered likely to die within 12 months [9, 10]. Box 1 identifies the mandated expectations in this guidance [10].

The majority of care received by patients during the last year of their life is in their home or, for many elderly people, in their care home. The fact that their illness is progressing and their functional status deteriorating often means however, that many patients will spend significant time in hospitals during their last year of life. It has been

estimated that 20% of hospital beds are occupied by patients near the end-of-life many of whom do not need, or want, to be there [11] and despite the majority wishing to die at home, almost 50% of patients still die in a hospital in the United Kingdom [12]. The lack of recognition of the fact that patients are nearing the ends of their lives and open discussion of this with the patients and their families is considered a major barrier in achieving better outcomes including enabling people to die with comfort and dignity, to be cared for where they would most want to [11, 13, 14] and fulfilling the many other "wishes" that are important to them.

Palliative care is more than just end-of-life or "brink-of-death" care. Some of the newest challenges are in providing effective support for those living with cancer, or other advanced illness, for long periods of time who are suffering from a complex mix of effects of the illness itself,

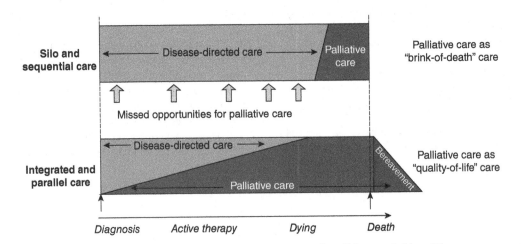

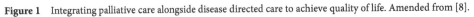

Figure 1   Integrating palliative care alongside disease directed care to achieve quality of life. Amended from [8].

the effects of the treatments for the disease and the psychosocial and psychospiritual impacts of facing not only the fear of recurrence, flare-ups, deterioration and death but also the ongoing symptoms such as fatigue, disability, and the change of role and social and family dynamics [15–17].

There are a broad range of challenges in delivering high-quality palliative, end-of-life, and terminal care including professional competence and confidence, teamwork, and organisational factors, and access to resources. Patients with advanced disease can present some of the most challenging ethical, physical, psychological, and social issues, and it is vital to have a grasp of the communication skills required to explore these issues effectively. It is also important to be able to identify when referrals to specialists and other services are needed.

This chapter outlines the principles that underpin effective care for people with advanced disease, provides some definitions and contexts and presents an overview of the attainment and assessment of quality in palliative care. It focusses mostly on the needs and care of adults although most of the principles are transferable to the care of children. The palliative care of children and young people has some very specific requirements and services and these are discussed in Chapter 15 (Palliative care for infants, children and young people).

Definitions and Explanations

Box 2:   Etymology

The word "hospice" originates from the Latin *hospes* meaning host; *hospitalis*, a further derivative, means friendly, a welcome to the stranger. The word *hospitium* perhaps begins to convey the vital philosophy of the hospice movement: it means the warm feeling between host and guest. Hence, a hospice denotes a place where this feeling is experienced, a place of welcome and care for those in need. The word "palliative" derives from the Latin *pallium*, a cloak. Palliation means cloaking over, not addressing the underlying cause but ameliorating the effects.

Hospice and Palliative Care

Much of our understanding and knowledge of the philosophy, science, and art of palliative care has developed and grown through the work of the hospice movement. Dame

Cicely Saunders worked with patients suffering from advanced cancer and undertook systematic narrative research to understand what patients were experiencing and needed. The bedrock of the hospice philosophy is that of patient-centred holistic care focusing on quality of life and extending support to significant family members:

> What links the many professionals and volunteers who work in hospice or palliative care is an awareness of the many needs of a person and his/her family and carers as they grapple with all the demands and challenges introduced by the inexorable progress of a disease that has outstripped the possibilities of cure [18].

Saunders opened the first Hospice in London in 1967 and since then services supporting people with terminal illness have spread across the world with more than 16,000 hospices or palliative care units. Although "hospice" has perhaps become thought of as a location of care, a place, it is much more than this and in essence is synonymous with palliative care. Both have a philosophy of care not dependent on a place or a building but on attitude, expertise, and understanding.

The term "palliative care" was coined by Canadian urological cancer surgeon, Balfour Mount, as a term to apply hospice principles more broadly including within the hospital and home settings. More recently, the term *specialist palliative care* has been used to represent those professionals and services that concentrate on this area of health care as their main role and expertise, recognising that almost all healthcare professionals provide elements of palliative care for patients as part of their practice.

Palliative care has been defined by the World Health Organisation as:

> "An approach that improves the quality of life of patients and their families facing the problems associated with life-threatening illness, through the prevention and relief of suffering by means of early identification and impeccable assessment and treatment of pain and other problems, physical, psychosocial and spiritual" [19 p. 84].

Palliative care [19]:
- provides relief from pain and other distressing symptoms;
- affirms life and regards dying as a normal process;
- intends neither to hasten nor postpone death;
- integrates the psychological and spiritual aspects of patient care;
- offers a support system to help patients live as actively as possible until death;

• offers a support system to help the family cope during the patient's illness and in their own bereavement;
• uses a team approach to address the needs of patients and their families, including bereavement counselling, if indicated;
• will enhance quality of life and may also positively influence the course of illness; and
• is applicable early in the course of illness, in conjunction with other therapies that are intended to prolong life, such as chemotherapy or radiation therapy, and includes those investigations needed to better understand and manage distressing clinical complications.

To this end palliative care is a partnership between the patient, their family carers, and a wide range of professionals. It integrates the psychological, physical, social, cultural, and spiritual aspects of a patient's care, acknowledging and respecting the uniqueness of each individual:

> You matter because you are you, and you matter until the last moment of your life. We will do all that we can to help you not only to die peacefully, but to live until you die [20].

End-of-life Care

End-of-life care can be a confusing term since it may be interpreted by patients, families and professionals as meaning someone is dying very soon, within days (see last days of life below). However, in health and care policy and practice standards such as for instance those of the UK National Institute for Health and Care Excellence (NICE) and the General Medical Council, end-of-life care is usually regarded as a focus on the last 6-12 months of life and refers to the care needed by everyone as they approach the end part of their lives [9, 21]. It is of course difficult to define the last 12 months of life prospectively and much thought has been given to how indicators may help identify people. Figure 2 shows an example developed in Scotland of how such indicators can be incorporated into guidance to help professionals and services identify people who are at risk of deteriorating and dying.

The End-of-Life Care strategy (EoLCS) in England and Wales defined a pathway to optimise the quality of care in the last months of life (Figure 3) [12]. Many other countries have had similar initiatives.

To ensure that "I can make the last stage of my life as good as possible because everyone works together confidently, honestly and consistently to help me and the people who are important to me, including my carer(s)." the UK National Palliative and End-of-Life Care Partnership has introduced six ambitions with six underpinning foundations (Figure 4) [22].

Last Days of Life and Terminal Care

When a patient becomes so unwell that they will die soon, that they are actively dying, this may be called terminal care or care in the last days of life. In some countries this is referred to as "brink-of-death" care. The standards of care needed at this time has been a focus of considerable attention and resulted in defining the priorities of care for the dying person in England (Figure 5) [23].

Care after Death and Bereavement Care

After a patient has died there is still much that needs attention. The persons' body will need care and preparation that is personalised to their religious, cultural, and pre-morbid instructions. The family and religious practitioners may wish to be involved in this to say goodbyes or in performing cleansing and dressing for burial or cremation.

Bereavement and grief are universal experiences but can have diverse impacts on individuals. The impact of the loss of a loved-one is life-long. It may cause immediate critical issues such as the care of a child and the grief may be problematic for some causing significant changes in wellbeing, mental health, and social and financial functioning. More information on this is available in Chapter 8 (Integrating new perspectives: Working with loss and grief in palliative care).

Specialist Palliative Care

Specialist palliative care came into focus with the founding of St Christopher's Hospice by Saunders. It was here that an approach was developed that formed the basis for the role of specialist services which include hospices, hospice at home, and hospital and community palliative care teams. These services provide:

• High-quality care for patients and their relatives, especially those with complex needs.
• A range of services to help provide optimum care: whether the patient was at home, in hospital, or required specialist in-patient care.
• Education, advice, and support to other professionals.
• Evidence-based practice.
• Research and evaluation.

The subsequent, mostly unplanned, often charitably funded, growth of specialist palliative care services has led

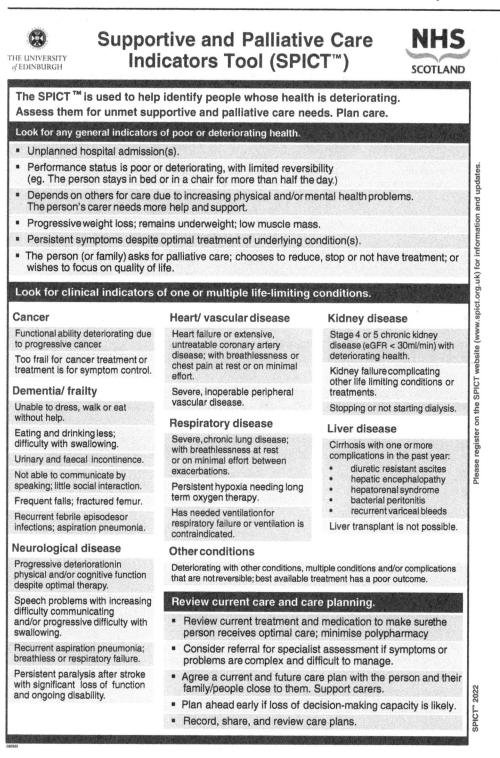

THE UNIVERSITY *of* EDINBURGH

Supportive and Palliative Care Indicators Tool (SPICT™)

NHS SCOTLAND

The SPICT™ is used to help identify people whose health is deteriorating. Assess them for unmet supportive and palliative care needs. Plan care.

Look for any general indicators of poor or deteriorating health.

- Unplanned hospital admission(s).
- Performance status is poor or deteriorating, with limited reversibility (eg. The person stays in bed or in a chair for more than half the day.)
- Depends on others for care due to increasing physical and/or mental health problems. The person's carer needs more help and support.
- Progressive weight loss; remains underweight; low muscle mass.
- Persistent symptoms despite optimal treatment of underlying condition(s).
- The person (or family) asks for palliative care; chooses to reduce, stop or not have treatment; or wishes to focus on quality of life.

Look for clinical indicators of one or multiple life-limiting conditions.

Cancer

Functional ability deteriorating due to progressive cancer

Too frail for cancer treatment or treatment is for symptom control.

Dementia/ frailty

Unable to dress, walk or eat without help.

Eating and drinking less; difficulty with swallowing.

Urinary and faecal incontinence.

Not able to communicate by speaking; little social interaction.

Frequent falls; fractured femur.

Recurrent febrile episodes or infections; aspiration pneumonia.

Neurological disease

Progressive deterioration in physical and/or cognitive function despite optimal therapy.

Speech problems with increasing difficulty communicating and/or progressive difficulty with swallowing.

Recurrent aspiration pneumonia; breathless or respiratory failure.

Persistent paralysis after stroke with significant loss of function and ongoing disability.

Heart/ vascular disease

Heart failure or extensive, untreatable coronary artery disease; with breathlessness or chest pain at rest or on minimal effort.

Severe, inoperable peripheral vascular disease.

Respiratory disease

Severe, chronic lung disease; with breathlessness at rest or on minimal effort between exacerbations.

Persistent hypoxia needing long term oxygen therapy.

Has needed ventilation for respiratory failure or ventilation is contraindicated.

Other conditions

Deteriorating with other conditions, multiple conditions and/or complications that are not reversible; best available treatment has a poor outcome.

Kidney disease

Stage 4 or 5 chronic kidney disease (eGFR < 30ml/min) with deteriorating health.

Kidney failure complicating other life limiting conditions or treatments.

Stopping or not starting dialysis.

Liver disease

Cirrhosis with one or more complications in the past year:
- diuretic resistant ascites
- hepatic encephalopathy
- hepatorenal syndrome
- bacterial peritonitis
- recurrent variceal bleeds

Liver transplant is not possible.

Review current care and care planning.

- Review current treatment and medication to make sure the person receives optimal care; minimise polypharmacy
- Consider referral for specialist assessment if symptoms or problems are complex and difficult to manage.
- Agree a current and future care plan with the person and their family/people close to them. Support carers.
- Plan ahead early if loss of decision-making capacity is likely.
- Record, share, and review care plans.

Please register on the SPICT website (www.spict.org.uk) for information and updates.

SPICT™ 2022

Figure 2   The supportive and palliative care indicators guidance (2019) used in Lothian National Health Service (NHS), Scotland. (Reproduced with permission from NHS, available at www.palliativecareguidelines.scot.nhs.uk).

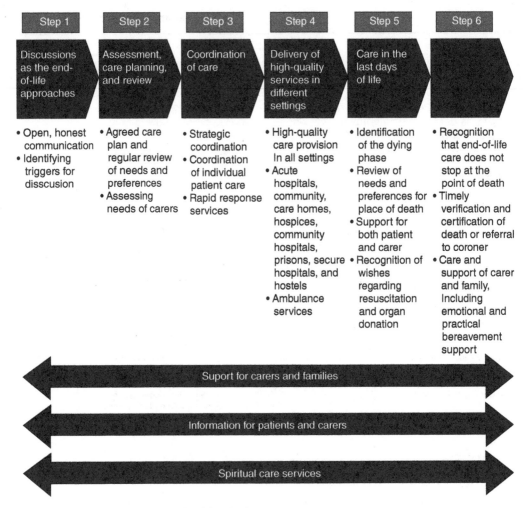

Step 1	Step 2	Step 3	Step 4	Step 5	Step 6
Discussions as the end-of-life approaches	Assessment, care planning, and review	Coordination of care	Delivery of high-quality services in different settings	Care in the last days of life	

• Open, honest communication • Identifying triggers for disscusion	• Agreed care plan and regular review of needs and preferences • Assessing needs of carers	• Strategic coordination • Coordination of individual patient care • Rapid response services	• High-quality care provision In all settings • Acute hospitals, community, care homes, hospices, community hospitals, prisons, secure hospitals, and hostels • Ambulance services	• Identification of the dying phase • Review of needs and preferences for place of death • Support for both patient and carer • Recognition of wishes regarding resuscitation and organ donation	• Recognition that end-of-life care does not stop at the point of death • Timely verification and certification of death or referral to coroner • Care and support of carer and family, Including emotional and practical bereavement support

Suport for carers and families

Information for patients and carers

Spiritual care services

Figure 3   The end-of-life care pathway. (Reproduced from [12]).

Six ambitions to bring that vision about

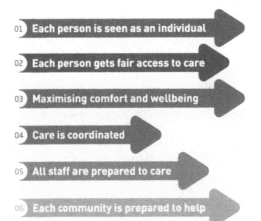

01 Each person is seen as an individual
02 Each person gets fair access to care
03 Maximising comfort and wellbeing
04 Care is coordinated
05 All staff are prepared to care
06 Each community is prepared to help

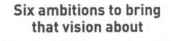

"I can make the last stage of my life as good as possible because everyone works together confidently, honestly and consistently to help me and the people who are important to me, including my carer(s)."

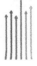

Figure 4   The ambitions of the National Palliative and End-of-Life Care Partnership in England [22].

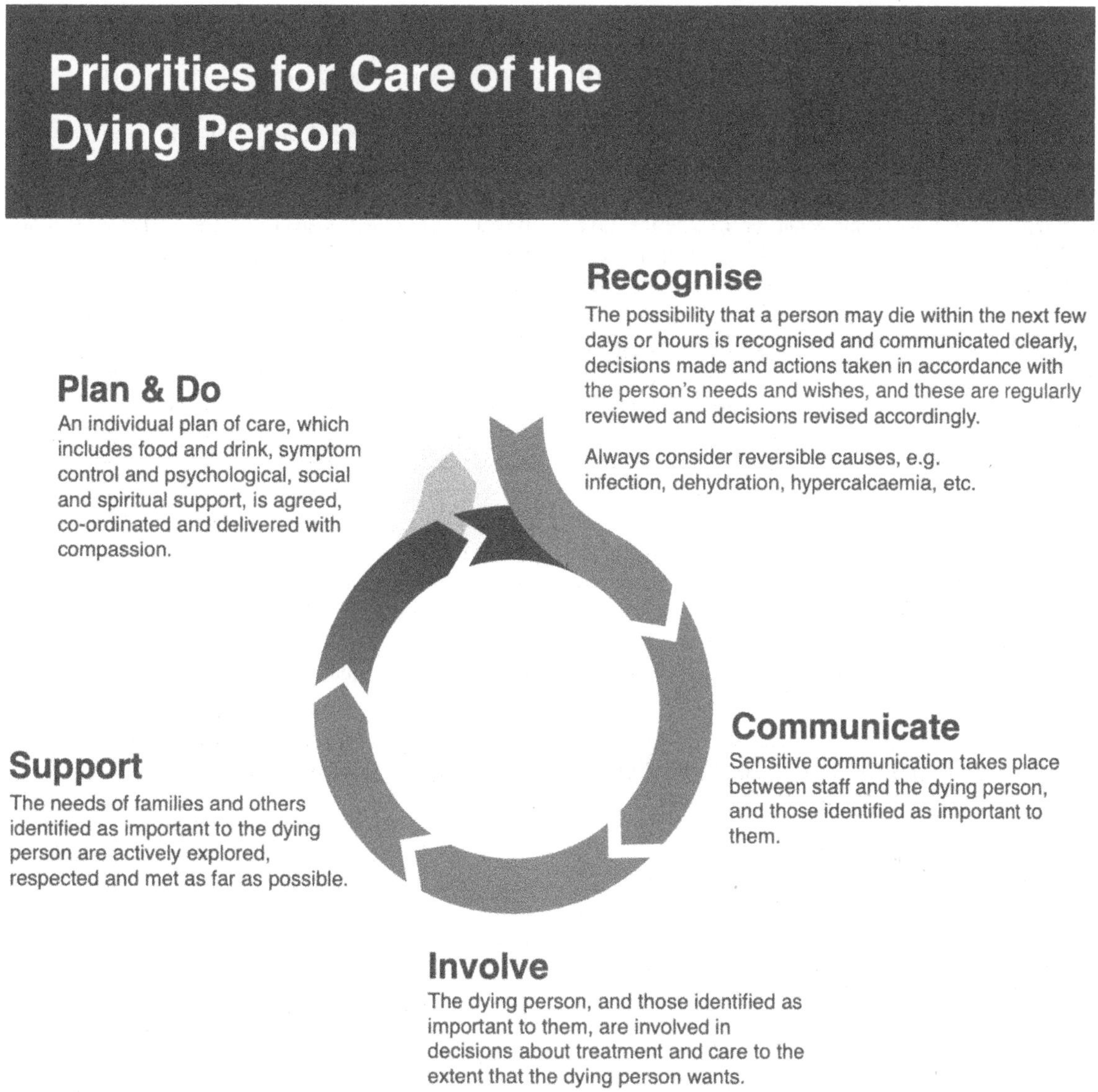

Priorities for Care of the Dying Person

Recognise

The possibility that a person may die within the next few days or hours is recognised and communicated clearly, decisions made and actions taken in accordance with the person's needs and wishes, and these are regularly reviewed and decisions revised accordingly.

Always consider reversible causes, e.g. infection, dehydration, hypercalcaemia, etc.

Plan & Do

An individual plan of care, which includes food and drink, symptom control and psychological, social and spiritual support, is agreed, co-ordinated and delivered with compassion.

Support

The needs of families and others identified as important to the dying person are actively explored, respected and met as far as possible.

Communicate

Sensitive communication takes place between staff and the dying person, and those identified as important to them.

Involve

The dying person, and those identified as important to them, are involved in decisions about treatment and care to the extent that the dying person wants.

Figure 5 The five priorities of care for the dying person [23].

to a wide variety of models of service provision, distribution, and funding, with some areas, and therefore patients, being better served than others.

Not everyone that dies will have such complex needs that they require direct contact with specialist palliative care services. In integrated services that provide high quality care for people at the end of their lives those that provide the direct contact are advised, supported, and trained by this small group of specialists.

Issues for Palliative Care Worldwide

Fifty-nine million people die across the world each year, 80% of deaths occurring in developing countries. The world population is estimated to increase by 50% in the next 50 years and almost all of this increase in population will be in the developing world. In addition, there will be a huge shift in age of the population with a two- to threefold increase in population aged over 60 years in both the developed and the developing world.

The 2018 the *Lancet* Commission on Palliative Care and Pain Relief stated that no other important health intervention is as lacking or inequitably distributed as pain relief, the pillar of palliative care [24]. It estimated that 45% of all deaths in 2015 (25 million people) experienced serious suffering, 80% of whom were in low income countries. Despite the 2014 World Health Assembly resolution calling for all member states to develop, strengthen, and implement palliative care services as part of universal health coverage [25], such services remain underdeveloped or non-existent in many parts of the world, 45% of countries having no access to palliative care [26]. The global burden of serious health-related suffering is projected to double by 2060 [27].

Although not enshrined in the Human Rights Act, most would agree that every individual has the right to pain relief and the International Association for the Study of Pain constructed a declaration to this effect in 2010. Inexpensive, effective methods exist to relieve pain and other symptoms but tens of millions of people die each year in unrelieved suffering. The *Lancet* Commission recommended that morphine be made available alongside an essential package

of other low cost drugs, medical equipment and human resources (Box 3). They call for all countries to ensure universal access to this Essential Package by 2030.

Under the international treaty, *Single Convention on Narcotic Drugs* [28], governments are responsible for ensuring that opioids are available for pain management. The 2021 report from the International Narcotics Control Board, marking sixty years of the treaty, showed that opioids are still not widely available for medical needs [29]. More than 90% of the global morphine is used in industrialised countries where 17% of the world's population live. Over 75% of the world population will have insufficient analgesia, or no analgesia at all if they suffer from pain.

The main impediments to opioid availability are government concern about addiction; insufficient training of healthcare professionals; and restrictive laws over the manufacture, distribution, prescription, and dispensing of opioids. There is also considerable prescribing reluctance on the part of the healthcare profession, due in part to concerns about legal sanctions. This is made worse by the burden of regulatory requirements, the often insufficient import or manufacture of opioids, and the fear of the potential for diversion of opioids for non-legitimate use.

Box 3:   The Essential Package of medications that need to be universally available [24]

Amitriptyline
Bisacodyl (Senna)
Dexamethasone
Diazepam
Diphenhydramine (chlorpheniramine, cyclizine, or dimenhydrinate)
Fluconazole
Fluoxetine or other selective serotonin-reuptake inhibitors (sertraline and citalopram)
Furosemide
Hyoscine butylbromide
Haloperidol
Ibuprofen (naproxen, diclofenac, or meloxicam)
Lactulose (sorbitol or polyethylene glycol)
Loperamide
Metoclopramide
Metronidazole
Morphine (oral immediate-release and injectable)
Naloxone parenteral
Omeprazole
Ondansetron
Paracetamol
Petroleum jelly

Unmet Need and Continued Suffering in the Developed World

The major challenge for those who seek to improve the care for patients with advanced disease is to ensure that all healthcare professionals consider palliative care an important part of the care of their patients, is a responsibility in their own role and that they have adequate skills, knowledge, and specialist support to undertake it effectively. This is of crucial importance in the 70% of the week that occurs "out-of-hours" when patients are especially vulnerable to the deficits in healthcare systems.

There are defined groups of patients who have poor outcomes, who underutilise specialist palliative care services, who have insufficient access to services and for whom service models need to develop to meet their needs in an appropriate way. Patients with illnesses other than cancer and those who are old and frail are considerably disadvantaged compared to those with cancer, and chapters later in this book discuss these issues in some depth and provide information on how to tackle them.

Health professionals over the world recognise the fundamental human right to die with dignity. However, the notion of what constitutes a "good death" may vary considerably between and within cultures. Additionally, while it has been shown that there are greater similarities than differences between cultures when living and dealing with illness such as cancer we know that it is more difficult for people from ethnically minoritised communities to access or obtain information, support, and services that will meet their needs. Issues of communication, applicability of information, organisational and staff attitudes, and discrimination are contributing factors across the spectrum of health and illness contexts, and having cancer is no exception to this experience [30, 31, 32]. Compounding this disadvantage and poor quality of life is that people from diverse ethnic communities are more likely to be poor and have financial and housing difficulties. Professionals need to tailor their care for patients with greater understanding of socio-cultural and spiritual contexts as well as to individual variations in concepts of disclosure and open discussion of deterioration and dying, patient autonomy and collective decision making, and preferences and wishes that constitute a good death.

Gatrad and colleagues [33] suggest that realising high-quality palliative care for all will need fundamental changes on at least three fronts:

1. Tackling institutional discrimination in the provision of palliative care.

2. Progress in incorporating transcultural medicine into medical and nursing curriculums.

3. A greater willingness on the part of health-care providers to embrace complexity.

Cicely Saunders developed the model of holistic care termed "Total Pain" which is explored further in Chapter 10 (Pain and its management). Using this model can help us see how marginalised groups of people may suffer more "social pain" than others. For example Gunaratunum has done much to help us understand more about migrant communities and the suffering that may be unfathomable to health professionals unless we open our minds to understand their life journey [34, 35].

Enabling People to Be at Home

The majority of people wish, ideally to die at home with the family around them. However, some people don't want this. For some leaving this memory or bad spirit for the family may be something they don't want. For others they only want to be at home if their symptoms are well managed and for many the prime consideration is whether their family can cope.

Death in the patient's preferred place of care can sometimes be used as a measure of quality of care and is quite a reductionist construct given that for many people the "choice" is so dependent on a number of variables (symptoms, family, money, services, and support) and how they play out. However, wherever the patient wants to be at the end they will spend a lot of time at home in the last months of their illness.

The key things that need to be in place to achieve the best possible care for people in the last months of life include:

• identifying people that are approaching the end-of-life (around 1% of GP list), maybe using the Supportive and Palliative Care indicators (SPICT) tool (Figure 2) and for the patient who has become very unwell, the "uncertain recovery" model such as AMBER Care can help integrate a palliative care approach [36].

• Information sharing, discussions and care planning for deterioration (steps 1-2 of the pathway in Figure 3);

• coordination of care, availability of medication and equipment, and rapid access to help and expertise (Ambitions statement 4, Figure 4);

• delivery of high-quality care by trained and competent practitioners in all service sectors. (Ambitions statement 5, Figure 4)

These facets of care are discussed in depth in other chapters of this book, and Chapter 20 (Care in the last days of life and after death) focusses specifically on enabling people to die in the place of their choice.

Thomas [37, 38] developed seven standards (Box 4) to help primary care providers and teams improve their

---

Box 4:   The seven "Cs": gold standards for palliative care in primary care

Communication: Practice register; regular team meetings for information sharing, planning, and reflection/audit; patient information; patient-held records.

Coordination: Nominated coordinator maintains register, organises meetings, audit, education symptom sheets, and other resources.

Control of symptoms: Holistic, patient centred assessment and management.

Continuity out-of-hours: Effective transfer of information to and from out-of-hours services. Access to drugs and equipment.

Continued learning: Audit/reflection/critical incident analysis. Use of continuing professional development time.

Carer support: Practical, financial, emotional, and bereavement support.

Care in the dying phase: Protocol-driven care addressing physical, emotional, and spiritual needs. Care needs around and after death acted upon.

delivery of palliative care. In partnership with Marie Curie these have been used to develop the "Daffodil" quality standards of the UK Royal College of GPs to help optimise the care of patients in their homes [39]. This is explored further in Chapter 4 (Palliative care in the community).

Communication with, and the quality of, out-of-hours primary care services is of critical importance in achieving the goals of care [40, 41]. In more closed health systems such as the hospice programme in the United States, achievement of care and death at home is almost a prerequisite criterion of entry to the programme and therefore self-fulfilling; however, 80% of deaths in America are in hospital and only 7% die at home under hospice care.

The Principles of Palliative Care

Knowing how to approach patients with advanced illness is the first step in achieving effective care. Six key principles underpin effective, holistic care:

1. Consider the patient and their family/carers as the unit of care while respecting patient autonomy and confidentiality and acknowledge and encourage their participation.
2. Perform a systematic assessment of physical, psychological, information, social, financial, cultural and spiritual needs.
3. Communicate findings to the patient, providing information and support at all stages.
4. Relieve the patient's symptoms promptly: *There is only today*.
5. Plan proactively and thoroughly for potential/anticipated future problems.
6. Use a team approach listening to suggestions and views and involving resources for extra support at an early stage.

What Do Patients and Their Carers Need?

The uniqueness of each individual's situation must be acknowledged and the manner of care adapted accordingly. The essence of what patients and their carers may need is outlined in Box 5.

It should be clear from this that communication skills (see Chapter 7: Conversations and communication) play a fundamental role in achieving good palliative care and quality of life for the patient:

> Almost invariably, the act of communication is an important part of the therapy; occasionally it is the only constituent. It usually requires greater thought and planning than a drug prescription, and unfortunately it is commonly administered in subtherapeutic doses [42].

Box 5:   The rights and needs of patients and their carers

Patients have a right to confidentiality, pain control, and other symptom management and, wherever possible, to choose the setting of death and the degree of family and professional involvement. They also have a right to deny the illness.

Information

The patient has a need to be offered sensitive, clear explanations of:

- the diagnosis and its implications;
- the likely effects of treatments on activities of daily living and well-being;
- the type and extent of support that may be required and how it may be addressed; and
- expected symptoms and what may be done about them.

Quality of life

The patient has a need for life that is as normal, congenial, independent, and as dignified as possible.

An individual's quality of life will depend on minimising the gap between their expectations and aspirations and their actual experiences. This may be achieved by:

- respect, as a person as well as a patient, from properly trained staff who see themselves as partners in living,
- effective relief from pain and other distressing symptoms,
- an appropriate and satisfying diet;
- comfort and consolation, especially from those who share the patient's values and beliefs and/or belong to the same cultural community;
- companionship from family and friends and from members of the care team;
- continuity of care from both the primary care team and other services;
- consistent and effective response to changes in physical and psychosocial discomfort; and
- information about support and self-help and other groups and services.

Support for carers

The patient's family or other carers have a need for support at times of crises in the illness and in their bereavement. These needs include:

- practical support with financial, legal, housing, or welfare problems;
- information about the illness (with the patient's consent) and the available support;
- respite from the stress of caring;
- involvement of carers in the moment of death and in other aspects of care;
- bereavement support; and
- special support where the patient's death may directly affect young children or where the patient is a child or adolescent.

Achieving Good Symptom Management

The management of any problem should be approached as follows:

- Anticipation
- Evaluation and assessment
- Explanation and information
- Individualised, personalised treatment
- Re-evaluation and supervision
- Attention to detail
- Continuity of care.

Anticipation

Many physical and nonphysical problems can often be anticipated and in some instances prevented. Failure to anticipate problems and to set up appropriate management strategies (e.g., who should they call?) is a common source of dissatisfaction for patients. Understanding the natural history of the disease with specific reference to an individual patient, awareness of the patient's psychosocial circumstances and identification of risk factors allows planning of care by the team. For an example of applying this in practice, see Box 6.

Evaluation and Assessment

An understanding of the pathophysiology and likely cause(s) of any particular problem is vital in selecting and directing appropriate investigations and treatment. Deciding what treatment to use is based on consideration of the evidence of the mechanism of the symptom and of the treatment's

---

Box 6: Applying an understanding of the natural history of a disease and psychosocial awareness to care planning

A 45-year-old woman has recently been found to have spinal metastases from her breast cancer. Potential issues that could be anticipated are:

- Pain – due to the bony origin; this may need non-steroidal anti-inflammatory drug (NSAID), opioids, and radiotherapy.
- Constipation – start laxatives when opioid is prescribed.
- Spinal cord compression – examine neurology if unsteady or complains of numbness.
- If she has young children – may need help, practically and in telling the children.
- Work – may she need financial and benefit advice?
- Hypercalcaemia – check blood if nauseated or confused.
- Psychospiritual – how is she coping with the impact?

---

efficacy, safety, and appropriateness in the situation. This is illustrated by the following specific examples:

- Sedation for an agitated patient with urinary retention is not as helpful as catheterisation.
- Antiemetics for the nausea of hypercalcaemia are important but so too is lowering the serum calcium (if appropriate).
- A patient who is fearful of dying may be helped more by discussing and addressing specific fears rather than taking benzodiazepines.
- Pain in a vertebral metastasis may be helped by analgesics, radiotherapy, orthopaedic surgery, transcutaneous electrical nerve stimulation, and acupuncture. A decision as to which to prescribe is made only by careful assessment.

Comorbidity is common and should always be considered. For example, it is easy (and unfortunately common) to assume that the pain in a patient with cancer is caused by the cancer. In one series almost a quarter of pains in patients with cancer were unrelated to the cancer or the cancer treatment [43].

The multidimensional nature of symptoms, such as pain, means that the use of drugs may be only one part of treatment. A holistic assessment is vital in enabling the most effective management plan. This includes eliciting the patient's concerns and focusing on their feelings.

Explanation and Information

Management of a problem should always begin with explanation of the findings and diagnostic conclusions. This usually reduces the patient's anxieties, even if it confirms their worst suspicions – a monster in the light is usually better faced than a monster unseen in the shadows. Further information may be useful to some patients. A clear explanation of the suggested treatments and follow up plan is important for the patient to gain a sense of control and security. Allow plenty of space for questions and check that what you meant to convey has been understood. Some real examples:

- Mr H, with advanced liver disease, was very anxious in the outpatient department. He told me he had developed a tender lump on his chest. On examination this turned out to be gynaecomastia, most probably, I thought, due to the spironolactone. With this explanation, and the relief of his anxiety, he chose to continue the drug rather than have recurrence of his ascites.
- Mrs S looked worried and was angry. We discussed the scan results she had had six months earlier, before her chemotherapy and surgery. "So what does that mean?" she asked. "I'm afraid that means the cancer cannot be cured,"

I said. She dissolved in tears and said "Thank you doctor. I have been thinking this, but no one would tell me."

Individualised Treatment
The individual physical, social, and psychological circumstances of the patient and their views and wishes should be considered in planning care. For example, lymphoedema compression bandages may be unused unless there is someone available to help the patient to fit them daily.

Treatment options need to be shared with the patient and their perspective on choices be explored. For example:
• Mr K developed arterial occlusion in his leg. Because of his other symptoms, he was thought to have recurrent bladder cancer, but this was not confirmed by scans. He needed to consider whether to have an amputation. It appeared most likely that he would die from his cancer within the next weeks to months. He decided that he would only have the amputation if he had six months or more to live and he declined the operation.

Re-evaluation and Supervision: Be Proactive
The symptoms of frail patients with advanced disease can change frequently. New problems can occur and established ones worsen. Interventions may be complex (many patients take more than 20 pills a day), and close supervision is vital to ensure optimum efficacy and tailoring to the patient. Family carers may take on a lot of new tasks including managing medicines and using equipment. Educating and empowering family carers to feel safe, listened to, and supported is vital for the patient's care but also the family carer wellbeing and bereavement. One key action is to make sure that family carers know how to safely dispose of medicines when they are no longer needed (take them to the pharmacy).

Attention to Detail
The quality of palliative care is in the detail of care. For example, it is vital to ensure that the patient not only has a prescription for the correct drug but also can obtain it from the pharmacy, have adequate supplies to cover a (long) weekend, and understand how to adjust it if the problem worsens.

Continuity of Care
No professional can be available for 24 hours, and 7 days a week, but patients may need support at all hours of the day. Transfer of information within teams and to those that may be called upon to provide care (e.g., out-of-hours services) is one way of ensuring continuity of care. Patient-held records, clear plans in nursing care records at the patient's house, team handover/message books, and formalised information for out-of-hours services [44] are all ways to achieve this.

Limits of Symptom Control
There is always something more that can be done to help a patient, but it is not always possible to completely relieve symptoms. Specialist advice should usually have been sought for help in the management of intractable symptoms. This extra support is in itself an important way of helping the patient.

In such situations an acceptable solution must be found to provide adequate relief of distress for the patient. For the management of a physical symptom and sometimes of psychological distress, this may be a compromise between the presence of the symptom and sedation from medications. It is hard for a team to accept suboptimal relief of symptoms, and discussions with the patient and the family may be very difficult. It is important for the team to remember the great value of their continuing involvement to the patients and their carers, to acknowledge how difficult the situation is, and not to abandon the patient because it is painful and distressing for the professionals:

> Slowly, I learn about the importance of powerlessness.
> I experience it in my own life and I live with it in my work.
> The secret is not to be afraid of it—not to run away.
> The dying know we are not God.
> All they ask is that we do not desert them [45].

Attaining Quality in Palliative Care

The quality of palliative and end-of-life care is an area of increasing focus. Discussion of treatment benefits and burdens and of end-of-life choices is an important feature of quality in advanced disease.

The National Institute for Health and Clinical Excellence (NICE) in the United Kingdom has developed Quality Standards for end-of-life care for adults [46] and for the care of adults in the last days of life [47]. The four statements of quality for priority areas for improvement in care in the last days of life are shown in Box 7. The NICE quality standards for end-of-life care for infants, children and young people are shown in Box 8 [48].

Box 7:   Quality standards for Care of adults in the last days of life [47]

Statement 1 Adults who have signs and symptoms that suggest they may be in the last days of life are monitored for further changes to help determine if they are nearing death, stabilising, or recovering.

Statement 2 Adults in the last days of life, and the people important to them, are given opportunities to discuss, develop, and review an individualised care plan.

Statement 3 Adults in the last days of life who are likely to need symptom control are prescribed anticipatory medicines with individualised indications for use, dosage, and route of administration.

Statement 4 Adults in the last days of life have their hydration status assessed daily, and have a discussion about the risks and benefits of hydration options.

Box 8:   Quality standards for end-of-life care for infants, children, and young people [48]

Statement 1 Infants, children, and young people with a life-limiting condition and their parents or carers are involved in developing an advance care plan.

Statement 2 Infants, children, and young people with a life-limiting condition have a named medical specialist who leads and coordinates their care.

Statement 3 Infants, children, and young people with a life-limiting condition and their parents or carers are given information about emotional and psychological support, including how to access it.

Statement 4 Infants, children, and young people with a life-limiting condition are cared for by a multidisciplinary team that includes members of the specialist paediatric palliative care team.

Statement 5 Parents or carers of infants, children, and young people approaching the end-of-life are offered support for grief and loss when their child is nearing the end of their life and after their death.

Statement 6 Infants, children, and young people approaching the end-of-life and being cared for at home have 24-hour access to both children's nursing care and advice from a consultant in paediatric palliative care.

The End-of-life care strategy in England and Wales has defined an array of quality outcomes markers [49]. Similar initiatives are in place in many countries across the world [50-53].

Audit of Quality

Various measures of outcomes in palliative care have been developed [54] and the Australian palliative care sector is world leading in using routine clinical assessment information for measurement and benchmarking of outcomes of specialist care [55]. The National Audit of Care at the End-of-Life (NACEL) examines and benchmarks care in community and acute hospitals in England and Wales through retrospective patient case note reviews, organisation self-assessment questionnaires and survey of experience of bereaved family. In 2019–2020 audit 6823 casenotes were reviewed in 239 hospitals. This indicated, for example, that 74% of families felt the quality of care provided to the patients was good, excellent or outstanding [56].

The experiences of patients is often gathered by proxy, through seeking the feedback of bereaved relatives such as in the national survey of bereaved people (VOICES) survey [57]. Recently, the "Care of the Dying Evaluation" has been tested across a number of countries to develop a common, core international questionnaire (i-CODE) and in time data set [58].

Conclusion

The majority of people die with a progressive illness and most will benefit from integrating palliative care alongside other care and treatments. As illness progresses the need for symptom management and the balancing of the burdens and benefits of treatments increases. Sharing information with patients and their families about their illness is pivotal to enabling them to make decisions and accessing care and support that is right for them. There are huge deficits worldwide in providing adequate pain relief and inequities within countries of access to services and in achieving the best outcomes for patients and the families.

This Handbook will help you know more about what to do to care for your patients and aims to improve outcomes and reduce the inequities for our patients who are diverse in their social-cultural and medical contexts but all of whom need holistic, personalised, compassionate, and competent care.

References

1. Gott, M., Seymour, J., Ingleton, C. et al. (2011). That's part of everybody's job: the perspectives of health care staff in England and New Zealand on the meaning and remit of palliative care. *Palliative Medicine*. doi: 10.1177/0269216311408993.
2. Oliver, D. (2016). David Oliver: end of life care in hospital is everyone's business. *BMJ* 354: i3888.

3. Connor, S. (ed.) (2020). *Global Atlas of Palliative Care at the End of Life*, 2e. London: Worldwide Palliative Care Alliance. http://www.thewhpca.org/resources/global-atlas-on-end-of-life-care

4. Redinbaugh, E.M., Sullivan, A.M., Block, S.D. et al. (2003). Doctors' emotional reactions to recent death of a patient: cross sectional study of hospital doctors. *BMJ* 327: 185.

5. Mitchell, G.K. (2002). How well do general practitioners deliver palliative care? A systematic review. *Palliative Medicine* 16: 457–464.

6. Gawande, A. (2015). *Being Mortal: Illness, Medicine and What Matters in the End*. London: Profile Books Ltd.

7. Clarke, R. (2021). *Breathtaking: Inside the NHS in a Time of Pandemic*. London: Little Brown Book Group.

8. Buss, K., Rock, L.K., and McCarthy, E.P. (2017). Understanding palliative care and hospice. *Mayo Clinic Proceedings* 92: 280–286.

9. General Medical Council. (2010). *Treatment and Care Towards the End of Life: Good Practice in Decision Making*. London: GMC.

10. Bell, D. (2010). GMC guidelines on end of life care. *BMJ* 340: c3231.

11. Lakhani, M. (2011). Let's talk about dying. *BMJ* 342: d3018.

12. Department of Health. (2008). *End of Life Care Strategy*. London: DH.

13. Boyd, K. and Murray, S.A. (2010). Recognizing and managing key transitions in end of life care. *BMJ* 341: c4863.

14. National Audit Office. (2008). *End of Life Care*. London: Stationary office.

15. Department of Health. (2011). *Improving outcomes: A strategy for cancer.*

16. Armes, P.J., Richardson, A., Crowe, M. et al. (2009). Patients' supportive care needs beyond the end of treatment: a prospective and longitudinal survey. *Journal of Clinical Oncology* 27: 6172–6179.

17. Fairhurst, J. (2021). PRosPer: cancer prehabilitation and rehabilitation. E-Leaning for Health.

18. Saunders, C. (1993). Foreword. In: *Oxford Textbook of Palliative Medicine* (ed. D. Doyle, G.W.C. Hanks, and N. Macdonald), v–viii. Oxford: Oxford University Press.

19. World Health Organisation. (2002). *National Cancer Control Programmes: Policies and Managerial Guidelines*, 2e. Geneva: World Health Organization.

20. Saunders, C. (1976). Care of the dying—the problem of euthanasia. *Nursing Times* 72: 1049–1052.

21. National Institute for Health and Care Excellence. (2019). End of life care for adults: Service delivery NG142. https://www.nice.org.uk/guidance/ng142. (accessed 12th May 2023).

22. National Palliative and End of Life Care Partnership Ambitions for Palliative and End of Life Care: a national framework for local action 2015–2020. https://www.england.nhs.uk/publication/ambitions-for-palliative-and-end-of-life-care-a-national-framework-for-local-action-2021-2026. (accessed 12th May 2023).

23. Leadership Alliance for care of Dying People (2014). One chance to get it right. London: UK Government. https://assets.publishing.service.gov.uk/government/uploads/system/uploads/attachment_data/file/323188/One_chance_to_get_it_right.pdf. (accessed 12th May).

24. Knaul, F.M., Farmer, P.E., Krakauer, E.L. et al. (2018). Alleviating the access abyss in palliative care and pain relief-imperative of universal health coverage: the *Lancet* Commission report. *Lancet* 391: 1391–1454.

25. World Health Organization. (2014). Strengthening of palliative care as a component of comprehensive care throughout the life course., Geneva.

26. The Worldwide Hospice Palliative Care Alliance. (2014). Global atlas of palliative care at the end of life. World Health Organization and The Worldwide Hospice Palliative Care Alliance, Geneva.

27. Sleeman, K.E., de Brito, M., Etkind, S. et al. (2019). The escalating global burden of serious health-related suffering: projections to 2060 by world regions, age groups, and health conditions. *The Lancet Global Health* 7: E883–E892.

28. United Nations. (1962). *Single Convention on Narcotic Drugs, 1961*. United Nations sales No. E62.XI.1. New York, NY: United Nations.

29. (2021). Celebrating 60 years of the single convention on narcotic drugs of 1961. INCB. United Nations Vienna.

30. Calanzani, N., Koffman, J., and Higginson, I. (2013). Palliative and end of life care for Black, Asian and minority ethnic groups. Marie Curie.

31. Islam, Z., Pollock, K., Patterson, A. et al. Thinking ahead about medical treatments in advanced illness: a qualitative study of barriers and enablers in end-of-life care planning with patients and families from ethnically diverse backgrounds. HS&DR 17/05/30 in press 2022.

32. Kai, J., Beavan, J., and Faull, C. Challenges of mediated communication, disclosure and patient autonomy in cross-cultural cancer care. *British Journal of Cancer* 2011; 1–7. doi: 10.1038/bjc.2011.318.

33. Gatrad, A.R., Brown, E., Notta, H. et al. (2003). Palliative care needs of minorities. *BMJ* 327: 176–177.

34. Gunaratnam, Y. (2013). *Death and the Migrant*. London: Bloomsbury.

35. Gunaratnam, Y. Case stories. http://www.case-stories.org. (accessed 12th May 2023).

36. Carey, I., Shouls, S., Bristowe, K., Morris, M., Briant, L., Robinson, C., Caulkin, R., Griffiths, M., Clark, K., Koffman, J., and Hopper, A. (2015 March). Improving care for patients whose recovery is uncertain. The AMBER care bundle: design and implementation. *BMJ Support Palliat Care* 5 (1): 12–18.

37. Thomas, K. (2003). *Caring for the Dying at Home: Companions on a Journey*. Oxford: Radcliffe Medical Press.

38. Thomas, K. (2003). The gold standards framework in community palliative care. *European Journal of Palliative Care* 10 (3): 113–115.

39. Royal College of General Practitioners. Daffodil Standards. https://www.rcgp.org.uk/daffodilstandards. (accessed 12th May 2023).

40. Fisher, R.F.R., Lasserson, D., and Hayward, G. (2016). Out-of-hours primary care use at the end of life. *BJGP* 66: e654–e660.

41. Brettell, R., Fisher, R., Hunt, H. et al (2018). What proportion of patients at the end of life contact out-of-hours primary care? *BMJ Open* 8: e020244.

42. Buckman, R. (1993). Communication in palliative care: a practical guide. In: *Oxford Textbook of Palliative Medicine* (ed. D. Doyle, G.W.C. Hanks, and N. Macdonald), 47–61. Oxford: Oxford University Press.

43. Twycross, R.G. and Fairfield, S. (1982). Pain in far advanced cancer. *Pain* 14: 303–310.

44. Coordinate my care (2017). https://www.england.nhs.uk/london/wp-content/uploads/sites/8/2020/03/CMCPatient Leaflet.pdf. (accessed 12th May 2023).

45. Cassidy, S. (1988). *Sharing the Darkness; the Spirituality of Caring.* London: Darton, Longman and Todd.

46. National Institute for Health and Care Excellence. (2021). End of life care for adults. Quality standard QS13.

47. National Institute for Health and Care Excellence. (2017). Care of dying adults in the last days of life. Quality standard QS144.

48. National Institute for Health and Care Excellence. (2017). End of life care for infants, children and young people. Quality standard QS160.

49. Department of Health. (2009). *End of Life Care Strategy: Quality Markers and Measures for End of Life Care.* London: DH.

50. Standards Review Group. (2018). National Palliative Care Standards 5e. Palliative Care Australia. https://palliativecare.org.au/wp-content/uploads/dlm_uploads/2018/02/PalliativeCare-National-Standards-2018_web-3.pdf (accessed 12th May 2023).

51. African Palliative Care Association. (2010). Standards for providing quality palliative care across Africa. APCA.

52. Ferrell, B.R., Twaddle, M.L., Melnick, A., and Meier, D.E. (2018 December). National consensus project clinical practice guidelines for quality palliative care guidelines, 4th edition. *Journal of Palliative Medicine* 21 (12): 1684–1689.

53. Canadian Hospice Palliative Care Association (CHCPA). (2013). A model guide to hospice palliative care: based on national principles and norms of practice.

54. Bausewein, C., Daveson, B., Benalia, H., Simon, S.T., and Higginson, I.J. (2009). Outcome measurement in palliative care. PRISMA.

55. Palliative care outcomes collaborative (2021). Patient outcomes in palliative care. https://documents.uow.edu.au/content/groups/public/@web/@chsd/@pcoc/documents/doc/uow269015.pdf. (accessed 12th May 2023).

56. National Audit of care at the End of Life (NACEL) (2019/20). (2021). Healthcare quality improvement partnership.

57. Office of National Statistics Statistical. (2015). National Survey of Bereaved People (VOICES): quality of care delivered in the last 3 months of life for adults who died in England.

58. Mayland, C.R., Gerlach, C., Sigurdardottir, K. et al. (2019). Assessing quality of care for the dying from the bereaved relatives' perspective: using pre-testing survey methods across seven countries to develop an international outcome measure. *Palliative Medicine* 33 (3): 357–368.

2

Patient and Public Involvement in Palliative Care

John Rosenberg and Kerrie Noonan

Introduction

The emergence of the modern hospice movement in the 1960s and 1970s spearheaded patient involvement through a model of care that placed *total care* at the centre of palliative care. With the explicit inclusion of the "family" in this focus, a holistic approach to assessment and management of those receiving palliative care embraced the physical, psychological, social, and spiritual components of care. Similarly, the modern hospice movement engaged local communities through volunteer programs, many of which are still running today. Indeed, as Small [1] says, "the modern hospice movement and palliative care deserve a central place in any history of public and patient involvement" [1 p. 29]. The presence of ordinary citizens in the everyday endeavours of hospice gave public voice to what had been previously hidden. Over time, this approach to the care of those living with life-limiting illnesses largely became integrated with mainstream healthcare, including its declaration as the discrete discipline of palliative medicine in 1987. This enabled the pre-existing processes for patient and public involvement found in healthcare to be applied to palliative care [1].

However, this institutional management of dying did not shift the focus of palliative care from those with advanced cancer. Non-malignant, life-threatening illnesses – such as motor neurone disease, cerebrovascular disease, AIDS, and dementia – were not considered to be within the remit of many palliative care services until relatively recently. Public and professional bodies representing those with specific diseases, including those above, were the avenue through which patient and public voices were heard. In many countries, mainstream palliative care services could not provide equitable access to care. While metropolitan-based services might include specialist palliative care, in regional, rural, and remote locations, it could be uncommon or completely absent, despite identified need. Interestingly, this was not simply a function of population density, as Randall, Rosenberg, and Reimer [2] explored, noting that comparable challenges to access to services were found in both the United Kingdom and Australia, despite their vastly different population densities. Indeed, even within large tertiary hospitals, where people were dying of non-malignant disease – sometimes in high acuity settings like Intensive Care or Emergency Departments – palliative care would not necessarily be referred in, or even have a presence in the hospital at all.

Three distinct barriers to patient and public participation in palliative care are identified in the literature: paternalism, gatekeeping, and inequity of access.

The 'Benign Paternalism' of Palliative Care

The motives for providing palliative care are well-intentioned and unquestionably find their origins in the desire to relieve suffering. Not simply a clinical exercise, palliative care practice is fundamentally interpersonal, and the patient voice in decision-making would be reasonably expected to be central to it. However, with mainstreaming and medicalisation, this is disputable. The term medicalisation has been defined as "the process whereby more and more of everyday life has come under medical dominion, influence and supervision" [3 p. 295]. Illich [4] had a more deterministic view of this kind of medical decision-making. He asserts that medicalisation creates the conditions that enable paternalism to be practiced and normalised in the medical system. He and others [3–6] view medicalisation as a form of social control, making it possible for

Handbook of Palliative Care, Fourth Edition. Edited by Richard Kitchen, Christina Faull, Sarah Russell and Jo Wilson.
© 2024 John Wiley & Sons Ltd. Published 2024 by John Wiley & Sons Ltd.

previously non-medical issues to be re-categorised as "deviant." Without medicalisation in a definitional sense, medical social control loses its legitimacy and is more difficult to accomplish [3]. The development of a technique of medical social control may precede the medicalisation of a problem, but for implementation some type of medical definition is necessary [3 p. 216]. Hence, we can see that diagnosing dying, categorising dying and viewing death as deviant (as in the medical construction of prolonged dying), and taking the position that everyone who is dying requires palliative care, is one way of bolstering medical social control and reinforcing the legitimacy of the biomedical model [7].

The term "benign paternalism" aligns the paternalism in palliative care to a compassionate rather than a malicious intent [8]. The goal of holistic care, for example, acknowledges the total experience of dying and attempts to address these elements of human suffering. Yet arguably, locating psychological, social, and spiritual care within the remit of palliative care can be seen as a "mechanism for extending medical control over dying" [9 p. 141]. Although well-intentioned, holistic models of care can decontextualise and medicalise experiences that are fundamentally experiential, contextual, and beyond the capacity of services to provide support for in most models of healthcare; critically, these experiences should be addressed within context.

The *Liverpool Care Pathway* was an example of the problems arising from the exclusion of patients and families in participating fully in end-of-life care decision-making. The original intent of the pathway was to ensure compassionate care at end-of-life. However, in 2014, the *Pathway* was the focus of a national enquiry in England because of reported abuses of power by medical practitioners, allegedly made worse by the pathway systems [10]. Subsequently, it was revealed that 50% of people had been placed on the *Pathway* without consent or without the knowledge of family members [11, 12].

Gatekeeping in Palliative Care

Gatekeeping is a strategy that is used by those with power and control to maintain the status quo [13]. One function of gatekeeping behaviour is to protect the system and to benefit the system the behaviour serves. This includes the delivery of health services and the production of knowledge [13, 14]. In palliative care, gatekeeping has been found to have a negative impact on participation in both research and community engagement activities [13, 15]. A recent review of gatekeeping behaviour in

palliative care research found the main reason patients and their families were excluded from research recruitment was the view that palliative care patients and their families are vulnerable and participation in research is a threat to patient well-being [16]. Further, the readiness or willingness of patients to participate was frequently assessed by healthcare providers or family members rather than asking the patient directly. In contrast, another study found that when patients are asked directly about having medical students involved in their care, patients responded extremely positively and welcomed the experience [17]. Importantly, patients were given the choice to decide.

Even where public participation is established, gatekeeping behaviours can be evident. An Australian project founded upon community-based participation in end-of-life care identified issues with gatekeeping by health professionals and other experts [13]. Community members, working on a variety of strategies that aimed to increase awareness and participation in palliative care, experienced this:

> Deliberate strategies of obstruction and misinformation were also used by other workers in the field, on occasion. In one example, a prominent worker in one community was repeatedly invited to meetings about the work. They never turned up. Then just as the work was getting media coverage and a particular strategy was about to be launched this person spoke out against the work at local meetings, questioned the legitimacy of the person leading the work, and told people that if they allowed this to continue, they were putting vulnerable people in danger [13 p. 31].

When health providers were perceived to view community efforts negatively or when people in the health system were actively working to maintain control, this behaviour was particularly damaging to community participation:

> It is when people … don't acknowledge that contribution or someone does the work and then they claim the credit, or they feel that you can't do it as a community group because it's their turf [13 p. 32].

Hard to Reach?

Palliative care service planning for populations within national or regional jurisdictions will sometimes designate subpopulations of patients as "vulnerable" or "targeted." Typically, these groups are marginalised by mainstream society, adding stigma to poor access to care; these groups might include people with severe, persistent mental illness; those experiencing homelessness; indigenous peoples; those from culturally and linguistically diverse origins; racial minorities; refugees; those identifying as LGBTQI +; those with disabilities; prisoners; and others [18]. Many current models of palliative care categorise these groups as "hard to reach" populations.

However, could it be that it is *healthcare services*, not populations, that are "hard to reach?" Palliative care has been criticised for continuing to reflect its origins in white, middle-class and religious settings where people with advanced cancer comprised more than 90% of the palliative care patient population. The term "hard to reach services" has been used by advocates in the disability sector to encourage palliative care services to alter their language to describe people who are living with disabilities and nearing the end of their lives; sometimes in supported accommodation, but certainly not always, and often subject to social stigma and disadvantage [19]. Similarly, the work of Stajduhar and colleagues with those experiencing homelessness strongly question the suitability of mainstream palliative care services to provide accessible and appropriate end-of-life care [20]. The work of Dr Naheed Dosani and his colleagues from Inner City Health Associates in the *Palliative Education and Care for the Homeless* (PEACH) project in Toronto, Canada, is a groundbreaking venture that fundamentally relies upon the participation of those who access the service from a place of profound disadvantage (for more information, gottohttps://www.icha-toronto.ca/programs/peach-palliative-education-and-care-for-the-homeless).

The hospice movement and palliative care have evolved through improved clinical practices, pain and symptom management, and research activities. However, the mainstreaming of palliative care brought its routinisation and over-medicalisation, impacting upon patient and public participation. It is in this context that new approaches to the provision of palliative care emerged, and where the primacy of the citizen – not simply the "patient" – and their community is promoted.

A New Paradigm: Public Health Palliative Care

Public Health Palliative Care is an umbrella term for a range of social and community-based interventions that are implemented alongside the medical and health services provided to people with a life-threatening illness. Until

relatively recently, public health has focused primarily on disease control and prevention. In the late twentieth century, public health approaches were addressing the health and well-being of whole populations. Early public health strategies focused on the reduction of mortality and morbidity of communicable diseases and strategies such as better sanitation and nutrition and did not address social determinants of health [21]. This included early intervention and prevention programs designed to modify the behaviour of individuals and change environments to enable health improvements [22]. Yet as early as 1978, the World Health Organization (WHO) asserted the right of all people to participate in the planning and delivery of their own health care [23].

Health Promoting Palliative Care

The WHO *Ottawa Charter for Health Promotion* [24] was considered the beginning of "new public health," signalling a shift away from a biomedical approach to disease prevention and toward a greater acknowledgement of the social determinants of health. To address this, the *Ottawa Chapter* identified five key action areas:

Building healthy public policy.
Creating supportive environments.
Strengthening community action.
Developing personal skills.

• Reorienting healthcare services toward prevention of illness and promotion of health.

These five action areas were adapted by Kellehear [25] to articulate *Health Promoting Palliative Care* (HPPC), which outlined a way for palliative care services to adopt health promotion principles and these key action areas. In essence, HPPC was an invitation to palliative care services to move upstream of direct patient care and to think beyond service delivery to the wider role that palliative care has in civic society. In this way, *Public Health Palliative Care* (PHPC) has become the term to describe this perspective and the practices that are derived from it.

In the past, "public health" and "palliative care" may have been viewed as contradictory concepts [26]. Yet there is now international agreement that the health and well-being of people with life-limiting illnesses can be improved with social and community interventions based upon the *Ottawa Charter* [24, 27]. PHPC acknowledges that health services (including palliative care) alone are not sufficient to provide holistic end-of-life care for individuals and their families, and that a

...conscious, planned and deliberate political and social set of actions taken by the key players in any community to enhance the support and wellbeing of everyone affected by ageing, dying, death, loss and caregiving [28 p. xiv].

This description captures the proactive, rather than reactive, approach by communities and healthcare services providing support to all those impacted with life-limiting illnesses.

Circles of Care

It has been suggested that about 95% of the care of dying people takes place away from healthcare systems [18]. Who, then, is participating in this care? In many cases, there is a constellation of people and organisations that provide this support, with or without the help of formal palliative care service providers. It is in this context that the application of HPPC can be understood. One model that can be useful is *Circles of Care* which can be used to identify the components of a whole-of-community approach to dying, caregiving, death, and grieving. The model places the person with a life-limiting illness at the centre of a constellation of support – first the patient's inner and outer support networks (family, friends), which is wrapped around by community (such as the patient's neighbours, local community groups), then service providers and service delivery [29]. The final circle is policy, acknowledging that these concentric circles of care exist within broader policy contexts, which equally inform how care and support can be given.

Involvement in Care

Framing of patient and public participation in a PHPC approach enables palliative care services to view patient and public participation as a partnership, rather than competing forces. If formal care providers and informal carers are equal partners in the demands of caregiving, then it is context that underpins services and identifies sources of support within and beyond social networks of care.

Formal care is provided by accredited health professionals (including doctors, nurses, and allied health professionals) and trained volunteers through the provision of healthcare or hospice services. Informal care, or the support from families, friends, work colleagues, community groups, faith communities, and other informal support networks, has long been recognised as sharing the demands of caregiving to both the dying person and their caregivers [30]. Informal care can be

viewed as social and interpersonal. It is a continuation of naturally occurring social networks that a person with a life-limiting illness and their family are already connected to. In this sense, informal care has a significant role in the life of a dying person because it is where people are doing their living and connecting while they are preparing for the end of their lives. These networks are the source of social support that is often quite "ordinary" – for example, keeping company, reading aloud, doing the shopping, babysitting, or providing transport for children to school or sports, housework, and food preparation. It may or may not include direct personal care, such as attending to hygiene, assistance with eating and drinking, or toileting.

Informal care happens alongside formal care, although it is not always recognised or valued in the same way as service delivery. This undervaluing has been a key issue for patient and public engagement. For example, how can palliative care services justify the broadening of service delivery to include public engagement when healthcare services are already under-resourced and stretched in providing clinical care? A PHPC approach argues that increased service delivery cannot solve or address social problems such as loneliness or the stigma that can be associated with end-of-life care. Social problems, as noted in the *Ottawa Charter* [23], cannot be tackled with medical or health interventions alone; they require a social response.

Increasingly, social media provides a platform for the voices of individuals experiencing the issues arising from dying, caregiving, death, and grief. Those who are – or become – public figures at such a time add a voice via social media that promote their and others' participation in the experience. For example, see Box 1 for the example of Jade Goody.

Box 1: Case Study: Jade Goody

Celebrity illnesses and deaths are one example of "lay experts" who live their dying and death in the public sphere. Popular culture and access to information via the internet and mass media provides deeply personal stories and insights into illness, dying, death, and grief. Jade Goody was diagnosed with cervical cancer during her participation on a reality TV program.

Goody's use of social and mainstream media while she was dying provided her with the status of *lay expert* and had the impact of creating a significant increase in cervical screening in Britain. This became known as the "Jade effect" [31].

Involvement in Communities

Key to engagement in palliative care is working alongside community members to encourage and enable participation. Community engagement is the process that enables communities and services to work together to understand, build capacity, and address issues to improve their experience of end-of-life and bereavement. It exists on a spectrum of engagement that extends from informing, consulting, co-producing, collaborating through to empowering, depending on a range of factors such as the degree of participation from the local community and the intention of the work [32]. This spectrum is based on Arnstein's *Ladder of Participation* [33], and "is designed to aid professional services and the communities they serve to embark on community engagement projects with an open awareness of the key components underpinning their success" [32 p. 5].

This spectrum provides palliative care services with a way of understanding the different levels of community engagement. All levels of engagement have an important role in patient and community participation, and this model encourages palliative care services to be aware of the role of patient and community participation. For example, providing information and consulting with citizens is a more passive form of engagement that aims to raise awareness and provide education. Community projects that are focused on collaboration and empowerment, however, are more likely to be led by community members who self-organise and design the interventions.

Critically, the language of engagement is itself problematic when understood from a perspective of power. Cormac Russell, a commentator based in the UK, addresses the question, "How do we get people to engage?" Russell tweets,

> With respect, you don't **get** ppl [people] to engage. You listen to what they are about enough to act on, and then support them to work with other to do what they care deeply about. It's not about getting ppl to do what we want. [33]

The issue here rests with the word "get." Palliative care services that are unsuccessful in their attempts to "get" communities to engage with them have an opportunity to rethink their place in this interaction. Of course, it depends upon the nature of the engagement – for example, providing information requires something different to a community-led initiative where the service is invited to contribute. However, wherever it sits on this continuum, engagement by services and communities in collaboration requires an informed and authentic understanding of the place each partner takes. This is especially so where services provide knowledge and skills about palliative care to a community initiative. This situation can directly challenge the service's power as "experts":

> ...the palliative care profession is confronted with the irony of relinquishing its "ownership" of the business of dying while leading communities to reclaim their principal role in the business of dying. The very services possessing the expertise to lead this shift in control are the same services that would be required to cede that control [8 p. 8].

Two examples where there is the imperative to engage in this way are referred to as *Compassionate Cities* and *Compassionate Communities*.

Compassionate Cities and Compassionate Communities

Compassionate Cities are:

> ... communities that publicly encourage, facilitate, supports and celebrates care for one another during life's most testing moments and experiences, especially those pertaining to life-threatening and life-limiting illness, chronic disability, frail ageing and dementia, grief and bereavement, and the trials and burdens of long-term care. [35 p. 1].

Compassionate Cities focus more on civil actions, including civic partnerships through the local government and other organisations, such as schools, places of worship, and trade unions. Typically, any organisation can lead or promote the *Compassionate Cities Charter* which articulates these elements in detail (https://www.phpci.org).

Compassionate Communities are described as:

> ...communities that develop social networks, social spaces, social policies and social conduct that support people through the many hours, days, weeks, months and sometimes years of living with a life-threatening or life-limiting illness, ageing, grief and bereavement, and long-term caregiving [27 p. xiv].

It can be seen how Compassionate Communities flourish where both the proximity of palliative care services to end-of-life issues, and the capacity, skills, and knowledge of

communities are part of the same endeavour. The core elements of Compassionate Communities are:
- Build capacity and death literacy through education and shared experiences.
- Value and focus on existing community strengths and assets.
- Recognise communities as the experts on their own lives and valuing them as key stakeholders, not just participants.
- Communities identify their needs and are empowered to lead the change.
- Focus on equity and inclusion with a broad understanding of health and wellbeing.
- Achieve sustainability through partnerships and shared leadership.
- Take a whole-of-community approach, recognising that palliative care and health services cannot do this alone.
- Think beyond individuals to include social and community networks.

(https://bc-cpc.ca/all-resources/community-organizations/compassionate-communities-toolkit/)

Compassionate Communities are often designed as programs or community development initiatives that bring together small groups of people with shared goals of developing ways to improve dying, death, and bereavement experiences. A critical, first step in this process is to identify what characteristics of Compassionate Communities already exist – what "assets" are in place upon which to build in conscious, deliberate ways?

Asset-Based Community Development

Asset-Based Community Development [ABCD] provides an approach that identifies the existing capacity of communities to support its citizens who are dying, caregiving, or grieving. Russell [36] describes six key building blocks that enable community mobilisation to address local issues. These are shown in Figure 1.

This approach need not be complicated. For example, Matthiesen and colleagues [37] utilised ABCD in rural

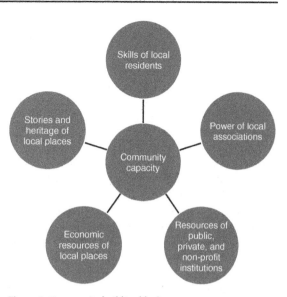

Figure 1 Community building blocks.

and urban communities in the northwest of England to establish a community-led initiative to raise awareness of end-of-life conversations and care, and determine local priorities to sustain them. This demonstrates its transferability across demographic and geographical regions; it has cross-cultural applicability and enables the expression of diversity. The freedom in ABCD processes lies in the local character it enables – members of the public participate in end-of-life issues in whatever ways are appropriate to them. This might include creative and arts-based initiatives, discussion groups, public forums, support networks, and information sources both hard copy and online.

Involvement in Services

The origins of the modern hospice movement demonstrate a longstanding practice of public participation in palliative care services. It was community activism that brought about the establishment of hospices and organised fundraising to maintain them. In many parts of the world, this remains the case where communities lobby successfully for a local community hospice. This original "reformist agenda" was unsurprisingly overtaken in the subsequent evolution of palliative care into mainstream healthcare [39] and in many jurisdictions, hospices are unsupported by government in favour of integrated palliative care services. Whether or not one is a more suitable alternative is

---

Box 2: Case example: The Scottish Partnership for Palliative Care

The Scottish Partnership has developed several programs and projects that provide an opportunity for health services and the general public to connect for the purposes of growing awareness about palliative care. Demystifying death day and the EASE course (End-of-Life Skills for Everyone) are examples of public participation programs [38].

another matter, however it is certainly true that community-based governance of a hospice is more accessible to citizens than informing the quality of care in monolithic healthcare systems.

A growing presence of active citizenry [1] as an expression of self-determination and influence has seen healthcare attempts to assimilate the "consumer voice" in its governance. This is increasingly the case in palliative care also. With changing attitudes towards the authority of experts and powerful health systems, patients and public (who are, after all, the same people) are asserting their demands that healthcare improve the quality of services and become more responsive, that they include users of healthcare and community stakeholders into the governance of services. In many jurisdictions, this is a mandated requirement. What might this look like in practical terms? The representation of community members on Boards or Advisory Committees, including those who are living with life-limiting illnesses or have been caregivers, demonstrates public participation in services.

Of course, the increasing influence of the public voice has also led to legislative reform in a number of jurisdictions where euthanasia has become legalised. Although the assertion of the palliative care sector in many places is that its remit does not include euthanasia, this distinction is not necessarily shared by the active citizenry – care at the end-of-life and euthanasia can both be viewed as end-of-life issues by many members of the public. In either case, public participation in advocacy and lobbying for legislative reform is a notable example of the influence the collective voice can have. Interestingly, in Belgium, it is a requirement that, following a request for medical assisted dying, palliative care assessment and interventions are mandatory in the attempt to relieve suffering.

Involvement in Research

In the past, there has been substantial resistance to the inclusion of palliative care patients in research, where they would be considered *too ill to talk* [39]. In this context, it has been asserted that clinicians can act as proxies for patients; that this could lead to undue influence of self-selecting proxies; that short life-expectancy disqualifies patients from meaningful participation; and that research too technical to impose upon seriously ill people. Sadly, this is an example of the kind of benign paternalism noted above, that has a protective intent but a silencing effect.

Two important considerations apply here. Firstly, it is held here that the voices of the "patient" and the public who

> **Box 3: Case example: The Death Literacy Index**
>
> The Death Literacy Index was developed following a decade of qualitative and quantitative research about end-of-life care networks. This 29-item survey tool that can be used in compassionate community projects to understand more about the strengths and challenges related to death literacy. The tool can be used for research, evaluation, and to facilitate community conversations. The DLI is an example of how end-of-life research with carers and community members can influence the development of participatory tools [30, 44].

are invested in end-of-life issues have primacy; this applies not only to the nature of the clinical care they receive, but in their choice to participate, or not, in research. This exercise of autonomy is susceptible to the influence of benign paternalism and gatekeeping, yet can be a matter of social justice. In reviews over the past decade or so, palliative care patients, caregivers and bereaved people have expressed a willingness to participate in research, seeing it as inherently valuable, and an opportunity to contribute for the betterment of others if not themselves [40, 41].

Secondly, the methodological approaches to research in palliative care require careful thought. Although clinical trials are conducted in palliative care populations, it is not a field that lends itself readily to research designs such as randomised controlled trials, for example. Indeed, a report in the Patient Experience Library [42] in the UK gives a cutting critique of evidence-based practice, which silences the patient voice as a source of evidence and privileges "hard" evidence, with a great risk of subsequent harm. Rather, where the voices of patient and public are sought, participatory research methods can be highly effective; they are an important part of the palliative care history and the current research landscape. For example, network mapping and social network analysis provide a rigorous research method to ABCD [43, 44]. Digital storytelling, such as photovoice, allows for narrative evaluation of experience and gives primacy to the lived experiences of ordinary citizens in their dying, caregiving, and grieving.

Conclusion

Public participation is a key factor in the emergence of the modern hospice movement and, to a lesser extent, the development of the healthcare discipline of palliative care. Patient participation is at the heart of holistic palliative care, yet its prevalence has something of a chequered history. With an increasingly aged population and changing expectations of the interaction between healthcare services and their clientele, there is an opportunity to fundamentally refashion approaches to patient and public involvement in palliative care. Patient and public involvement can be embedded into care, communities, services, and research.

The relatively recent emergence of Public Health Palliative Care provides approaches that enable patient and public voices to be heard. The *Ottawa Charter for Health Promotion* [24] and the *Circles of Care Model* [29] underpin engagement of health and palliative care services with the general public. It is this ordinary citizenry who can not only participate in end-of-life care support for its members but drive much of the social response to the complex issues that arise.

References

1. Small, N. (2012). Public and patient involvement in palliative care. In *Handbook of Palliative Care*, 3rd edition (ed. C. Faull, S. de Caestecker, A. Nicolson, and F. Black), 29–41. Hoboken NJ: John Wiley and Sons.
2. Randall, D., Rosenberg, J.P., and Reimer, S. (2017). Solid and liquid modernity: a comparison of the social geography of places to die in the UK and Australia. *Death Studies* 41 (2): 103–111.
3. Conrad, P. (1992). Medicalization and social control. *Annual Review of Sociology* 18: 209–232.
4. Illich, I. (1976). *Medical Nemesis*. New York: Pantheon.
5. Conrad, P. and Schneider, J.W. Newman, D.M and O'Brien, J. (1992). Medicine as an institution of social control. *Sociology: Exploring the Architecture of Everyday Life Readings* 191–199.
6. Zola, I.K. (1972). Medicine as an institution of social control. *The Sociological Review* 20 (4): 487–504.
7. Noonan, K. (2018). *Renegade Stories: A Study of Deathworkers Using Social Approaches to Dying, Death and Loss in Australia*. Doctoral thesis. Penrith: Western Sydney University.
8. Rosenberg, J. (2011). Whose business is dying? Death, the home and palliative care. *Cultural Studies Review* 17 (1): 15–30.
9. Howarth, G. (2007). *Death and Dying: A Sociological Introduction*. Cambridge: Polity.
10. Knights, D., Wood, D., and Barclay, S. (2013). The Liverpool care pathway for the dying: what went wrong? *British Journal of General Practice* 63 (615): 509–510.
11. Watts, T. (2012). End-of-life care pathways as tools to promote and support a good death: a critical commentary. *European Journal of Cancer Care* 21 (1): 20–30.
12. Neuberger, J., Guthrie, C., and Aaronovitch, D. (2013). More care, less pathway: a review of the Liverpool care pathway. *Department of Health*.
13. Horsfall, D., Psychogios, H., Rankin-Smith, H., Read, N., and Noonan, K. (2020). *Researching Compassionate Communities in Australia: A short-term longitudinal study [Internet]*. Available from: http://dx.doi.org/10.13140/RG.2.2.31469.67046
14. Velasco Garrido, M., Zentner, A., and Reinhard Busse, A. (2011). The effects of gatekeeping: a systematic review of the literature. *Scandinavian Journal of Primary Healthcare* 29 (1): 28–38.
15. Noonan, K., Leonard, R., and Horsfall, D. (2011). You can't do that! Researching alternate stories of community participation at end of life. *Third Sector Review* 17 (1): 75.
16. Kars, M.C., Van Thiel, G., van der Graaf, R., Moors, M., de Graeff, A., and Van Delden, J. (2016). A systematic review of reasons for gatekeeping in palliative care research. *Palliative Medicine* 30 (6): 533–548.
17. Arolker, M., Barnes, J., Gadoud, A., Jones, L., Barnes, L., and Johnson, M. (2010). "They've got to learn." A qualitative study exploring the views of patients and staff regarding medical student teaching in a hospice. *Palliative Medicine* 24 (4): 419–426.
18. Sallnow, L., Smith, R., Ahmedzai, S.H., Bhadelia, A., Chamberlain, C., Cong, Y., Doble, B., Dullie, L., Durie, R., Finkelstein, E.A., and Guglani, S. (2022). Report of the lancet commission on the value of death: bringing death back into life. *The Lancet* 399 (10327): 837–884.
19. Grindrod, A. (2021). Dying with disability: a disability and palliative care intersectoral partnership framework. *Research and Practice in Intellectual and Developmental Disabilities* 2021 8 (2): 138–151.
20. Stajduhar, K.I. (2020). Provocations on privilege in palliative care: are we meeting our core mandate? *Progress in Palliative Care* 28 (2): 89–93.
21. Laverack, G. (2017). The challenge of behaviour change and health promotion. *Challenges* 8 (2): 25.
22. Green, J. (2010). The WHO commission on social determinants of health. *Critical Public Health* 20 (1): 1–4.
23. World Health Organization. (1978). *The Declaration of Alma Ata*. Geneva: World Health Organization.
24. World Health Organization. (1987). *Ottawa Charter for Health Promotion*. Geneva: World Health Organization.
25. Kellehear, A. (1999). *Health Promoting Palliative Care*. Melbourne: Oxford University Press.
26. Rosenberg, J.P. and Yates, P.M. (2010). Health promotion in palliative care: the case for conceptual congruence. *Critical Public Health* 20 (2): 201–210.
27. Sallnow, L., Richardson, H., Murray, S.A., and Kellehear, A. (2016). The impact of a new public health approach to end-of-life care: a systematic review. *Palliative Medicine*. Vol. 30, SAGE Publications Ltd. 200–211.
28. Wegleitner, K., Heimerl, K., and Kellehear, A. (2016). Preface. In: *Compassionate Communities: Case Studies from Britain and Europe* (ed. K. Wegleitner, K. Heimerl, and A. Kellehear), xii–xvii. Abingdon: Routledge.
29. Abel, J., Walter, T., Carey, L.B., Rosenberg, J., Noonan, K., Horsfall, D. et al. (2013). Circles of care: should community

development redefine the practice of palliative care? *BMJ Supportive & Palliative Care* 3 (4): 383–388.

30. Horsfall, D., Noonan, K., and Leonard, R. (2012). Bringing our dying home: how caring for someone at end of life builds social capital and develops compassionate communities. *Health Sociology Review* 21 (4): 373–382.

31. Ashton, D. (2014). The expertise of illness: celebrity constructions and public understandings. In: *The Social Construction of Death* (eds. L. Van Brussell and N. Carpentier), 114–134. London: Palgrave Macmillan.

32. Sallnow, L. and Paul, S. (2014). Understanding community engagement in end-of-life care: developing conceptual clarity. *Critical Public Health* 25 (2):1–8.

33. https://twitter.com/CormacRussell/status/1515378190 998515714.

34. Abel, J. and Kellehear, A. (2021). *The Compassionate City: A Charter of Actions*, new edition. https://www.phpci.org/news/2021/1/17/compassionate-cities-charter-2021-update.

35. Russell, C. (2022). *Asset-Based Community Development (ABCD): Looking Back to Look Forward*. eBook Partnership.

36. Matthiesen, M., Froggatt, K., Owen, E., and Ashton, J.R. (2014). End-of-life conversations and care: an asset-based model for community engagement. *BMJ Supportive & Palliative Care* 4 (3): 306–312.

37. Patterson, R.M., Gibb, C. and Hazelwood, M.A. (2022 February). End of life aid skills for everyone in Scotland. *Palliative Care and Social Practice* 16: 26323524221076511.

38. Small, N. and Rhodes, P.J. (2000). *Too Ill to Talk? User Involvement and Palliative Care*. Psychology Press.

39. Bloomer, M.J., Hutchinson, A.M., Brooks, L., and Botti, M. (2018). Dying persons' perspectives on, or experiences of, participating in research: an integrative review. *Palliative Medicine* 32 (4): 851–860.

40. White, C. and Hardy, J. (2010). What do palliative care patients and their relatives think about research in palliative care?—a systematic review. *Supportive Care in Cancer* 18 (8): 905–911.

41. Patient Experience Library. (2020). *Inadmissible evidence. The double standard in evidence-based practice, and how it harms patients*. https://www.patientlibrary.net/cgi-bin/download/file/227119.

42. Leonard, R., Horsfall D., and Noonan, K. (2015). Identifying changes in the support networks of end-of-life carers using social network analysis. *BMJ Supportive & Palliative Care* 5 (2): 153–159.

43. Leonard, R., Horsfall, D., Rosenberg, J., and Noonan, K. (2020). Carer experience of end-of-life service provision: a social network analysis. *BMJ Supportive & Palliative Care* 10 (2): e20–.

44. Leonard, R., Noonan, K., Horsfall, D., Kelly, M., Rosenberg, J.P., and Grindrod, A., Rumbold, B., and Rahn, A. (2021). Developing a death literacy index. *Death Studies* 46 (9):1–3.

3 Equity, Diversity and Inclusion in Serious Illness

Noura Rizk, William E. Rosa and Liz Grant

Introduction

Social justice advocate and global health pioneer, Dr. Paul Farmer, asked, "If health is a human right … who is considered human enough to have that right?" [1]. There is possibly no better starting point for a chapter on inequalities than this reflection. The question does not ask how disparities can be eradicated or what solutions are needed to enhance optimal health and social care services, but simply and quite boldly: Who is considered human enough to be afforded the right to health?

When applied to the palliative and the end-of-life context, the question might be posed: Who is considered human enough to have their suffering relieved and their death dignified? Again and again, society is forced to reckon with the fact that our legacy is not defined by how well we attend to the needs of our healthiest populations, but how committed we are to providing compassionate and humanising care for the sickest and most disenfranchised among us. Who is considered human enough to have that right?

This chapter aims to summarise the background literature on inequalities in palliative care as they relate to broader health and social care considerations; offer a principle-based approach to promoting equity across the serious illness continuum; and identify steps towards inclusive palliative care for several historically excluded and at-risk groups. Although we attempt to provide a comprehensive review of inequalities, we acknowledge that we may likely and inadvertently leave out mention of groups actively facing bias or fall short in attempts to be inclusive. Thus, we offer this chapter as a starting point for scholarly discourse.

Background

Although palliative care is considered a right to the highest standards of mental and physical health, and a fundamental aspect of universal health coverage per Sustainable Development Goal 3, only 12% of the current global palliative care need is currently being met [2]. In fact, despite more than 61 million people worldwide experiencing an estimated six billion days of serious health-related suffering (SHS) annually, about two-thirds of countries have no or extremely limited provision of palliative care and over 80% have low to non-existent access to opioids for pain relief [3, 4]. The lionshare of unalleviated SHS impacts seriously ill individuals and families living in low- and middle-income countries (LMICs) – the poor, the overlooked, and the unseen – those who have been historically considered not human enough to have unfettered rights to health, to dignity, and to palliative care. Over the next four decades, the global burden of SHS is expected to escalate about 87%, disproportionately disadvantaging those in LMICs among other at-risk groups (e.g., older people over age 70) [5].

In addition to quantifying the global burden of SHS and designing an essential package of physical and human resources that could be costed and disseminated to bridge palliative care delivery gaps around the world, The Lancet Commission on Global Access to Palliative Care and Pain Relief highlighted the global pain divide that keeps people with life-limiting illnesses and injuries in LMICs suffering needlessly. Using opioid access as a tracer for palliative care and pain relief provision, the Commission calculated that 50% of the world's poorest populations live in countries that receive less than 1% of the annual opioid analgesics distributed worldwide. Conversely, the richest 10% of the

Handbook of Palliative Care, Fourth Edition. Edited by Richard Kitchen, Christina Faull, Sarah Russell and Jo Wilson.
© 2024 John Wiley & Sons Ltd. Published 2024 by John Wiley & Sons Ltd.

world's population live in countries that receive nearly 90% of the annual distributed opioid morphine equivalent.

The Commission wrote, "Poor people in all parts of the world live and die with little or no palliative care or pain relief. Starting into this access abyss, one sees the depth of extreme suffering in the cruel face of poverty and inequity ... The fact that access to such an inexpensive, essential, and effective intervention is denied to most patients in LMICs ... is a medical, public health, and moral failing and a travesty of justice" [6 p.1391]. This 90/10 pain divide is reflective of a dire human divide: those considered human enough to have their pain and symptomatic distress adequately managed and those not considered human enough to have their suffering relieved. This travesty is rooted in imbalanced science that fails to prioritise disparities research in palliative care and pain relief [6].

In addition to those who are living in poverty, countless historically excluded and systematically marginalised groups living in all countries have faced bias, stigma, and suffering in the absence of person-centred and holistic palliative care access that seeks to enhance the quality of living and dying. COVID-19 has exacerbated SHS and health outcomes for many at-risk people, including the incarcerated, persons with disabilities, persons experiencing homelessness, those with substance use disorder, and sexual and gender minorised populations, and racial, ethnic, and cultural minority groups, among others [7].

Defining "Palliative Care": A Critical Endeavour

The International Association for Hospice and Palliative Care sought to update and improve the 2002 World Health Organisation (WHO) definition of *palliative care* through a consensus-based approach, embedding choice, equality, and diversity and engaging the expertise of experts from countries of all income levels. The provision of palliative care services for children, older persons, and vulnerable populations, as well as equitable access to controlled essential medicines for pain relief and palliative care (e.g., opioids, benzodiazepines) are incorporated in this definition:

> the active holistic care of individuals across all ages with severe health related suffering, because of severe illness and especially of those near the end of life. It aims to improve the quality of life of patients, their families, and their caregivers [8 p.761]

- *Suffering is health-related when it is associated with illness or injury of any kind.*
- *Health-related suffering is serious when it cannot be relieved without medical intervention and when it compromises physical, social, spiritual, and/or emotional functioning because of severe illness.*
- *Severe illness is a condition that carries a high risk of mortality, negatively impacts quality of life and daily function, and/or is burdensome in symptoms, treatments, or caregiver stress [8 p.761].*

The new definition challenged the unintentional discriminating factors which traditionally meant that palliative care was understood to be about alleviating suffering only at the end-of-life and often only for patients with cancers. It also sought to speak to the huge local and global disparities in the access to and quality of palliative care determined by, for example, age, disease type, ethnicity, religion, social class, and geography. It highlighted it as an "active" process that is rooted in relationship at the individual and community level.

As the renewed definition of palliative care suggests palliative care is both multi-dimensional and complex. As previously mentioned, the availability of and accessibility to quality palliative care is integral to achieving universal healthcare coverage (UHC) [9]. Importantly, holistic palliative care should be responsive to:

- the different stages of illness as experienced by patients;
- the differing needs associated with various illnesses;
- patients' and their families' and carers' cultural, social, spiritual beliefs about illness and death.

This consensus-based definition is a key tool to advance a unified and coherent approach to evidence-based advocacy so that all stakeholders across sectors are clear on the purpose, aims, utility, value, and anticipated outcomes of palliative care [5].

Palliative care should be fully integrated throughout the life course and care continuum. This integration requires all health professionals to be trained in generalist palliative care skills, including the ability to recognize when specialist palliative consultation is needed across the health system it can be provided as a standalone intervention or in conjunction with disease-modifying treatments. Palliative care does not suddenly start and curative care suddenly end. As Boyd et al. have shown the journey of care is rarely linear, but rather there are ups and downs, patients become very ill, improve, decline, then improve again – a circular and often unpredictable trajectory [10].

Over the past two decades, major inequalities in the development and delivery of palliative care have been identified beyond the Lancet Commission. These include inequalities in the following domains:
- early and timely identification of the need for palliative care
- availability, accessibility, and appropriateness of palliative care
- comprehensiveness of care capable of embracing different and hidden facets of physical, psychological, social, and spiritual need
- services that discriminated, often with unconscious bias, on the basis of race, age, social status
- culturally, traditionally, and religiously inappropriately designed care
- a lack of understanding of the reach and purpose of the services
- a lack or reduced opportunities to negotiate services that meet changing needs

Inequalities do not just randomly happen, they reflect structural injustices. Inequalities can affect not only the patient and their family network, but also other informal carers and service providers. Understanding the processes that inform and perpetuate these inequalities and identifying their etiologies can provide guidance on how to dismantle them and reshape systems rooted in equity, inclusion, and social justice. Such process mapping can also help to identify those areas that may be outside of the realm of policy makers, palliative care practitioners and primary care providers to change – areas where wider societal change is a prerequisite to improving health outcomes for all sections of society.

The Environment that Breeds Inequalities

There are multiple ways of looking at how national health and social care systems are established, sustained and managed. One way is to understand how inter-related and frequently interlocked structures inform units of care delivery, and consequently, engender an environment where inequalities at all levels of care provision can emerge. Marmot's initial report on the social determinants of health, *Closing the gap in a generation: Health equity through action on the social determinants of health* [11] put into the public, and the public health domain what Tudor Hart [12], and countless other protagonists of "community care" had been saying for years, namely that well-being owes far less to health services than to

the systems and structures in which these health services functions. Marmot's updated report, *Health Equity in England: The Marmot Review ten years on* [13], showed that this last decade has been marked by deteriorating health and widening health inequalities throughout England. Understanding how the societal determinants of health and the determinants of the health system sit together provides a critical matrix to understanding, addressing, and unveiling the sources of inequalities. When applied to the provision of palliative care, we see that it is a set of different interlocking and interconnecting structures which together determine how palliative care is delivered and received. Box 1 provides an overview of these structures:

Box 1: Structures shaping care

Institutional structures: The way that care systems are built and maintained. This includes both the physical space and place of care, and also the delivery processes and the packages of care managed by institutions. Once in place, packages of care, like buildings, are often difficult to deconstruct and reshape.

Educational structures: The way that skills are taught and transferred, the premises on which healthcare teaching is delivered, the foundational knowledge base which determines the type of care that is presented as the standard "normative" care within communities and national systems.

Economic structures: The way in which care is costed, and the drivers to greater cost efficiency and productivity. Alongside the very direct care costings economic structures determine the benefit systems, and drive decision making for carers, and for relatives. Once a night-time carer's allowance has been put in place, or a benefit granted, few feel able to make changes.

Societal structures: The ways in which society establishes its norms and values. There is an overriding emphasis on unity within our health systems, with established patterns and processes and systems of healthcare which veer away from complexity and multi-dimensional "untidy" diverse approaches to care, and encourage an endless move towards uniformity.

Identity structures: Potentially the most fluid of all of the structures, they also can be the most set in stone. Identity structures refer to the way that each of us, experience and interpret the world around us, influenced by religious, social, emotional beliefs and traditions, family and cultural normative behaviours and expectations.

A Principle-Based Approach to Palliative Care Equity

Perhaps the best way of understanding and tackling inequalities is to first focus on a set of principles that encapsulate the best in palliative care and to explore situations in every day service where these principles have been compromised.

Principle One: Palliative care is reflective of different communities' meta-narratives on death and dying

The Lancet Commission on the Value of Death recently sought to bring focus to the interrelated social, economic, cultural, religious, and political factors that inform how death, dying, and grief are engaged across various contexts and in the global village as a whole. The narratives of individuals with advanced, progressive illnesses and their families – the narratives that define and shape the cultures of marginalised groups within our increasingly multicultural societies – are harder to hear and often overshadowed by a dominant voice rooted in colonisation and white supremacy [14]. And, again, the most disadvantaged suffer most from imbalances in suffering, dying, and grieving.

Truth-telling narratives in serious illness are often pushed aside by a death-defying, death-ignoring meta-narrative focused on cure and life-sustaining interventions, explicitly valuing quantity of life over quality. All the grand religious traditions recognised the inspiration of the sacred beyond the grave, the possibilities of passing places between this world and the "next," or another unseen parallel space, and acknowledged that the essence of life was that it was physically finite, yet spiritually eternal. Aging and death were understood and accepted within the religious and social frameworks that constituted a community's culture and traditions.

The Value of Death Commission [15] highlighted the complexity of world views which disregarded people's perspectives and ancient connections with nature and knowledge. They set out to describe a "realistic utopia" on how and what dying "could be." Their five principles of the realistic utopia call for a world where: (1) the social determinants of death, dying, and grieving are tackled; (2) dying is understood to be a relational and spiritual process rather than simply a physiological event; (3) networks of care lead support for people dying, caring, and grieving; (4) conversations and stories about everyday death, dying, and grief become common; and (5) death is recognised as having value.

The Commission noted the changing narrative across the world to explain and indeed manage life's beginnings and endings, recognising that a major consequence is an uncertainty of talking about death and dying. This has been coupled with a continued expectation that success lies in cure and fending off death rather than in ensuring that those with life limiting illnesses can have a good death. Who suffers the most in such situations? Is it the patient receiving aggressive treatments when treatments are potentially harmful? Or the family hanging onto hope that death is still somewhere in the future and thus failing to say goodbye properly? Or the clinician who feels that they have failed when nature has taken its course? All of these have been challenged with the unpredictability brought about by the pandemic, with its battle imagery of fighting against COVID-19 and the deep seated desire, and societal pressure to "win" over COVID-19.

Principle Two: Palliative care is responsive and adaptive to a person's beliefs, tradition, language, culture, and way of life

Fewer opportunities to openly discuss death and dying is a degradation of health professionals' expertise and ability to actively respond to religious, spiritual, and cultural community needs. Investments have been made by the National Health Service (NHS) in establishing ethnic sensitivity, cultural awareness, and competency trainings, and developing a fairness culture within the health service. Respect for the religious and spiritual beliefs of others is now core to care and an essential competency.

But for many patients such respect for their beliefs has not resulted in recognition of their particular spiritual issues and needs, nor has it been translated into the empathic engagement needed to have open, honest, and transparent dialogue with clinical teams [16].

In studies conducted in Edinburgh with health professionals, we uncovered considerable anxieties about discussing and supporting the spirituality of others with differing beliefs.

Members of minority ethnic communities have found themselves struggling to access care and to find support that respects and honours their particular traditions and views, and this has had significant negative consequences for those nearing death and for their families. Equitable palliative care must ensure that all patients and their families are able to carry out the traditions and rituals important to them, in a space and place where they feel comfortable and respected (Box 2). COVID-19 and isolation from family, faith communities, and social support systems has elevated the risk for spiritual distress, spiritual injury, and spiritual crisis [17]. Every health professional is accountable for spiritual care assessments for seriously ill

Box 2: Cross cultural care

Daniel was admitted with advanced carcinoma of the lung.

He is 42 years old and of Nigerian origin but has lived away from Nigeria for many years. He was originally admitted for uncontrolled and severe pain, but his condition has rapidly deteriorated and he is now bedbound. He has a large family and an argument has developed between the patient's family and a care assistant looking after him. The family brought in some food that they wished the patient to have and the care assistant has said they are unable to use facilities to heat the food due to health and safety regulations. The care assistant is very unhappy about Daniel's relatives being disruptive – particularly by praying "too loudly."

The case is discussed at the multidisciplinary team (MDT) meeting, and one of the nurses caring for Daniel explains that his family members are scared about what is happening to him. They believe that if he has the right food to eat, he will become stronger and will be able to have more treatment to cure his cancer. She has spoken to Daniel separately who wants to go along with whatever his family members want, although he is aware that he is dying and wants to go back to Nigeria to die. The team agrees that the doctor, the nurse, and the social worker caring for Daniel will hold a family meeting to ensure an environment of cultural safety and cultural humility is nurtured.

Following the meeting, the ward agrees to let Daniel's family prepare his meals; they also look into the possibility of him flying to Nigeria, including access to palliative care services in the country.

individuals and their loved ones – which should consistently occur upon intake, during care transitions and changes in clinical status, and certainly in advance of the time surrounding dying and death.

Inequalities in care can arise specifically because of migration. While UK systems of palliative care are, broadly speaking, individual rather than family focused, there is a latent expectation within the health service that family support will be available to "fill the gaps" in care. For those who lack easily accessible community or family support, such as those who have recently arrived in the UK, particularly from circumstances of violence, armed conflict, or imminent threat, this can result in care failures, patient harm, and negative clinical outcomes. Patients newer to the system frequently lack awareness of what services are available and lack an understanding of the cost of services, risking their socioeconomic wellbeing and stability.

Thoughtful and sensitive communication with patients and relatives is an essential aspect of person-centred,

high-quality, and holistic palliative care provision. Alongside those who struggle to communicate in English because it is a second or third language, many patients (even those who speak English as their mother tongue) feel they lack the "medical English speak" to communicate properly with doctors and nurses, or to question their palliative care plans.

Additionally, it is important to engage the services of an interpreter and include them as part of the multi-disciplinary team where possible. Allowing family members to interpret can lead to nondisclosure of potentially important information. There may also be a role for interpreters in promoting cultural understanding and insight for the care professionals beyond language interpretation [18]. Chapter 7, Conversations and Communication, provides practical guidance on working with interpreters to facilitate good communication.

Principle Three: Person rather than disease-focused palliative care

The COVID-19 pandemic has shifted national and global attention from the commonly categorised "palliative care diseases" (e.g., cancers, heart failure, human immunodeficiency virus (HIV) in many regions in Africa). Cancer in the United Kingdom has a well-understood "public story" incorporated within its narrative. It is a death conversation, even if the threads of that conversation are about "fighting death," "not giving in," and "not losing the battle."

In 2008, Murray and Sheikh [19] argued that health professionals and systems must apply the lessons learned from cancer to the growing number of people dying from non-malignant illnesses. Those living with advanced diseases, dementia, organ failure, or physical frailty still have far fewer services available that are much less likely to deal with all dimensions of need. Many palliative care services are still designed in traditional, disease specific ways thus reducing the opportunity of accessing benefits to properly and effectively addressing their symptoms. Having a disease that is not boxed into a set time, with a set prognosis and expected clinical picture, creates health service difficulties as palliative structures are set up to manage, and be managed within a pre-determined and often erroneous time line. The disease one lives and dies with can in some cases be financially crippling, leading families into a spiral of poverty.

Several tools, such as the Supportive and Palliative Care Indicators Tool (SPICT) (see Chapter 1: The Context and Principles of Palliative Care), have been developed in the UK to challenge the inequalities due to types of and access to care. These tools inherently emphasise the need for health professionals to engage the concept of palliation in practice as they make care decisions with patients [20]. One question remains a useful indicator of access: Would you be surprised if this person died within the next year? If the answer is "no," Boyd and colleagues argue, consideration should be given to placing such patients, irrespective of diagnosis, onto a palliative/supportive care register. Box 3 provides a small case study of good practice in decision-making. Rather than providing a definitive prognostication index, this approach enables the practitioner to adjust the focus of care from curative/life prolonging to supportive/palliative care and to ensure that they consider the likely needs of the patients and provision of care, ensuring that patients are able to achieve excellence in end-of-life care, including discussions around advanced care planning, decisions around cardio-pulmonary resuscitation (CPR) and to prevent unnecessary/unwanted hospital admissions.

Box 3:   Holistic decision making

Tom, a 74-year-old man with chronic obstructive pulmonary disease (COPD) has been increasingly breathless for the past two years and is now house-bound due to breathlessness on exertion. Tom has reported moderate to severe pain of unknown etiology in his lower back, likely due to overall deconditioning and debility. He lives with his wife Pauline who is 72 years and is his main carer. Pauline is also unwell, suffering from diabetes and chronic leg ulcers. They are receiving some assistance from social services who help with shopping and cleaning, but despite this are still struggling to manage. The district nurses visit regularly and suggest referring Tom to the local hospice for assistance with symptoms of breathlessness and pain. Tom and Pauline are reluctant for referral to the hospice as they see the service as being only for patients with advanced cancer who are dying. After some further discussion with the community respiratory nurse – who they know well – they agree to a joint visit from the palliative care community nurse together with the respiratory nurse.

After undertaking a holistic assessment of Tom's and his wife's needs, the palliative care nurse refers Tom to the physiotherapist for advice on non-pharmacological management of his breathlessness while starting him on oral morphine to control his symptoms more quickly. She refers him to day care which he will be able to attend once a week in order to give his wife caregiver respite. She also arranges for the occupational therapist to visit to assist with adaptations to their home to enable Tom and Pauline to care for themselves more easily. The palliative care nurse and respiratory nurse arrange to visit again in two weeks' time to review the situation.

Principle Four: Palliative care is initiated at the most appropriate time for the patient

The most impactful way to reduce inequalities in access to and in management of the complexity of all pain and suffering is to ensure that palliative care starts not at the end point just before death, but at the stage the patient, their carers, and health workers recognise that the person is confronting an illness that is, ultimately, life-limiting. Consulting and involving palliative care for the "actively dying" patient is a disservice to the dying one who may have unmet needs, the loved ones who may be struggling with anticipatory grief, and the ethics of "do no harm." But knowing how, what, and when to provide such care remains difficult for many practitioners. Too early, and angst is exacerbated, especially in a pervasive culture that is socially death-denying; too late, and blame is apportioned for delays in starting to administer palliative care. In a curative focused environment, where hope is pinned to retaining life at all costs, there is often a huge reluctance among practitioners to raise discussions about death and dying.

Universally accessible and publicly provided palliative care that is integrated as a component of comprehensive health coverage should ideally start at the time of serious illness diagnosis, work in tandem with disease-modifying treatments, ensure holistic care for patients during the time surrounding death, and continue to support bereaved loved ones. This ongoing and evolving model of palliative care involvement allows access to needed services as new symptoms arise and the patient condition ebbs and flows. The changing nature of the emphasis on what palliative care is and does, creates a much more fluid space for developing equitable, inclusive services. Moving from the construction of palliative care as disease-focused towards a more patient-focused construction that is determined by the patient's experience of suffering creates new opportunities for palliative care professionals to intervene. While the cancer journey facilitates a conversation about palliation, other diseases such as COPD provide no such ready trigger. Longitudinal studies from Edinburgh's Primary Palliative Care Research Group, working with people with end-stage COPD identified the way in which COPD was a "disease with no beginning," "a middle that is a way of life," and "an unpredictable and unanticipated end." However, if the integrated model is achieved, there is no need for palliative care intervention at beginning, middle, or end, but rather a continuous and evolving relationship-based model that allows for palliation and whole-person/whole-family support throughout the experience of illness, dying, death, and grief.

Pinnock et al. provide a telling description of the difference in approach to patients with COPD which has a fundamental influence on equity. In contrast to consultations with people with cancer where there was often a more natural discussion on death, a familiar and comfortable pattern of consulting with a patient with a chronic illness prevented initiating an unlooked for discussion about the future:

"Interviewer: I was going to ask you whether you have talked to him at all about what might happen in the future and how things might progress?
GP: No, not really. He usually has got his own [agenda in the consultation]. It's more reassurance about how he is and chatting generally and he just likes a bit of social discourse I think." [21 p.7]

Has it changed in this past decade? Prior to the pandemic the response is likely to be no, the pockets of excellence, and the aspirations for good conversations around dying, are held in tension with unprecedented rise in demand on General Practice.

Principle Five: The most equitable palliative care is fluid and adapts to suit the changing physical needs of patients and their carers

Palliative care needs to recognise both the linear journey element of living in the face of death (i.e. the inevitability of death) and the potential circular nature of this journey (the lack of certainty on timing of death, the ups and downs of the disease journey, and the remissions and relapses). The majority of health services are constructed along linear models, and once patients are on the conveyer belt of a linear approach to care it is extremely difficult to move off it.

Inequalities result, in part, when the care being given is not the care needed. There are various reasons why both health professionals and patients struggle to make the care changes that would better serve the emerging needs related to life-limiting and serious illness. Patients can lack the right information about the nature of the care they can expect to receive, especially patients not familiar with the health system, or they may lack the confidence to challenge the nurse or the doctor when prescriptions are repeated, or advice given that was suitable a year ago, but has been overtaken by events. Patients may fear that describing an improvement may result in care being withdrawn, or a change in the routine of care. Patients and their loved ones may be uninformed or incorrect in their conceptions of palliative care, their rights to holistic treatment, and their opportunities to have psychosocial, spiritual, and cultural care needs addressed beyond pain management. Box 2

captures a respectful and cohesive approach to inclusively manage a potentially divisive cultural and social issue.

Those least likely to challenge the routine are those most at risk of receiving a form of care that does not actually meet their current needs. Alongside the multiple patient-initiated reasons for continuing with the status quo there are an equally large number of reasons that are linked to professional reluctance or indecision around change, such as nurses feeling inhibited to speak out in support of change, especially if senior medical leadership has made difficult to reverse decisions, such as social care benefits, introduction of meals on wheels, or intensive homecare. Health professionals that are not trained in palliative care can also hold misconceptions of the aims and benefits of palliative care that prevent them from involving these services. This lack of education permeates the health professions and widens disparities between who is able to access needed services and who continues to suffer without the ethical relief of distress.

Principle Six: Palliative care is accessible and responsive to those who have been marginalised at interpersonal, institutional, systemic, and structural levels.

There are multiple reasons why some people exist on the margins of society or have been pushed to the edges of society. These include, for example, individuals with severe and/or untreated mental health challenges, pronounced learning or physical disabilities, and persons experiencing homelessness and substance use disorder, among others.

Providing equitable and inclusive palliative care to persons who have been disenfranchised is challenging, not least because palliative care, as a service, is dependent on the concept of continuity of health care. Current palliative care referral structures require practitioners to establish beginnings, to identify changes that transition a person from one form of palliative care to another form of specialist palliative care often with new people and new approaches. Much palliative (and indeed health) care assumes a stable address for identification and billing, as well as safe discharge planning; the availability of the patient to attend appointments; and the ability to be in the "right place" at the "right time" for the service to function.

Take persons experiencing homelessness for example. Barriers include:
- Unstable living conditions and situations complicated by potential lack of safety and estranged relationships with family
- Lack of identification or other pertinent documentation

- Untreated medical conditions and potentially under addressed daily needs
- Experiences of stigma, bias, and judgment within an inflexible health system
- Nature of receiving palliative care in homeless hostels with the extra burden of care placed on hostel staff.

Suggestions to improving access to care for those who are homeless have been identified (Box 4).

A number of new initiatives have been undertaken to improve access to palliative care for persons experiencing homelessness. A UK model embedding palliative care teams (nurses and social workers) within homeless hostels for two half-days a month to support and train hostel staff improved outcomes. The model fostered collaborative learning between the hostel staff and palliative care specialists, where hostel staff felt more confident, recognised their roles and were able to identify opportunities to seek the needed health or social care for their residents. Equitable access to primary care, nevertheless, remained a challenge for many of the reasons mentioned above [22].

Palliative care provision for incarcerated persons is also an area of great inequality in care provision. A European Association for Palliative Care (EAPC) Taskforce set up in 2017 mapped palliative care provision in prisons in Europe, where England and Wales were the only countries to have some designated palliative care units within prisons, the limited availability was an indicator for inequitable care [23]. A recent Scottish study that explored the role of hospices in supporting patients in prison showed that only 30% of the hospices were providing direct care to patients with palliative care needs in prison, while 65% of hospices were sharing advice to prison healthcare teams in order to support prisoners with their end-of-life needs. Key challenges have been identified [24], including the lack of preparation to support people if they were given compassionate release, and the prison environment making it difficult for people to receive controlled medication and medical equipment [25] "now, there wasn't an option for

her to die in the prison … you wouldn't have been able to fit all the equipment we needed into her room … it would have been a fire risk, because you couldn't get a bed through the door if a fire was to start in the prison. So, it was just no, no, she wouldn't have been able to die there" [25 p.569].

Principle Seven: Palliative care has no age barriers

The majority of palliative care services have been established with a specific population in mind, an adult population, often between the ages of 40–70, the majority of whom have a diagnosis of cancer. Children's palliative care has made huge advances in recent years leading to it being recognised as a speciality in its own right. Resources such as the International Children's Palliative Care Network speak of the shift in perspectives [26]. NICE developed a guide specifically for End-of-Life care for infants, children, and young people with life-limiting conditions: planning and management in 2016 and the UK charity Together for Short Lives has developed resource guides to support families of children during preference and choice of care.

Older people who have additional minoritised identities (e.g., Indigenous groups, racially or culturally marginalised) are at increased risk of being overlooked and experiencing harm. Health professional education at all levels and system-wide policies must be accountable for creating care environments for older people that are culturally safe, respectful, and invested in the ideal of a "longevity society" where older people thrive as full members of society [27].

Getting the place of care right for frail older persons is challenging. The COVID-19 pandemic exacerbated what was already an inequitably funded, and unequal system of care. The diversity of the services offered within care homes, the complexity of the needs of residents almost all of whom are living with frailty has led to inequalities in access to appropriate palliative care. The British Geriatiric Society report notes 400,000 older people live in care homes in the UK a number projected to rise by 127% within the next 20 years [28]. Most of those living in care homes are in their last two years of life. Though care home staff are skilled at reducing the risk of falls, care residents are three times more likely to fall than others of the same age living in their home [29]. Are care homes set up to provide comprehensive palliative care services? Staff in care homes may be less aware of the need for palliative care and the requirements to consider issues such as end-of-life care planning. Frequently there is little discussion with the patient and their relatives about what should happen if the patient's

---

Box 4:   Improving care for those who are homeless

- Building trust between homeless and health professional, removing stigma, and careful listening.
- Linking and developing partnerships between community and health services, allowing more flexibility.
- Training of health and social professionals to understand experiences and lives of homeless people.
- Provision of community palliative care beds within homeless hostels.

condition changes or their condition deteriorates unexpectedly. There is a disparity in the standard of palliative care between those with a diagnosis of cancer and those with other chronic, life-limiting conditions such as dementia. The long period of decline that the frail elderly experience often does not fit with a hospice care model. Until recently, the palliative care community had relatively little dialogue with geriatricians, many of whom provide holistic care, although as the 2018 Care Quality Commission report found there is limited emphasis on planning for dying [30]. It is not uncommon that end-of-life care for the frail elderly is triggered by crises admissions followed by weekend and night-time referrals to community crises care teams to provide a care cover until "something can be done, somewhere can be found" for the patient. Several educational programmes to improve palliative care in UK care homes were implemented which have been assessed as having a positive impact on care staff skills and communication including "The Six Steps to Success," NHS England – North West » Six Steps to Success in End-of-Life Care; "PACE (Palliative Care Across Europe)" final1-pace-impactpublication.pdf (europa.eu); "the Namaste programme" Namaste Care Programme | The End-of-Life Partnership (eolp.co.uk) and "Needs Round," an approach delivered in Australia that incorporates clinical triage, person centred planning and case-based education has been tailored to UK context [31]. Also see Chapter 16: Frailty, Dementia and Multi-Morbidity.

Principle eight: Palliative care is inclusive of all historically excluded groups

Historically excluded groups have experienced marginalisation structurally and systemically due to power imbalances and deliberate injustices that degrade their humanity due to race, culture, ethnicity, sexual orientation, or gender identity, among other identities. The rights of lesbian, gay, bisexual, transgender, and queer/questioning individuals (LGBTQ+) have been recognised by several legislatives in the UK including the Equality Act (2010), Gender Recognition Act (2004), the Civil Partnership Act (2004) and Same-Sex Marriage in 2014. However, the LGBTQ+ community still has negative experiences when accessing health and social services – ranging from sanctioned discrimination and violence, to homophobia and transphobia, to stigma and disenfranchised grief and bereavement for the spouses, chosen families, and social supports of LGBTQ+ patients. Understandable distrust of the health system, coupled with potential abandonment from faith communities and families of origin and broader social

marginalization and mistreatment, leads to worse health outcomes among these populations. The underassessment of LGBTQ+ identity and specific health needs, preferences, and concerns, as well as services not recognising the sanctity and validity of minoritised sexual orientations and gender identities create barriers during treatment in addition to the exclusion of spouses and partners from important conversation regarding care. The chosen families of LGBTQ+ individuals often shoulder the added burden of fear and worry of mistreatment alongside their grief in the serious illness context [32].

The first studies exploring the health experiences of the LGBT community with advanced illness when accessing healthcare in the UK highlighted barriers to access and offered a set of recommendations to improve care. These included recommendations at: individual level such as the avoidance of heteronormative assumptions and language, sensitivity to sexual orientation, acknowledgement of preferences regarding disclosure of sexual identity and gender history, sensitive exploration of relationships and partners with care, and the inclusion of partners and significant others in the conversations about care.

At the service level, recommendations included clarity of policy and procedures regarding discrimination, the inclusion in training about LGBT communities, and LGBT visibility, visual indicators such as signs of inclusivity e.g., the rainbow, and active partnerships with LGBT communities [33]. These have progressed to become more inclusive in order to create culturally safe healthcare environments for LGBT persons and their families (both chosen and biological).

Research conducted by Jones and colleagues in the US points to people of less well represented racial and ethnic groups having more severe pain, less advance directive completion, more in-hospital deaths with higher frequency of aggressive medical treatment, less palliative care consultation, and often experience both implicit and explicit bias and discrimination [34]. Palliative specialists around the world are calling for transformations of clinical practice, research, education, and policy to dismantle racist structures and reshape care environments that readily address the social determinants of health and the global historical narrative of racism, that has had intergenerational and multidimensional impact. Jones et al. identified a top ten list of pointers in delivering care that was antiracist, many of the pointers are applicable in UK settings [35]. Investments are needed to forge race-conscious palliative care systems informed by socially just research and practice models [36].

Principle nine: Palliative care adapts to change, embeds quality and effectively utilises modern technology in response to changing contexts

Palliative care professionals are trained to address and lead complex decision-making in times of clinical uncertainty. They are skilled and proactive in managing severe deterioration that accompanies different disease trajectories. However, the COVID-19 pandemic shocked all health systems and changed the very nature of palliative care access and provision. Looming front and centre in the examination of inequalities and the systems of provision for palliative care in the UK and globally is the impact of the pandemic. With the onset of the pandemic, palliative care rapidly moved in many countries from being both a discrete specialist led service and a service working to support non-specialist delivery in the hospital and community sectors, to a system that was being integrated into specialist, emergency, intensive care in a dynamic, rapidly transitioning uncertain period. Attempting to meet the changing and urgent needs of patients and those of staff unprepared for the weight of suffering and death put new pressures on palliative care (Chapter 23: Creating space, clarity, and containment in order to sustain staff: managing the emotional impact of palliative care work, focusses on supporting staff). As public health guidance required people to remain in isolation with limited physical contact, palliative care services adapted and responded in creative ways extending outreach services, training to non-specialists, employing technology for communication and developing strategies to promote staff well-being [37]. These critical lessons of rapid change, flexibility, training of staff and repurposing plans to meet ever growing demands and these may be valuable to carry forward.

Box 5 includes transcripts from palliative care teams in the UK and Europe on the implementation of digital solutions to support communication between patients and families [37].

However, inequalities in the use of the communication technology were present when access to equipment was limited and existing information technology systems were fragile. In addition, people with either communication difficulties, severely unwell or older adults often struggled [37]. Using technology as a communication mechanism is dependent on having access to, and being able, familiar and comfortable with using technologies. And while health facilities may have been able to offer inclusive design technologies, the cheapest most commonly used technologies were often not suitable for families and carers who had hearing, sight or touch disabilities. Digital equity is a priority for the modernisation and advancement of palliative care.

Some of the many challenges to discussions about patient preference and advance care planning between healthcare workers, the patient and family were exacerbated further during the pandemic. With extreme patient isolation from family and from professionals, uncertainty in response to treatment, increased workload on staff and more limited choices of discharge, it became more challenging to have meaningful discussions regarding individualised care and share the information across services [38].

International Dimensions and Palliative Care Integration into Humanitarian Relief Services

There is a huge need for palliative care in all countries, especially in low-and-middle income countries (LMICs). While palliative care is recognised as an integral component of healthcare and a marker of quality within a health care system by WHO, many health systems continue to fail to meet the mark. The second edition of the Economist Intelligence Unit Quality of Death Report show high income countries at the top of the ranks and disparities in the quality of death between less and more wealthy countries continue to widen. The scarce availability and access to pain medication, limited training programmes and resources, as well as the lack of basic service infrastructure hinders palliative care development.

However, exceptional efforts by lower income countries like Panama, Mongolia, and Uganda have given promise. The positive impact that contributed to rapid access of care was contributed to the integration of palliative care into primary settings, collaborative work in development of teaching programmes and innovative means to make medication and care affordable. Furthermore, home and community-based care may be key in bridging inequities to care present in rural areas [39].

Box 5:   The use of digital tools to support communication between patient and families

"The iPads which we managed to raise through charity donations – through the use of our Face Book page – are now available on all wards with the support of our IT team and information governance teams have allowed many families to speak or even just see their loved ones." [37 p.825]

"On the COVID unit we only allowed 2 visitors for 30 min to say goodbye to a dying patient. We invested a lot in virtual saying goodbye with Jitsi which IT installed on special laptops for this. We have a very good team of psychologists and chaplains that were available 24/7 to give support to the COVID team and helped with the virtual goodbye saying." [37 p.822]

As highlighted in Chapter 1: The Context and Principles of Palliative Care, the Lancet Commission on Palliative Care and Pain Relief estimated that 80% of people who experienced serious health-related suffering in 2015 were from LMICs [3], where palliative care is underdeveloped and healthcare systems are overwhelmed. Shifting towards low-cost solutions such as the introduction of an essential package of medication and medical equipment safely prescribed at the primary care level as well as developing the competencies of healthcare workers is paramount.

Palliative care needs were seen to exacerbate further or be left neglected when responding to complex humanitarian crisis such as during displacement of individuals, at refugee camps, disease outbreaks, and at mass casualty events where people are triaged based on their odds of survival [40]. Box 6 illustrates some complex humanitarian setting scenarios where palliative care is indicated.

Box 6:   Palliative care scenarios in the settings of humanitarian crises

"Scenario 1: Mass casualty triage.

Following an earthquake resulting in hundreds of deaths and severe damage to local infrastructure, the wounded are presenting to an emergency field hospital. Medical staff are triaging people to different areas for immediate life-saving care, less serious injuries, and those whose injuries are too severe to survive and are deemed unsalvageable. One such young man has a severe crush injury. He is confused and agitated, complaining of thirst, and moaning in pain." [41 p.2]

"Scenario 2: End-stage disease.

An NGO is responsible for care provision in a refugee camp bordering a country with ongoing and evolving civil war. A woman who was forced to flee two weeks ago arrives with her teenage son. Prior to fleeing she was receiving hemodialysis for end-stage renal disease. The camp does not have access to dialysis, and the physician assessing her expects she will deteriorate and die within the coming few weeks with the limited available care." [41 p.2]

"Scenario 3: Incurable condition.

An Ebola Treatment Centre has been established to care for patients at a time when the case fatality rate approaches 60%. All care is provided in full Personal Protective Equipment, minimizing time and contact with patients. A woman from an outlying area has been admitted to the Centre. Family members are not allowed to enter the Centre due to concerns of contagion and she has had no contact with family since her arrival. Despite supportive treatment she is deteriorating rapidly with a dire prognosis. While experiencing ongoing diarrhoea and vomiting, she is delirious, distressed, and calling out for loved ones." [41 p.2]

The WHO has established a guide to integrating palliative care in response to humanitarian emergencies [42] and palliative care has been added as an essential concept of health in the latest edition of The Sphere Handbook [43]. Models of effective integration of palliative care in humanitarian care teams can be found in Jordan, Bangladesh and India, and these models push the boundaries of traditional palliative care to meet the bespoke needs of the different experiences. For example a clinician working at a medical unit at Za'atari camp in Jordan, provided spiritual therapy and prescribed higher doses of pain medicine to Syrian refugees after having received palliative care training. The following quotes the experiences of a 34 year old female with advanced cancer who was living at Za'atari camp:

Every day that I don't see [the palliative team] and the pain comes, I enter a different world. I can't talk with anyone or contribute anything. It's very difficult. But the mobile medical team drives me whenever I need it. Whenever they don't come, I go to the clinic and I take pills and if there's a vacation, then they give me the shot and the pills for the day of the vacation. Thankfully, I take them and I can sleep and eat. They changed my life a lot [44 p.26].

Adaptive models of the palliative provision, by training and supporting workers on site can challenge inbuilt inequalities [45]. As Farzana Khan explains in her analysis of the needs of those in refugee settings, reaching beyond the visible to hear the complexity of need is important:

Mojidor is a 10-year old Rohingya boy with bone cancer living in Cox's Bazar refugee camp, Bangladesh. When he was diagnosed at the camp field hospital, Mojidor and his mother cried all night fearing he would soon die. Mojidor has two little sisters. His father is missing. We found Mojidor in a tent lying on a mat, unable to move or walk because of his pain. In the past, Mojidor was a typical football-loving boy. His nickname was 'bhuissya' meaning 'buffalo'. We started pain treatment, and now Mojidor can walk and even smiles a little [45 p.4].

Armed conflicts are increasingly dangerous and violent as militarised violence has become more sophisticated and treacherous. The 2022 Russian invasion of Ukraine has shocked systems everywhere with the murder, sexual assault, and displacement of thousands of Ukrainian citizens. In these dire times with accompanying dire consequences, it is critical that the value of alleviating suffering and dignifying death be prioritized and kept central to emergency planning and response interventions.

Box 7 sets out a set of steps urgently required to alleviate suffering and care for these with palliative needs [46].

Box 7:   Recommendations for alleviating suffering in war

Urgent Recommendations	• Prioritise humane, dignified, and compassionate care for the dying even in the face of conflict as outlined in the Sendai Framework for disaster Risk Reduction
	• Leverage multidisciplinary academic, clinical, and policy stakeholders to partner with civilians and community-based networks to create safe, supportive spaces to discuss anticipatory grief and fear, and provide psychosocial and spiritual support for the dying and the grieving
	• Strengthen and extend existing bereavement support systems and services that bridge transitional care gaps between health systems and communities
	• Relay the experiences of families and children confronting death and dying to provide realistic understanding of the consequences and harms of militarized violence
	• Provide telehealth supports within and outside of conflict regions to provide psychosocial, spiritual, and bereavement supports
	• Triage serious health-related suffering in both community- and hospital-based settings to ensure timely and strategic responses to the dying processes of those with life-threatening illness
	• Create pathways for controlled essential medicines access (i.e., opioids) to manage pain and other distressing symptoms at EOL
Ongoing Recommendations	• Identify war and violence as a social determinant of dying, death, and grief, creating future crises standards of care that include attention to EOL and bereavement
	• Address war as an integral component of the death system that mediates life and death in the presence of threat, danger, and violence
	• Continue to relay the stories of death and dying in the face of war in academia and lay media to reveal the dehumanizing truths of EOL and grief amid violence
	• Highlight stories of marginalized groups within conflict regions, including the incarcerated, refugees, homeless, cultural, and ethnic minorities, children, women, and the elderly, to address the intersectionality of violence and structural discrimination
	• Continue to support policies and practices to actively dismantle racism, bias, and neo-colonialist structures that devalue the living and dying of human beings across cultures and contexts
	• Advocate for integrated palliative care models in all countries to ensure suffering is alleviated across the serious illness continuum in both times of peace and war
	• Increase death literacy and global collective action toward health and social equity, freedom, and the right to a sacred dying and death

---

Prior to the war, opioid availability and palliative care access in both Ukraine and Russia were unacceptably low given the estimated SHS in both countries. Given the increased pain and trauma inflicted by war, there are undoubtedly countless Ukrainians and Russian suffering without critical access to analgesics and other symptom relieving essential medicines.

To tackle the discrepancies and gaps in care a global network of palliative care researchers and specialists have come together under the banner of PallCHASE, (Pallchase.org – Palliative Care in Humanitarian Aid Situations and Emergencies) [47]. Its aim is to see a world where everyone affected by humanitarian situations or emergencies who is experiencing serious health-related suffering has access to palliative care.

Conclusion

The barriers to accessing palliative for those who are the most poor and who are suffering the most are without doubt, "the most disfiguring inequity in health care today" [48]. This lack of inclusion into services or failure to find and refer to the most appropriate service is often not through intention, but through lack of knowledge, a loss as to what to do next, a failure of systems and service design. Getting end-of-life care "right" lies at the heart of what it means to be an equitable society and thus prioritising this area needs no apologies.

References

1. Farmer, P. (2003). *Pathologies of Power: Health, Human Rights, and the New War on the Poor*. Berkeley, CA: University of California Press.
2. UN high-level political meeting on UHC. (2019). 1966 international covenant; and WHPCA Global Atlas 2d ed.
3. Knaul, F.M., Farmer, P.E., Krakauer, E.L., De Lima, L., Bhadelia, A., Kwete, X.J., Arreola-Ornelas, H., Gómez-Dantés, O., Rodriguez, N.M., Alleyne, G.A., and Connor, S.R. (2018 April 7). Alleviating the access abyss in palliative care and pain relief—an imperative of universal health coverage: the Lancet Commission report. *The Lancet* 391 (10128): 1391–1454.
4. WHPCA Global Atlas 2d ed.
5. https://pubmed.ncbi.nlm.nih.gov/33944616.
6. Knaul, F.M., Rosa, W.E., Arreola-Ornelas, H., and Nargund, R.S. (2022). Closing the global pain divide: balancing access and excess. *The Lancet Public Health* 7 (4): e295–e296. doi: 10.1016/S2468-2667(22)00063-9.
7. IAHPC briefing notes.
8. Radbruch, L., De Lima, L., Knaul, F., Wenk, R., Ali, Z., Bhatnaghar, S., Blanchard, C., Bruera, E., Buitrago, R., Burla, C., and Callaway, M. (2020). Redefining palliative care—a new consensus-based definition. *Journal of Pain and Symptom Management* 60 (4): 754–764.
9. World Health Organization (2018). United Nations Children's Fund Declaration of Astana. https://www.who.int/docs/default-source/primary-health/declaration/gcphc-declaration.pdf (accessed 29 March 2021).
10. Boyd, K., Mason, B., Kendall, M. et al. (2010). Advance care planning for cancer patients in primary care: A feasibility study. *British Journal of General Practice* 60: e449–e458.
11. CSDH (2008). Closing the gap in a generation: health equity through action on the social determinants of health. Final Report of the Commission on the Social Determinants of Health. Geneva: WHO. https://www.who.int/publications/i/item/WHO-IER-CSDH-08.1 (accessed 9 August 2022).
12. Tudor Hart, J. (1971). The inverse care law. *The Lancet* 297: 405–412.
13. Marmot, M., Allen, J., Boyce, T., Goldblatt, P., and Morrison, J. (2020). *Health Equity in England: The Marmot Review ten Years On*. London: Institute of Health Equity.
14. https://ecancer.org/en/journal/editorial/121-decolonizing-end-of-life-care-lessons-and-opportunities#.Ymqakyx11NE.twitter.
15. Sallnow, L., Smith, R., Ahmedzai, S.H. et al. (2022). Report of the Lancet Commission on the Value of Death: bringing death back into life. *The Lancet* 399 (10327): 837–884. doi: 10.1016/S0140-6736(21)02314-X.
16. Irajpour, A., Moghimian, M., and Arzani, H. (2018). Spiritual aspects of care for chronic Muslim patients: a qualitative study. *Journal of Education and Health Promotion* 7: 118. Published 2018 Sep 14. doi: 10.4103/jehp.jehp_199_17.
17. Ferrell, B.R., Handzo, G., Picchi, T., Puchalski, C., and Rosa, W.E. (2020). The urgency of spiritual care: COVID-19 and the critical need for whole-person palliation. *Journal of Pain and Symptom Management* 60 (3): e7–e11. doi: 10.1016/j.jpainsymman.2020.06.034.
18. Norris, W.M., Wenrich, M.D., Nielsen, E.L. et al. (2005). Communication about end-of-life care between language-discordant patients and clinicians: insights from medical interpreters. *Journal of Palliative Medicine* 8: 1016–1024.
19. Murray, S.A. and Sheikh, A. (2008). Care for all at the end of life. *BMJ* 336: 958–959.
20. Lilyman, S. and Bruce, M. (2016). Palliative care for people with dementia: a literature review. *International Journal of Palliative Nursing* 22: 76–81.
21. Pinnock, H., Kendall, M., Murray, S.A. et al. (2011). Living and dying with severe chronic obstructive pulmonary disease: multiperspective longitudinal qualitative study. *BMJ* 342: d142.
22. Armstrong, M., Shulman, C., Hudson, B., Brophy, N., Daley, J., Hewett, N., and Stone, P. (2021). The benefits and challenges of embedding specialist palliative care teams within homeless hostels to enhance support and learning: perspectives from palliative care teams and hostel staff. *Palliative Medicine* 35: 1202–1214.
23. Turner, M., Chassagne, A., Capelas, M.L., Chambaere, K., Panozzo, S., Teves, C.M., and Riegler, E. (2021). Mapping palliative care provision in European prisons: an EAPC task force survey. *BMJ Supportive & Palliative Care* 0: 1–7. doi: 10.1136/bmjspcare-2020-002701. Published Online First: 22 April 2021.
24. http://globalpalliativecare.org/covid-19/uploads/briefing-notes/briefing-note-palliative-care-for-detainees-in-custodial-settings.pdf.
25. Mcparland, C. and Johnston, B. (2021). Caring, sharing, preparing and declaring: How do hospices support prisons to provide palliative and end of life care? a qualitative descriptive study using telephone interviews. *Palliative Medicine* 35: 563–573.
26. http://www.icpcn.org (accessed 9 August 2022)
27. Rosa, W.E., Bhadelia, A., Knaul, F.M., Travers, J.L., Metheny, N., and Fulmer, T. (2022). A longevity society requires integrated palliative care models for historically excluded older people. *The Lancet Healthy Longevity* 3 (4): e227–e228.
28. BGS. (2021). Ambitions for change: Improving healthcare in care homes. Available at BGS Ambitions for change - Improving healthcare in care homes.pdf (accessed 9 August 2022).
29. BGS (2020). End of life care in frailty: care homes. https://www.bgs.org.uk/resources/end-of-life-care-in-frailty-care.homes (accessed 29 March 2021).
30. Limb, M. (2018). Care Quality Commission finds growing inequalities in access to health and social care in England.
31. Macgregor, A., Rutherford, A., Mccormack, B., Hockley, J., Ogden, M., Soulsby, I., Mckenzie, M., Spilsbury, K.,

Hanratty, B., and Forbat, L. (2021). Palliative and end-of-life care in care homes: protocol for codesigning and implementing an appropriate scalable model of Needs Rounds in the UK. *BMJ Open* 11: e049486.

32. Rosa, W.E., Banerjee, S.C., and Maingi, S. (2022). Family caregiver inclusion is not a level playing field: toward equity for the chosen families of sexual and gender minority patients. *Palliative Care and Social Practice* 16: 26323524221092459. Published 2022 Apr 19. doi: 10.1177/26323524221092459.

33. Bristowe, K., Hodson, M., Wee, B., Almack, K., Johnson, K., Daveson, B.A., Koffman, J., Mcenhill, L., and Harding, R. (2018). Recommendations to reduce inequalities for LGBT people facing advanced illness: ACCESSCare national qualitative interview study. *Palliative Medicine* 32: 23–35.

34. Jones, T., Luth, E.A., Lin, S.Y., and Brody, A.A. (2021). Advance care planning, palliative care, and end-of-life care interventions for racial and ethnic underrepresented groups: a systematic review. *Journal of Pain and Symptom Management* 62 (3): e248–e260. doi: 10.1016/j.jpainsymman.2021.04.025. https://pubmed.ncbi.nlm.nih.gov/33984460.

35. Jones, K.F., Laury, E., Sanders, J.J. et al. (2022). Top ten tips palliative care clinicians should know about delivering antiracist care to Black Americans. *Journal of Palliative Medicine* 25 (3): 479–487. doi: 10.1089/jpm.2021.0502.

36. Sanders, J.J., Gray, T.F., Sihlongonyane, B., Durieux, B.N., and Graham, L. (2022). A framework for anti-racist publication in palliative care: structures, processes, and outcomes. *Journal of Pain and Symptom Management* 63 (3): e337–e343. doi: 10.1016/j.jpainsymman.2021.10.001.

37. Dunleavy, L., Preston, N., Bajwah, S., Bradshaw, A., Cripps, R., Fraser, L.K., Maddocks, M., Hocaoglu, M., Murtagh, F.E., Oluyase, A.O., Sleeman, K.E., Higginson, I.J., and Walshe, C. (2021). 'Necessity is the mother of invention': specialist palliative care service innovation and practice change in response to COVID-19. Results from a multinational survey (CovPall). *Palliative Medicine* 35: 814–829.

38. Bradshaw, A., Dunleavy, L., Walshe, C., Preston, N., Cripps, R.L., Hocaoglu, M., Bajwah, S., Maddocks, M., Oluyase, A.O., Sleeman, K., Higginson, I.J., Fraser, L., and Murtagh, F. (2021). Understanding and addressing challenges for advance care planning in the COVID-19 pandemic: an analysis of the UK CovPall survey data from specialist palliative care services. *Palliative Medicine* 35: 1225–1237.

39. Aregay, A., O'connor, M., Stow, J., Ayers, N., and Lee, S. (2020). Strategies used to establish palliative care in rural low- and middle-income countries: an integrative review. *Health Policy and Planning* 35: 1110–1129.

40. Powell, R.A., Schwartz, L., Nouvet, E., Sutton, B., Petrova, M., Marston, J., Munday, D., and Radbruch, L. (2017). Palliative care in humanitarian crises: always something to offer. *The Lancet* 389: 1498–1499.

41. Hunt, M., Nouvet, E., Chénier, A., Krishnaraj, G., Bernard, C., Bezanson, K., de Laat, S., and Schwartz, L. (2020 October 28). Addressing obstacles to the inclusion of palliative care in humanitarian health projects: A qualitative study of humanitarian health professionals' and policy makers' perceptions. *Conflict and Health* 14: 70. doi: 10.1186/s13031-020-00314-9. PMID: 33133234; PMCID: PMC7592183.

42. WHO. (2018). Integrating palliative care and symptom relief into primary health care: a WHO guide for planners, implementers and managers. Geneva, World Health Organization.

43. SPHERE Association. (2018). The sphere handbook: humanitarian charter and minimum standards in humanitarian response Geneva, Switzerland.

44. Pinheiro, I. and Jaff, D. (2018). The role of palliative care in addressing the health needs of Syrian refugees in Jordan. *Medicine, Conflict, and Survival* 34 (1) .1–38

45. Khan, F. and Dogherty, M. (2018). Neglected suffering: the unmet need for palliative care in Cox's Bazar. London, United Kingdom.

46. Rosa, W.E., Grant, L., Knaul, F.M., Marston, J., Arreola-Ornelas, H., Riga, O., Marabyan, R., Penkov, A., Sallnow, L., and Rajagopal, M.R. (2022 April 16). The value of alleviating suffering and dignifying death in war and humanitarian crises. *The Lancet* 399 (10334): 1447–1450.

47. PallCHASE | The University of Edinburgh.

48. Horton, R. (2018). Offline: "A sea of suffering". *The Lancet* 391: 1465.

4 Palliative Care in the Community

Matthew Doré, Catherine Millington-Sanders, Rachel Campbell, Paul Thomas, Laura Calamos, Rachael Marchant, Carolyn Doyle, Rachel Lukwago, Karen Hodson, and Susan van Beveren

Introduction

It's so much easier to suggest solutions when you don't know too much about the problem.

— Malcolm Forbes

It is easy to forget that dying at home, apart from in the past 50 years, used to be the norm in the United Kingdom (UK). The debate in the early 1960s was around the lack of availability of hospital beds for dying patients, particularly the old [1, 2]. At that time, it was recognised that death could not always be effectively managed at home, and admission for symptom control and nursing care was sometimes necessary.

Although admissions to hospital have increased in frequency in recent decades, even now patients in their last year of life spend much of their time at home. However, admissions to hospitals accelerate towards the end-of-life (Figure 1). Prior to the COVID-19 pandemic, more than half of deaths occurred in hospital and more than a third of patients died in community settings, either at home (20%) or in care homes (16%) [3].

In 2020 the COVID-19 pandemic correlated with approximately 76,000 excess deaths in England and Wales compared to the numbers anticipated pre-pandemic. Of these excess deaths more than half (41,000) occurred at home and in care homes [5]. For the first time ever, people aged over 85 were more likely to die in a care home than in hospital. Clearly the pandemic has been exceptional and complicates predictions for future years. Despite this, it is clear that with an ageing population and the recent data regarding place of death, the background trend is that increasingly people are dying in the community, and particularly in care homes. Indeed, it is predicted 76% of all deaths in England and Wales will occur in care facilities, hospices, and at home by 2040 [6].

This chapter explores palliative care in the community and the new developments that aim to improve its quality and extend its provision to all patients, irrespective of diagnosis and location. We of course understand a balance is needed between the safety net of expert medical in-patient facilities, but here we focus on growing and supporting the community in holistic end-of-life care as well as considering the benefits of primary care networks evolving into neighbourhood teams, as described in the Fuller Stocktake report [7]. In addition, we emphasise the need to partner with communities, building on the national "Ambitions for Palliative and End-of-Life Care" and Ambition 6: Each community is prepared to help [8]. We settle on an overall vision of strong partnership working between generalists and specialists in order to facilitate planned, palliative, and end-of-life care as a desirable and natural community event.

Ethos – What Is a Healthy Death?

A sum can be put right: but only by going back till you find the error and working it afresh from that point, never by simply going on.

— C.S. Lewis, The Great Divorce

The 2022 Lancet Commission [9]: The Value of Death: bringing death back into life argues that since 1950 dying in the UK has become overly medicalised and needs to be rebalanced.

At the core of this rebalancing must be relationships and partnerships between people who are dying, families, communities, health and social care systems, and wider civic society [7 p.838].

Handbook of Palliative Care, Fourth Edition. Edited by Richard Kitchen, Christina Faull, Sarah Russell and Jo Wilson.
© 2024 John Wiley & Sons Ltd. Published 2024 by John Wiley & Sons Ltd.

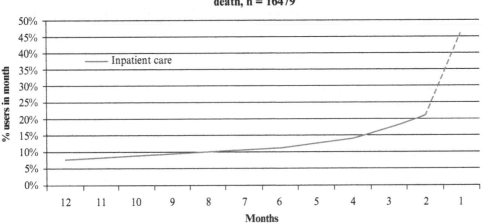

% people using inpatient and social care in months before death, n = 16479

Figure 1   Hospital admissions at end-of-life [4].

A clear focus of community palliative care is to nudge palliative care back to the social and human event it used to be, i.e., to de-medicalise dying. Indeed, dying is a natural event, a family event, a community event, and a part of all our individual lives. This holistic concept of death as not just physiological but social, relational, and spiritual within a culture and community and has led to the concept of the "Healthy Death".

The root of the concept of a "Healthy Death" is found in several different concepts of "health";-

1. MacIntyre's idea of *narrative unity* [10]: Health is the ability to tell our life stories as integrated wholes.
2. Antonovski's idea of salutogenesis [11]: Health is the ability to retain a sense of coherence despite severe stress.
3. The Alma Ata Declaration (1978): Health is a complete state of physical, mental, and social well-being, and not merely the absence of disease [12].

When we consider these models of "health" in the context of death, and into the community context, personal narrative continues in those the individual is connected to after death. This often gives meaning, purpose, and satisfaction to life. Fundamentally a healthy death, like a healthy life, is to create a meaningful story [13].

In a modern Western context, many are used to thinking of death in a negative way and do not know how to approach it in a positive way. In particular, many carers, families, and communities have little or no experience of a positive approach, and if they attempt this it can be viewed with suspicion by those who expect this stage to be relentlessly unhappy. Inexperience can cause missed opportunities to do good and minimise harm. End-of-life is full of potential for positive experiences, especially when difficulties are accepted, not avoided. The end-of-life period can teach people to live in healthy ways, as well as die in healthy ways. Difficulties are inevitable – the whole range of bio-psycho-social-spiritual difficulties. These difficulties need a whole community structure around them to help guide the person and families through. Professional help may be needed but is a lot less effective without the background wisdom of the community to support.

Everyone involved needs opportunities to learn how to do this well, including how to use opportunities of the moment to develop the positive coherence of someone's life, including its end. The dying person should be encouraged to contribute – in ways that are both realistic and enhancing.

The core caring team (that normally includes family members, friends, and professionals) need examples, guidance and support to address the needs of the dying person whilst highlighting the positive coherence of their life story, building the community that relates to them, and developing skills that might also help them later in life. This concept of integrating the community to support those that are dying underpins the public health approach to palliative care – this is in a nutshell the *Compassionate Communities* model.

Public Health Approach to Palliative Care – Compassionate Communities

Then an old sage remarked: 'It's a marvel to me that people give far more attention to repairing results than to stopping the cause, when they'd much better aim at prevention.

Let us stop at its source all this mischief,' cried he, 'come, neighbours and friends, let us rally; if the cliff we will fence, we might almost dispense with the ambulance down in the valley.'
– Joseph Malins, The Ambulance Down in the Valley

A public health system includes primary care and community teams, secondary/tertiary care (hospitals & hospices), and social care support and care homes. However, we are also aware of those wider population health initiatives such as reducing health inequalities and improving social determinants of health, good housing, employer wellbeing programmes, clean water, and health and safety. In policy there are measures such as education, community development, and social ecology which all feed into public health.

Not only does a public health view examine the patterns of disease, illness, disability, or injury across a population, but it also plans a whole population approach to their prevention, harm-reduction, and necessary treatment and care. Indeed, public health has now extended beyond simply preventing disease to a more active "health promotion". This is in efforts to include health and well-being and community involvement in healthcare.

For the last 50 years, palliative care has been viewed as primarily a profession-led concern, a medical speciality. The NHS, and our modern Western culture, see the professionals as central to the care of dying, the bereaved, and their families.

Compassionate communities' ethos is one in which we see palliative care being embedded in every aspect of the community, as opposed to sitting atop and providing a service [14] – making community a partner and participant rather than a targeted service need. The individuals in the community surrounding the dying patient are more than bystanders at the end-of-life and they must be far more than volunteers managed by a health service.

Many of the dying and grieving processes occur across the wide civic and local community settings. It is in that broader and longer experience, across those multiple settings, that we must recognise and promote true holistic palliative care provided by its own community.

If we don't do this, we risk imposing both our subconscious prerogative of what we think dying should look like, misunderstanding cultural, religious, and spiritual needs; we risk medicalising the non-medical and because we are a

limited resource, we would risk intermittent reactionary medical consultations disjointed from the lived reality. There will always be a clear place for in-patient hospices, and taking over complex care when needed; however if our true aim is to make dying a normal, and not a frightening prospect, we need to create a system which supports, aids, and signposts society in this normal and natural process. Thus, it is by understanding and acting with, and alongside, community and wider civic partners that palliative care will be able to begin to address its vision of true holistic care.

For unless clinical forms of palliative care are able to connect with public health concerns that take them beyond a narrow focus on health services and symptom science, the problem of care of the dying, the bereaved, and caregivers will continue to resemble models of late care and crisis management [15 p.2].

The keys to accomplishing this vision are outside our comfortable face-to-face patient care; rather they are found in building partnerships in the community, social care professionals, policy development and health services restructuring.

Over recent years we have gradually realised and acknowledged the various challenges the diverse and minority areas of society have in accessing palliative care services. Whether consciously or unconsciously barriers to access palliative care services are well documented, for example, for people from ethnic and religious minorities, lower and middle income sectors, and the marginalised in prisons or living on the streets, and to others whose identities are hidden from us.

Any hope in addressing these issues is likely to lie in the development of our care models in conjunction with hearing from diverse voices within the community and its wide array of services. We cannot be everywhere, we cannot commission specialist services focusing on one group to such a degree that we neglect others. Nor can we assume services meet the needs of all who may benefit. The vision of whole population, whole life, whole death palliative care needs a public health approach (For further detail on bereavement see Chapter 8: Integrating new perspectives: Working with loss and grief in palliative care).

How Can We Help to Bring About a Healthy Death?

"Faith" is a fine invention
When Gentlemen can see –
But Microscopes are prudent
In an Emergency.

— Emily Dickinson

The Lancet Commission [9] describes five principles of its vision for death and dying:

1. The social determinants of death, dying, and grieving are tackled
2. Dying is understood to be a relational and spiritual process rather than simply a physiological event
3. Networks of care lead support for people dying, caring, and grieving
4. Conversations and stories about everyday death, dying, and grief become common
5. Death is recognised as having value

As previously outlined, these principles require society to understand the limitations of the purely medical approach and ways to overcome them. These principles can help structure the ways in which we can practically apply the concept of a "Healthy Death" and create a compassionate community.

Key principles include:
Acknowledgement of how difficult and skilled caring is, especially as one approaches end-of-life.
Guidance to collaborate and explore with patients and carers to think through their own plans (rather than dogmatically adopt protocols or just defer to others).
Development of the skills of those involved that helps them to feel confident and creative – empowered to do things themselves, without automatically deferring to "expert" help.

Dr Clare Fuller, a palliative care practitioner for nearly 30 years, then herself becoming a carer, described practical things that already exist that can help an individual who is dying [16]:

1. **Proactive Planning** – "What Matters Most" conversations, Advance care planning, Advance statements, Power of Attorney, Care escalation plans, DNACPR, ReSPECT, Decision support (See Chapter 9: Recognising deterioration, preparing, and planning for dying for explanation of these topics)
2. **Community Care** – Involvement of primary care, community care, palliative care, voluntary care
3. **Clear Explanations** – How the system works, what to do when things happen in the middle of the night, how to detect deterioration.

Some specific practical examples and suggestions of how these areas can be addressed include:

- **Involve Children.** Especially with practical tasks
- **Social Events.** A sequence of gatherings, parties – dancing, singing

- **Rota of Visitors.** Sitting, holding a hand, playing music, reading stories
- **Plan the Funeral.** Recognising that an individual comes through sharing memories, photographs, food, music and other details of a full life that are unique to us all.
- **Anticipate the Memorial.** Plan for a time in the future when some of the grief and practical considerations have settled, to come together and remember a whole life story again, as a community [9].
- **WhatsApp Group/Facebook/Twitter/social media.** To encourage positive conversations in the community. Sharing stories, planning sometimes, finding connection.
- **Practical Help.** Food, take children on holidays and sleep-overs.
- **Memory Box/Letters.** For reading once died, or significant birthdays/events.
- **Life Story.** Write a booklet or make a film of the person's life.

Recognising the Role and Needs of Families and Unpaid Carers

Family and unpaid carers offer vital support for people living with advanced serious illnesses, disabilities, and for those approaching the end-of-life. Achieving end-of-life care at home is heavily dependent on their contributions [17]. However, this caregiving role is associated with substantial emotional, social, financial, and physical morbidity and even mortality [18]. Evidence suggests that good support for example via informal support and social networks can positively affect caregiver physical and mental health outcomes [19, 20].

Thoughtful multi-disciplinary team approaches which enable consistent identification of family and unpaid carers are essential in order to trigger assessment of each caregiver's needs. An example of a validated assessment tool is Carers Support Needs Assessment Tool Intervention (CSNAT-I), aimed to help identify and prioritise the areas in which the caregiver requires further support; divided into those that enable the caregiver to care and those that enable more direct support for themselves [21]. Further to assessment, processes should be in place to sign-posting caregivers to access formal and informal information and support within the system and community.

How Can Professionals Help?

The focus on late dying and early bereavement has led to a dominance of medical, nursing and psychological professions and services with small recognition and far fewer resources invested in the longer, more crucial journey of care provided by communities – neighbourhoods, schools, workplaces, faith groups, local governments, social media, friendship networks [15p.1].

The Provision 21 of the Health and Care Act 2022 outlines commissioning hospital and other health services in England [15]. An important amendment submitted by Baroness Ilora Finlay now crucially includes provision of palliative care and mandates for:

1. Palliative care in every setting
2. Twenty-four hours a day, seven days a week (24/7) access to palliative care beds, and advice and support for professionals, patients, and carers.
3. Readily available supply of the key medications, equipment, and staff
4. Systems to share key information across the key stakeholders
5. Promotion and recording of what matters most conversations
6. Ongoing quality improvement and research to ensure that services are innovative and responsive to changing needs and evidence

There have been many community-based initiatives to try and improve end-of-life care, from recognition and advance care planning through to care in the last days of life. Professionals are cautioned to embed themselves in the community, acting in our expert areas, but never taking over, being a resource, but never dictating, being reliable and responding but not ruling. Facilitating a solution, but not always being the solution. We educate, advise, signpost, and support as a hub of knowledge.

Below are some helpful initiatives and examples for various professionals. There is significant variation of resources and community models of palliative care across the UK. As with all initiatives we must be mindful of imposing a service upon a community, as opposed to working alongside and in conjunction with as part of a wider framework supporting community palliative care.

Primary Care

NHS England has described primary care services to include general practice, community pharmacy, dental, and optometry services [22]. However, primary care in reality evolves in response to both the commissioning and community needs, shifting from historically medical

models, embracing partnership working to help improve the health and well-being of the local population. Multidisciplinary teams continue to facilitate collaboration for example with voluntary sector organisations expanding the reach into and with communities for example with schools, places of worship, and businesses.

General practice accounts for the bulk of primary care services and is delivered on the basis of "registered lists" of patients for individual practices. However, general practice is wider than just GPs; it includes a growing range of practice staff such as nurses, paramedics, clinical pharmacists, social prescribers, link workers, receptionists, and practice managers, as well as community-based staff.

General Practice plays a key role in the delivery of end-of-life and bereavement care and is ideally placed to reduce variation in care, regardless of diagnosis, age, ethnic background, sexual orientation, disability, or social circumstances. The majority of people receive palliative care in the community, led by primary care and community nursing services. Only a small proportion require specialist hospice care input and these are still more likely to be complex cancer cases rather than other illnesses or frailty.

An average individual GP with a list size of 2,000 will have around 20 patient deaths in a year.

Only about two of these will be sudden as a result of acute disease with no previous chronic condition or as a result of an accident, the vast majority dying from chronic illness of some form:

- Five deaths will be from cancer.
- Six from organ failure including heart failure, chronic obstructive pulmonary disease, and renal failure.
- Seven will be from diseases of old age, frailty, and dementia [23].

Three typical trajectories are described to enable early palliative care, of functional decline towards the end-of-life: rapid, intermittent, and gradual [24].

Early identification of people with palliative care needs is an essential trigger to activate enablers of consistent personalised care and support planning for all those who may benefit from planned end-of-life care, such as: Multidisciplinary team reviews, compassionate conversations about "What Matters Most" to the person and their carers as well as documentation of these conversations in order to ensure cross-sector health and care professionals are aware of the person's preferred priorities of care. Ideally people are able to input into their own record so their wishes are clear.

There is variation in access to primary care as well as experience and health outcomes for some people and groups compared to the rest of the population [25, 26]. Robust systems for hearing the voices of these people and groups such as practices working with their patient participation groups or with Healthwatch, and voluntary, community, and social enterprise sector partners are essential to ensure services are developed according to the diverse palliative care needs of the local population. This should extend to people and groups who might not be registered or "visible" to the NHS.

Primary Care Networks

Primary Care Networks (PCNs) were developed in England to bring general practices together to work at scale, aligning ways of working between different organisations to enhance their effects on the health and care of the local population, each covering populations of 30,000–50,000 people. PCNs and equivalent, in other nations, could develop strategies for Healthy Deaths by promoting *community-oriented integrated practice* [27] – a way to practice which develops multidisciplinary teams skilled at whole system operating.

Routinely gathered data aligned to PCN areas could help to evaluate different approaches. Learning from structured approaches to collaboration for end-of-life care and palliative care could inform shared care for other complex issues, like diabetes – to help people know how to enhance health as well as treat diseases, in populations as well as individuals [28].

The Daffodil Standards for General Practice – UK General Practice Standards for Advanced Serious Illness and End-of-Life Care

The Royal College of General Practitioners and Marie Curie developed a population-based quality improvement programme, the Daffodil Standards [29]. The Standards provide a free, evidence-based framework to help practices self-assess and consistently offer the best end-of-life and bereavement care for patients. The Standards involve the entire practice team and enable practices to be proactive in end-of-life care.

The Standards can be applied to the whole practice population i.e. those affected by end-of-life care and bereavement or practices can choose to focus on a particular Standard of interest or a cohort of people, e.g., for older people in care homes [30].

There are eight Standards:

1. Professional and competent staff
2. Early identification
3. Carer Support – before and after death
4. Seamless, planned, coordinated care
5. Assessment of unique needs of the patient
6. Quality care during the last days of life
7. Care after death
8. General Practice being hubs within Compassionate Communities

The simple three-level approach covers:

Level 1: Core Essentials – Focusing on internal practice systems to enable consistency of care, for example, helping practices confirm practice leadership, communicate the vision with the whole team to improve end-of-life care and review the consistency of practice processes, such as coding. There are free templates to enable retrospective death audits and prospective MDT analysis.

Level 2: Enhanced – Improving communication, shared planning, and compassionate care, by reflecting on the data collected teams self-assess against good practice evidence. Once areas of improvement have been confirmed, SMART goals can be set and reaudited at an agreed time.

Level 3: Advanced – Coproduction of care and compassionate communities encourages practices to work with other practices for example within a primary care network or federation. There are also tools to work with patient participation groups.

The Daffodil Standards were launched in 2018 and are recognised by the Care Quality Commission in England, as well as being relevant to general practice in the devolved nations of the UK [31].

Pharmacists as Part of Primary Care and Community Teams

Community pharmacy teams are valuable members of primary care and community teams, helping to gather and respond to information from patients or more often their carers. People often visit a pharmacy for information about self-care, medicines optimisation, and troubleshooting around prescriptions, such as ensuring people understand the use of different medicines and what side effects to look out for. In recent years, the development of clinical pharmacists in practices also offer expert guidance.

Families also see the pharmacy team after death when returning unused medication and therefore have a role in offering a compassionate bereavement response as well as sign-posting people to support.

For people living with life-limiting conditions who are approaching the end-of-life, it is particularly important to have timely access to medicines and clinical support from pharmacy teams. Both community and practice clinical pharmacists, are well placed to support regular reviews of medicines in order to optimise symptom control, minimise burden from side-effects and ensure that any medicines no longer required, are deprescribed with appropriate guidance.

Anticipatory prescribing approaches, to ensure symptom control in the last days of life vary across UK. Facilitation of rapid and efficient access to medicines for patients in the community is vital to minimise crisis and stress for patients, carers, and staff. However, there is no nationally recommended model and access continues to vary across the UK [32]. It is helpful for professionals to familiarise themselves with local pathways to access end-of-life care medication both in and out of hours; access to shared clinical records further improve patient outcomes [33].

Daffodil Standards for Community Pharmacies

The Royal Pharmaceutical Society in partnership with Marie Curie developed Standards for community pharmacies. These launched in 2022 and plan to align with the Daffodil Standards for General Practice and aim to support community pharmacy teams to undertake simple quality improvement measures and build on the care they already provide to people affected by advanced serious illness and end-of-life care [34].

Community and District Nursing Integrating with Social Care Teams

In order to coordinate end-of-life care in the community, interprofessional collaboration is important, particularly with increasing complexity of patients' needs. Community nursing is a vital partner in the primary care multi-disciplinary team and contact between the patient and community nurses in the last three months of life is associated with less admissions and A&E attendances [35]. This care is often coordinated by a District Nurse.

Community nursing includes nurses from differing fields of practice, and differing levels of experience, which support the complexity of need that may arise when people are approaching end-of-life. District Nurses are registered nurses, who have completed a university based programme in specialist practice, caring for people in the community environment. Using their advanced skills, district nurses lead and direct community teams in the delivery of high quality and compassionate end-of-life care. District Nurses are well placed to identify people early with palliative care needs for people already on their case load as well as assessing, care planning and facilitating treatment of symptoms. They also have significant experience of how to navigate the system and planning ahead to enable people to access the right help at the right time.

As out-of-hours makes up to three times that of in-hours work, out-of-hours practitioners need to be thoughtfully integrated with day-time services so people become confident that they have 24/7 support for palliative care (as emphasised in the Health and Care Bill 2022 (England)) [22].

In some areas there are specific schemes for out-of-hours specialist palliative care, especially regarding subcutaneous breakthrough medications, however in most of the UK this role is taken by out of hours GP and community nurse service.

It has been estimated that around 40% of District Nurses' work is devoted to caring for patients with palliative care needs [36], and District Nurses themselves describe palliative care as being a central part of their work [37] especially considering their principal role to be that of coordinator of care [38, 39]. Patients and carers have identified that district nurses are the professionals who have the greatest regular contact with palliative care patients in the community [40]. District Nurses have reported their work as being emotionally stressful, time consuming, and unpredictable. Although District Nurses see their role in community palliative care as vital, they fear that this is not well recognised by their managers [41].

District nurses are clearly a central, and necessary professional lynchpin in community care. Their role, similar to other professionals, straddle both active practical interventions (such as syringe drivers, wound and catheter care) to the more supportive, explorative and holistic signposting and enabling. District nurses, however, are absolutely front-line in the judgement of balance between supporting the patient, family, and community to lead in care, against that of professionals taking over aspects of care. This tension is where humble wisdom of the individual circumstances is necessary and important. Holistic care and compassion lie at the heart of the district nurse role, balancing "caring in the moment" alongside "future care planning". For this to be effective, communication and involvement with the patient, family and MDT is critical [42].

Thus, it is particularly important to encourage and enable close and supportive relationships within multiprofessional teams working together in conjunction for the patient and their family. Both for better supported working relationships, and also shared decision-making on the degree of intervention, support, empowering, signposting needed for the patient, family, and community.

Training of district nurses in palliative care was a key policy of the NHS Cancer Plan in which £6 million was invested in a training programme delivered by the 34 English cancer networks. This was the largest and most focused programme of its kind in palliative care and the evaluation reported that following training, the confidence of district nurses increased, particularly for those with little previous training in palliative care or no formal district nurse qualification. However, there was no change in either carer satisfaction or GP assessment of district nurse knowledge or skills [43].

Together with social care colleagues, community nurses hold invaluable knowledge about people and those important to them; supporting teams to think beyond the medical model.

The Care Act 2014 places responsibilities on social workers to provide information and advice to enable people to "make good decisions about care". This gives social workers a supportive and understanding role as the person comes to terms with what is happening to them or someone close to them. In this way social workers are well suited to respond to various challenges associated with living with a terminal illness and when approaching the end-of-life. A social worker trained in palliative care, being a part of the community, seeing the person as an individual, helping find joint solutions, looking at the whole person, family and circumstances is the ideal.

Social care is often an under-acknowledged and poorly valued profession in both professional circles and wider society, however this is grossly unfounded as it holds a central role in community, holistic palliative care, especially in signposting and co-ordinating care with their unique perspective. Their role in referral to other services like financial support, help with housing, advocacy, and working with schools or employers are often as alleviating (or more so) to anxiety, stress and worry than any medication would be.

Working with families is key to social work at the end-of-life. They understand the vulnerability of carers and the wider family situation and are therefore a resource of advocacy, assessment, and negotiation in managing risk positively to enable "what matters most" conversations with patients and families. Indeed, at times when there are divergent or conflicting perspectives on the needs of the dying person, social workers are vital in their skills in mediation and negotiation.

Importantly, social workers generally work with individuals and groups who are materially disadvantaged, marginalised, and excluded from mainstream society and working with cultural, ethnic, and economic diversity, family and support networks, bereavement, interventions across the lifecycle, interdisciplinary practice and therefore have insight, links and can navigate the various services and systems.

Care Home and Domiciliary Care Staff

Arguably the most significant group of professionals in palliative and end-of-life care for people living in a care home or in their own home are professional carers. These frontline staff are frequently under-appreciated and poorly remunerated professionals. Sometimes, the only human contact people receive is from carers. If there was any profession which understands the situation in its holistic context these carers are often the most informed. We recommend that carers are involved at multidisciplinary meetings, and multiprofessional teams improve communication with professional carers.

Care homes are grouped into residential and nursing homes. The former is supported by community nursing teams and the latter typically employ their own nursing staff. The proportion of people dying in a care home is an increasing trend, likely a feature of our ageing population. The majority of deaths occurring in nursing home facilities are to people who are over 85-years-old, with an average length of stay of less than a year. Many residents have multiple comorbidities, and indeed around 70% of care home residents have dementia [44]. Specialist palliative care community teams continue to mainly see people with cancer diagnoses and complex symptoms; their presence in care homes is traditionally a lot less than in other settings. In the future, exploring and resourcing joint models of working and training between specialist palliative care, primary care teams and care homes will be important to improve residents' experiences of symptom control and quality of deaths as well as helping care home staff to feel well-supported to care for their dying residents. Care home staff can feel unsupported to look after residents at the end-of-life [45]. In addition, palliative care education needs to embrace frailty issues, such as, dementia, prescribing and deprescribing.

For people living in a care home or on their own at home, professional carers become an integral part of their family, community, and professional team caring for them. It is thus essential that they are involved and fully aware of the plan of care and the needs and wishes of the person concerned to act in-part as their advocate and voice. Many care homes and domiciliary care providers will contribute to some degree of advance care planning with people, to help them understand their needs and wishes. In 2020, NHS England's Long Term Plan committed to roll out the 'Enhanced Health in Care Homes model by 2024, focusing on proactive, personalised care. Key features to reduce variation in care include; a named clinical lead for each care home; regular MDTs to drive weekly care home rounds as well as every resident having a holistic assessment of needs and a resulting personalised care and support plan, within seven days of admission or readmission. The Daffodil Standards for General Practice, complemented this approach by developing specific resources and tools to enable quality improvement in practices, to support delivery of end-of-life care in Older People's Care Homes [30].

Allied Health Professionals (AHPs) and Pastoral, Spiritual, and Religious Support

AHPs encompass a broad range of professionals, including physiotherapists, occupational therapists, dieticians, speech and language therapists, psychologists. In the community, the role these professionals play is often under-recognised and commonly the primary solution in supporting patients, particularly when understanding "what matters most" and maintaining their wish to stay at home. For example, through providing equipment, assistance with medication, physiotherapy, and occupational therapist's strategies to manage symptoms, management of swallow or feeding difficulties or through additional resources and support. Furthermore, the role AHPs provide in educating and supporting carers and family in delivering care in the community is a valuable asset in rehabilitative palliative care and helping people live as well as possible in familiar surroundings [46].

A challenge is AHP cover across the UK is variable with differing access to services and provisions across all the professional groups in each area. A role AHPs in particular avail is their ability to navigate the local system, understanding how to work collaboratively in order to maximise access to skills, resources, and equipment. This is often time critical and is invaluable to enable well-planned end-of-life care in the community.

Existential or spiritual pain can cause great distress to the person who is living with a terminal illness and/or dying as well as the family, friends, and the wider community. True holistic care embraces and enquires about people's pastoral, spiritual, religious, and cultural needs, enabling people to process their existential questions, concerns, and experiences, often tapping into deeply held beliefs about themselves, the world and their place in it. For some this may involve religious practice and rituals which are often critical to understand and respect. However, assumptions cannot be made, and only by asking "what matters most" about people's beliefs, can we help them receive the support they most need. For our increasingly diverse population many have no affiliation or connection to organised faith or belief groups. Whilst hospitals and hospices often have Chaplains or Pastoral Teams who provide such person-centred support for the dying person and their families, there is often patchy provision of an equivalent for community-based care or care home facilities. There is an increasing need for skilled Pastoral and Spiritual Support Practitioners to work within community MDT's facilitating the development of connections, networking and training among local faith, belief and cultural leaders to enhance and engage more fully the invaluable support they can offer within communities, particularly for people affected by end-of-life care and bereavement.

What Can Communities Do?

*No man is an Island, entire of itself; every man
is a piece of the Continent, a part of the maine;*
— No Man is an Island, John Donne

It is clear a "Healthy Death" isn't achievable in individual isolationism. In the same way that it takes a village to raise a child, it takes a community to nurture a death.

There is a growing movement across the UK to pursue initiatives to form "Healthy Deaths" at scale. The COVID-19 pandemic made people acutely aware of the importance of collaboration, support, and guidance when facing death. Indeed, our very own mortality has recently been brought to the fore, which has acted counter to the previously hidden and unspoken nature of dying in the West.

In the UK, the 2019 NHS Long Term Plan [47] provides a great opportunity to systematically develop collaboration. The plan describes a vision for integration of effort:

> We will give people more control over their own health and the care they receive, encourage more collaboration between GPs, their teams and community services, as 'primary care networks', to increase the services they can provide jointly, and increase the focus on NHS organisations working with their local partners, as 'Integrated Care Systems', to plan and deliver services which meet the needs of their communities[48 p.2].

This long-term view, in conjunction with the Health and Care Bill 2022, and NICE guidance for end-of-life care [49], makes palliative care a commissioned necessity, encourages co-ordinated multi-practitioner care, with access to specialist skills when needed. Along with the growing movement of a public health approach to palliative care or "Compassionate Communities", a fertile ground is created for a purposeful "Healthy Death" narrative to be widely formed into fruition.

All of this can take many forms and will be bespoke to the individual patient, their families, the community in which they live and the services available to them. Ensuring these systems of support are interconnected and easily signposted is vital.

A Structured Non-Biased Process or Resource to Outline Local Services

Working together is important as is the recognition that everyone is a service and everyone is a signpost. In order to empower people and communities to understand where and how to find help and support, commissioned and non-commissioned resources should be mapped and shared as a "directory of resources" for people and professionals to easily access, by local areas. When an online resource is generated this can include maximising shared community spaces, such as social meeting spaces, places of worship, parks and gardens, and hospices. It can involve disease specific support groups, psychological and mental health groups, other community clubs, sports groups, the library, neighbours and religious organisations. The inter-connectedness of these networks is upheld by the individuals within these communities who bring their own experience and skills, professional and non-professional; these may include friends, neighbours, family, members of a support group, counsellors, and religious leaders.

Education and Training

End-of-life care core skills education and training framework was developed in partnership by Health Education England, Skills for Health, and Skills for Care [50]. The framework divides key skills and knowledge into three tiers to help support the provision of high-quality, person-centred care for terminal patients and their families. This guidance aims to support employers to improve the consistency in training and assessment of cross-sector multi-professionals.

The majority of end-of-life care in the community, is and will be delivered by generalist staff, without specialist palliative care qualifications [51]. Focussed multi-professional, end-of-life care education and training is undoubtably essential to improve the delivery and experiences of care as well as reduce inequalities. There are multiple challenges associated with delivering end-of-life care training in a meaningful way to enable improved outcomes of patients and families. High-quality training therefore needs to be multifaceted in design and tailored to the needs of staff. Organisational culture of person-centred end-of-life care is another important consideration to enable continued positive behaviour change.

End-of-Life Care for All (e-ELCA) is a freely accessible e-learning programme aimed to enhance the training and education of NHS staff, hospice workers and social care staff as well as volunteers involved in delivering end-of-life care [52]. The programme was commissioned by the Department of Health to support the implementation of the Department of Health's 2008 national End-of-Life Care Strategy. The modular online training format, allows participants to build on their skills, at their own pace and relevant to their learning needs, and is available to all generalist staff.

There is a plethora of training providers offering end-of-life care training, for example local community training hubs and hospices and training as well as national providers such as charities and independent education providers.

Local Hospice Providers

Most hospices have training and education departments and are fantastic sources of expertise and knowledge to help build skills and confidence in community generalist teams. Many have links with engagement and research teams with the benefit of appraising end-of-life care training outcomes. Working together to deliver training programmes brings the advantage of building local relationships and shared understanding of system challenges and opportunities.

National Providers

Recognised charities in end-of-life care, such as Marie Curie, Sue Ryder, Macmillan, and Together for Short Lives, are excellent hubs of knowledge and training for staff, patients, and families. Disease specific, ageing-well and bereavement-care charities also offer important resources to support sign-posting, referral pathways and education for staff and people within communities. (For further detail on children and young people see Chapter 15: Palliative care for infants, children and young people).

Recognised Palliative Care Education and Training Certificates and Programmes

Many of these require funding either by commissioners or directly by providers. These range from improving generalist skills through to enabling those with a special interest and specialist expertise.

Examples include:

- The European Certificate in Essential Palliative Care is a respected qualification following an eight-week online facilitated learning course for multi-professionals with assessment by a reflective portfolio, examination and viva.

- The Cardiff University, Palliative Medicine for Health Care Professionals, MSc – this in-depth course is over three years as part-time distance learning.

- The Gold Standards Framework (GSF) was developed in 1998 and played an important role in focusing and improving end-of-life care in primary care. GSF principles have been integrated within primary care, supported by inclusion as part of the original GP Contract Quality Outcomes Framework supporting the basic need for GP practices to have palliative care registers and regular EOLC multi-disciplinary team meetings. GSF have grown as an independent end-of-life care training provider supporting accreditation programmes to different sectors such as care homes and hospitals. GSF continue to encourage providers to improve end-of-life care, to provide more proactive person-centred coordinated care, with more people identified to be in their last year of life offered advance care planning discussions and enabled to live well and die well in the place and manner of their choosing with effective communication and collaboration with care home sector.

Developing Communities of Practice to Support Peer Learning

Project ECHO is a worldwide movement providing an online learning and support methodology. It supports knowledge sharing between members from health and social care professions and facilitates the exchange of specialist knowledge and best practice to help build skills and confidence. Use of Project ECHO continues to grow in the UK, supporting hospices and the wider palliative care sector to operate as effectively as possible [53].

Conclusion

We cannot direct the wind, but we can adjust the sails.
— Dolly Parton

Presently, the natural evolution of palliative care has resulted in a system which is more individualistic rather than population based. This is no bad thing in-and-of-itself; however, it does have some consequences. Good intentions have resulted in a predominate focus on the dying individual (opposed to the wider needs of carers and communities), is overly concerned with measurable outcomes, e.g., pain measurement and preferred place of death (opposed to framing how to shape healthy deaths that develop positive, meaningful stories), and is overly reliant on the skills of palliative care specialists (opposed to

empowering carers and communities to confidently lead a co-ordinated approach to healthy deaths at scale).

This medical evolution of palliative care we naturally find ourselves in – "treat the patient in front of you rather than the population behind" has in-part led to the inequalities of access and sections of poor provision we have seen and demonstrated. In future, we need to evaluate models of care in order to properly develop and our services, trained workforce and communities to reach all people with palliative care needs. Fourth generation evaluation, based on relativism, offers a robust approach to work with stakeholders including the local population and consider the gaps and unmet need in order to define the course and actions to be followed [54].

Indeed, many recent movements have recognised these issues. We are in a privileged position to start to build better. The pandemic has shed light on more collegiate working and reshaping of services, the inequalities are increasingly being recognised, we have realised our services are limited and our role should empower as much as enable the carers and communities we live in.

Policies within geographic areas that could help people to learn how to support healthy deaths at scale:

- A Compassionate Communities, public health approach should be formed and nurtured across a geographical area to create a belonging.

- A narrative of everyone is a service and everyone is a signpost to others.

- Integrate primary, secondary, community, and social services to support Healthy Deaths – linked to the same geographic areas, including relevant organisations such as schools and pharmacies and enhance a sense of belonging with a family's local groups and faith or spiritual communities.

- Provide structured guidance and responsive support nurturing the ethos of Healthy Deaths. This should include localities offering a fully mapped "directory of services" to support professionals and their communities.

- Routinely embedding the language of "What Matters Most" and considering future care planning from birth to death. Training all professionals to ask about and contribute to care planning documentation over time whilst also acting as a signpost to any relevant support and services.

- Support Self-Care, Shared-Care, and Networks of Carers – to develop "bottom-up" locality-based, team-working to address complex issues. This could be seen as a form of local participatory democracy, with embedded community-developers, valuable for many issues other than end-of-life. Informal and practical help by neighbours and scheduled help by volunteers (like shopping) all contribute to keeping a household routine in place even as care needs shift over time.

• Embed freely accessible quality improvement programmes, such as the Daffodil Standards, to continuously drive improvements and improve equity for people affected by serious illness and end-of-life care.

• Assess and address education and training needs for community generalist staff and primary care networks to reach the complex and diverse palliative care needs of the people they care for. This includes specific needs of staff caring for specific communities, such as, those working in care homes.

• Services to develop processes and systems to systematically hear the voices of people within the communities they serve, in order to understand how to evolve services to meet the palliative care needs relevant to the diversity within the local population.

• Routinely teach fourth generation evaluation – so researchers, practitioners, citizens, and educationalists come to understand approaches to inquiry that illuminate inter-connected and dynamic phenomena as well as individual facts.

• Reducing unnecessary medicalisation, increased community leadership, and greater coordination across community settings where people are experiencing living with care-giving roles, illness, dying and grief such as in schools, universities, faith groups and businesses to get involved, and make collaboration for health a normal, expected part of end-of-life. And then it could become an expected role of citizens throughout life.

We think of a Healthy Death as a positive story, co-created from many contributions. The patient, the family, the wider community, as well as relationships with professionals. Palliative care can help facilitate this story. Our role is embedding the knowledge and skills across the population, to demonstrate deaths normality, to share care, to utilise resources, and to enable consistency of care to individuals, at scale. A collective narrative bringing value to the patient and community.

You do not have to be good.
You do not have to walk on your knees
for a hundred miles through the desert, repenting.
You only have to let the soft animal of your body
love what it loves.
Tell me about your despair, yours, and I will tell you mine.
Meanwhile the world goes on.
Meanwhile the sun and the clear pebbles of the rain
are moving across the landscapes,
over the prairies and the deep trees,

the mountains and the rivers.
Meanwhile the wild geese, high in the clean blue air,
are heading home again.
Whoever you are, no matter how lonely,
the world offers itself to your imagination,
calls to you like the wild geese, harsh and exciting –
over and over announcing your place
in the family of things'

– Wild Geese, Mary Oliver

References

1. Hughes, G.H. (1961). 453. London, Calouste Gulbenkian Foundation, 1960. 63 pp. *Nursing Research* 10 (2): 122.
2. Wilkes, E. (1965). Terminal cancer at home. *The Lancet* 285 (7389): 799–801.
3. Abi-Aad, G. (2017). End of life care. Available at: https://www.kpho.org.uk/__data/assets/pdf_file/0006/72375/End-of-Life-Care-2017.pdf (accessed 19 August 2022).
4. Bardsley, M., Dixon, J., and Georghiou, T. (2010). *Social Care and Hospital Use at the End of Life*. London: Nuffield Trust.
5. Office for national statistics. (2021, May 07). Office for national statistics. Retrieved 19 05 2022, from Deaths at home increased by a third in 2020, while deaths in hospitals fell except for COVID-19: https://www.ons.gov.uk/people populationandcommunity/birthsdeathsandmarriages/deaths/articles/deathsathomeincreasedbyathirdin2020whiled eathsinhospitalsfellexceptforcovid19/2021-05-07 (accessed 19 August 2022).
6. Etkind, S.N., Bone, A.E., Gomes, B., Lovell, N., Evans, C.J., Higginson, I.J., and Murtagh, F.E.M. (2017). How many people will need palliative care in 2040? Past trends, future projections and implications for services. *BMC Medicine* 15 (1): 1–10.
7. Next steps for integrating primary care: Fuller Stocktake report NHS England and NHS Improvement May 2022. https://www.england.nhs.uk/wp-content/uploads/2022/05/next-steps-for-integrating-primary-care-fuller-stocktake-report.pdf (accessed 02 February 2023).
8. National Palliative and End of Life Care Partnership (2021 May). CD Ambitions for palliative and end of life care: a national framework for local action 2021-2026. https://www.england.nhs.uk/wp-content/uploads/2022/02/ambitions-for-palliative-and-end-of-life-care-2nd-edition.pdf (accessed 02 February 2023).
9. Sallnow, L., Smith, R., Ahmedzai, S.H., Bhadelia, A., Chamberlain, C., Cong, Y., … Wyatt, K. (2022). Report of the lancet commission on the value of death: bringing death back into life. *The Lancet* 399 (10327): 837–884.
10. Mckenzie, G. (1983). MacINTYRE, A.:" After virtue: a study in moral theory. *Australasian Journal of Philosophy* 61 (a).
11. Antonovsky, A. (1987). *Unraveling the Mystery of Health: How People Manage Stress and Stay Well*. Jossey-bass.

12. World Health Organization (1978). Declaration of alma-ata (No. WHO/EURO: 1978-3938-43697-61471). World Health Organization. Regional Office for Europe. https://www.euro.who.int/__data/assets/pdf_file/0009/113877/E93944.pdf (accessed 19 August 2022).

13. Thomas, P. (2022). Facilitating healthy deaths at scale. *British Journal of Community Nursing* 27 (9): 432–435.

14. Abel, J. (2018). Compassionate communities and end-of-life care. *Clinical Medicine* 18 (1): 6.

15. Kingston, H., Millington-Sanders, C., and Abel, J. (2022). Clinical practice methods combined with community resources. *Oxford Textbook of Public Health Palliative Care*, 155.

16. Fuller, C. (2021). End-of-life care: perspective of a relative rather than a professional. *British Journal of Community Nursing* 26 (4): 176–178.

17. Stajduhar, K., Funk, L., Toye, C. et al. (2010). Part 1: home-based family caregiving at the end of life: a comprehensive review of published quantitative research (1998–2008). *Palliative Medicine* 24: 573–593.

18. Schulz, R. and Beach, S.R. (1999). Caregiving as a risk factor for mortality: the caregiver health effects study. *JAMA* 282 (23): 2215–2219. doi: 10.1001/jama.282.23.2215.

19. Götze, H., Brähler, E., Gansera, L. et al. (2014). Psychological distress and quality of life of palliative cancer patients and their caring relatives during home care. *Support Care Cancer* 22: 2775–2782.

20. Lee, K.C., Chang, W.C., Chou, W.C. et al. (2013). Longitudinal changes and predictors of caregiving burden while providing end-of-life care for terminally ill cancer patients. *Journal of Palliative Medicine* 16: 632–637.

21. Norinder, M., Årestedt, K., Axelsson, L., Grande, G., Ewing, G., and Alvariza, A. (2023). Increased preparedness for caregiving among family caregivers in specialized home care by using the Carer Support Needs Assessment Tool Intervention. *Palliative & Supportive Care* 1–7.

22. Health and Care Act 2022 UK Public General Acts, 2022 c. 31. https://www.legislation.gov.uk/ukpga/2022/31/contents/enacted (accessed 19 August 2022).

23. Murray, S.A. and Sheikh, A. (2008). Care for all at the end of life. *BMJ* 336 (7650): 958–959.

24. Murray, S. Palliative care from diagnosis to death. *BMJ* YouTube. Freely accessible https://youtu.be/vS7ueV0ui5U (accessed 21 August 2022).

25. Equalities and health inequalities references: The Marmot Review (2010). *Fair Society, Health Lives*. London: The Marmot Review. (accessed 21 August 2022).

26. Care Quality Commission and Ending, A.D. (2016). Addressing Inequalities in End of Life Care. *London, UK: Care Quality Commission*.

27. Thomas, P., Calamos, L., Chandok, R., and Colin-Thomé, D. Developing community-oriented integrated practice. https://www.healthmatters.org.uk/Library/coip_0322.pdf (accessed 15 January 2023).

28. Unadkat, N., Evans, L., Nasir, L., Thomas, P., and Chandok, R. (2013). Taking diabetes services out of hospital into the community. *London Journal of Primary Care* 5 (2): 87–91. Available at: https://www.ncbi.nlm.nih.gov/pmc/articles/PMC3960647 (accessed 19 August 2022).

29. Daffodil standards for general practice: the RCGP and Marie Curie UK general practice core standards for advanced serious illness and end of life care. https://www.rcgp.org.uk/daffodilstandards (accessed 21 August 2022).

30. Daffodil Standards – Older people in care homes focus. https://www.rcgp.org.uk/learning-resources/daffodil-standards/older-people-care-homes (accessed 21 August 2022).

31. Millington-Sanders, C. and Noble, B. (2018). New UK general practice core standards for advanced serious illness and end of life care. *British Journal of General Practice* 68 (668): 114–115. (accessed 21 August 2022).

32. Ogi, M., Campling, N., Birtwistle, J. et al. Community access to palliative care medicines—patient and professional experience: systematic review and narrative synthesis. *BMJ Supportive & Palliative Care* Published Online First: 28 March 2021. doi: 10.1136/bmjspcare-2020-002761 (accessed 21 August 2022).

33. Latter, S., Campling, N., Birtwistle, J. et al. (2020). Supporting patient access to medicines in community palliative care: on-line survey of health professionals' practice, perceived effectiveness and influencing factors. *BMC Palliative Care* 19: 148. doi: 10.1186/s12904-020-00649-3. (accessed 21 August 2022).

34. Royal pharmaceutical society: new end of life care standards. https://www.rpharms.com/recognition/setting-professional-standards/daffodil-standards (accessed 29 August 2023).

35. Leniz, J., Henson, L.A., Potter, J. et al. (2022). Association of primary and community care services with emergency visits and hospital admissions at the end of life in people with cancer: a retrospective cohort study. *BMJ Open* 12: e054281. doi: 10.1136/bmjopen-2021-054281.

36. Audit Commission for Local Authorities and the National Health Service in England and Wales (1999). First assessment: a review of district nursing services in England and Wales. Audit Commission.

37. McHugh, G., Pateman, B., and Luker, K. (2003). District nurses' experiences and perceptions of cancer patient referrals. *British Journal of Community Nursing* 8 (2): 72–79.

38. McIlfatrick, S. and Curran, C.I. (2000). District nurses perception of palliative of palliative care services: part 2. *International Journal of Palliative Nursing* 6 (1): 32–38.

39. Bliss, J. (2000). Palliative care in the community: the challenge for district nurses. *British Journal of Community Nursing* 5 (8): 390–395.

40. Beaver, K., Luker, K.A., and Woods, S. (2000). Primary care services received during terminal illness. *International Journal of Palliative Nursing* 6 (5): 220–227.

41. Burt, J., Shipman, C., Addington-Hall, J., and White, P. (2005). Palliative care: perspectives on caring for dying people in London.

42. Walshe, C., Payne, S., and Luker, K. (2012). Observing district nurses roles in palliative care: an understanding of aims and actions. *BMJ Supportive & Palliative Care* 2: A2–A3.

43. Shipman, C., Burt, J., Ream, E., Beynon, T., Richardson, A., and Addington-Hall, J. (2008). Improving district nurses' confidence and knowledge in the principles and practice of palliative care. *Journal of Advanced Nursing* 63 (5): 494–505.

44. Seymour, J.E., Kumar, A., and Froggatt, K. (2011). Do nursing homes for older people have the support they need to provide end-of-life care? A mixed methods enquiry in England. *Palliative Medicine* 25 (2): 125–138.

45. Macgregor, A., Rutherford, A., McCormack, B. et al. (2021). Palliative and end-of-life care in care homes: protocol for codesigning and implementing an appropriate scalable model of Needs Rounds in the UK. *BMJ Open* 11: e049486. doi: 10.1136/bmjopen-2021-049486. (accessed 14 May 2023).

46. Rehabilitative palliative care enabling people to live fully until they die A challenge for the 21st century. Hospice UK. 2015 publication. https://professionals.hospiceuk.org/docs/default-source/What-We-Offer/Care-Support-Programmes/rehabilitative-palliative-care/rehabilitative-palliative-care-enabling-people-to-live-fully-until-they-die.pdf? (accessed 21 August 2022).

47. National Health Service. (7 January 2019). NHS long term plan. https://www.longtermplan.nhs.uk. (accessed 21 August 2022).

48. National Health Service (7 January 2019). NHS Long term plan – A summary. https://www.longtermplan.nhs.uk/wp-content/uploads/2019/01/the-nhs-long-term-plan-summary.pdf.

49. (16 October 2019). End of life care for adults: service delivery NICE guideline [NG142] Published. https://www.nice.org.uk/guidance/ng142 (accessed 21 August 2022).

50. Health Education England, Skills for Health, Skills for Care End of Life Care Core Skills Education and Training Framework. www.skillsforhealth.org.uk/services/item/536-end-of-life-care-cstf-download (accessed 21 August 2022).

51. Shipman, C., Gysels, M., White, P. et al. (2008). Improving generalist end of life care: national consultation with practitioners, commissioners, academics, and service user groups. *BMJ* 337: a1720.

52. End-of-life care for all e-learning programme. https://www.e-lfh.org.uk/programmes/end-of-life-care (accessed 21 August 2022).

53. Project ECHO. Hospice UK https://www.hospiceuk.org/innovation-hub/support-for-your-role/networks-communities/project-echo (accessed 21 August 2022).

54. Guba, E. and Lincoln, Y. (1989). *Fourth Generation Evaluation*. London: Sage.

5 Hospital Palliative Care

Paul W. Keeley

Introduction

Palliative care is an approach that improves the quality of life of patients and their families facing the problem associated with life-threatening illness, through the prevention and relief of suffering by means of early identification and impeccable assessment and treatment of pain and other problems, physical, psychosocial and spiritual [1].

The World Health Organisation (WHO) definition of palliative care is at pains to avoid any statement or implication about where palliative care should be undertaken, precisely because the authors of the definition were clear that palliative care could and should be undertaken in any clinical context. Not merely that but the definition goes on to state that:

> [Palliative care] uses a team approach to address the needs of patients and their families, including bereavement counselling, if indicated.

Palliative care is not a solitary pursuit. A team approach and especially a multidisciplinary approach, is essential. Hospital palliative care teams are significant in the history of palliative care in that it was precisely the suffering of dying patients in hospital that had been highlighted in the immediate post-war period that prompted the development of the hospice movement and palliative care [2, 3]. The development of hospital palliative care teams, soon after the emergence of the first modern hospices, was the beginning of addressing unmet palliative care needs in patients failed by the health system of the mid-twentieth century and especially the hospitals.

This chapter will explore the role of palliative care teams in the context of hospitals. Within this we will explore the generic features of palliative care that are applicable everywhere and go deeper into those features of hospital palliative care that will have most impact on patients and practitioners and which are most germane to the practice of palliative care within hospitals. The history of modern health-care systems can seem at times like a constant reordering of the relationship between hospital and community provision. It seems likely for the foreseeable future – unless there is some major revolution in health care – that hospitals as they exist just now as providers or secondary and tertiary care are likely to be with us for some time. Palliative care will need to continue to adapt itself to hospital care in order to ensure that the best care is offered to those with palliative care where they are rather than where we (or they) might like them to be.

The chapter will therefore cover what a hospital palliative care team does, the roles within them and the interactions between palliative care teams and those with whom they need to interact to provide the best care possible for patients. The chapter touches upon not just *what* palliative care teams do in hospitals but also *how* they undertake their work. This involves an approach to quality improvement, advance care planning and broadening access to palliative care for hospital patients.

A Very Short History of Hospital Palliative Care Teams

While the history of modern palliative care is traced to the foundation of St Christopher's Hospice in London by Dame Cicely Saunders, other pioneers of the specialty built on this and developed other models. The Canadian surgeon, Dr Balfour Mount had visited St Christopher's Hospice in 1973 and rather than develop the same model of a free-standing hospice, established a ward providing similar services within

Handbook of Palliative Care, Fourth Edition. Edited by Richard Kitchen, Christina Faull, Sarah Russell and Jo Wilson.

an established hospital, the Royal Victoria Hospital, Montreal. At the same time he eschewed the word "hospice," and instead coined the term *Palliative Care* [4, 5]. A little after this, in 1976, the first hospital palliative care team was established in the UK at St Thomas's Hospital in London, acting as a liaison, advisory team [6].

Even the most vocal of critics, who had referred to the hospices as "too good to be true and too small to be useful" called for the integration of "palliative care support units offering consultations, home care services, and a few beds for the most difficult cases … in all the places where the serious dying is done: in the front line of the dull old NHS" [7]. While the author's desire that hospices should "wither" didn't come true, the emergence of palliative care teams in hospitals did continue and expand over the coming decades. There was a recognition early on that the hospital palliative care team may face particular challenges and stresses which were different from those encountered in the setting of a hospice where the culture and support may be different from that of the hospital team [8].

The expansion of palliative care services was rapid thereafter, with 324 hospital-based teams by 2004 [4]. There is now wide acceptance, at least within the UK, of hospital-based teams, though often medical staff may have posts with sessional input to both hospice and hospitals. Differing models exist, in terms of the types of service offered in hospitals across the world and there are marked discrepancies in the provision of hospital palliative care services in different parts of the world. In the United States, for example, there are quite marked variations across states in the provision of palliative care in hospitals, dependent in part on the type of hospital (public and not-for-profit hospitals are much more likely to have a programme than for-profit hospitals, for example) and the geographical location in the country (the north east and pacific being more likely than south west and south east central states) [9].

Barriers to Access

The presence of palliative care teams in hospitals is not enough, of itself, to ensure that patients with palliative care needs have those needs met. While there is now ample evidence that palliative care is of benefit from early in the course of incurable disease, there remain barriers to the incorporation of palliative care within the care offered to patients in hospital [10]. These barriers – cultural, attitudinal, structural, and organisational – exist within hospitals and work to the detriment of the care of patients with palliative care needs.

The early involvement of specialist palliative care aimed at enhancing quality of life has demonstrable benefits in terms of patient satisfaction, concordance with patient wishes and reductions in anxiety and depression [11]. Perhaps as important, early incorporation of palliative care into clinical care brings with it benefits in terms of survival and the reduction of health-care costs [10, 12, 13].

The barriers to access are manifold and relate to knowledge, attitudes, and orientation on the part of clinicians and relatives and referrers (Figure 1). In many areas of the world there may be little or no service available for clinicians to refer to. Even within the well-developed health services in the wealthy countries, the availability of palliative care services can be patchy [14]. It may simply be that there are few if any palliative care services to refer to. Where services do exist, potential referrers may be unaware of their presence, having never encountered them in their specialist rotations or posts, or because those services in the case of hospices may be at a distance from acute hospital services [15]. What is key is that hospital palliative care teams have an educational and service obligation to ensure that among potential referrers there is a knowledge of how and when to refer and what the criteria for referrals should be. Moreover, clinicians who are members of specialist palliative care teams – whether based in hospital or hospice – have a duty to ensure that they have or establish good ongoing relationships with clinical networks, founded on mutual respect, with ease of access for advice and become embedded in structures of referral and support.

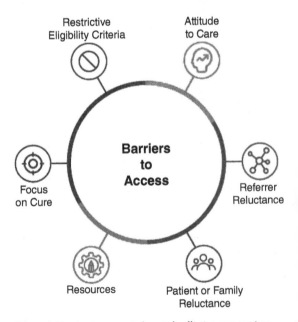

Figure 1 Barriers to access to hospital palliative care services.

Referrers may have a misplaced fear of upsetting patients, may see referral as an admission of professional failure or an abandonment of a patient they have known since diagnosis into the care of others. Families or patients may themselves be resistant to referral. They may see referral to palliative care as almost hastening the death in itself or there may a fear of diminishing the patient's sense of hope.

For older people a number distinct barriers have been identified in the provision of palliative care in hospital. These include attitudinal differences to the care of older people, a focus on curative treatments within hospitals and a lack of resources. There are evidently differing understandings of whose responsibility it is to provide palliative care for older people, and uncertainly over the roles of specialist and generalist palliative care providers in acute hospitals [16].

One of the key points to note is the fact that, given the nature of palliative care as a specialty, that the reach of hospital specialist palliative care teams (HSPCTs) is unlikely to be sufficiently wide to ensure that the needs of all patients with advanced disease are going to be met by those teams – even if it were possible to fund diverse and well-staffed teams. It is arguable that it would not necessarily be desirable that a HSPCT delivers *all* the palliative care that is required. There is an argument that part of the role of a HSPCT is as a leaven within the hospital, encouraging and facilitating good generalist palliative care among their clinical colleagues. By analogy, it would not be functionally possible for a hospital to ensure that every single patient with chronic obstructive pulmonary disease were managed, or even seen by a respiratory team. In the same way, not every patient with advanced incurable disease will require the input of a member of the HSPCT [17].

The Features of a Hospital Palliative Care Team

The models or ideals for teams tend to come from the realm of the business world. Teams should have the characteristics of working with a high degree of interdependence, sharing authority and responsibility, being accountable for collective performance and working towards a common goal and shared rewards. This seems to be a reasonable definition that would fit palliative care teams as well as teams in business [18].

When we think of the range of activities of palliative care services (patient assessment, clinical management, and engagement and communication with professionals, patients and families) it is evident that palliative care multi-professional teams should have a range of responsibilities spread across the different roles (Figure 2). Team members bring their skills and experiences as individuals as well as in their professional role. For example, diagnostic assessment and prescribing skills may be provided by the medical team and those in advanced practice roles. Holistic, psychological, and spiritual assessment and interventions can be provided by a range of clinical roles including psychologists, social workers and chaplaincy. Extended team members may also include family support workers and volunteers meeting the specific needs of patients and their families. There are crossovers in skills and it is important for a team to have a range of skills and experience as it is impossible for one individual to meet all the needs of patients and their families. Palliative care is based on the principle of multi-professional working. There are risks to concentrating skills on one particular person. Solo work risks isolation, idiosyncratic management, lack of professional growth and burnout [19, 20].

Palliative care teams then are a group of people with a full set of complementary skills working together to complete the task of providing or facilitating good palliative care within, in the case we are discussing, a hospital setting. In general, teams tend to be have "core" members, typically doctors (senior specialists, doctors in specialist training) and clinical nurse specialists, with the extended team being drawn from other specialties/professions such as pharmacy, chaplaincy, physiotherapy, and occupational therapy, or clinical psychology and with access to the skills of other teams (for example psychiatry) less able to offer comprehensive palliative care services.

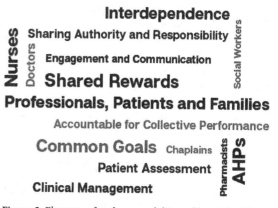

Figure 2 Elements of and responsibilities of hospital palliative care teams.

Teams tend to produce better results in both qualitative and quantitative terms (frequency of visits etc.). Care receiver satisfaction with a team is influenced favourably by collaboration, conflict resolution and cohesive functioning. Combined skills generally produce better decisions and improved outcomes. Effectiveness of service provision is improved by regular audit and other QI work against agreed national and international standards. Individual practitioners may be prone to burnout and poor decision-making [21].

Interaction with Other Teams

Models of hospital palliative care teams will vary across hospital and national settings – from established integrated inpatient units with outreach and liaison to small, part-time arrangements with a solely advisory role. The perception of the palliative care team within the hospital is a significant one to bear in mind in ensuring effectiveness. Tellingly the first teams were self-perceived as a new model of "hospice" rather than as an integral part of the hospital teams [22]. Indeed, it is quite revealing that the language used in the early descriptors was that of a "terminal care" team. While it is evident that palliative care teams from an early stage were heavily involved in the hospital care of patients with cancer, it was only by the mid-1990s that attention was being drawn in the literature to the needs of patients with non-malignant disease in hospitals [23].

What is evident is that while the historic focus of palliative care has been on cancer-related death and the palliative needs of cancer patients, the growing awareness of the needs of patients from both within and outwith palliative care means that focus and attention of palliative care teams must be towards the palliative care needs of patients rather than their diagnoses.

There has been a growing realisation over recent decades that the palliative care needs of patient groups other than those with cancer are unmet and are deserving of equal attention as patients with cancer. The danger, of course, is that there becomes an arms war of competitive need, notwithstanding the fact that specialties outwith palliative care have noted the palliative care needs of their patients. Subsequent to this, many teams have worked collaboratively to map and define these needs in a consistent and methodologically sound way, to seek therapeutic strategies for addressing them and promoted service developments to meet them [24–26].

Heart failure, respiratory disease, end-stage renal disease and neurological diseases all have a significant claim to the resources of palliative care team on the basis that they have significant symptom needs and, in many cases, a worse prognosis than many cancers [27]. The problem for palliative care teams in approaching the needs of patients with non-malignant disease will be the fact they may have less predictable illness trajectories, making prognosis, and advance care planning more difficult. Likewise, patients with non-malignant disease may be under-recognised by referrers as suitable for referral to palliative care and may have symptom clusters for which palliative care has a threadbare evidence base [28, 29].

Assessment of Patients

In considering patients with palliative care in a non-palliative care setting, it is important to again look at the WHO definition of palliative care:

> Palliative care is an approach which improves the quality of life of patients and their families facing the problems associated with life-threatening illness through the prevention and relief of suffering by means of early identification [1].

The important part of the definition here is the *impeccable assessment and treatment of pain and other problems physical, psychosocial, and spiritual* [1].

While those working in palliative care will be familiar with the definition, it is important to pick up on that palliative care looks to provide relief from pain and other distressing symptoms. Palliative care integrates psychological and spiritual aspects of care, uses a team approach to address the needs of patients and their families, and aims to enhance quality of life. This is done in conjunction with other therapies that are intended to prolong life such as chemotherapy or radiation therapy, and includes those investigations needed to better understand and manage distressing clinical complications.

The reason for highlighting these points are, these are all integrated elements into holistic assessment, and this is key to understanding their relationship to palliative care as being holistic in its aims as a speciality. The WHO definition of palliative care relates in an interesting way and dovetails with the WHO definition of health, which states that "health is a state of complete physical, mental, and social well-being and not merely the absence of disease or infirmity" [30]. It is important to point out the shift from a pre-war definition of health as the absence of disease and infirmity to much more positive view, but also interestingly that in looking at health in the second half of the twentieth century, clinicians were looking towards health being a holistic matter, not merely involving the physical, but also maintaining that mental and social well-being was important as well in clinical care.

Against this backdrop of a changing understanding of the different elements of health and disease and a more holistic view, Cicely Saunders developed the idea of "Total Pain." Her research using opioids in the early 1950s led to a realisation from her studies of dying hospice patients that pain wasn't merely a physical phenomenon, but there were elements of both psychological, social, and spiritual elements that were at play that led to her coining the phrase of "Total Pain" [31].

This entails consideration of the more existential aspect of suffering as part of the experience of dying patients and of ill patients as a whole. The WHO definiton was developed in large part by Robert Twycross's who had worked with Cicely Saunders in the early day of St Christopher's. Twycross advanced the concept further in the WHO definition by incorporating the need for "impeccable assessment and treatment of pain and other problems, physical, psychosocial and spiritual" [1].

This becomes a theme within palliative care in its development and the fact that there's a recognition that in suffering and in symptoms, there are a range of influences, physical, psychological, and social, as well as spiritual involved in suffering. It's important that those are assessed as part of addressing the problems that are at play within patients with advanced, incurable disease. Saunders' view of pain, having all of these elements at play and using pain as a model for the rest of human suffering was important as a development because this was in sharp contrast to the previous biomedical model that was reductionist and saw the whole of suffering as relating to the body rather than the more numinous elements of human experience.

Meeting the needs of those suffering with life-limiting illness will mean addressing all of those elements of that suffering in an assessment, incorporating all of the different elements of care. It may be difficult, if not impossible, to achieve the "impeccable" assessment aspired to by the WHO definition, but the aspiration, within the limits of the practically achievable, is still of value. It will be seen as evidence that suffering is multifactorial and involves different elements of the human character and different facets of human life. The biomedical model, concentrating on the merely physical and the physiological, will be inadequate for that unless it incorporates the physical, psychological, the spiritual, and the social.

There will of course be a tension between the time and resource demands of a busy palliative care service and the need for holistic assessment. The environment of an acute hospital may not afford the ability to assess patients as holistically as in the setting, say, of a hospice. Hence there will need to be a balance between the comprehensiveness of the assessment, the incorporation of information already available from other clinicians who have already cared for or have clinical responsibilty for the patient and the realities of work in a busy clinical environment where it may not be practically possible to replicate the holistic assessment that *may* be feasible in a hospice.

For the most part, assessments will take the form of the traditional history, examination and investigations of the biomedical model of care augmented, to a greater or lesser extent, by psychiatric or psychological assessment, a review of the patient's family and social support and framework of spiritual or existential beliefs, practices, and concerns. There have been attempts to systematise these assessments either for clinical practice or for research. These incorporate the preparation, history taking and physical examination before explaining, planning, and closing a consultation considering the patient's and the family's individual wishes and goals.

There have been attempts over the years to systematically look at the holistic assessment of supportive and palliative care needs. A number of holistic assessment tools have been developed. These include the Oncology Clinic Patient Checklist, The Palliative Care Assessment Tool Supportive Care Needs Survey (long form and short form), The Distress Management Tool, Symptoms and Concerns Checklist, Initial Health Assessment Form Problems and Needs in Palliative Care Instrument Sheffield Profile for Assessment and Referral for Care, and the Needs at the End-of-Life Screening Tool [32]. These had between 12 and 138 items for each of the tools assessed - a very wide range. Twelve items for a particular assessment tool might seem very small, 138 seems unwieldy and impractical, and some are used for particular groups such as cancer patients. All of them, in their own way and in the settings or functions for which they were designed are useful and validated, however, none of them seem to have demonstrated an improvement in quality of life [33]. One further example not highlighted by Ahmed and colleagues in their systematic review has found some clinical use in the United Kingdom as part of the Gold Standards Framework. This tool, applies a mnemonic PEPSICOLA to the holistic assessment of patients and is shown in Figure 3 [34, 35].

A holistic assessment is necessary for palliative care teams to give some degree of structure to encounters, to encourage the provision of holistic care and to ensure the

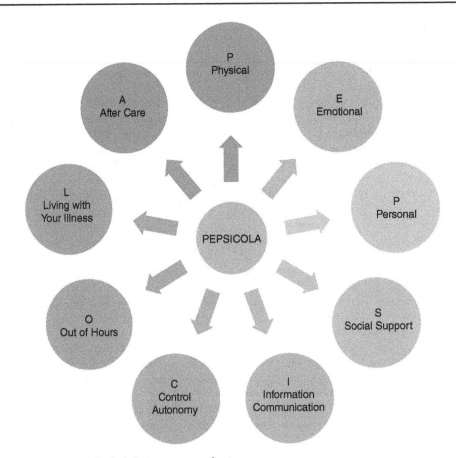

Figure 3 PEPSICOLA mnemonic for the holistic assessment of patients.

collection of comprehensive patient information to facilitate effective advance care planning. A holistic assessment should concentrate on the impact on daily living, function and quality of life. In addition to the physical, social, psychological, and spiritual, Ahmed and colleagues also incorporated a significant point, which is an ethical one. The background information and assessment preferences are significant in that they place the patient at the centre of the assessment, thus respecting autonomy. The background information about what patients want and what their needs are and what they want assessed in the first place, as well as managed, should be a significant feature of the assessment.

While it may not be feasible to undertake the kind of holistic assessment that may be more typical of a hospice admission in one session in the context of hospital palliative care, it may be possible to glean the same or similar information. An alternative would be to undertake the assessment over a number of sessions. As with hospice or community work it is sometimes difficult to gain a holistic picture in one single sitting and it's very unlikely that a patient will give a whole picture of their life in the process of one single clinical encounter. An assessment of needs should be seen as patient led or patient centred, should be seen as continuous and supplement, but not replace, day-to-day assessment.

With particular reference to advance care planning, summary records of assessments should be first agreed with patients so that they know the information on which decisions are being made, both by them and by health-care professionals, and that this should be documented and easily accessible for other health-care professionals. The assessment should then perhaps best be done by different members of the clinical team or teams looking after a patient and can be incorporated at a range of different points during either their hospital stay or in multiople encounters in clinic.

Holistic assessments then are an essential part of the work of hospital palliative care teams. As key feartures they will incorporate the physical, emotional, psychological, social, and spiritual needs of patients and may borrow from assessments developed for a variety of clinical purposes. They may not feature the extensive complete assessment undertaken at admission to some inpatient specialist palliative care units due to the demands of time and balancing a larger patient number in an acute, non-specialist palliative care environment. However, it may be that with assesments collated over team by different members of the team using complementary skills, it may be feasible to assemble the relevant clinical information needed to make clinical judgements as part of patient-centred care and plan care holsitically in line with patient needs and wishes.

Choice of Place of Death

The place of the patient in health policy – particularly in a centralised health economy such as the United Kingdom has, until relatively recent years been somewhat peripheral. The policy shifts of the 1980s with an emphasis on patient choice, brought with it, at least ostensibly a move to the considerations of the patient being at the heart of policy. Palliative care, with an explicit patient-centric focus has sought to promote patient choice at the heart of this issue. While it is certainly the case that the majority of patients consistently express the view that they would like to die at home [36], it is also the case that most patients do not and indeed end up dying where they would explicitly rather not die – in hospital [37].

From relatively early on in the history of hospital palliative care teams it became apparent that there was a dissonance between the expressed choice of patients for place of death and where they actually ended up dying. For those with access to palliative care services, preferred place of death could be achieved in a majority of patients, but a number of factors could be identified as confounding intentions, like unexpected deterioration in clinical condition, difficulties coping for families and carers and delayed or late presentation precluding appropriate transfer [38].

There exists a tension for palliative care teams in hospital. The aim of patient-centred care should be to respect the expressed wishes, where possible of patients, to facilitate the death they want, where they want it. While this will be, for many, home, for others a number of factors will come into play – the feasibility of getting home if particularly dependent or if support is not available in their particular setting – meaning that hospital may be their place of death. The task and energy of the palliative care team then is to ensure the best quality of death in hospital.

Audit and Quality Improvement

Clinical audit is a quality improvement process that seeks to improve patient care and outcomes through systematic review of care against explicit criteria…Where indicated, changes are implemented…and further monitoring is used to confirm improvement in healthcare delivery [39].

Quality improvement refers to the use of systematic tools and methods to continuously improve the quality of care and outcomes for patients [40]. It is arguable, of course, that the whole project of the specialty of palliative care is a global quality improvement (QI). Looking at the history of palliative care, which grew from an increasing recognition of the failures of health care as it existed at the time in the care of the dying, it is easy to see that the efforts Cicely Saunders and the early pioneers of palliative care in symptom control, holistic assessment, psychological, spiritual, and social care and the development of services all served to improve the quality of living and dying with advanced incurable disease. It should come as second nature, therefore, to palliative care professionals to engage in work towards further enhancing the care of patients with palliative care needs by improving the clinical processes around care. A self-critical attitude and a degree of humility in assuming that we do not always offer the gold standard of care, even in highly specialised settings like hospices will foster a culture that constantly aims to offer consistent improvements in care through audit and quality improvement work.

The audit process is cyclical. The first task is to identify the clinical practice to be examined, whether identified as an issue of importance or a problematic concern. Having identified the clinical issue to be studied or analysed, finding best clinical standards allows a benchmark against which current or historic practice can be measured. The best practice can be in the form of a local, national, or international clinical guideline for a particular clinical practice or activity. The next task will be the collection, either retrospective or prospective, of data measured against the accepted criteria or standard. Such has been the involvement over the years of palliative care professional in audit and QI work that there exist many validated audit tools to facilitate audit without palliative care teams needing to invent their own [41, 42].

Audit becomes quality improvement when the cycle is complete and where the changes resulting from the identification of variation from best practice noted in audit become an action to change and improve practice. This comprises the plan, do, check, act cycle (Figure 4) [43].

That audit and quality improvement enhances the quality of care of patients with palliative care needs has been borne out by a number of studies [44–47]. But while there is much audit activity undertaken in palliative care as in many other areas of health care, it must be borne in mind that the audit process should ideally be a constant process of quality improvement. At times audit may not result in positive change and it is important to recognise the factors within the audit cycle that may contribute to this. Often a key and missing stage may be the fact that teams do not identify the underlying reasons for failing to meet particular standards and in avoiding this key point may avoid the at times challenging structural change required to implement meaningful quality improvement [47].

It is evident that audit and quality improvement are significant challenges for palliative care teams in all global settings, including areas of the world where resources are limited (indeed it is arguably more so given that effective audit and quality improvement, should in theory, produce the utilitarian effect of promoting the best and most effective services within the limits of the available resources). While the general principles of audit and quality improvement remain the same whatever the clinical environment, there are particular contextual and local issues in particular settings. The combination of local knowledge and the experience of international collaborative organisations in

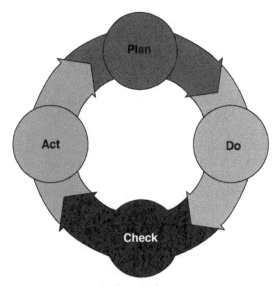

Figure 4 Plan, Do, Check, Act cycle.

deploying resources and proficiency in service evaluation and large-scale audit may be particularly useful in developing countries [48].

Differences from Other Settings

Palliative care seems to have struggled with a sense of identity over the first 40 years of its existence. At significant points over that time there has been a number of supposed existential crises about the nature of palliative care. There does indeed seem to be a crisis of confidence about the specialty, about what it should do, where it should direct its efforts or even whether the word "palliative" should be abandoned as unhelpful [49]. Palliative care within hospitals is an adjustment of an approach that should be applicable everywhere. The significant challenges to the application of palliative care are those of philosophy and environment. Hospices are specifically designed to allow an environment of peace and a routine that allows space for the spiritual and the emotional, with room for families and loved ones that may not be feasible in hospitals. Similarly, the approach within hospitals of interventions which may no longer be appropriate at the end-of-life may be in conflict with the goals of good palliative care. In both cases, the continuing task of the hospital palliative care team will be one of negotiation and advocacy on behalf of patients and relatives in terms of the provision of adequate or appropriate space for them, and with other teams to adjust their approach to the goals of good palliative care (the avoidance of unnecessary interventions, effetivepalliation and addressing psychological and spiritual needs).

Ultimately the adaptability of palliative care has allowed it to be delivered across a number of settings (particularly across hospice, hospital, and community). The maintenance of the distinction between these settings and the approaches to them creates a degree of tension perhaps, with hospitalists and primary care practitioners maintaining the distinctiveness of their roles while at the same time the palliative care approach being seen as a continuing unifying presence. Unitary schemes of training, offering balanced experience between training environments across all palliative care settings should be encouraged to ensure this continuing approach.

Team Roles

Clinical

The most obvious and central role of the palliative care team in the hospital is clinical. While the particular settings of palliative care teams in different hospitals (large teaching hospital or district general hospital) will often define differing roles and responsibilities or emphases, it is clear that the palliative care team has a clinical orientation (sometimes to the detriment of other roles). So it is that whatever the setting, the palliative care team is likely to have a clinical workload. Similarly, the orientation of a particular hospital setting will necessarily set the perspective and the limits of a team seeking to meet the palliative care needs of patients in hospital.

The setup of each hospital will of course determine the orientation of the team and the skillset required by its members. For example, the orientation, workload, and skillset of a palliative care team in a district general hospital differs from that in a large teaching hospital or tertiary specialist unit (for example a specialist cancer hospital). While it may seem obvious or trivial to mention this, it has significant implications for training, staffing, and development. For example, a team in a large teaching hospital with specialist teams for the management of complex cancers will need not only experience and confidence in managing these cancers and their complications, but also the ability to manage such patients in the setting of the intensive care unit where they may spend time during their illness. This will bring with it the necessity to take on and accommodate the ethical and technical issues at stake, which may be at variance with encounters elsewhere in the hospital. Similarly, the presence of members of a palliative care team in a disease clinic (for example for multiple sclerosis or lung cancer) emphasises both the integration of palliative care into the normal care and enhances opportunities for earlier and more effective intervention. In every hospital there will of necessity be a reorientation to the ethos of differing departments with which palliative care teams may need to engage, from gerontologists who may have an instinctive understanding and wide experience of natural death in hospital to a plastic surgery unit oriented to cure who may have few deaths a year. In addition to the differing specialties encountered, teams will have to accommodate changing configurations over years and decades as hospitals and health services reorganise and reconfigure. A constant awareness of the organisations in which teams work, their strategic direction, and the wider context of health care is a perennial task for hospital palliative care teams.

The initial role of palliative care teams in hospitals seemed to be to overtly missionary – to bring the ideas developed in hospices into a hospital setting. David Clark tells us that "Hospice ideals and practices began to be disseminated into other settings from the 1970s" [4] while Dunlop and Hockley assert that palliative care teams would not be where they were "had it not been for the therapies and insights developed within the modern hospice setting" [6]. This is undoubtedly true but presents only part of the story.

A more balanced view from the past 45 years of palliative care teams would be that of adapting the palliative care approach to the hospital and using and adapting it in conjunction with the teams with which they have had to collaborate. More importantly, rather than adopting a missionary or evangelical stance in developing palliative care for patients in hospitals, it has been more productive to integrate into other hospital care teams. What is evident is that the early and systematic integration of teams brings significant benefits for patients [50].

Education and Teaching

The setting of the hospital palliative care team will undoubtedly have a bearing on the teaching they can undertake and the impact they can make on other teams. Palliative care education is likely to make its greatest impact where it reaches the greatest number of those who are likely to have the greatest bearing on the care of patients with palliative care needs. In highly specialised hospital environments (for example, tertiary cancer centres) a focus on the education of cancer specialists in a range of roles (specialist nurses, doctors, and allied health professionals) is going to be important.

In truth there is an educational role to every single encounter between the hospital palliative care team and other teams. This is particularly true of the encounter between the team and less experienced professionals on wards. There is always a thirst for knowledge about palliative care, which can seem to have esoteric knowledge in areas of symptom control and communication. Taking time with more junior members of staff to go through a management plan for a patient, to get them to attend a bedside or clinic consultation and witness the communication skills developed over years of significant conversations can have a lasting, if not life- or career-changing impact if done with consideration and the aim of allowing the other member of staff to grow and thrive.

Research

There are a number of structural, cultural, and ethical reasons why palliative care research has perhaps taken a back seat compared to the educational and clinical roles that hospital palliative care has established in the decades of its existence. One of the most obvious is financial, whereby, certainly in the United Kingdom, a significant proportion of the funding of core services in hospices are through charitable fundraising. The obvious corollary of this is that were core services fully funded by government, the fundraising of palliative care organisations could be then directed towards funding research [51]. That is not to say that there are not laudable examples of charitable funding of research through organisations such as Marie Curie and Macmillan. There are other reasons for the sometimes infuriatingly limited evidence base of palliative care. Research within palliative care can be challenging because of a degree of logistic and ethical issues around dealing with patients. By their very nature, patients with advanced life-threatening disease are notably frail and this presents a problem of recruitment and attrition in palliative care trials. There are similarly ethical issues in conducting trials at the end-of-life and ethics committees are understandably cautious about trials involving this group of patients [52].

There is however, some cause for optimism. Research in palliative care is steadily increasing and this will bring with it the benefits of a critical mass of research-skilled palliative care clinicians able to collaborate to bring about good-quality, and impactful research. This will bring with it the prospect of larger scale, multi-centre national and international studies. Disciplinary backgrounds including basic scientists, social scientists, and clinicians are required for effective collaboration [53]. Research collaboration with existing networks and using the research training that exists within universities and other educational institutes to acquire generic skills will be essential for future research advances.

Leadership

The history of palliative care has been one from the beginning of challenging existing models of care and developing new ones across a range of different settings. In addition to outlining the roles of clinical, education, teaching, and research outlined above, Cicely Saunders highlighted the dynamism of early pioneers and the fact that palliative care would have to engage with differing health sectors so that it would be able to:

> hold its position between specialist teams with continually developing expertise and the general challenge to all that patients should have skilled attention to the end of their lives, whatever their disease or disability. [54, p. 12]

Leadership presents a problem in palliative care where a particular health organisation may be served by a variety of agencies independent of each other. In the United Kingdom, for example, the integration and

coordination necessary for effective change may be difficult where a population is served by a health board or trust for hospital inpatients, an independent hospice and an entirely separate community team, each with different management structures and sources of funding. Similarly, sustainable development across sectors may again be difficult when reliant on charitable funding.

Perhaps, however, the greatest feat of leadership we can undertake is simply doing our job. The everyday work of a palliative care teams incorporates each of the elements outlined above: we teach, we inquire, we lead others by breaking through decision-sclerosis and encouraging realistic decision-making with patients' values at their core. It is easy to forget at times how the mere presence of a specialist palliative care team has a significant but imperceptible effect on the culture of clinical practice, acting as a leaven on the culture within a hospital.

How Effective are Palliative Care Teams?

The question of the effectiveness of hospital palliative care teams is an unusual one that has occupied inordinate attention in the literature of palliative care [55–57]. Specialisation has been a feature of medicine that gained increasing momentum in the nineteenth century and has accelerated into areas of sub-specialisation. There will always be the tension within health care – nursing, medicine, and allied health professionals – in the holism of the generalist and the need for highly specialised knowledge of some conditions. Palliative care straddles an uncomfortable balance between a generalist subject – everyone dies and every hospital contains dying patients – and the fact that the specialty has accrued, over the half century of its existence, a valuable body of knowledge and skills which it can apply in a hospital setting.

As has been outlined, palliative care professionals attempted to ensure the provision of palliative care in a hospital setting. Unlike more established specialties, in an era where there is a demand for evidence of effectiveness to justify the allocation of resources, palliative care has felt the need to assess its own contribution in terms of patient outcomes. Assessing the effectiveness of palliative care teams is methodologically difficult as the interventions are often complex and have multiple variables which are difficult to adjust for. The methodology of systematic reviews and randomised controlled trials may just not be adequate to demonstrate the complex interventions – pharmacological, psychological, social, and spiritual – that palliative care teams provide.

It is important however, to bear in mind, despite attempts to make the measurable important (and indeed the important measurable), it is evident that palliative care teams are an essential part of hospital care and will be an integral part of that care as long as patients die in hospital. There are evidently clear clinical elements to care that palliative care teams are demonstrably able to positively impact. The concentration on effectiveness should move away from a need to justify the presence of palliative care teams in hospital towards demonstrating particular, well-defined impacts where trial methodology can be used to provide evidence for service funders and providers to develop hospital palliative care teams. The presence of a palliative care team as a resource for other teams in multidisciplinary work, education, and training (placements and formal teaching for example) cannot be overemphasised.

Multidisciplinary Team Work

In the context of hospital palliative care team, multidisciplinary team (MDT) work has two aspects that deserve consideration. It should go without saying that the hospital palliative care team itself should be multidisciplinary. The history of palliative care is that of a multidisciplinary endeavour and it is hard to conceive of an arrangement whereby a HSPCT could successfully consist of anything other than members from diverse range of professions.

Quite what the optimal composition of a HSPCT should be is a matter of debate [58]. The constituents of most teams will reflect historic funding arrangements whereby funding has allowed the staffing of members initially – often in the form of sessional input from hospices or pump-priming from charitable foundations in order to make a case of more permanent funding. The growth of teams tends to have been organic and opportunistic (making use of funding growth, in the UK, for example, as part of the NHS Cancer Plan of 2000) [59]. There have been explicit attempts, however, to give some shape to the constituent members of palliative care teams:

> The multi-disciplinary palliative care team should contain trained specialist medical and nursing staff, social workers, physiotherapists, occupational therapists and should relate to other disciplines such as dietetics and chaplaincy [60, p. 16].

This list is not exhaustive (and does not, disappointingly, include specialist pharmacist input) but does at least give some indication of the range of skills required, particularly in large hospitals to meet the palliative care needs in a holistic way. Each member of the team should ideally input regularly in MDT meetings to ensure care is optimised and the skills of each member of the team is appropriately brought to bear on the care of patients. Similarly, there may be differing points at which the differing skillsets may be required – diagnostic or prescribing at one stage in a patient's illness, discharge planning or rehabilitation at others, but it is unlikely that the experiences of a particular patient with palliative care needs throughout their hospital stay will not need the input of more than one member at some stage.

The second important, and indeed, increasingly important facet of multidisciplinary work relates to palliative care input to wider multidisciplinary team working. For a range of chronic conditions, initially in the case of cancers and now increasingly in non-malignant disease, management decisions are taken collectively by properly constituted MDTs. Multidisciplinary teams in cancer have certainly demonstrated better clinical and process outcomes for cancer patients and represent an attempt at holistic care for patients, in which palliative care has a key role to play ensuring effective communication between team and patient [61].

The Future

Palliative care professionals more than most, understand the inherent difficulties in predicting the future. It is difficult enough on the level of an individual patient – how much more difficult is it to predict the future of health care and society at large. Changes within health care have been rapid and unpredictable. Palliative care has been remarkably adaptable in its ability to adjust to its application from its origins in hospices to its work across community and hospital settings. As with any human endeavour, palliative care has a patchwork of successes and failures. The spectacular rise and fall of the Liverpool Care Pathway is a case in point [62]. The conjunction of ethical concerns met a perfect storm of press interest and political zeitgeist which resulted in perhaps a chastening downfall which after 50 years of success gave palliative care its first large-scale hubristic reverse [63].

The fear of setbacks should not deter innovation in health care. The development of new services and treatments is hardly a smooth succession of unerring success. The constant creative tension between maintaining underlying clinical and ethical principles and the vision of improving the lot of patients with end-stage incurable disease is challenging, and unless humans become immortal, these we will have with us always. What our patients die of or with, will however change, and palliative care professionals will have to adjust themselves to differing disease trajectories and symptoms clusters, to differing treatments with differing adverse effects and differing patient, family, and professional expectations. The hospital of the future may itself be very different from that just now and we must adapt similarly to that change, as we must to perhaps to the changing roles of doctors, nurses, and other health professionals with regard to training and professional responsibilities.

While it is clear that no professional is clairvoyant and able to see into the future, it is incumbent on hospital-based teams to have a clear awareness of the past and a keen eye upon the current changes in the nature of diseases and their treatment, our patients' experiences of those diseases and their families' needs. It requires an active research community to work in areas of symptom control and the qualitative aspects of patients' experience to illuminate future care and for palliative care organisations to collaborate with public health bodies and health planners to plot the future as far as this is possible.

We owe the dying and those facing incurable progressive disease no less.

Acknowledgement

Many thanks to Ruairidh Keeley for producing Figures 1, 2, and 4.

References

1. World Health Organization. National cancer control programmes: policies and managerial guidelines, 2nd ed. Geneva: World Health Organization, 2002.
2. Hinton, J.M. (1963 January 1). The physical and mental distress of the dying. *Quarterly Journal of Medicine* 32 (1): 1–21.
3. Exton-Smith, A.N. (1961 August 5). Terminal illness in the aged. *The Lancet* 278 (7197): 305–308.
4. Clark, D. (2007 May 1). From margins to centre: a review of the history of palliative care in cancer. *The Lancet Oncology* 8 (5): 430–438.
5. Mount, B.M. (1976 July 17). The problem of caring for the dying in a general hospital; the palliative care unit as a possible solution. *Canadian Medical Association Journal* 115 (2): 119.
6. Dunlop, R.J. and Hockley, J.M. (1990). *Hospital-Based Palliative Care Teams.* Oxford: Oxford University Press.
7. Douglas, C. (1992 February 29). For all the saints. *British Medical Journal* 304 (6826): 579–580.
8. Beszterczey, A. (1977 November). Staff Stress on a newly-developed palliative care service: the psychiatrist's role. *Canadian Psychiatric Association Journal* 22 (7): 347–354.
9. Dumanovsky, T., Augustin, R., Rogers, M., Lettang, K., Meier, D.E., and Morrison, R.S. (2016 January 1). The growth of palliative care in US hospitals: a status report. *Journal of Palliative Medicine* 19 (1): 8–15.
10. Temel, J.S., Greer, J.A., Muzikansky, A., Gallagher, E.R., Admane, S., Jackson, V.A., Dahlin, C.M., Blinderman, C.D., Jacobsen, J., Pirl, W.F., and Billings, J.A. (2010 August 19). Early palliative care for patients with metastatic non–small-cell lung cancer. *New England Journal of Medicine* 363 (8): 733–742.
11. Higginson, I.J. and Evans, C.J. (2010 September 1). What is the evidence that palliative care teams improve outcomes for cancer patients and their families? *The Cancer Journal* 16 (5): 423–435.
12. Connor, S.R., Pyenson, B., Fitch, K., Spence, C., and Iwasaki, K. (2007 March 1). Comparing hospice and nonhospice patient survival among patients who die within a three-year window. *Journal of Pain and Symptom Management* 33 (3): 238–246.
13. Morrison, R.S., Dietrich, J., Ladwig, S., Quill, T., Sacco, J., Tangeman, J., and Meier, D.E. (2011 March 1). Palliative care consultation teams cut hospital costs for Medicaid beneficiaries. *Health Affairs* 30 (3): 454–463.
14. Hui, D., Elsayem, A., DeLa Cruz, M., Berger, A., Zhukovsky, D.S., Palla, S., Evans, A., Fadul, N., Palmer, J.L., and Bruera, E. (2010 March 17). Availability and integration of palliative care at US cancer centers. *JAMA* 303 (11): 1054–1061.
15. Hawley, P. (2017). Barriers to access to palliative care. *Palliative Care: Research and Treatment* 10: 1–16.
16. Gardiner, C., Cobb, M., Gott, M., and Ingleton, C. (2011 March 1). Barriers to providing palliative care for older people in acute hospitals. *Age and Ageing* 40 (2): 233–238.
17. Quill, T.E. and Abernethy, A.P. (2013 March 28). Generalist plus specialist palliative care—creating a more sustainable model. *New England Journal of Medicine* 368 (13): 1173–1175.
18. Katzenbach, J.R. and Smith, D.K. (2005 July 1). The discipline of teams. *Harvard Business Review* 83 (7): 162.
19. Cooper, R.J. (2009 November 1). Solo doctors and ethical isolation. *Journal of Medical Ethics* 35 (11): 692–695.
20. Bush, J. (2020 April). Engaging the solo practitioner to reduce errors and burnout. *Journal of Medical Regulation* 106 (1): 16–21.
21. Fernando, G.V. and Hughes, S. (2019 September 2). Team approaches in palliative care: a review of the literature. *International Journal of Palliative Nursing* 25 (9): 444–451.
22. Bates, T., Hoy, A.M., Clarke, D.G., and Laird, P.P. (1981). The St. Thomas' Hospital terminal care support team—a new concept of hospice care. *Lancet* 2: 1201–1203.
23. Gannon, C. (1995 May 27). Palliative care in terminal cardiac failure. Hospices cannot fulfil such a vast and diverse role. *British Medical Journal* 310 (6991): 1410.
24. Davidson, P.M., Paull, G., Introna, K., Cockburn, J., Davis, J.M., Rees, D., Gorman, D., Magann, L., Lafferty, M., and Dracup, K. (2004 January 1). Integrated, collaborative palliative care in heart failure: the St. George Heart Failure

Service experience 1999–2002. *Journal of Cardiovascular Nursing* 19 (1): 68–75.

25. Rocker, G.M., Simpson, A.C., and Horton, R. (2015 September 1). Palliative care in advanced lung disease: the challenge of integrating palliation into everyday care. *Chest* 148 (3): 801–809.

26. Hepgul, N., Gao, W., Evans, C.J., Jackson, D., vanVliet, L.M., Byrne, A., Crosby, V., Groves, K.E., Lindsay, F., and Higginson, I.J. (2018 March 1). Integrating palliative care into neurology services: what do the professionals say? *BMJ Supportive & Palliative Care* 8 (1): 41–44.

27. Traue, D.C. and Ross, J.R. (2005 November). Palliative care in non-malignant diseases. *Journal of the Royal Society of Medicine* 98 (11): 503–506.

28. Fallon, M. and Foley, P. (2012). Rising to the challenge of palliative care for non-malignant disease. *Palliative Medicine* 26 (2): 99–100.

29. Johnson, M. and Fallon, M. (2013). Just good care? The palliative care of those with non-malignant disease. *Palliative Medicine* 27 (9): 803–804.

30. World Health Organization. (1946 June 19–22). *Preamble to the Constitution of the World Health Organization as Adopted by the International Health Conference.* New York: World Health Organization.

31. Clark, D. (1999 September 1). "Total pain," disciplinary power and the body in the work of Cicely Saunders, 1958–1967. *Social Science & Medicine* 49 (6): 727–736.

32. Aslakson, R., Dy, S.M., Wilson, R.F. et al. (2017). *Assessment Tools for Palliative Care. Agency for Healthcare Research and Quality (US).* Rockville, MD: PMID: 28837305.

33. Ahmed, N., Ahmedzai, S.H., Collins, K., and Noble, B. (2014 September 1). Holistic assessment of supportive and palliative care needs: the evidence for routine systematic questioning. *BMJ Supportive & Palliative Care* 4 (3): 238–246.

34. The Gold Standards Framework. A programme for community palliative care. https://goldstandardsframework.org.uk (accessed 5 April 2021).

35. Thomas, K. (2003). *Caring for the Dying at Home: Companions on the Journey.* Abingdon, Oxon: Radcliffe Medical Press.

36. Hoare, S., Morris, Z.S., Kelly, M.P., Kuhn, I., and Barclay, S. (2015 November 10). Do patients want to die at home? A systematic review of the UK literature, focused on missing preferences for place of death. *PloS One* 10 (11): e0142723.

37. Gomes, B., Higginson, I.J., Calanzani, N., Cohen, J., Deliens, L., Daveson, B.A., Bechinger-English, D., Bausewein, C., Ferreira, P.L., Toscani, F., and Meñaca, A. (2012 August 1). Preferences for place of death if faced with advanced cancer: a population survey in England, Flanders, Germany, Italy, the Netherlands, Portugal and Spain. *Annals of Oncology* 23 (8): 2006–2015.

38. Dunlop, R.J., Davies, R.J., and Hockley, J.M. (1989 July). Preferred versus actual place of death: a hospital palliative care support team experience. *Palliative Medicine* 3 (3): 197–201.

39. NICE. (2002). *Principles for Best Practice in Clinical Audit.* Abingdon: Radcliffe Medical Press.

40. Jabbal, J. (2017). *Embedding a Culture of Quality Improvement.* London: King's Fund.

41. Hearn, J. and Higginson, I.J. (1999 December 1). Development and validation of a core outcome measure for palliative care: the palliative care outcome scale. Palliative Care Core Audit Project Advisory Group. *BMJ Quality & Safety* 8 (4): 219–227.

42. Edmonds, P.M., Stuttaford, J.M., Penny, J., Lynch, A.M., and Chamberlain, J. (1998 July). Do hospital palliative care teams improve symptom control? Use of a modified STAS as an evaluation tool. *Palliative Medicine* 12 (5): 345–351.

43. Berk, M., Callaly, T., and Hyland, M. (2003 May). The evolution of clinical audit as a tool for quality improvement. *Journal of Evaluation in Clinical Practice* 9 (2): 251–257.

44. Benitez-Rosario, M.A., Castillo-Padrós, M., Garrido-Bernet, B., and Ascanio-León, B. (2012 October 1). Quality of care in palliative sedation: audit and compliance monitoring of a clinical protocol. *Journal of Pain and Symptom Management* 44 (4): 532–541.

45. Tsai, L.Y., Li, I.F., Liu, C.P., Su, W.H., and Change, T.Y. (2008 September). Application of quality audit tools to evaluate care quality received by terminal cancer patients admitted to a palliative care unit. *Supportive Care in Cancer* 16 (9): 1067–1074.

46. Morita, T., Fujimoto, K., Namba, M., Sasaki, N., Ito, T., Yamada, C., Ohba, A., Hiroyoshi, M., Niwa, H., Yamada, T., and Noda, T. (2008 January). Palliative care needs of cancer outpatients receiving chemotherapy: an audit of a clinical screening project. *Supportive Care in Cancer* 16 (1): 101–107.

47. Crombie, I.K. and Davies, H.T. (1993). Missing link in the audit cycle. *Quality in Health Care* 2 (1): 47.

48. Selman, L. and Harding, R. (2010 January). How can we improve outcomes for patients and families under palliative care? Implementing clinical audit for quality improvement in resource limited settings. *Indian Journal of Palliative Care* 16 (1): 8.

49. Watt, C.L., Downar, J., Ahmedzai, S., Baldwin, D., Currow, D., and Clark, D. (1993). Whither the hospices? In: *The Future for Palliative Care: Issues in Policy and Practice* (ed. D. Clark), 167–177. Milton Keynes, Bucks, England: The Open University Press.

50. Vanbutsele, G., Pardon, K., Van Belle, S., Surmont, V., DeLaat, M., Colman, R., Eecloo, K., Cocquyt, V., Geboes, K., and Deliens, L. (2018 March 1). Effect of early and systematic integration of palliative care in patients with advanced cancer: a randomised controlled trial. *The Lancet Oncology* 19 (3): 394–404.

51. Foley, K.M. (2005 November 1). The past and future of palliative care. *The Hastings Center Report* 35 (6): S42–S46.

52. Addington-Hall, J. (2002 September). Research sensitivities to palliative care patients. *European Journal of Cancer Care* 11 (3): 220–224.

53. Kaasa, S., Hjermstad, M.J., and Loge, J.H. (2006 December). Methodological and structural challenges in palliative care research: how have we fared in the last decades? *Palliative Medicine* 20 (8): 727–734.

54. Saunders, C. (2000 August 1). The evolution of palliative care. *Patient Education and Counseling* 41 (1): 7–13.

55. Bajwah, S., Oluyase, A.O., Yi, D., Gao, W., Evans, C.J., Grande, G., Todd, C., Costantini, M., Murtagh, F.E., and Higginson, I.J. (2020). The effectiveness and cost-effectiveness of hospital-based specialist palliative care for adults with advanced illness and their caregivers. *Cochrane Database of Systematic Reviews* (9): CD012780.

56. Oluyase, A.O., Higginson, I.J., Yi, D., Gao, W., Evans, C.J., Grande, G., et al. (2021). Hospital-based specialist palliative care compared with usual care for adults with advanced illness and their caregivers: a systematic review. *Health Services and Delivery Research* 9 (12).

57. DePalma, R., Fortuna, D., Hegarty, S.E., Louis, D.Z., Melotti, R.M., and Moro, M.L. (2018 September). Effectiveness of palliative care services: a population-based study of end-of-life care for cancer patients. *Palliative Medicine* 32 (8): 1344–1352.

58. Kousaie, K. and von Gunten, C.F. (2017). Models of palliative care team composition: nurse practitioneronlyversus interdisciplinary teams that include specialist *physicians. Journal of Palliative Medicine.* Dec 1; 20 (12):1313-.

59. Department of Health. (2000). *The NHS Cancer Plan: A Plan for Investment, a Plan for Reform.* London: Department of Health.

60. Department of Health. (1995). *A Report by the Expert Advisory Group on Cancer to the Chief Medical Officers of England and Wales. A Policy Framework for Commissioning Cancer Services – The Calman–Hine Report.* London: Department of Health.

61. Prades, J., Remue, E., Van Hoof, E., and Borras, J.M. (2015 April 1). Is it worth reorganising cancer services on the basis of multidisciplinary teams (MDTs)? A systematic review of the objectives and organisation of MDTs and their impact on patient outcomes. *Health Policy* 119 (4): 464–474.

62. Neuberger, J., Guthrie, C., and Aaronovitch, D. (2013). *More Care, Less Pathway: A Review of the Liverpool Care Pathway.* London: Department of Health.

63. Seymour, J. and Clark, D. (2018). The liverpool care pathway for the dying patient: a critical analysis of its rise, demise and legacy in England. *Wellcome Open Research* 3: 15.

6

Ethics in Palliative Care Practice

Derek Willis

I cannot teach anybody anything, I can only make them think

Socrates

Introduction

One chapter in a book cannot hope to cover all that ethics is and the application of ethics to the practice of palliative care. All it can try to do is raise some questions, challenge you to think, and point the reader in the direction of sources and opinions that may be helpful or interesting for further reading. I hope that what is in this chapter will challenge you to grapple more with ethics in your own practice and encourage you to explore this world in more depth.

Ethics and ethical discussions have grown in both their volume and complexity over the past 10 years, particularly within health care. To some this branch of philosophy is an interesting subject—but, in their opinion, it is a diversion away from the "proper" science-based aspects of medicine, which have a solid evidence base. When one considers what medicine involves, balancing of harms and benefits, societies and the distribution of resources in those societies, how to conduct useful research, for example, it seems clear that ethics is not an "optional extra," but something that all practitioners should have some knowledge about. In fact, it could be argued, that we are all ethicists and philosophers at heart anyway—we just do not recognise that we do this as part of living generally and health care practice specifically. This is important to state at the outset, as

sometimes it can seem that palliative care has a monopoly on ethical issues. There is no getting away from the fact that, given the type of patients requiring palliative care and stage of illness that they are at, that there are ethical issues that are especially relevant to the specialty. Also, the practice of palliative care recognises that the physical is not the only aspect that is important regarding patient care. Holistic care, which is at the heart of palliative care, would necessarily include respecting that person as a moral agent and allowing them to express their moral choices i.e. treating them ethically and allowing them to be ethical in their behaviour.

Ethics is generally split into three areas of study—applied ethics, moral philosophy, and metaethics. In this chapter we will look at some aspects of the first two areas. I will define the area of metaethics and have provided some further reading at the end of the chapter if the reader is interested. While a fascinating subject, metaethics is beyond the scope of this chapter to cover in detail.

The difference between these branches of ethics can be illustrated by comparing it to a game—such as a game of rugby. Applied ethics are what we define as ethically right with regards to a specific subject, e.g., is euthanasia morally justifiable? To use our rugby analogy,[1] it describes what happened in a particular game of rugby—did the players play by the rules and was it a "good game" of rugby? So, in the clinical example of euthanasia—do I think that this is a particular harm or inherent good such that it should be available for people? Moral philosophy is describing what the rules are that we use to reach decision in applied ethics—in our rugby game example it is what the rules of scrums, conversions, and tries are. To return

---

[1] This helpful analogy is used in the helpful book Metaethics: An Introduction by Andrew Fisher [1]. I am not sure if this is his metaphor/idea, but this is where this author first saw it.

Handbook of Palliative Care, Fourth Edition. Edited by Richard Kitchen, Christina Faull, Sarah Russell and Jo Wilson.
© 2024 John Wiley & Sons Ltd. Published 2024 by John Wiley & Sons Ltd.

to euthanasia I may have used the argument that this is wrong because killing is wrong. By using the argument of the wrongness of killing what branch of moral philosophy or what rule or moral reasoning am I using to back this stance? Metaethics is describing what we are doing when we "do ethics" e.g., do the rules we use mean anything? Do they describe something that is true or is it a social construct? In our rugby example it is pundits talking about rugby as a wider subject—commentating on movements within the game and the politics of it. To summarise

Applied Ethics	Specific game	Specific real world ethical issue
Moral theory	Rules e.g., scrum	Specific Moral philosophy e.g., deontology
Metaethics	Pundit's discussion	What do we mean by ethical rules

What Do We Mean by Ethics?

Ethics as a branch of philosophy is not peculiar to medicine itself. Trying to define exactly what ethics is and what the study of ethics involves can sometimes be quite tricky. However, as is often the case with most philosophy, going back to the Greek fathers of the subject can provide us with guidance. The Greek philosophers (particularly Socrates, Plato, and Aristotle) defined ethics as an attempt to describe what the "good life" was and is. Such a life would encompass not only what a good person is and the good things that such a person would do, but also what their life and character should be. Such a good life would be embodied in a person whose life is enriched and "flourishing." While a good life might be difficult to talk about in a multi-cultural environment with many competing ideas of what the "good" should be—it is not too difficult to see how this can be translated across to the practice of a profession. Bioethics (the ethics of health-care practice) is the discussion and the description of what it means to be a good health-care professional—be this doctor, nurse, physio etc. So, this definition of ethics is not merely describing what good actions are, but rather what an ethical practitioner should be and what ethical practice looks like. Therefore, bioethics encourages us not just to think of single health-care practitioners and what their behaviour and character should be, but also what we expect from groups of practitioners. In other words, what makes a good nurse as well as what makes that individual nurse good.

One of the things that can put people off the subject of ethics are the words and descriptions that are often used.

These can seem confusing and feel arcane—with long discussions over what the words mean in the first place. As has already been argued, we are all, to a lesser or greater degree, amateur ethicists. As people, we frequently have to weigh outcomes, decide what are right and wrong actions in our everyday living. What moral philosophies seek to do is to try and describe how they observe people making moral decisions and attempt to define them. They are stepping back and looking at how we make decisions. They then define what ought to happen as well as what does happen. To use technical language, ethics is both descriptive and prescriptive. A further word that is used when defining how someone should act is that that we are describing what "normative" behaviour should be.

I now turn to definitions of what a few of the words used in bioethics mean and what the various moral philosophers' stances are. I hope this will provide readers with a road map, so as you study and read further you have a clearer understanding of the terminology and technical language. I hope this will help you to decide what your own rule book is and how you decide what is right concerning ethical dilemmas. I will then turn to some of the issues within applied ethics in palliative and end-of-life care that are current at the time of writing and I will use case scenarios to try and illustrate the issues involved.

The Three Main Moral Philosophical Standpoints

Case 1

Imagine that you are shopping with a very close friend. The person that you are with is trying some new clothes on. There is no possible universe in which what they are wearing looks good on them and they are asking you directly whether they look good in it. What do you do?

Before you read on it would be useful for you to write down or think about what your instant response to this imagined situation would be and why you respond in the way you do

It maybe that you feel that to tell a lie to this person would be wrong. After all, your close friend is asking you a direct question. So, in this circumstance it maybe that you think that to obey the rule "Never tell a lie" would be appropriate. The outcomes of what you say (or do) are less important than obeying this rule. The branch of moral philosophy that would agree with this approach is called **deontology**. Those who hold to deontology would say that in every situation that obeying the rule, in this case to not lie, is the right thing to do. The Greek word that deontology is derived from, deon, is often incorrectly translated as rule. It is probably more likely to be the Greek word for duty. It is easy to see how monotheistic religions may find this thinking attractive, obeying divine rules or commandments—but it is also possible to have a humanist or atheist deontological world view. An example of a secular deontologist is Kant. Kant is very definite in his view that the only thing that we can be guaranteed about is that actions are wrong in and of themselves. He claims we can never be sure of outcomes.

It could be however, that you decided that it was better to look at what the outcomes of lying might be. It might be that you felt that telling a lie is not an absolute rule that one must follow—rather it is the outcome of a lie that makes it right or wrong. What one must do, by this viewpoint, is weigh-up the harms and benefits of a particular action, and act such that you maximise the beneficial outcome. Telling a lie to your friend could be outweighed by not hurting their feelings by being honest. So, telling a lie may be the right thing to do. This view of looking at moral situations as being justified by their outcomes is called **consequentialism.** The most commonly held consequentialist standpoint is **utilitarianism.** For the utilitarian, the outcome that one must aim for is the maximisation of happiness. So, a utilitarian would say that the right course of action is one where the maximum amount of happiness is produced, or the least amount of harm.[2]

It might be that you looked at our original case and were more concerned about the kind of character that you are and that it might not be actions that define what is right but the character of the person doing them. So, in case 1, it could be argued that it is wrong to be the kind of person who tells a white lie. In this situation the motivation of lying should be considered in justifying the action. Does a "virtuous" friend tell lies to another friend who has asked a direct question expecting honesty? This rather more nebulous view of looking at morality or defining goodness is often called **virtue theory**. People who agree with virtue theory/virtue ethics would state that people generally are not all that concerned about absolute actions but are more bothered about the motivation, personality, and character of the person that is doing them.

Virtues in these circumstances are not "moral" virtues—but rather the characteristics of a person that makes them function as a good person—back to our Greek idea of the good life. Socrates and Plato talk of the Greek traditional virtues of wisdom, piety, courage, justice, and moderation—although Plato does drop piety as a virtue in his later writings. Aristotle talks about virtue as being a "golden mean" between the excess and deficiency (both described as vices) of a characteristic. So, for example, Aristotle seeks to define what a good soldier is and in doing this identifies the virtue of courage as being integral to this definition. The vice of courage is cowardice—the deficiency of courage—we would not expect a good soldier to be someone who runs away from a fight. The excess of courage is foolhardiness—picking a fight for the sake of it—not knowing when to surrender. Therefore, the golden mean of courage is avoiding cowardice and foolhardiness and finding the mean of these vices. Twentieth century philosophers (e.g. Foot and McIntyre) have rediscovered the idea of virtue and taken it from its Greek origins. They would argue that virtue theory's emphasis on character helps to find a way forward between the impasse of deontologists' and consequentialists' argument regarding rules or outcomes as the right measurement of morality. They are also argued as being particularly relevant to those roles we term professions. Defining a professional role requires us to define the virtues which the role would demand and ensuring that professionals display those characteristics.

Summary

- Deontology thinks that obeying rules and following duties is the correct way to behave ethically
- Utilitarianism states that the "rightness" of actions lies in the amount of happiness they promote
- Virtue theory emphasises the role of character in ethical discourse.

Principlism

Two moral philosophers who wanted to try and create some middle ground between these various ways of moral theory created a system of thought called **principlism**. Beauchamp

---

[2] There are two types of utilitarianism that are put forward—act and rule. Bentham is said to be an act utilitarian—someone who states that all actions must be weighed by the harm and happiness they produce in determining the right thing to do. Mill is described by some as saying certain rules (e.g. justice) are good not because they are rules but because of their outcome. One can therefore follow specific rules and be a utilitarian.

and Childress[3] suggested that there are four principles within medical ethics which are a good starting point for discussing ethical problem relating to a clinical issue. These would not solve moral problems, rather they aim to give a starting point for discussion. These four principles are:

a) **Autonomy:** looking at and respecting a patient's ability to make their own decisions for themselves. It can be taken that autonomy is synonymous with individuality. But this stance ignores the fact that we are a community and you expressing your autonomy may inhibit someone else's autonomy. It can also be argued that groups of people have autonomy e.g. a professional group deciding what the scope of their practice is. Autonomy therefore is often a balancing act between these autonomies rather than automatically following an individuals' choices per se.

b) **Beneficence:** to always act in the patient's interest—to do good for the patient.

c) **Non-Maleficence:** to never do anything that would cause harm to the patient

d) **Justice:** a more communitarian view which is trying to either make sure that everyone has an equal share or where inequality exists to instigate some measure to try and rectify this.

Principlism is probably the most widely used and taught ethical system within Western health care. Sometimes people criticise principlism as trying to provide answers where actually the four principles themselves generate more questions than they answer. I would argue that the main reason for the usefulness of principlism is precisely because of that, that it is an approach that helps to define what the main questions are that need answering in a particular situation.

Summary

- Principlism advocates 4 "pillars"—autonomy, beneficence, non-maleficence and justice, and involves applying these pillars to ethical situations.

Consent and Advance Consent

Much that is written with regards to ethics within palliative care tends to concentrate on "single issue" ethical problems—is euthanasia right or wrong—do we have to be always truthful to patients regarding their diagnosis? It could be argued that there is one overarching or one "meta" question that encompasses all the ethical issues that arise in palliative and end-of-life care. I would contend that much of what is at the heart of such ethical discussions, in palliative care practice relates to consent from patients and the limits and abilities of a patient to make consent for themselves. It is also an issue about which all the various "tribes" of ethics have something to say.[4]

Deontologists would state that respecting the rule/duty of consent is important, but that other rules and duties may "trump" it for that individual patient. The utility of consent and promoting it for the maximum number would be important for a utilitarian. For a virtue theorist consent would be valuable as it is what virtuous health-care practitioners promote and the good character of such a practitioner should be one that informs and promotes choice by the patient.

This is not to state that choice is not a concern of any health-care practitioner outside of palliative care. Health care, in whatever context, has consent at its heart. However, the types of consent that are involved with life limiting illness and end-of-life care have some distinctions when compared with that in general health care. We call on patients to make consent regarding their future self and we are often balancing harms and benefits where cure is not the aim of a procedure. It also calls into question what the limit of consent is specifically how much a patient can ask or require of a health-care practitioner.

Advance Care Planning

Case 2

Jane has a diagnosis of widespread metastatic breast cancer. She is undergoing palliative chemotherapy which she feels is important as she wants as much time as possible with her family. She knows that her time is short—but she is very clear that she does not want to die at home. It is important to her that her children should not associate the family home with her death and that they should not see their mum there. She wants to record this wish so she can be taken from her home, preferably to a hospice when she starts to die.

---

[3] Principlism is described in the Book Principles of Biomedical Ethics [2]. One of the authors is a utilitarian and the other a deontologist, People who advocate using principlism use the fact that two philosophers from different philosophical tribes have agreed on them. They would state that this demonstrates that people with different moral rules can agree on them.

[4] There is much that is useful regrading "general" consent contained in the GMC document [3]. These guidelines recommend partnership between clinician and patient and this is a good model to use irrespective of the context of the consent that is being sought.

Consent in the specific area of future planning—the type of preferences that Jane in our case above wants to record—has become more discussed and advocated during the COVID-19 pandemic. Advance care planning (ACP) is a system which, put simply is asking what patients' future preferences for treatment and care are and documenting them. This can be used if the patient later becomes unable to tell their health-care practitioner what they are—obviously if a patient is able to communicate an ACP is not needed. For the purposes of this section, ACP is trying to define what treatments a patient would like and what treatments they would not want to have in the future. Positive wishes are those I would want given to me (e.g. I would like antibiotics) and negative wishes are those I would not like (e.g. I would not like to go to hospital). Within a legal framework, due to legal precedent, we have more ability to have our negative wishes (not to be treated) respected than to be able to insist on positive treatments (what I would want). This is based on the premise that non-consensual treatment i.e. not having consent is deemed to be assault. Where this assault leads to harm the legal wrong is termed "battery." No such defined legal category exists for not respecting future positive wishes. In other words—just because I want something does not make a practitioner duty bound, by law, to respect this.[5]

One question that is raised is what the "good" of ACP is—given that the circumstances under which an ACP is brought into force are generally when the patient is unaware. It begs the question how a patient can benefit from something that they do not know has been respected. Champions of ACP would give a form of a deontological argument. They would argue that involving the patient in discussions of future care plans are a good in themselves—irrespective of outcome or a patient's knowledge of them being followed. The "good" of ACP for the patient lies in the conversation itself. With regards to respecting future wishes the family and health-care practitioners are the beneficiaries, not the patient. The family and health-care team know they are doing what the patient would ask of them if they were able to do so. Therefore, ACPs are good both in themselves and from their outcomes. That is not to say that ACPs are without their pitfalls.

> **Case 3**
>
> *Samyal is a foundation doctor. He has been told by his consultant that he needs to fill in a Treatment Escalation Plan form for Jack, a patient who has metastatic prostate carcinoma. Samyal has been told that under no circumstances must Jack be admitted into hospital. Jack initially agrees but then asks if it means he can have no antibiotics intravenously for the recurrent chest infections that he gets.*

There is a danger that ACPs can be seen as a way of discriminating against patients with a palliative diagnosis or those who are elderly. One could argue Case 3 is an example of this happening. It is perfectly reasonable for a patient who has a palliative diagnosis to be admitted to hospital as part of their symptom control. Many patients who have a palliative diagnosis have reversible symptomatology e.g. pain from spinal cord compression requiring radiotherapy and admission to hospital in these circumstances could be appropriate. Of course, all this is different if the patient themselves is refusing admission.

One of the other dangers is to imply that patients cannot change their minds after their ACP has been written. This is to argue that an ACP discussion is one event—when as is the case for consent for some medical procedures,[6] it is ongoing discussion that needs revisited and "checked" regularly. It could be argued that to try and make decisions for our future selves is difficult. How do we know what we will really want in circumstances that we cannot imagine or have not experienced yet? However, we ask people to do this all the time. For example, our children make decisions about GCSE's and A levels, decisions based on thoughts regarding future careers which the young person may find that they do not want to do in the future. Consenting to an operation is asking someone to imagine whether the future self who has an operation is better off than the future self who does not want it. In other words, making decisions for our future self is what we do as part of life and part of health care anyway. In that sense there is nothing "special" about ACP. Decision-making is not paralysed because we might be somebody different later in life in

---

[5] For more details on positive and negative freedoms and rights in law look at Isaiah Berlin—political philosopher—who first coined this term. A summary of his argument can be found in Positive and Negative Liberty [4].

[6] The dialogue leading to a decision continued 1—GMC (gmc-uk.org) [3]—useful guidance concerning "ongoing consent".

those, yet unknown, circumstances. Decisions are reached with the knowledge and opinions that we have regarding ourselves as we are at this moment.

Therefore the "good" of an advance care plan is having the discussion with the patient in the first place and seeking their consent. Just as we routinely check that patients still feel the same about receiving treatments such as chemotherapy, so too patients who have an ACP with wishes recorded have not written something in stone. ACP should not be a single episode of consent, but an ongoing discussion about what the patient's priorities are and whether these have changed. People are able and indeed do change their minds about their negative and positive treatment wishes as their circumstances change. I line with any "tool"—there is potential for misuse or misapplication. This is not the fault of the tool per se—more the fault of the practitioner that is using and applying it.

Summary

- ACPs are good to the patient by virtue of having the conversation with the patient in the first place.

- Respecting a patient's preferences are good to the relatives, carers, and health-care professionals of that patient.

- ACPs are an ongoing discussion and should not be used as a "blanket" way of barring certain groups from hospital admission.

Decisions about Cardio-pulmonary Resuscitation

Case 4

Helen has just had a conversation with her patient, Mrs Davies, which did not go well. Mrs Davies has widespread metastatic breast cancer with bone and brain metastases. The medical team feels that when Mrs Davies stops breathing or when her heart stops, trying to resuscitate her would be unsuccessful and just cause her harm. They therefore want to put a do-not-resuscitate order in place. Helen thought that Mrs Davies understood that resuscitating her with her advanced disease would be unsuccessful. When Helen asked Mrs Davies if she wanted to be resuscitated Helen was surprised that her patient said yes. Helen does not know what to do—as she and her medical team are convinced that not resuscitating is not in Mrs Davies' best interest.

GMC guidance describes two types of circumstance where a Do Not Cardio-Pulmonary Resuscitate Order (DNACPR) is written—one where the patient refuses consent for this to happen in the future, the other where the medical team feel that the treatment will not work and would cause significant harm to the patient if conducted.[7] In this sense there is nothing "special" about such orders. All treatments involve patients making decisions of whether they consent to them and for a medical team weighing harms and benefits of treatments. It is important to note that DNACPR orders only come into play when the patient dies. There is therefore nothing active that the medical team has done to bring about the death of the patient—by not resuscitating they are either respecting a patients' wishes or are not attempting a treatment which will be unsuccessful or both. Despite there being much helpful guidance on how to conduct DNACPR discussions—situations like Case 4 can often arise.[8] The medical teams do not want to provide a treatment which the patient wants. Some of the reasons that this type of impasse can arise are:

a) **A patient has an unrealistic expectation of the success of CPR**. In circumstances where a patient has a sudden arrest with no other underlying disease CPR has a high success rate. The type of patients seen in palliative care, where DNACPR orders are written, have advanced disease and a poor prognosis. Resuscitation in these circumstances is unlikely to be successful. It is often the case that patients feel that CPR is equally successful in all circumstances. This lack of knowledge may be why there was a difference in attitude between Mrs Davies and Helen.

b) **The way the question is asked gives a false expectation of success.** If a patient is asked if they would like to be resuscitated it may sound as if the medical team are asking for withdrawal of a treatment that may work. If the question is more accurate and asks if the patient wants to be spared having either an unsuccessful treatment, a treatment that may only cause them harm or if they want to be kept at home, then a different response is often given by the patient. The health-care team need to be clear that they are describing what the benefits of treatment are. In end-of-life care with patients who have advanced disease there are arguably no benefits. Patients are not often clear about this because of the form of words that health-care practitioners use to inform them.

---

[7] GMC guidance [5].

[8] The National Resuscitation Council provide a lot of helpful guidance specifically in filling in their recommended RESPECT form but also in having DNACPR discussions more widely [6].

c) **The conversation is had as a consent discussion rather than as an information giving discussion**. Some of this confusion of the type of "informing" conversation that is required comes from a misunderstanding of the legal case known as the Tracey judgement.[9] The family of Mrs Tracey brought a case against a Cambridge hospital as the family felt that the medical team should have discussed the DNACPR order they put on their mother, who was suffering from both end stage lung cancer and the effects of a road traffic accident. The judgement found that the ITU team were not wrong to have made a do not resuscitate order on the lady, Mrs Tracey; they were wrong not to have told her. This was not a conversation asking for the patient's consent—rather a discussion telling her that this decision was being reached. Distress of the patient was not enough to not discuss with her as having difficult/distressing conversations are part of health-care practice. Patients do have the right to seek a second opinion and the decision should be reached by a Multi-Disciplinary Team. If there is still disagreement, there is helpful advice provided further by the GMC in the "treatment at the end-of-life booklet" paragraph 47–49 [5].

Summary

- CPR in patients with advance disease in the palliative/end-of-life stage of their disease is mostly unsuccessful.
- A DNACPR discussion should be had with the patient if it would not cause them harm.
- DNACPR is a medical decision—but this should be made by an MDT and a patient can have access to a second opinion.

Assisted Dying, Suicide, and Euthanasia

In the previous parts of the chapter, it has been presumed that consent of a patient is an inherent good. Assisted dying or assisted suicide (AS) directly pose two ethical questions which challenge this stance on consent: whether patients can validly consent to something that is meant to harm them and whether there is a limit to what a patient can ask of a health-care professional.

Case 5

Dr Todd is a GP who seeing her last patient of the day. John has motor neurone disease and seemed to be doing well. John seems in a lot of distress at this consultation and Dr Todd wants to know why this is so. John tells her that his finding life a burden, that he feels he is causing distress to his family and he wants to go to Dignitas in Switzerland, an organisation which provides assisted dying to certain patients. John says that his computer has broken down and wants Dr Todd to look up the details on her computer. Dr Todd is concerned—if she does this could this be viewed as assisting John's suicide?

The moral philosopher Mill in his book *On Liberty* which informs the ethical foundation of a lot of democratic Western political theory and thought, insists that governments cannot intervene in anything that a person validly consents to[10]—even if the person is consenting to something that harms him or her. Some of this argument contributed to a change in legal and societal attitude towards harm of suicide. Suicide, which previously was classed as illegal is now decriminalised in the UK and many countries in the world—hence people are no longer prosecuted for trying to commit suicide. Assisting someone to commit suicide is still illegal and it is this part of the law that proponents of assisted dying/suicide seek to get changed. But why assisted suicide and not looking to legalise euthanasia itself?

Some would argue that there is a distinction between assisting and doing. Doing would be that we "actively" cause the person's death while assisting is helping create the circumstances under which someone else can do it themselves. So, "doing" would be me pushing you off a cliff, "assisting" would be me driving you up to a cliff from which you jump yourself. Or to use the clinical situation directly, assisting would be me driving you to Dignitas in Switzerland and doing would be me actively injecting you with a lethal injection of drug intended to end someone's life.[11]

The UK and many other countries draw a legal line regarding suicide in that it is illegal for someone else to "assist" a person to kill themselves. For example, if Dr Todd looks up the website of Dignitas for John this could be regarded by English law as assisting. This is particularly

---

[9]Legal reference: Tracey v Cambridge Uni Hospital NHS Foundation Trust & Ors [2014] EWCA Civ 822 [7].

[10] The only purpose for which power can be rightfully exercised over any member of a civilised community, against his will, is to prevent harm to others. His own good, either physical or moral, is not a sufficient warrant. He cannot rightfully be compelled to do or forbear because it will be better for him to do so, because it will make him happier, because, in the opinions of others, to do so would be wise, or even right JS Mill [8].

[11] APM Physician Assisted Dying Web Materials—APM Online. Free to non-members, a useful resource with multiple articles discussing subject of assisted suicide [9].

true for health-care practitioners—relatives who assist are judged on a case-by-case basis.

This is not to say that there are no critics of the claimed ethical difference between assisting and doing. Some of these arguments are similar in nature to the alleged distinction between withdrawing and withholding. It is perceived that there is a difference between actively withdrawing treatment and passively withholding. However, in both situations an active decision is reached to do, or not do an action—therefore many contend there is no moral difference between the two. Some would say that this is similar to assisted dying and euthanasia—in both an active decision is involved in doing an action—the type of action is, it is argued by some, irrelevant. Also, in both assisted dying and euthanasia, the intention is to end the patient's life—i.e. the outcome is the same and another person is still involved in bringing this about. Those who argue this claim there is therefore no moral difference between assisted dying and euthanasia.

The binary distinction between assisting and doing could also be accused of falling apart when it is a health-care professional who is involved, and it becomes a medically assisted suicide. If I am providing you with a lethal cocktail of medication, which you drink, is there still a definitive distinction of doing vs assisting? Proponents would still say "yes" and that there is a definite moral distinction between medical assisted suicide and euthanasia. Others would counter this argument by pointing out that if a clinician has prescribed something, then they must have some responsibility for the outcomes. For instance, if a patient takes an antibiotic, they are known to be allergic to, that I have prescribed I would still have responsibility for the allergic reaction even though it is the patient who took the medication.

Some readers of this chapter may already be in a country where medically assisted suicide is legal and that they are required to prescribe and administer lethal medications. This circumstance poses the question of whether health=care professionals are permitted to withdraw consent for procedures where there may be moral difficulties for them personally in taking part in them. Conscientious objection by health-care professionals is accepted for interventions such as termination of pregnancy, and it is argued could be extended to include involvement in assisted suicide. Recent case law in the UK has narrowed the scope of what such objection might be, objection cannot be just supporting terminations and providing the circumstances

under which it can occur—it can only apply to the actual act of doing a termination. One case relates to midwives who were responsible for running a ward where terminations occurred[12] and another to a medical secretary who refused to type a referral letter for a termination.[13] It has now been clarified that the only thing that a health-care practitioner can object to is being actively involved in a procedure. As I have argued, the distinction between assisted suicide and euthanasia rests on claiming that has no "doing." If this is the case, it can be argued that there is nothing to object to in assisted suicide[14] and therefore conscientious objection cannot be used by health-care practitioners with regards to assisted suicide.

The beginning of the chapter looked at principlism and specifically the duty of health-care professional to not cause harm to their patients. To assist in ending someone's life, to many in the specialty feel like a line that cannot be crossed. It is an interesting conundrum for health-care professionals who are both members of a society and members of a professional body. It may be that as member of society they feel that assisted suicide should be legal—but do not feel that their profession should administer it. Some may feel that it is wrong for society and profession—others right in both areas. The fact that professionals have foot in two camps often makes their response more complex.

Summary

- The debate around assisted suicide will continue.
- The important factors while reading around this subject are to clarify what the words used mean i.e., what do assisted dying and euthanasia involve and are they distinct.
- Also, each of us need to decide what questions and answers go to make up our response to the debate? For example, should health-care professionals ever be involved in a procedure meant to harm a patient, how much harm can a patient consent to?

Conclusion

I hope that this brief journey through some of the principles of moral philosophy and their application in case scenarios has pointed you in the "right" direction to help you

---

[12] Legal reference: Doogan & Anor v NHS Greater Glasgow & Clyde Health Board [2013] ScotCS CSIH 36 [10].

[13] Legal reference: Janaway v Salford Health Authority (1989) AC 537 [11].

[14] For a fuller discussion of this argument look at the paper: Willis D and George R Conscientious Objection and Physician Assisted Suicide [12].

understand more about this area and as the quote at the beginning of the chapter stated—made you think. Socrates, one of the founding fathers of philosophy, felt that writing anything down was counterproductive. For him to discover what the good life involved, was an active process of going to the marketplace and talking and asking questions to discover the answer to this. Ethics was, and is, a practical, doing subject as well as a cerebral exercise. I hope that as practitioners who serve patients who pose complex ethical dilemmas for us, we continue to discuss and hammer out what a "good" palliative care practitioner should be.

Acknowledgements

This chapter is dedicated to the memory of the Rev Margaret Woodlock-Smith—without whom there would have been no Prof Willis. With thanks to Prof Rob George for helpful comments on an early draft of the chapter.

References

1. Fisher, A. (2011). *Metaethics: An Introduction*. Routledge.
2. Beauchamp, T.L. and Childress, J.F. (1994). *Principles of Biomedical Ethics*, 4e. Oxford University Press.
3. General Medical Council. Decision making and consent—the dialogue leading to a decision continued. https://www.gmc-uk.org/ethical-guidance/ethical-guidance-for-doctors/decision-making-and-consent/the-dialogue-leading-to-a-decision-continued-1 (accessed 14 January 2021).
4. Stanford Encyclopedia of Philosophy. Positive and negative liberty. https://plato.stanford.edu/entries/liberty-positive-negative (accessed 14 January 2021).
5. General Medical Council. Treatment and care towards the end-of-life. https://www.gmc-uk.org/-/media/documents/treatment-and-care-towards-the-end-of-life—english-1015_pdf-48902105.pdf (accessed 21 January 2021).
6. Resuscitation Council UK. ReSPECT Resources. https://www.resus.org.uk/respect/respect-resources (accessed 14 January 2021).
7. Tracey v Cambridge Uni Hospital NHS Foundation Trust & Ors. (2014). EWCA Civ 822.
8. Mill, J.S. (1982). *On Liberty*. Penguin Classics.
9. Association for Palliative Medicine. APM physician assisted dying web materials. https://apmonline.org/news-events/apm-physician-assisted-dying-web-materials (accessed 21 January 2021).
10. Doogan & Anor v NHS Greater Glasgow & Clyde Health Board. (2013). ScotCS CSIH 36.
11. Janaway v Salford Health Authority. (1989). AC 537.
12. Willis, D. and George, R. (2018). Conscientious objection and physician assisted suicide: a viable option in the UK? *BMJ Support Palliat Care* 9 (4): 464–467.

Useful Sources

General Medical Council—Ethical guidance for doctors—GMC (gmc-uk.org)

Nursing Council—The Code: Professional standards of practice and behaviour for nurses, midwives and nursing associates (nmc.org.uk).

Philosophy bites http://philosophybites.com—a useful online collection of interviews with philosophers, free to access and a lot of ethical debate and moral philosophy covered in the site.

Stanford Encyclopaedia of Philosophy a useful online resource peer reviewed, regularly updated and thorough articles.

Useful texts

Sandel M *Justice What's the Right Thing to Do?* Penguin Books 2008.

Sandel is a political philosopher so this is not a bioethics book. However, he has the best and clearest description of Kant I have found and is very readable. There is a lot of moral philosophy, but little medical application in it.

Glover J *'Causing Death and Saving Lives'* Penguin Books 1990.

I do not agree with a lot of his conclusions—but well written and well argued with regards to assisting suicide, euthanasia, and killing.

JS Mill *Utilitarianism* Oxford University Press.

A collection of his original articles (he published these in a newspaper as separate articles).

Crisp R *Routledge Philosophy Guide to Mill on Utilitarianism* 1997.

Guide to Mill—advanced for this chapter but interestingly written.

Foot P *Natural Goodness* Clarenden Press 2003.

Modern take on virtue theory—Foot is the easiest to read of the modern virtue theorists.

Plato *The Republic* Penguin Classics.

Easier to read then Aristotle—effectively a play script. Contains the seeds of the ideas of virtue theory.

Aristotle *Nicomachean Ethics* Oxfords Worlds Classics.

Listed for completeness—hard to read but worth trying!

Conversations and Communication

Sarah Russell

To listen and to see me as a person, not just a name on a piece of paper

[1, p. 159]

Introduction

Conversations matter in palliative and end-of-life care. From the diagnosis of a life-limiting illness to the recognition that death is approaching, people face a myriad of discussions with health and social care providers, families, and friends. Some conversations are weighing up the benefits, risks, and consequences of investigations and treatment; others concerned with withdrawing and withholding treatment; or about preferred place of care when they are dying. Conversations can include communicating uncertainty as well as recognising physical deterioration and functional decline. Some discussions revolve around the inevitability of death and what a persons' future end-of-life choices and preferences are (advance care planning). Discussions may take place with families when the person is too unwell to speak, and/or when death is approaching. Conversations can be an expression (a safe space to say or hear unsafe things) of the emotional, psychological, social, and spiritual impact of living with the knowledge of certain death at an uncertain time in the future.

This chapter explores the principles, benefits, and challenges of good communication in palliative and end-of-life care. The aim is not to provide readers with a "one size fits all" model for conversations, but rather why good communication matters and examples of useful resources and models.

Why Communicate Well?

Communicating well is an essential part of palliative, end-of-life and patient-centred care [2]. While people may feel uncomfortable talking about their end-of-life wishes, not talking about them denies them the opportunity to fully participate in discussions and decisions about their current and future care [3]. Each person should be seen as an individual (Figure 1). People want the opportunity to engage in conversations about their future death and the care that they would want [4].

Communicating well has benefits [6], and effective communication is one of the conditions for a good death [7]. Good communication engenders meaningful and trusting relationships between healthcare professionals and patients, as well as increasing patient satisfaction, understanding, adherence, recall, and health outcomes [2, 8, 9]. Effective communication facilitates accurate identification of problems resulting in better symptom control, treatment assessment, physical, functional, psychological wellbeing, and functioning [6, 9]. Furthermore, advance care planning is more effective with accompanying communication skills and trust building processes [10]. Honest, clear sensitive conversations do not necessarily remove hope or increase distress [10], as good communication can improve the ability

> I and the people important to me, have opportunities to have honest, informed, and timely conversations and to know that I might die soon. I am asked what matters most to me. Those who care for me know that and work with me to do what's possible [5, p. 18]

Figure 1 Ambition one: each person is seen as an individual.

Handbook of Palliative Care, Fourth Edition. Edited by Richard Kitchen, Christina Faull, Sarah Russell and Jo Wilson.
© 2024 John Wiley & Sons Ltd. Published 2024 by John Wiley & Sons Ltd.

to cope with prognosis, prepare and plan for death [1, 11]. Disclosure of psychological concerns is likely to be improved with good communication resulting in better emotional health, resolution of symptoms and pain control, and a beneficial effect on patient outcomes and satisfaction [12].

There is a need to improve communication [13], with persistent evidence that poor communication is a regular source of patient, family, and clinicians' dissatisfaction about end-of-life care, particularly in hospitals [14, 15]. Poor communication leads to a failure from health-care practitioners to recognise or agree to patients' concerns, underrate distress, miss opportunities to improve patient self-management, increase psychological morbidity, and underestimate information needs [8]. Problematic communication can contribute to increased health-care professional stress, high malpractice claims, emotional burn out, low personal accomplishment, lack of job satisfaction and high psychological morbidity [16].

Blocks and Barriers to Communication

Good communication is hampered by blocks and barriers to discussions. Blocks to communication include verbal and non-verbal behaviours that inhibit conversations. Barriers to communication can include individual and organisational reasons why practitioners do not communicate well (Figure 2). Verbal communication is concerned with speech units and listening strategies [17]. Non-verbal communication (NVC) is a communication behaviour without linguistic content [18]. NVC is present even in silence, can be responsible for communicating attitudes and emotions [18], reinforce or contradict verbal comments altering the meaning of a message actions and outcomes [19]. NVC includes kinesics (gestures, facial expressions, and gaze patterns), proxemics (body posture, position, territoriality, personal space), and touch [20].

Principles and Benefits of Good Communication

Considering how we carry out conversations, and what those discussions contain, enables better person centred and rewarding discussions for patients, families, and clinicians. While there is multiplicity of communication definitions and inconsistency as to what exactly constitutes a communication skill [10], communication can be described as the

> efficient transmission of information, including verbal communication, such as speech units and listening strategies, and non-verbal communication, such as gestures and expressions, eye contact and body language. [17, p. 1]

However, communication is more than just the transmission of information. Back [9] points out that palliative care communication is

> a two-way, relational process that is influenced by context, culture, words, and gestures, and it is one of the most important ways that clinicians influence the quality of medical care that patients and their families receive. [9, p. 866]

Blocking Behaviours (Verbal and non-verbal behaviours)	
Clinician-led conversations rather than patient led, lack of eye contact, unfriendly or inappropriate body language, missing or avoiding cues in conversations, interruptions and interrupting, noise, not considering the cultural, language, literacy, or communication needs of the person, lack of pauses or silences, premature or false reassurance. Jollying along, inappropriate use of humour, not attending to the way a person expresses themselves.	Multiple questions, closed questions, leading questions, focussing on only one aspect of the conversation (e.g. just physical), switching topic, focus, or person. Use of jargon, not paying attention to the emotional, psychological, or spiritual aspects, not exploring the person's goals, concerns, hopes, fears, and expectations. Appearing judgemental, defensive, unconcerned. Not agreeing the focus of the conversation and summarising at the end.
Barriers to Communication (Individual, Organisational, Societal)	
• Lack of skills, competence, knowledge, confidence in communication skills • Fear of being blamed, taking away hope or eliciting a reaction that one is not sure how to respond to, not knowing what to say. • Expressing own emotions, thoughts, and awareness of death • The work environment not enabling conversations (e.g. privacy, noise, capacity, and time challenges)	

Figure 2 Examples of blocks and barriers to communication [1, 21–23].

Active listening or giving the person your full attention and listening empathically can provide an avenue for expression and reassurance [24]. The benefits of facilitative behaviours, attitudes, and traits of; empathy, genuineness, respect, unconditional positive regard, and reflexivity regularly feature in the communication skills research literature [10]. Sensitive truth telling, balancing hope and honesty is also present [25]. Clinicians are valued who listen, show empathy and honesty, encourage questions, clarify, and negotiate individual's information needs and level of understanding, as well as take a personalised approach to a persons' individual information preferences and differences in reactions to prognostic communication [25, 26]. Kathryn Mannix [27] reminds of the importance of the relevance of getting

> alongside another person and gain their confidence and trust, to begin the process of discovering their current position. [27, p. 4]

Furthermore, while the terms compassion, sympathy, and empathy are often used interchangeably in clinical practice, there are reminders to consider each construct separately [28] (Figure 3).

Communication Skills Training and Education

An individual's communication skills are not innate or fixed characteristics [29, 30], and good interpersonal skills alone are not a substitute for strong health-care communication [29, 30]. Most approaches to teaching communication in health care incorporate cognitive, affective, and behavioural components [6], and ongoing communication skills training (CST) plus reflection is necessary to transfer (and sustain) skills in practice [31, 32]. CST should be based upon sound educational principles including reflective practice with the opportunity to practice skills, directly observe patient encounters, use of experiential, interactive learning, and role-play scenarios which reflect the specific nature of the actual real-life practice interactions [29–31].

There are a wide variety of CST models and approaches. These range from verbal or written feedback, video, or audio recordings of simulated or real encounters, observation of practice, small group or one to one learning as well as being incorporated into degree or diploma studies, short sessions under one hour, a few hours, one, two, three, five-day workshops, and the use of actors as simulated patients [6, 29, 30]. CST can also be discipline or role specific, multi-disciplinary, have a focus on E-learning or blended learning (face-to-face training and online education) [6]. CST should foster:

> self-awareness and situational awareness related to emotions, attitudes, and underlying beliefs that may impact communication, as well as awareness of implicit biases that may affect decision making. [29, p. 42]

There is evidence that CST helps practitioners to be less likely to give facts only without individualising their responses to the patient's emotions or offering support [6]. However, the evidence remains unclear if the effects of CST are sustained over time, if consolidation sessions are necessary, which types of CST programmes are most likely to work and the benefits of CST on practitioner burn out [6]. Furthermore, patients and families are infrequently involved in developing or evaluating training programmes [31] and this should be addressed in the design and evaluation of CST programmes.

Facilitative Communication Skills

Facilitative communication skills are conversation catalysts with a variety of specific behaviours and characteristics [1]. They include conveying interest in the conversation and person through verbal and nonverbal behaviours e.g., physical position, facial expression, not being distracted. Also relevant is clarifying the purpose of the conversation e.g., *what shall we start with … today we are … what do you want to discuss?* Consider the tone, speed, volume, and pitch of your voice (paralanguage), language (English as first language or not as well as literacy), cultural norms for

---

Sympathy: an unwanted, pity-based response to a distressing situation, characterized by a lack of understanding and self-preservation of the observer.

Empathy: an affective response that acknowledges and attempts to understand individual's suffering through emotional resonance.

Compassion: enhances the key facets of empathy while adding distinct features of being motivated by love, the altruistic role of the responder, action, and small, supererogatory acts of kindness.

Figure 3 The constructs of sympathy, empathy, and compassion [28, p. 437].

that person or the cultural background they belong to as well as individual sensory needs (e.g., sight, hearing, speech, touch). Checking joint understanding of the purpose or goal of the conversation is important, as are open questions, inviting the person to express their concerns, questions, or thoughts e.g., *how are you today?*. Questions that focus on specific aspects e.g., *can you tell me what has been happening in the last few ...* or *you mentioned earlier about ... can you tell me more?* help to facilitate conversations.

Other characteristics include a psychological focus on questions rather than just physical emphasis e.g. *You mentioned ....,* as well as empathic statements and prompts to encourage further expressions or questions e.g., *What I'm hearing is ... have I got that right?,* nods, *umms, say more and go on.* Screening questions enable exploration to ensure all concerns have been mentioned e.g., *is there something else/anything else that we should discuss ... what have we not talked about?* Prioritising questions help maintain a focus on the individual e.g., *what is the most important thing for you right now?* or *you mentioned several things ... what would be most helpful to start with?* Summarising the discussion is useful to conclude and signpost to agreed next steps.

The use of pauses and silence enable, encourage, and facilitate the person to say more, clarify their thoughts or express their feelings. Silence is an underused skill despite there being evidence that connectional silences (pauses in conversations of two seconds or more) are associated with improved decision-making and patients' quality of life [33]. Basset et al [34] reminds that silence is an element of care fostering a connection that goes beyond the power of words. Silence has the potential to support therapeutic communication by facilitating listening, bearing witness, conveying empathy, and providing a consoling presence [34]. Moreover, silence can indicate a mental shift from doing something for the patient to a focus on being with [35]. Silence is a purposeful intervention rather than simply an absence of speech [34].

Specific Considerations

Not everyone is likely to receive good care because of diagnosis, age, ethnic background, sexual orientation, gender identity, disability, or social circumstances [13]. It is not possible to list all the considerations for every scenario or group of people, however it is relevant to highlight a few ones. The core principles of facilitative communication remain.

Hearing and Sight Loss

Few studies have examined hearing and sight loss in palliative and end-of-life care with some evidence that people with sensory loss report less satisfaction with communication and symptom control [36]. Reducing background noise, assessing the environment, increasing visual signage, considering sign language, visual/audio aids and providing sensory competence education to staff about the communication needs of patients or family members with sensory loss is important [36, 37].

Dementia

For people living with dementia, the

> ability to communicate with others (expressive aphasia) and to receive the communication of others (receptive aphasia) becomes increasingly difficult as the condition progresses. [38, p. 6]

Considerations of loss of capacity to make decisions in the future, imagine and envisage a future self can be problematic [38, 39]. Decision-making may be left to families and practitioners when the person does not have capacity to decide for themselves [38–40]. A recent applied model for making decisions towards the end-of-life [40] shows promise providing a framework for conversations and supporting decisions by carers. Figure 4 illustrates some conversation considerations for people living and dying with dementia.

Intellectual Disability

Chapter 19 (Palliative Care for People Living with Mental Illness and People with Intellectual Disabilities) covers in detail this specific consideration. Noorlandt et al. [42] however, point out that people with intellectual disabilities are often not actively involved in end-of-life decision-making processes due to communication challenges, assumptions of lack of capacity, and that they will not be able to carry out difficult conversations. People with severe or profound disability are also more likely to need support in conversations including different types of written material or ways to facilitate communication. A recent shared decision-making conversation aid developed through a Delphi panel shows promise with four themes, who are you, illness/end-of-life, making choices, and application [42].

Piers et al. [41]	Russell [23]	Harrison-Denning[38, 39]
Start early in the disease	Be prepared for parallel advance care planning – or when different members of the family or team are at different stages of their thinking and actions	It may take longer to process what you are saying – give the person sufficient time to respond
Evaluate mental capacity including fluctuating capacity	Be person-centred. How does the person like to make decisions, who else might need to be involved?	
Adjust communication style and content to the persons own level and rhythm	Consider the physical environment: noise, distractions, and a temperature that is too high or too low can be confusing	Ensure the space chosen to have the conversation is quiet and calm
		Be aware and maximise upon your non-verbal communication. Use active listening
		Focus on one question at a time
	When is the best time of day to carry out conversations: when is the person most alert and comfortable? Fatigue or hunger may inhibit conversations	Face the person directly and make good eye contact, ensure you give every opportunity to understand you are focussed on them
	Do not see every conversation as a decision and document-making one. Sometimes, the conversation is a contemplative one – a time for the person to share what matters to them, what is bothering them or what they want to do next	Use short, clear sentences that are free of clinical jargon. Use language and words that are familiar to them
Cover values, fears, and what is important to the person, as well as specific decisions	Encourage the person to talk with their family or friends; there may be important things they want to say to each other	Find out what their values and preferences are, what is important to them, their history, likes, strengths, beliefs etc.
Consider the role and importance of those close to the person with dementia including surrogate decision maker		They may or may not wish their family carer/member to be present; ensure you ask
When it is difficult or no longer possible to communicate verbally, keep a connection to the person	Be prepared for many conversations. This may be due to short-term memory loss, fatigue, or the desire of the person to talk about something that matters or worries them. See multiple conversations as an opportunity to connect and engage	Use other ways to communicate if helpful, written word, pictures etc.
Be attentive to their emotions, non-verbal communication and their behaviour	Be opportunistic: sometimes fundamental care can trigger conversations, for example reminiscence activities may be the catalyst for someone to remember a funeral in the past and think about their own, similarly helping someone bath and dress can make them realise their increased dependency on you and what that means for them	
	Do not be afraid of emotions such as tears or anger, see it as providing them with a safe space to express themselves	
The values, wishes, or care goals of the person need to be documented, including information transfer to other teams and services	When appropriate, offer to help document decisions and involve and inform others when relevant, such as the multi professional health and social care team. Make sure you know what documentation you use in your organisation and that the documents that have been produced make sense. Have a system to inquire again about a person's wishes and decisions to check they are still what they want	
End-of-life decision-making should be implemented, including the use of the best interests process, and consultation with the people close to the person as well as health-care practitioners needs to take place		

Figure 4 Recommendations for conversations for people living with dementia.

Culture, Ethnicity, and Language

Consideration must be given to the different cultural, ethnic, and linguistic needs of people as well as practitioners confidence, knowledge, and skills in providing culturally sensitive end-of-life care for ethnic minority patients [43]. This can include accommodating different beliefs about the sanctity of life, death, and dying, considering individual autonomy and family dynamics, language difficulties, formal or family interpreters, understanding spiritual and religious practices, the challenge of some groups accessing the health system and the impact of migration experiences [43, 44].

The use of formal interpreters is recommended. A 2016 systematic review regarding black and minority ethnic groups report that family members (including children) were often used as interpreters to deliver information about prognosis, diagnosis, and assess symptom management [45]. When professional interpreters were not used, there was inadequate understanding about diagnosis and prognosis during goals of care conversations, and patients had worse symptom management at the end-of-life, including pain and anxiety [45].

The 2018 report, *Care committed to me. Delivering high quality, personalised palliative and end-of-life care for Gypsies & Travellers, LGBT people and people experiencing homelessness* [46] provides recommendations to improve personalised end-of-life care for Gypsies and Travellers, LGBT people and people experiencing homelessness. There are several recommendations relevant to how and what conversations may contain or how they are experienced (Figure 5).

Virtual Communication

Prior to the COVID-19 pandemic, telemedicine (e.g., video and telephone consultations) was still emerging as part of routine palliative and end-of-life care [49], with arguments that palliative care was "too high-touch to be delivered via telehealth" [50, p. 17]. The pandemic identified the necessity and potential of virtual consultations, assessments, and conversations. There are challenges e.g. accessibility and preference disparities, logistical and technological barriers, as well as cultural and personal preferences. However, telemedicine enabled the reduction of exposure risk to vulnerable patients, their families and the

Gypsies, Roma, and Travellers (GRT)	• Hospitals and hospices generally rely on written distribution of information. This shows a presumption about literacy levels. • Positive and clear communication (without the use of jargon, which can be intimidating) would change the experience of hospital/end-of-life care. • Families may be wary of disclosing their Gypsy/Traveller identity for fear of discrimination, but this means that staff might not be aware that additional support might be required (e.g., access to literature). • End-of-life rituals are very important to Gypsy and Traveller communities. Funeral poverty can also be an issue. • There is cultural resistance to discussing end-of-life care or long-term illness in general. • A negative experience with a hospice/hospital/service will be shared among the communities. • Consider "The care I provide" and "The care I commission."
Homelessness	• In view of uncertainty and complexity, shift the focus from trying to identify people at the end-of-life and make the point at which someone's health is a cause for concern the trigger for action [47]. • Parallel planning–incorporating uncertainty and promoting well-being, dignity, and choice. • The importance of training hostel staff on communications skills and end-of-life care conversations. • Hostel staff upskilling palliative care staff and supporting people experiencing homelessness. • Consider "The care I provide" and "The care I commission."
Lesbian, gay, bisexual, transgender (or trans), queer people (LGBTQ)	• Consciously engage and be visible in LGBTQ inclusive practice and language, education, policy, and practice development and delivery. • Make existing services accessible and inclusive. • Consider "The care I provide" and "The care I commission." • It is highly recommended to read *Recommendations to reduce inequalities for LGBT people facing advanced illness* [48]

Figure 5 Communication considerations. Adapted from Tackling Inequalities in End-of-Life Care for Minority Groups VCSE Health and Wellbeing Alliance Project Group 2018 [46]

workforce as well as offering an effective, accessible, acceptable, and cost-effective alternative to face-to-face contacts [51, 52]. Helpful guides and resources being produced include:

Academic Health Science Network www.ahsnnetwork.com/helping-break-unwelcome-news A variety of resources.

Real Talk Training http://www.realtalktraining.co.uk

Giving news of a death to a loved one: Telephone call checklist for health-care staff

Evidence based advice for difficult conversations

Prompt list for phone and in-person urgent conversations about withdrawing or withholding life-sustaining treatments in UK critical care

A-Z index of digital flashcards covering a wide range of topics www.cardmedic.com/flashcards

Royal College of Nursing Having courageous conversations by telephone or video during the COVID-19 pandemic www.rcn.org.uk

Stanford Medicine, Serious Illness Programme A Resource for Conducting Conversations Virtually http://med.stanford.edu/advancecareplanning

The University of Edinburgh Supportive and Palliative Care Indicators Tool (SPICT): www.spict.org.uk Talking with people over the phone.

University of Oxford, Department of Psychiatry Helpful resources including animation and guide on informing of a death over the phone. www.psych.ox.ac.uk/research/covid_comms_support

Communication Resources

Self-awareness and understanding of one's own communication skills enhance the confidence and competence of clinicians in discussions. There are a variety of communication models and resources available drawn from expert opinion, best practice, or the evidence base [32]. While "one size does not fit all," and skills used should be individualised to each person and conversation, there is a common emphasis on a person-centred approach which explores their perspective, conveys visible empathy, in both information giving and the hearing of their story, as well as summarizes and plans at the end of the conversation [32]. These resources can be used to help identity the need for conversations or provide a guide for discussions (Figure 6).

Conversation Trigger Cards and Tools

There are online and/or physical tools to trigger discussions e.g., conversation cards, games, and website guides (Figure 7), with emerging evidence that they do have a place in advance care planning and end-of-life conversations [66]. The Dying Matters website https://www.hospiceuk.org/our-campaigns/dying-matters hosted by Hospice UK also has a number of useful resources as well as local, regional, national, or international websites.

AFIRM is an acronym which provides professional carers with a framework to guide informal conversations and uses these as opportunities to pick up on any underlying apprehensions or queries the person with dementia (and/or their family member) may have. Acknowledge the person's concern or questions. Find out what the person knows about the condition. Immediate concern(s) addressed by providing adequate information within the scope of your work. Respond to subsequent questions by providing accurate information within the scope of your work. Meeting suggested to discuss their concerns with significant people [38, 39].	**AMBER care bundle** https://www.guysandstthomas.nhs.uk/our-services/palliative-care A hospital tool for managing uncertain recovery over the next two months. It includes the development and documentation of a medical plan, consideration of outcomes, resuscitation and escalation status and daily plan revisiting. Assessment Management Best practice Engagement Recovery uncertain The emphasis on "clinical uncertainty" prompts health-care professional awareness of often-overlooked patients [57]. However, to be successfully normalised in clinical practice, the wider context in which AMBER operates should be considered [58].

Figure 6 Communication resources examples.

Calgary-Cambridge [53]

A generic model for structuring a consultation.

Initiating the session: establish initial rapport; identify reason for consultation with open questions; listen without interrupting; confirm and screen for further problems; negotiate agenda.

Gathering information: explore patient's problems; open to closed questions; listen attentively; facilitate patient responses; pick up cues; clarify unclear statements; summarize periodically; use clear questions; establish sequence of events; explore patient's ideas, concerns, expectations, and feelings.

Providing structure: summarize appropriately, signpost, use logical sequence, keep to time.

Building a relationship: appropriate non-verbal behaviour; develop rapport, use empathy, provide support; involve patient.

Explanation and planning: correct amount and type of information; aid recall and understanding; shared understanding; shared decision-making.

Closing and planning: forward planning; summary; final check.

PREPARED

Prepare for the discussion

Relate to the person

Elicit patient and caregiver preference

Provide information

Acknowledge emotions and concerns

Realistic hope

Encourage questions

Document

There is evidence that this model is helpful in communication skills training [54].

Listen [27]

Opening the box

Towards change

Building bridges

Towards connection

REAL Talk

https://www.realtalktraining.co.uk

Resources supporting experiential and reflective learning, focused on a range of communication problems and practices, for trainees from a wide range of backgrounds [30].

Psychosocial Assessment and Communication Evaluation (PACE)

An interventional tool that has the potential to improve communication, information consistency, and family perceptions of symptom control [59]. Commenced within 24 hours of admission and continued use until discharge. A documented script includes:

- Family details including key relationships
- Social details
- Patient Preferences
- Communication and information
- Any other concerns/issues
- Communication update to family

Five questions [60]

1. What is your understanding of your current health or condition?
2. If your current condition worsens, what are your goals?
3. What are your fears?
4. Are there any trade-offs you are willing to make or not?
5. What would a good day be like?

Five Recommendations for communicating with patients or family members about illness progression and end-of-life [61]

1. Ascertain patient or family member's perspective before offering your own.
2. Where possible, mirror the language of the patient or family.
3. Create opportunities to discuss the future.
4. Be clear about uncertainty.
5. Display sensitivity.

REDMAP Framework

www.spict.org.uk **or** www.ec4h.org.uk

A 6-step guide to future care planning conversations with people whose health is deteriorating and their families, which can be used in a variety of settings.

Ready—Expect—Diagnosis—Matters—Action—Plan

Figure 6 (*Continued*)

SAGE & THYME

www.sageandthymetraining.org.uk

A mnemonic that provides a memorable structure for conversations.

Setting create privacy and a comfortable environment.

Ask about their concerns

Gather all the concerns

Empathy, respond sensitively

Talk, discuss their worries

Help, find out who can help

You, establish what they can do themselves

Me, establish what you can do for them

End the conversation

A promising model for improving communication skills when working with cancer patients [55].

Shared decision-making using DECIDE from NHS Scotland

www.ec4h.org.uk

Define decision

Explain situation

Consider options

Invite views

Decide together

Evaluate Decision

SPIKES [56]

Originally intended as a protocol for breaking bad news.

Setting: includes privacy, involving significant others, listening mode, and body language.

Perception: the "before you tell, ask" principle; you should glean a fairly accurate picture of the patient's perception of their medical condition.

Invitation: check how much patient wants to know about diagnosis and treatment; obtaining overt permission respects the patient's right to know (or not to know).

Knowledge: give information at patient's pace using the same language as them; "chunk and check."

Empathy: listen for, identify, acknowledge and validate emotions.

Strategy and Summary: summarize discussion, give chance for questions or concerns; clarify next steps.

Serious Illness Conversation Guide (SICG):

www.ariadnelabs.org/serious-illness-care

A structured conversation guide part of the Serious Illness Care Programme from Ariadne Labs. Provides a framework to structure meaningful, realistic, and focused conversations about a patient's wishes, fears and worries for the future with their illness [62].

Includes:

- Set up the conversation
- Assess understanding and preferences
- Share prognosis
- Explore key topics
- Close the conversation
- Document your conversation
- Communicate with key clinicians

There is evidence that SICG helps to promote patient-centred health care that aligns with patient values and wishes [63].

Talk CPR

www.talkcpr.wales

Training tools to encourage conversations about CPR for people affected by life-limiting and palliative illnesses.

The Second Conversation Project

www.rcplondon.ac.uk/projects/
second-conversation-improving-training-around-end-life-care-conversations

Encourages junior clinicians to return to a conversation started by their seniors. It gives patients, carers, and family members the time and space to reflect on information they have received, while providing doctors in training with a valuable educational opportunity that builds their skills and confidence in handling end-of-life care discussions. Of most value to newly qualified doctors and worked well on wards where length of stay was longer, and end-of-life conversations frequently happen [64].

University of Edinburgh and NHS Scotland: Supportive and Palliative Care Indicators Tool (SPICT)

www.spict.org.uk

Identifies people with one or multiple advanced conditions who are at risk of deteriorating and dying. It offers case-by-case assessment and advice on communication and how to record plans for holistic, palliative care needs. Use as a guide to recognise that somebody has an advanced progressive illness, rather than as a prognostication tool [14].

VITAL Talk [65]

www.vitaltalk.org

1. Serious illness communication skills training and resources based upon three principles:Dealing with emotion is more important than giving lots of information
2. Information is best delivered in small packets that start with a headline
3. Patient values should be at the heart of medical treatment plans

Figure 6   (*Continued*)

Fink Advance Care Planning CardsTM Developed in the UK. Includes a deck of cards divided into four categories (how I like to talk about things, who and what matters to me, advance care planning/still to do, and as I die/celebrating my life). Cards are used to start, share, or continue advance care planning conversations. www.finkcards.com	*Grave Talk CardsTM* A resource from the Church of England (UK) of 50 unique cards for use in small groups, each with a thought-provoking question to get the conversation started. Topics covered include: Life, Death, Society, Funerals, Grief. Also used in death café scenarios. www.chpublishing.co.uk/books/9780715147030/grave-talk-cards
Marie Curie Talkabout Conversation CardsTM Developed in the UK. Conversation cards designed to help share wishes and learn more about family and friends. www.mariecurie.org.uk	*Talking Mats™* Developed in Scotland, an image-based aid to support people with communication difficulties to communicate effectively about things that matter to them. A Talking Mat has been developed to support advance care planning and help people to think ahead and plan for the future. www.talkingmats.com/category/advance-care-planning
The Conversation ProjectTM An initiative of the Institute for Healthcare Improvement www.theconversationproject.org	
Conversation startersTM Conversation starters for advance care planning from Speak Up (Canada). www.advancecareplanning.ca/resource/conversation-starters	*Dying to Talk CardsTM* Online card game developed in Australia (guided by Coda Alliance's Go Wish card game) to help talk about wishes and preferences for care at the end-of-life. www.dyingtotalk.org.au/card-game
Go Wish CardsTM A deck of 36 cards developed by the CODA alliance in the USA to help start end-of-life discussions. www.codaalliance.org/go-wish	*DöBra cardsTM* Swedish adaptation of the GoWish cards www.dobra.se/en/dobra-toolbox/dobra-card-game
My Gift of Grace or HelloTM A conversation game (USA) with 47 Question Cards, and 32 Thank You Chips. Players have a chance to share their answers to the same question, trading chips as part of the game play. www.mygiftofgrace.com	*Heart2Hearts: Advance Care Planning CardsTM* Developed in the USA, a deck of cards invented to provide 52 conversation starters about end-of-life health-care issues. www.discussdirectives.com/heart2hearts-acp.html
The Conversation GameTM Originally developed by the CODA Alliance (USA). Includes a deck of 36 cards and instruction leaflet. Objective is to be an easy and entertaining way to think and talk about how you want to be treated if you became seriously ill. www.conversationsforlife.co.uk	

Figure 7 Examples of conversation trigger cards and tools.

Summary

Conversations matter in palliative and end-of-life care. There are many resources, models, and frameworks to aid practitioners in person centred discussions. One size does not meet all and an individualised approach should always be taken. As practitioners we have the responsibility to pay attention to our skills, ability, competence in, and reflection on conversations in order to provide, facilitate and enable the best possible palliative and end-of-life experience to people and those that matter to them.

References

1. Russell, S. (2016). Advance care planning and living with dying: the views of hospice patients. Doctoral Thesis, University of Hertfordshire (accessed 19 February 2022).
2. Kaasa, S., Loge, J.H., Aapro, M., Albreht, T., Anderson, R., Bruera, E., Brunelli, C., Caraceni, A., Cervantes, A., Currow, D.C., and Deliens, L. (2018 November 1). Integration of oncology and palliative care: a Lancet Oncology Commission. *The Lancet Oncology* 19 (11): e588–e653.
3. NHS England and NHS Improvement. (2022). Personalised palliative and end-of-life care. www.england.nhs.uk/eolc/personalised-care (accessed 19 February 2022).

4. The Choice in End of Life Care Programme Board. (2015). What's important to me. A review of choice in end-of-life care. London: The Choice in End of Life Care Programme Board. www.gov.uk/government/publications/choice-in-end-oflife-care (accessed 19 February 2022).

5. National Palliative and End of Life Care Partnership. (2021 May). Ambitions for palliative and end-of-life care: a national framework for local action 2021–2026.

6. Moore, P.M., Rivera, S., Bravo-Soto, G.A., Olivares, C., and Lawrie T.A. (2018). Communication skills training for healthcare professionals working with people who have cancer. *Cochrane Database of Systematic Reviews* (7): CD003751. DOI: 10.1002/14651858.CD003751. 4.

7. Sallnow, L., Smith, R., Ahmedzai, S.H., Bhadelia, A., Chamberlain, C., Cong, Y., Doble, B., Dullie, L., Durie, R., Finkelstein, E.A., and Guglani, S. (2022 February 26). Report of the Lancet Commission on the Value of Death: bringing death back into life. *The Lancet* 399 (10327): 837–884.

8. King, A. and Hoppe, R.B. (2013 September). "Best practice" for patient-centered communication: a narrative review. *Journal of Graduate Medical Education* 5 (3): 385–393.

9. Back, A.L. (2020 March 20). Patient-clinician communication issues in palliative care for patients with advanced cancer. *Journal of Clinical Oncology* 38 (9): 866–876.

10. Beavan, J., Fowler, C., and Russell, S. (2011). Communication skills and advance care planning. In: *Advance Care Planning in End of Life Care*, (eds. Keri Thomas and Ben Lobo) 1st edition, 261–276. Oxford University Press.

11. Temel, J.S., Greer, J.A., Muzikansky, A., Gallagher, E.R., Admane, S., Jackson, V.A., Dahlin, C.M., Blinderman, C.D., Jacobsen, J., Pirl, W.F., and Billings, J.A. (2010 August 19). Early palliative care for patients with metastatic non-small-cell lung cancer. *New England Journal of Medicine* 363 (8): 733–742.

12. Maguire, P., Faulkner, A., Booth, K., Elliott, C., and Hillier, V. (1996 January 1). Helping cancer patients disclose their concerns. *European Journal of Cancer* 32 (1): 78–81.

13. Care Quality Commission. (2016 May). A better ending: addressing inequalities in end-of-life care. Care Quality Commission, London.

14. Bailey, S.J. and Cogle, K. (2018 October). Talking about dying: how to begin honest conversations about what lies ahead. London: Royal College of Physicians.

15. Royal College of Physicians. (2021 February). Acute care resource end-of-life care in the acute care setting. Royal College of Physicians, London. 2018 February.

16. Feinmann, J. (2002 November 16). Brushing up on doctors' communication skills. *The Lancet* 360 (9345): 1572.

17. Mata, Á.N., de Azevedo, K.P., Braga, L.P., de Medeiros, G.C., de Oliveira Segundo, V.H., Bezerra, I.N., Pimenta, I.D., Nicolás, I.M., and Piuvezam, G. (2021 December). Training in communication skills for self-efficacy of health professionals: a systematic review. *Human Resources for Health* 19 (1): 1–9.

18. Knapp, M.L. and Hall, J.A. (2010). *Nonverbal Communication in Human Interaction*, 7e. Boston: Wadsworth Publishing.

19. Banerjee, P., Verma, N., Mohan, C., Rustagi, S.M., Nair, B.T., and Rautela, A. (2021 July 1). Listening between the lines: introduction of a module for teaching nonverbal communication skills to MBBS students. *Archives of Medicine and Health Sciences* 9 (2): 264.

20. McCorry, L.K. (2011). *Communication Skills for Health Care Professionals*, 1e. Wolter and Kluwer Publishing.

21. Parry, R., Land, V., and Seymour, J. (2014 December 1). How to communicate with patients about future illness progression and end of life: a systematic review. *BMJ Supportive & Palliative Care* 4 (4): 331–341.

22. Pollock, K. and Wilson, E. (2015 July 1). Care and communication between health professionals and patients affected by severe or chronic illness in community care settings: a qualitative study of care at the end of life. *Health Services and Delivery Research* 3 (31).

23. Russell, S. (2018 September 2). Challenges of advance care planning for those with dementia. *Nursing And Residential Care* 20 (9): 451–455.

24. Gravier, S., Burney, S., and Radermacher, H. (2019). Reflective practice in palliative care. *InPsych the Bulletin of the Australian Psychological Society Limited* 15–19. 19InPsych-June-Palliative-care_p14-19.pdf (caresearch.com.au).

25. Clayton, J.M., Hancock, K., Parker, S., Butow, P.N., Walder, S., Carrick, S., Currow, D., Ghersi, D., Glare, P., Hagerty, R., and Olver, I.N. (2008 July). Sustaining hope when communicating with terminally ill patients and their families: a systematic review. *Psycho-Oncology: Journal of the Psychological, Social and Behavioral Dimensions of Cancer* 17 (7): 641–659.

26. van der Velden, N.C., Meijers, M.C., Han, P.K., van Laarhoven, H.W., Smets, E., and Henselmans, I. (2020 May). The effect of prognostic communication on patient outcomes in palliative cancer care: a systematic review. *Current Treatment Options in Oncology* 21 (5): 1–38.

27. Mannix, K. (2021). *Listen: How to Find the Words for Tender Conversations*. Dublin, Ireland: William Collins, Harper Collins Publishers.

28. Sinclair, S., Beamer, K., Hack, T.F., McClement, S., Raffin Bouchal, S., Chochinov, H.M., and Hagen, N.A. (2017 May). Sympathy, empathy, and compassion: a grounded theory study of palliative care patients' understandings, experiences, and preferences. *Palliative Medicine* 31 (5): 437–447.

29. Gilligan, T., Coyle, N., Frankel, R.M., Berry, D.L., Bohlke, K., Epstein, R.M., Finlay, E., Jackson, V.A., Lathan, C.S., Loprinzi, C.L., and Nguyen, L.H. (2018 February 1). Patient-clinician communication: American Society of Clinical Oncology consensus guideline. *Obstetrical & Gynecological Survey* 73 (2): 96–97.

30. Parry, R., Whittaker, B., Pino, M., Jenkins, L., Worthington, E., and Faull, C. (2021). Realtalk evidence-based communication training: development of a conversation analysis-based intervention designed to be delivered by

clinical trainers. doi: 10.21203/rs.3.rs-969047/v1 (accessed 27 February 2022).

31. Brighton, L.J., Koffman, J., Hawkins, A., McDonald, C., O'Brien, S., Robinson, V., Khan, S.A., George, R., Higginson, I.J., and Selman, L.E. (2017 September 1). A systematic review of end-of-life care communication skills training for generalist palliative care providers: research quality and reporting guidance. *Journal of Pain and Symptom Management* 54 (3): 417–425.

32. Russell, S. (2018). Communication skills and advance care planning. In: *Advance Care Planning in End of Life Care*, (eds. Keri Thomas, Ben Lobo, and Karen Detering), 2nd edition, 259–271. Oxford University Press.

33. Gramling, C.J., Durieux, B.N., Clarfeld, L.A., Javed, A., Matt, J.E., Manukyan, V., Braddish, T., Wong, A., Wills, J., Hirsch, L., and Straton, J. (2021 November 6). Epidemiology of Connectional Silence in specialist serious illness conversations. *Patient Education and Counseling* 105 (7):2005–11.

34. Bassett, L., Bingley, A.F., and Brearley, S.G. (2018 January). Silence as an element of care: a meta-ethnographic review of professional caregivers' experience in clinical and pastoral settings. *Palliative Medicine* 32 (1): 185–194.

35. Tornøe, K.A., Danbolt, L.J., Kvigne, K., and Sørlie, V. (2014 December). The power of consoling presence-hospice nurses' lived experience with spiritual and existential care for the dying. *BMC Nursing* 13 (1): 1–8.

36. Carpenter, J.G., Ersek, M., Nelson, F., Kinder, D., Wachterman, M., Smith, D., Murray, A., and Garrido, M.M. (2020 April). A national study of end-of-life care among older veterans with hearing and vision loss. *Journal of the American Geriatrics Society* 68 (4): 817–825.

37. Queen, S.E. (2021). Optimizing communication in palliative and hospice care: a toolkit for audiologists. CUNY Academic Works. https://academicworks.cuny.edu/gc_etds/4233 (accessed 27 February 2022).

38. Harrison Dening, K., Scates, C., McGill, G., and De-Vries, K. (2019 June). A training needs analysis of admiral nurses to facilitate advance care planning in dementia. *Palliative Care: Research and Treatment* 12: 1178224219850183.

39. Harrison Dening, K., Sampson, E.L., and De Vries, K. (2019 February). Advance care planning in dementia: recommendations for healthcare professionals. *Palliative Care: Research and Treatment* 12: 1178224219826579.

40. Davies, N., De Souza, T., Rait, G., Meehan, J., and Sampson, E.L. (2021 May 27). Developing an applied model for making decisions towards the end of life about care for someone with dementia. *PloS one* 16 (5): e0252464.

41. Piers, R., Albers, G., Gilissen, J., De Lepeleire, J., Steyaert, J., Van Mechelen, W., Steeman, E., Dillen, L., Vanden Berghe, P., and Van den Block, L. (2018 December). Advance care planning in dementia: recommendations for healthcare professionals. *BMC Palliative Care* 17 (1): 1–7.

42. Noorlandt, H.W., Korfage, I.J., Tuffrey-Wijne, I., Festen, D., Vrijmoeth, C., van der Heide, A., and Echteld, M. (2021 November). Consensus on a conversation aid for shared decision making with people with intellectual disabilities in the palliative phase. *Journal of Applied Research in Intellectual Disabilities* 34 (6): 1538–1548.

43. Islam, Z., Taylor, L., and Faull, C. (2021 Nov). Thinking ahead in advanced illness: exploring clinicians' perspectives on discussing resuscitation with patients and families from ethnic minority communities. *Future Healthcare Journal* 8 (3): e619.

44. Green, A., Jerzmanowska, N., Green, M., and Lobb, E.A. (2018 September). "Death is difficult in any language": a qualitative study of palliative care professionals' experiences when providing end-of-life care to patients from culturally and linguistically diverse backgrounds. *Palliative Medicine* 32 (8): 1419–1427.

45. Silva, M.D., Genoff, M., Zaballa, A., Jewell, S., Stabler, S., Gany, F.M., and Diamond, L.C. (2016 March 1). Interpreting at the end of life: a systematic review of the impact of interpreters on the delivery of palliative care services to cancer patients with limited English proficiency. *Journal of Pain and Symptom Management* 51 (3): 569–580.

46. Tackling Inequalities in End of Life Care for Minority Groups VCSE Health and Wellbeing Alliance Project Group. (2018). Care committed to me. Delivering high quality, personalised palliative and end-of-life care for Gypsies & Travellers, LGBT people and people experiencing homelessness: a resource for commissioners, service providers, and health care and support staff. London: Hospice UK, on behalf of the Tackling Inequalities in End of Life Care for Minority Groups VCSE Project Group.

47. Shulman, C. and Hudson, B.F. (2018 February 19). Palliative care for homeless people. [Powerpoint presentation]: Homeless Link and Hospice UK. Homelessness and end-of-life care workshop.

48. Bristowe, K., Hodson, M., Wee, B., Almack, K., Johnson, K., Daveson, B.A., Koffman, J., McEnhill, L., and Harding, R. (2018 January). Recommendations to reduce inequalities for LGBT people facing advanced illness: ACCESSCare national qualitative interview study. *Palliative Medicine* 32 (1): 23–35.

49. Collier, A., Morgan, D.D., Swetenham, K., To, T.H., Currow, D.C., and Tieman, J.J. (2016 April). Implementation of a pilot telehealth programme in community palliative care: a qualitative study of clinicians' perspectives. *Palliative Medicine* 30 (4): 409–417.

50. Stockdill, M.L., Barnett, M.D., Taylor, R.A., Dionne-Odom, J.N., and Bakitas, M. (2021 February 1). Telehealth in Palliative Care: communication strategies from the COVID-19 pandemic. *Clinical Journal of Oncology Nursing* 25 (1).

51. Qian, A.S., Schiaffino, M.K., Nalawade, V., Aziz, L., Pacheco, F.V., Nguyen, B., Vu, P., Patel, S.P., Martinez, M.E., and Murphy, J.D. (2022 January 5). Disparities in telemedicine during COVID-19. *Cancer Medicine* 11 (4):1192–201.

52. Sutherland, A.E., Bradley, V., Walding, M., Stickland, J., and Wee, B. (2021 December 1). Palliative medicine video

consultations in the pandemic: patient feedback. *BMJ Supportive & Palliative Care* 11 (4): 404–405.

53. Kurtz, S., Silverman, J., Draper, J., van Dalen, J., and Platt, F.W. (2017 December 21). *Teaching and Learning Communication Skills in Medicine*. CRC press.

54. Clayton, J.M., Butow, P.N., Waters, A., Laidsaar-Powell, R.C., O'Brien, A., Boyle, F., Back, A.L., Arnold, R.M., Tulsky, J.A., and Tattersall, M.H. (2013 March). Evaluation of a novel individualised communication-skills training intervention to improve doctors' confidence and skills in end-of-life communication. *Palliative Medicine* 27 (3): 236–243.

55. Griffiths, J., Wilson, C., Ewing, G., Connolly, M., and Grande, G. (2015 October 1). Improving communication with palliative care cancer patients at home—a pilot study of SAGE & THYME communication skills model. *European Journal of Oncology Nursing* 19 (5): 465–472.

56. Baile, W.F., Buckman, R., Lenzi, R., Glober, G., Beale, E.A., and Kudelka, A.P. (2000 August). SPIKES—a six-step protocol for delivering bad news: application to the patient with cancer. *The Oncologist* 5 (4): 302–311.

57. Koffman, J., Yorganci, E., Murtagh, F., Yi, D., Gao, W., Barclay, S., Pickles, A., Higginson, I., Johnson, H., Wilson, R., and Bailey, S. (2019 October). The AMBER care bundle for hospital inpatients with uncertain recovery nearing the end of life: the ImproveCare feasibility cluster RCT. *Health Technology Assessment (Winchester, England)* 23 (55): 1.

58. Johnson, H., Yorganci, E., Evans, C.J., Barclay, S., Murtagh, F.E., Yi, D., Gao, W., Sampson, E.L., Droney, J., Farquhar, M., and Koffman, J. (2020 September 16). Implementation of a complex intervention to improve care for patients whose situations are clinically uncertain in hospital settings: a multi-method study using normalisation process theory. *PloS one* 15 (9): e0239181.

59. Higginson, I.J., Koffman, J., Hopkins, P., Prentice, W., Burman, R., Leonard, S., Rumble, C., Noble, J., Dampier, O., Bernal, W., and Hall, S. (2013). Development and evaluation of the feasibility and effects on staff, patients, and families of a new tool, the Psychosocial Assessment and Communication Evaluation (PACE), to improve communication and palliative care in intensive care and during clinical uncertainty. *BMC Medicine* 11 (1): 1–14.

60. Gawande, A. (2014). *Being Mortal: Medicine and What Matters in the End*, 1e. New York: Metropolitian Books, Henery Holt and Company.

61. Ekberg, S., Parry, R., Land, V., Ekberg, K., Pino, M., Antaki, C., Jenkins, L., and Whittaker, B. (2021 December). Communicating with patients and families about illness progression and end of life: a review of studies using direct observation of clinical practice. *BMC Palliative Care* 20 (1): 1–2.

62. McGlinchey, T., Mason, S., Coackley, A., Roberts, A., Maguire, M., Sanders, J., Maloney, F., Block, S., Ellershaw, J., and Kirkbride, P. (2019 December). Serious illness care Programme UK: assessing the "face validity," applicability and relevance of the serious illness conversation guide for use within the UK health care setting. *BMC Health Services Research* 19 (1): 1–9.

63. Beddard-Huber, E., Gaspard, G., and Yue, K. (2021). Adaptations to the serious illness conversation guide to be more culturally safe. *International Journal of Indigenous Health* 16 (1).

64. Mathew, R., Weil, A., Sleeman, K.E., Bristowe, K., Shukla, P., Schiff, R., Flanders, L., Leonard, P., Minton, O., Wakefield, D., and St John, K. (2019 June). The Second Conversation project: improving training in end-of-life care communication among junior doctors. *Future Healthcare Journal* 6 (2): 129.

65. Back, A., Tulsky, J.A., and Arnold, R.M. (2020 June 2). Communication skills in the age of COVID-19. *Annals of Internal Medicine* 172 (11): 759–760.

66. Gazarian, P.K., Cronin, J., Dalto, J.L., Baker, K.M., Friel, B.J., Bruce-Baiden, W., and Rodriguez, L.Y. (2019 March 1). A systematic evaluation of advance care planning patient educational resources. *Geriatric Nursing* 40 (2): 174–180.

8 Integrating New Perspectives: Working with Loss and Grief in Palliative Care

Nikki Archer and Linda Machin

Introduction

It's so hard when you go in to visit them. You can feel the tension. It's there but invisible. Roger just avoids talking about things. I think he knows what is happening but doesn't want to talk. Elizabeth is making plans for when she is not here. She got upset the other day talking about the life they've shared. He was like "come on we need to be strong". I just smiled and got on with what I needed to do. He knows she is dying but he just copes by getting on with the practicalities. I felt helpless and didn't know what to say.

Joyce, Staff Nurse.

Working with dying, death, and bereavement is a central part of palliative care. The ability to deal sensitively with the consequent, often complex, and demanding landscape of loss and grief is the basis for providing high quality palliative care. However, it is a challenging area of practice which remains largely invisible, unplanned for, and misunderstood [1–3].

This chapter addresses the centrality of loss and grief, generated by dying, death, and bereavement. It sets out a practice framework for the Bereavement Pathway in palliative care [4], that incorporates the theory and practice of the Range of Response to Loss model (RRL) [5] and a family systems approach [6]. The chapter has three sections:
1. Understanding loss and grief. This section explores loss and grief as fundamental, human experiences and introduces the RRL model as a contemporary framework for understanding and assessing the spectrum of reactions and coping responses prompted by grief.
2. Loss and grief in palliative care. This section explores the palliative care context of dying, death, and bereavement,

defined as the Bereavement Pathway. This pathway is explored along with the losses these experiences incur for patients, carers, and practitioners. A family systems approach is used to engage with the relationship dynamics of those at the centre of receiving and delivering palliative care.
3. Integrating new perspectives into palliative care practice. The final section describes how the new perspectives, described in sections 1 and 2, might be integrated into palliative care and a case study is presented to exemplify how these ideas might be used in practice.

Understanding Loss and Grief

What Does Loss Look Like?

Anything that you have you can lose; anything you are attached to, you can be separated from; anything you love can be taken away from you. Yet, if you really have nothing to lose, you have nothing. [7, p. 211].

Loss is a universal human experience woven into everyday life. Experiences of loss can be both:
• part of the common journey through life e.g., leaving school, moving house, retirement, timely death.
or arise
• from more particular individual circumstances e.g., relationship changes and loss such as separation and divorce; health changes and losses, such as disability and illness; unfulfilled hopes such as childlessness; social or economic disadvantage such as unemployment, poverty; untimely bereavement [2, 5].

The impact of the worldwide COVID-19 pandemic has introduced a new and extensive range of losses into life and these include [8] the loss of everyday normal activities:
• loss of connectivity with others
• loss of finances and jobs

Handbook of Palliative Care, Fourth Edition. Edited by Richard Kitchen, Christina Faull, Sarah Russell and Jo Wilson.
© 2024 John Wiley & Sons Ltd. Published 2024 by John Wiley & Sons Ltd.

- loss of safety and security
- loss of opportunity for marking key life events
- loss through death of a family member.

Everyone is faced with managing and integrating a wide range of change and loss into their lives. Some people manage this well, while others struggle. The impact of a loss and the ability to manage it will depend upon the nature and visibility of the loss, personal and circumstantial factors, and the way these might promote resilience or result in vulnerability. The culture within which a loss occurs can be the context of effective support or the context of misunderstanding and unavailable support. While some losses can be remedied, for many, including death, dying, and bereavement there is no possible reversal, only an adjustment to the reality of what has been lost [5]. Death, dying, and bereavement are usually seen as the hardest and greatest losses which we face within our lives [9].

What is Grief?

Grief is an experience prompted by a significant loss and is uniquely and individually expressed through the reactions to it and the adjustments which must be made to its consequences [3, 10]. Grief is not just an emotional phenomenon, but it impacts on all dimensions of experience: physical, cognitive, behavioural, spiritual, and social (see Figure 1). The wider culture, including ethnicity, race and belief systems, and more immediate social context, within which a loss occurs, shape perceptions about the relative significance of a loss and how people respond to it [3, 11]. For instance, an older Indian widow with a strong belief in an afterlife is likely to respond very differently to the experience of a terminal illness, from the way a young Western atheist does, who believes strongly in control of one's own life and that there is no afterlife. How an individual, and their family network makes sense of the

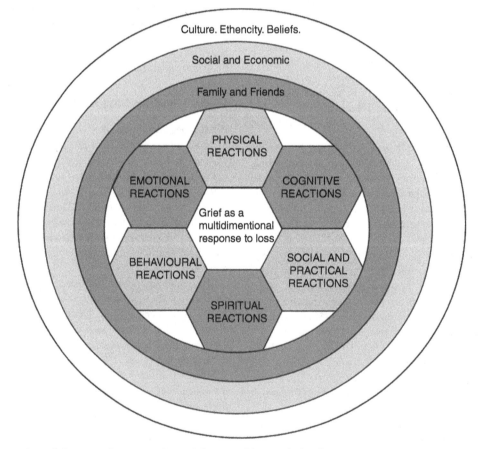

Figure 1   Grief: a multidimensional response to loss and the external factors which influence it.

experience of loss will be significantly influenced by the culturally derived and personally developed, life perspectives.

The nature and level of distress experienced within the different domains (see Table 1) will range in intensity from little or none, to heightened suffering that can lead to depression, anxiety, panic, social isolation, and existential and spiritual crisis [12].

What are the Risks? What Does Resilience Look Like?

The experiences of loss can have a profoundly negative impact on the lives and wellbeing of individuals, families, and the wider community. For a proportion of grieving people these negative outcomes will include emotional distress, anxiety, and depression [14]. It has been estimated that:

- Around one in four palliative care patients will experience these more severe levels of emotional and psychological distress [15] in response to the losses associated with their illness.
- Evidence has shown the negative impact of losses associated with caring for family members at end-of-life including depression and anxiety [16, 17].
- An estimated 10–15 per cent of bereaved people will be affected by complex grief with increased risk of depression, anxiety, substance abuse, suicidal thinking, and abnormalities in immune functioning [18]. The characteristics of Complicated Grief [19] or Prolonged Grief Disorder [20]

are persistent yearning for the deceased; prolonged and persistent negative cognitive, emotional, and behavioural symptoms; difficulty in functioning in work and social relationships; a sense of meaninglessness and disruption in beliefs which are present for at least six months.

However, the nature and diversity of grief reactions, are often misunderstood and many normal reactions or "symptoms" e.g. being emotional, wanting to talk about the illness or the deceased are seen as indications of not coping or of mental-health difficulties. This risk of pathologising grief ignores new understandings and insight about the human capacity for resilience in the face of loss [21]. Most people, although challenged by the impact of loss and their experience of grief, do possess sufficient inner resourcefulness or resilience to manage and get through traumatic and disturbing loss events. Resilience is characterised by qualities of flexibility and courage, by a capacity to make sense of experience and to retain some positivity, set alongside the availability and the willingness to access support [5, 22, 23]. These characteristics will be evidenced where people are able to effectively balance the emotional component of grief with ongoing life demands [24]. In the face of testing life experiences opportunities for growth in psychological, social, and spiritual maturity are possible [22, 25, 26] but there will be a journey to take in achieving resilience, which may be punctuated with periods of vulnerability.

There are numerous factors which have been identified as promoting adaptive grief responses or exacerbating

Table 1   How people react to loss [13].

Dimension	Reactions people experience in response to loss
Emotional	Numbness, sadness, anger, fear, relief, irritability, guilt, loneliness, apathy, longing, anxiety, meaninglessness, apathy, abandonment, envy.
Physical	Hyperactivity or underactivity, physical distress, chest pain, abdominal pain, headaches, nausea, panic attacks, changes in appetite and weight, fatigue, sleeping problems, restlessness, insomnia, crying and sighing, menstrual irregularities, sensitivity to noise, shortness of breath, and tightness of throat.
Cognitive	Worry about own/other's reactions. Attempts to rationalise and make sense of the loss. Thoughts focus on loss or work hard to think about other things. Difficulty in concentrating.
Social and practical	Avoid contact with others, lack interest in contact with others, struggles to be on own, engages with available support network. Social support unavailable.
Behavioural	Forgetfulness, slowed thinking, dreams about the loss, wandering aimlessly, crying, outward expressions of varied emotions, adapt behaviour to respond to others needs, need to share narrative of what has/is happening.
Spiritual	Existential questions raised, reappraisal of purpose and meaning of life, belief systems challenged or reaffirmed, searching for answers and reasons for the loss, meaning making.

distress (see Table 2). The complex interplay of risk and resilience is part of each grief experience. Even where there are multiple risk factors some people will be able to accommodate their loss effectively. While for others where there are fewer indications of risks, loss is experienced as distressing and debilitating grief [5, 27]. Where the risk includes complex mental-health issues, including potential self-harm or suicide further prompt assessment and referral to mental-health specialist will be required.

Theories Which Have Helped Us Understand Grief

Over the last one hundred years, grief theories, along with the extensive literature and research associated with them, have provided a conceptual base for understanding the nature of dying and bereavement. Early theoretical perspectives were influenced by Freud's psychodynamic school of thought [32]. The clinical work undertaken by Kubler-Ross [33] with dying patients and Bowlby's evolving ideas about the nature of human attachment [34] led to notions of stages or phases of grief. These theories focused on grief as an intrapsychic, time-bound experience with a bias towards a predominantly emotion-focused view of grief. The absence of, or too much, emotional expression of grief was seen as problematic. Implicit in this notion is that there is a predictable, ideal way for grief to be experienced, expressed, and worked through. The limitations of these perspectives have been widely recognised over 20 years and yet they remain embedded as the dominant discourse within western clinical healthcare practice [35–37]. Continued reliance

on these "traditional" conceptualisations means practitioners risk pathologising and undermining natural resilience [38].

Contemporary theories have brought a new focus to address the limitations of earlier ideas, and to give fuller recognition to the importance of cultural determinants of grief and insight into the nature of resilience. The Dual Process Model of grief emerged from research which sought to test the validity of the traditional "grief work" hypotheses [24]. It proposes that adaptation to grief consists of a two-dimensional process: loss orientation, with a focus on the distress of grief, and restoration orientation, attending to ongoing life demands. The ability to move or oscillate between the two modes is seen as necessary for successfully adapting to loss. Further explanations and discussions of grief theory have been published [36, 39].

The Range of Response to Loss Model (RRL): A Framework for Practice

The RRL model developed by Machin, was conceptualised as a result of listening to grieving people in practice and research [5, 40]. It provides a framework in which grief is conceptualised as a two-dimensional process. In the first of these dimensions, initial intuitive **grief reactions** are triggered and can be seen expressed in a range from:

• An **overwhelmed** reaction, where the distress of grief dominates

to

• A **controlled** reaction, where emotion is suppressed or avoided, and the focus is on ongoing life demands.

Table 2   Factors identified as promoting adaptive grief responses or exacerbating distress.

Factors increasing the risk of negative outcomes following loss [27–30]	Factors which support resilience following loss [22, 23, 31]
Other concurrent stresses and losses within the family (poor housing, debt, relationship issues)	Absence of concurrent stresses
History of multiple losses – previous experiences of death and loss how have these been managed? Quantity of losses which have been managed and personal resourcefulness or capacity for managing the loss	Positive life perspectives and personal resourcefulness
Strong dependency issues, difficult relationships	Previous positive experiences of managing loss
Pre-existing mental illness	Capacity to make sense of experiences
Untimely deaths	Culturally sensitive available support
Perceived lack of social support	Capacity to access available support
The nature of the death (in bereavement) *e.g. Traumatic/unexpected*	

These core grief reactions reflect the emotional and cognitive tensions prompted by loss and reflect language heard in practice and everyday life, for example:

• *It's just so overwhelming, I can't stop myself from crying and thinking about what has happened all of the time.*
• *I just need to stay strong and be there for the children, I've got to manage looking after them, I can't let him down.*

The second dimension of the RRL is described as a **coping response**, in which there is a conscious process involving facing the loss and managing its consequences. The ability to balance the overwhelmed and controlled reactions and to respond effectively to the reality of the changed life situation, is seen as an indication of resilient coping i.e., emotions are accepted and faced, and the practical consequences of loss are approached with realism and a sense of engagement. In contrast, where the capacity to balance feelings and functioning is impeded or absent and managing the changed life situation is problematic, vulnerability is indicated. Figure 2 shows the RRL model, and the two-dimensions integrated to provide a framework for practice. It is important to recognise that the concepts in the model are influenced by the wider context of culture, circumstances, and personal factors. Factors which will affect the propensity for vulnerability and resilience.

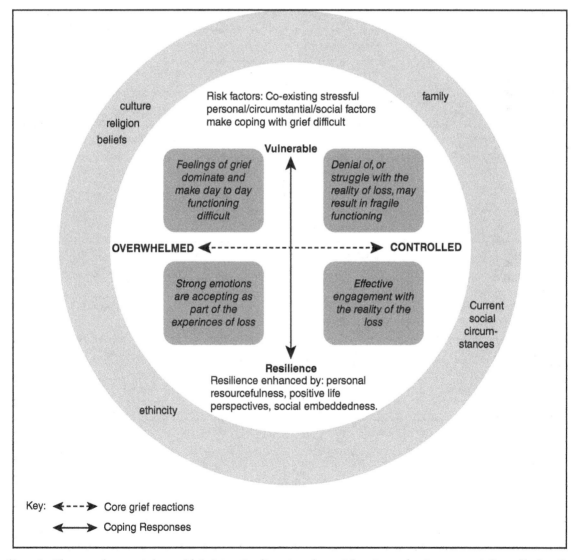

Figure 2   *The range of response to loss model: the interacting dimensions of core grief reactions and coping responses, influenced by the wider cultural context* [5].

The concepts in the RRL model are echoed in other theories particularly those influential theories used in palliative and bereavement care i.e. attachment theory [41] and the Dual Process Model [24].

The RRL is increasingly being used within palliative care settings as a framework to help practitioners identify individual and family responses to loss. A measure which is based on the RRL, is the Adult Attitude to Grief Scale (AAG) providing a tool for understanding the individual dynamics of a person's grief [5, 40]. The AAG is a validated nine statement, five-point Likert tool which provides a grief-specific measure of vulnerability and resilience [42].

Interest and enthusiasm, within palliative care psychosocial services, for the practice usefulness of the RRL model and the AAG scale in bereavement support, has led to the development of two pre-bereavement measures. These are the Attitude to Health Change scales (AHC), one for use with patients and one for use with their carers or family members. The AHCs help to provide practitioners with a measure for assessing patient and carer support needs and is a tool which also facilitates conversations about the experience of life limiting illness. Research is being undertaken to validate the AHCs. The concepts in the RRL are reflected in the AAG and AHC statements (see Table 3).

Table 3   Comparing the AHC statements (one for patients and one for carers) with the AAG statements [5].

3(i)	Overwhelmed reactions	
AHC (patient)	AHC (carer)	AAG
I find it difficult to switch off thoughts about my health	I find it difficult to switch off thoughts about ......'s health	For me, it is difficult to switch off thoughts about the person I have lost
I often feel emotional about my health e.g. fearful, anxious, sad	I often feel emotional about ....'s health e.g. fearful, anxious, sad......	I feel that I will always carry the pain of grief with me
My illness makes it harder for me to make sense of life	.........'s illness makes it harder for me to make sense of life	Life has less meaning for me after this loss

3(ii)	Controlled reactions	
AHC (patient)	AHC (carer)	AAG
I believe I should be brave when facing my illness	I believe I should be brave when facing ......'s illness	I believe I must be brave in the face of loss
It is important for me to keep my feelings about my health under control	It is important for me to keep my feelings about ......'s illness under control	For me, it is important to keep my grief under control
I try to focus on day to day life rather than my health	I try to focus on day to day life rather than ......'s health	I think it is best just to get on with life in spite of this loss

3(iii)	Resilient coping response	
AHC (patient)	AHC (carer)	AAG
I am able to face up to the feelings I have about my illness	I am able to face up to the feelings I have about ......'s illness	I feel able to face the pain which comes with grief
I feel emotionally strong enough to cope with my illness and its consequences	I feel emotionally strong enough to cope with ......'s illness and its consequences	I feel very aware of my inner strength when faced with grief
I believe that I will come to accept my illness and its consequences	I believe that I will come to accept......'s illness and its consequences	It may not always feel like it but I do believe that I will come through this experience of grief

Loss and Grief in Palliative Care

The Journey from Diagnosis to Bereavement

From the moment someone has a life-limiting diagnosis which confronts them with the real possibility of their own death, they and their family and friends are likely to experience a normal reaction of shock and psychological distress [25, 28]. From this point each patient will travel their own unique palliative care journey, accompanied by family members and practitioners. All will be challenged by fundamental life and death questions and multiple losses. Along with the loss of or reduced physical functioning, will be loss and change of social roles and personal identity [39]. Such latter losses are often unrecognised and unacknowledged or "disenfranchised" [25] even by practitioners [3]. Individual grief response to these losses will be unique to each patient and carer, influenced by personal, cultural and health care setting, and involving a period of adjustment to the changes each loss brings [3, 28]. Most people find an inner resilience enabling them to cope with the consequences of illness induced losses, but some people will experience more severe and prolonged distress [28, 43].

There are many rich personal narratives offering insight into the experiences of grief encountered by people who are dying and have been bereaved. In her recent biography Sarah Harding [44] wrote about her experiences of having terminal cancer:

It sometimes surprises me, the things that really get me down while living with this illness. Of course, there's the obvious stuff, like thinking about my own mortality, and the relentless treatment and the pain that often comes with it....It might seem odd to worry about not having children when I don't even know how much of a life I have left, but it's there ... That treatment, harsh as it is, will have killed any chance I might have had. It's making me cry just thinking about it.
Sarah Harding, Girls Aloud 2021 p. 169

Grief is often seen as a reaction only to bereavement, but the wider significant losses faced by patients (and their carers), need to be seen as grief-producing and recognised as such in palliative care [10, 39]. Sometimes these losses have misleadingly been described as "anticipatory grief," rather than seen as the "here and now" grief of life limiting illness [45, 46]. All practitioners are challenged to work alongside and in response to the losses and griefs of patients and their family carers, when delivering palliative care.

The Bereavement Pathway

The Bereavement Pathway [4] was developed as part of a UK Department of Health funded project to address the challenge of ensuring continuity of care between end-of-life and bereavement services. It identifies the Bereavement Pathway as being from the point of diagnosis along a continuum through end-of-life care and into bereavement, making the important link between pre and post death experiences. The original purpose of the pathway was to recognise and bring together the multiple services and aspects of support required for people and families facing or following bereavement. It usefully provides a framework for identifying and conceptualising the continuum of losses experienced along this pathway (Figure 3).

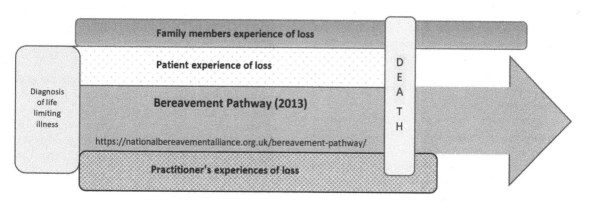

Figure 3   The Bereavement pathway and experience of loss in palliative care.

The Bereavement Pathway – A Journey of Losses for Patient, Carer, and Practitioner

Loss and change for the dying person along the Bereavement Pathway may include [39, 47–49]:

• loss of personal and social identity arising from loss of health and functional abilities, loss of social status and roles, loss of employment, loss of a sense of self, etc.

• dealing with, and empathy for, the losses being experienced by family and friends.

• confronting impending death, the loss of everything in the present and the future, which had made meaning of life. Family members are likely to have similar challenges as they too adapt to both their own losses and those of the dying person. These may include [50]:

• potential loss and change in personal health, employment, identity, social connections, finance, as the result of being a carer.

• dealing with and empathy for the losses being experienced by the dying person and other family members.

• adjusting to continual changes in the caring role.

• confronting one's own mortality.

Loss and change for family/friends post bereavement may include [51]:

• managing their experience of the death of a significant relative/friend.

• loss of the relationship and the social significance of that role.

• changes in lifestyle: financial, housing, social activity.

The family experience of dying and bereavement is a complex one. Throughout the Bereavement Pathway each family member, including the person who is dying, will be dealing with the impact of each loss and their own grief response [52]. During the COVID-19 pandemic separation from a dying relative or friend has heightened distress. This together with depleted social support at the time of the funeral and in subsequent weeks has intensified the experience of grief for many people.

Practitioners who provide care for patients and families along the Bereavement Pathway will also be facing losses. Loss and change for practitioners may include [47, 53]:

• Dealing with, sympathy/empathy for the dying person, their carers, family, and friends.

• Being the bearer of "bad news," challenged by a sense of powerlessness, not being able to "do" anything to make things better.

• Identification of personal experiences with the losses being experienced by the patients and family.

• Confronting one's own mortality.

A Family Systems Approach to Practice

Experiences of death, dying and bereavement happen within a family context. How family members manage the impact of loss and grief can have positive or negative consequences for a patient's general well-being and symptom control [54]. It is imperative, therefore, that practitioners incorporate a family approach to understanding and working with loss and grief [55]. This approach needs to include all the interacting personal and circumstantial factors within the family group, including for children, young people and family members with learning disability and impaired cognition [56, 57].

Culture shapes how individuals and families grieve and make meaning out of the experiences of illness, death, and bereavement [58]. Cultural attitudes are formed to reflect race, ethnicity, religion, and beliefs, and will contribute to how grief is defined and what are seen as acceptable responses to it. Other social factors too, such as, gender, age, class, and economic status will play a part in determining how grief is experienced and expressed. Sometimes cultural beliefs and practices are readily adopted by an individual, their family, and the wider community and this will provide an uncontentious supportive base within which to cope with loss and its consequences. In other situations, incongruity between the individual lived experience, family members and cultural norms and beliefs, create tensions for the individual and the wider social network. Awareness of these dynamics and alertness to their impact on patients and family members is central to offering sensitive and culturally appropriate support in palliative and bereavement care.

Alongside use of the RRL theoretical framework, adopting a family systems approach can provide a holistic approach to practice across the Bereavement Pathway.

Integrating New Perspectives into Palliative Care Practice

Grief is something which needs to be fully understood, supported, and assessed by practitioners as an integral part of delivering good palliative and end-of-life care. Good communication skills, cultural awareness and a broad understanding of loss and grief underpin practice. The RRL, and where appropriate use of the AHC and AAG, provide a simple explanation of the nature of loss and a language for describing and discussing it within a professional context.

The Role of the Practitioner: Core Skills

A person-centred approach to communication, is an underlying principle for working with loss and grief. This requires:

- An empathic and compassionate attitude complemented by good listening and communication skills to support grieving people.
- The ability to identify, through sensitive assessment, when people are vulnerable to the negative outcomes of grief.
- The ability to enhance, rather than undermine or pathologise, inherently resilient responses.
- Adopting a family systems perspective.

A three-tier communication skills framework for palliative care practitioners offering different levels of care [59, p. 121]:

- Level 1: communication skills: everyone working in palliative care should possess a basic level of skills which communicate compassion and understanding. Ability to give and receive information, allow discussion and expression of feelings, support and encourage resilience, and undertake assessment.
- Level 2: basic counselling skills: practitioners working within palliative care who have developed basic skills to facilitate greater awareness and understanding to support and encourage resilience.
- Level 3: qualified/experienced counselling: offering a trusting confidential relationship over time helping people with complex needs.

Ensuring culturally sensitive practice requires that practitioners have [60]:

- An inquisitive nature, an interest in finding out about the life perspectives of the individual and not making assumptions.
- An understanding of their own culture and responses to loss and how this can impact on how comfortable they feel supporting someone whose experiences are culturally different.

The Role of the Practitioner: Using the RRL as a Framework for Practice

Often the psychological and emotional care aspects of assessment and care planning are approached with no rationale, frame of reference or model to guide what is considered [28]. The theoretical principles of the RRL, and the AAG/AHC scales, can provide a framework which supports practitioners to:

- Use the Range of Response to Loss model as a "compass" for understanding grief and how it is likely to be expressed. Listening to the way in which people share their experiences offers indicators to their loss response. Table 4 outlines the narrative framework for understanding how the story of loss might be told within the RRL framework.
- Guide them in their support of patients and carers to see (i) how they might listen to and accept as normal the overwhelmed or controlled reactions to the losses they are facing and (ii) help them explore the practical, emotional, and social ways of coping with their illness or bereavement. (This may sometimes require calling on specific support from psychosocial practitioners).
- Consider using the AAG and AHC for more in-depth assessment and as tools to create opportunity for therapeutic conversations. Use of these tools requires practitioners have an understanding of their appropriate use in practice. For further information, see https://mapping-grief.care

This RRL framework helps practitioners recognise and understand the reactions and responses to the varied loss experiences along the Bereavement Pathway, supports identification of those at risk of poor outcomes, and enhances resilience.

The level of support needed across the Bereavement Pathway is set out in the NICE guidance [61] and the Public Health Model of Bereavement Care [62]. Both advocate a three-tiered component framework for the provision of support, which aligns with the three tier communication skills frame [59], for practitioners working in palliative care:

- **Component 1:** A high proportion of people (50–60%) with low vulnerability will require little formal support [62]. Acknowledging their grief, providing information about the normality of their grief and resources available, is an appropriate level of practitioner intervention. Generally, people can deal with their grief using support from their existing networks, including from family, friends, people in their broader community and the general support provided as an integral part of palliative care.
- **Component 2:** Some people (an estimated 30–40%), experience some level of difficulty and a measure of vulnerability [62]. They require some additional support, requiring basic counselling skills on a one-to-one basis or through group and peer support.
- **Component 3:** Few people (10%–15%), have more complex needs, with a high or severe level of vulnerability [62]. They will require more intensive interventions such as skilled counselling or mental-health support.

Distinguishing these different levels of support is essential for providing appropriate and effective care. All

Table 4   Narrative indicators of responses to loss [60].

Narrative process	Range of response to loss		
	OVERWHELMED	CONTROLLED	RESILIENT
Tell me about the loss.	Story of loss told in detail. Emphasis on the awfulness and impact of the loss.	Story of loss told with minimal detail. Emphasis is on fact.	Able to share coherent story of loss giving attention to both positive and challenging aspects.
Impact on you?	The engulfing nature of the feelings are described and expressed.	Strong desire to have control. Bravery dominates and painful emotions are minimised.	Pain of the loss is balanced by a positive sense of personal resourcefulness.
How are you managing	Lack of hopefulness about the situation and a sense of meaninglessness.	Desire to divert from the painful elements of loss and need to demonstrate strength and stoicism in meeting adversity.	Hopefulness and a sense of optimism combined with sense of meaning and personal strength.
Link to AAG/ AHC concepts	Disturbingly intrusive. Unremittingly painful. Robbing life of meaning.	Valuing stoicism. Denial of or covering distress. Focus on day-to-day living.	Courage in facing the loss. Sense of personal resourcefulness. Hopefulness.

practitioners need to be able to assess, give recognition to and provide assurance of the normality of grief to those people with lower-level needs (level 1), for those who need some additional but straightforward support this may be integrated into the practice care role (level 2) and for those with more complex grief (level 3) know where to refer to more specialist help e.g. psychosocial family support service within palliative care, or external mental-health services [2, 59, 62].

A Case Study
Illustrating the Use of the Range of
Response to Loss Model in Practice

The case study below illustrates how the RRL framework can be incorporated into practice.

CASE STUDY

Roger is 47 and his wife Elizabeth is 48; they have two daughters, Marie and Jayne who are in their early 20's. Elizabeth was diagnosed with Motor Neurone Disease four years ago. Her condition has deteriorated and she now requires support with all of her activities of daily living, including communicating.

Roger has recently made the decision to give up his job as director of a large electrical engineering business. Although they have a small family network, Elizabeth has a strong network of friends who visit regularly. Elizabeth knows she is dying – she has spoken openly about this, expressing her thoughts and feelings, wishes for the future, and has planned for not being part of her daughters' future lives by leaving gifts for future life milestones. Although she does not have a conventional religious faith she has spoken about her own parent's death and how she believes that they will be reunited one day. At times she has been extremely expressive of her emotions which have ranged from anger, sadness, and despair. Roger's reactions and responses are very different. He finds it difficult to talk with Elizabeth about what is happening, he prefers to focus on being positive and encouraging the family members to "be strong" and not upset each other. He focuses a lot on the practical aspects of her condition and care. He has undertaken copious amounts of research and frequently seeks information. He says that he knows Elizabeth is dying but feels they should not waste time and energy on things which cannot be changed. Often this difference in approach creates tensions between the two which Elizabeth finds emotionally difficult and frustrating. This can lead to periods of anxiety and breathlessness as she is worried that he is not coping as he does not talk about things. **He is worried that she is not coping when she becomes emotional.**

Assessment: starting points – practitioners should consider:

Background factors:
- Culture, ethnicity, religion.
- Current circumstances e.g., roles and responsibilities, relationships, support networks, health, employment.
- Previous experience of dealing with loss situations (observed), personal strength/vulnerability.

The case study demonstrates how family cultural differences and background might be influencing the responses to loss shown by Roger and Elizabeth. Roger's belief in being strong for others, apparent lack of social support and recent concurrent losses of his job and associated status are all likely to be influencing his response. This contrasts to Elizabeth who can make meaning out of her experience, drawing on her previous experiences of loss and support network.

Which grief reactions and coping responses can be observed, using the RRL as a guide? (See Figure 2).
- What are Elizabeth's and Roger's immediate and instinctive reaction to loss, overwhelmed, or controlled?
- Do you see evidence of resilience? An ability to manage both the feelings and day-to-day functioning.
- Is there evidence of vulnerability? Think about what the nature of this vulnerability is.

Some practice conclusions from the case study:

- **Elizabeth** has moved beyond her immediate reactions and the distress (understandable and normal), and her illness has changed to a position where she is coping with its consequences; accepting her feelings and addressing the reality of her situation evidenced through the plans she is making for the family – a demonstration of resilience.
- **Roger's** core reactions are controlling, and these are expressed by avoidance of his own feelings about Elizabeth's illness. Avoidance continues as a way of coping which does not allow for real engagement with either the emotional or practical consequences of Elizabeth's illness – a demonstration of vulnerability.
- **The difference in coping style between Elizabeth and Roger** contributes to tension in their relationship.

The practitioner needs to consider:
- What might the challenges be for how you respond to a patient or carer who deals with situations differently from the way you do?
- Is your natural style of reacting or coping with loss more like Elizabeth or Roger? How might this support or challenge how you respond?

- How might I work with Elizabeth and Roger?

What might support for Elizabeth include? What might support for Roger include? Might I enable them to recognise each other's needs?

Being empathic with a person's instinctive grief reactions and coping style is important in helping them feel respected and understood. This will help develop rapport between the practitioner and the patient/carer/bereaved. It is the starting point for engaging with the more difficult adjustments to reality which are being faced. Helping in this process of adjustment involves:
- for those overwhelmed by grief finding new strategies for coping with day-to-day life.
- for those controlling their grief, finding a safe space in which to face painful feelings [63].

What does this approach mean for Elizabeth and Roger?
- Elizabeth has, for the moment, moved into a positive coping phase but may return to a more emotion focused reaction (overwhelmed) as her illness progresses. At this point she will need space and support in facing up to the losses resulting from changes or deterioration in her health. For practitioners this will mean a willingness to acknowledge and empathise with her emotional responses which may, for a time take precedence over finding ways of reasserting her resilience.
- Roger's need for control is unlikely to make it easy for him to address feelings directly. Recognising and empathising with this starting point will help build a relationship of trust in which Roger might begin to feel safe opening up about his feelings. This can sometimes happen almost as an afterthought as a person, in passing, acknowledges the reality of their unspoken distress.

In palliative care, the fluctuations in loss and grief across the Bereavement Pathway means that there will be a continuous need for assessment and review.

Attention to the Family System

The case study illustrates both the individual and family experience of grief. The difference in coping between Roger and Elizabeth is creating tension within the family system. Figure 4 depicts Elizabeth's and Roger's family relationships and how this can be represented in the RRL framework. Practitioners play an important role within the tripartite system of family, carer, and practitioner. This can be a positive role facilitating open communication and understanding between family members. The challenge for practitioners is significant but the rewards in alleviating the tension that Joyce observed (at the beginning of the chapter) will be significant and

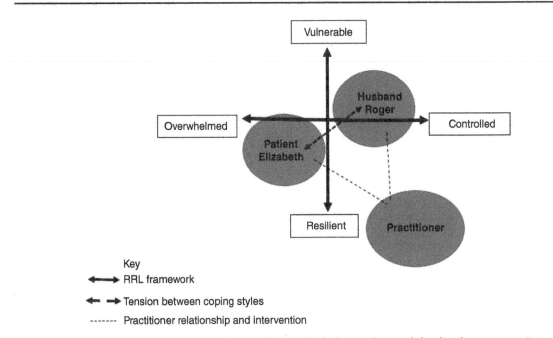

Figure 4   Case study: understanding a system approach and the RRL Elizabeth spans the overwhelmed/resilient categories. Roger is controlled/vulnerable. The practitioner role is attempting to maintain a controlled/resilient perspective.

important for Roger when he ultimately has to deal with Elizabeth's death.

Using the AAG and AHC for Assessment and Therapeutic Support

Where a patient/carer/bereaved person is showing heightened vulnerability, for example like Roger in the case study, further support may be required. When referral to a level 3 practitioner is thought to be required, the reasons this might be helpful should be discussed with the patient/carer and their agreement obtained to access more specialist help. The AAG or AHC can be used for deeper more focused work with patients, carers, or bereaved relatives. A training framework and induction into the use of the AAG and AHC is available. For further information on using the AAG as an assessment tool see https://mapping-grief.care.

What Support Might the Practitioner Need?

The challenging nature of working with multiple and diverse grief responses to loss is reflected in Joyce's quote at the beginning of the chapter. It is essential that healthcare organisations take responsibility to ensure that practitioners who are working with palliative care patients and their families are provided with regular and appropriate opportunities for clinical supervision or informal opportunities to debrief, reflect, and receive support.

Conclusion

The experiences of death, dying, and bereavement challenge fundamental beliefs and attitudes to what it means to be human, resulting in considerable levels of potential disorientation and distress or for positive personal growth [23]. We have explored these experiences through the lens of loss and grief along the Bereavement Pathway recognising grief as the normal response to loss. Although the full impact on long-term vulnerability and resilience has yet to be established, it is clear that there will be implications for practice approaches in both end-of-life care and bereavement care [64]. The ability to understand and support the diverse grief responses, enhance resilience, and identify those who are vulnerable to the negative impact of the experiences of loss and grief, is an important, but often hidden aspect of palliative care which practitioners can find challenging [1, 2]. The RRL provides a conceptual framework which can underpin practice when working with patients and family members facing death, dying, and bereavement. This approach along with addressing loss and grief from both an individual and wider family perspective, is being adopted in a number of hospice settings. Where this is being used the experience demonstrates the value of this method of engaging with patient and carer needs across the Bereavement Pathway.

References

1. Pearce, C., Honey, J.R., Lovick, R. et al. (2021). A silent epidemic of grief: A survey of bereavement care provision in the UK and Ireland during the COVID-19 pandemic. *BMJ Open* 11.
2. Breen, L.J. and Aoun, S.M. (2018). Bereavement care. In: *Palliative Care Nursing. Principles and Evidence for Practice*, 3e (ed. C. Walshe, N. Preston, and B. Johnston), 322–339. London: Open University Press.
3. Thompson, N. (ed.) (2002). *Loss and Grief: A Guide for Human Services Practitioners*. Basingstoke: PALGRAVE.
4. Bereavement Services Association and Cruse Bereavement Care. (2013). *Bereavement care service standards*. Available from: https://nationalbereavementalliance.org.uk/bereavement-pathway (accessed 3 November 2022).
5. Machin, L. (2014). *Working with Loss and Grief: A Theoretical and Practical Approach*, 2e. London: Sage.
6. Altschuler, J. (2005). Illness and loss within the family. In: *Loss, Change and Bereavement in Palliative Care* (ed. P. Firth, G. Luff, and D. Oliviere), 53–65. Maidenhead: Open University Press.
7. Kalish, R. 2016. Death, grief and caring relationships. In: *Grief is a Journey. Finding Your Path through Loss* (Cited by K.J. Doka), 211. New York: Atria.
8. Zhai, Y. and Du, X. (2020). Loss and grief amidst COVID-19: A path to adaptation and resilience. *Brain, Behavior and Injury* 87: 80–81.
9. Folkman, S. (2001). Revised coping theory and the process of bereavement. In: *Handbook of Bereavement Research* (ed. M.S. Stroebe, R.O. Hansson, and H. Schut), 563–584. Washington DC: American Psychological Association.
10. Doka, K.J. (ed.) (2007). *Living with Grief before and after the Death*. Washington DC: Hospice Foundation of America.
11. Quinn, A. (2005). The context of loss, change and bereavement in palliative care. In: *Loss, Change and Bereavement in Palliative Care* (ed. P. Firth, G. Luff, and D. Oliviere), 1–18. Maidenhead: Open University Press.
12. Holland, J.C., Andersen, B., Breitbart, W.S. et al. (2010). Distress c guidelines in oncology. *Journal of the National Comprehensive Cancer Network* 8 (4): 448–485.
13. Worden, J.W. (2009). *Grief Counselling and Grief Therapy*, 4e. New York: Springer.
14. Stroebe, M.S., Hansson, R.O., Schut, H., and Stroebe, W. (2008). Bereavement research: Contemporary perspectives. In: *Handbook of Bereavement Research and Practice. Advances in Theory and Intervention* (ed. M.S. Stroebe, R.O. Hansson, H. Schut, and W. Stroebe), 3–25. Washington: American Psychological Association.
15. Snowden, A., White, C.A., Christie, Z. et al.(2011). The clinical utility of the distress thermometer: A review. *British Journal of Nursing* 20 (4): 220–227.
16. Stajduhar, K., Funk, L., Toye, C. et al.(2010). Part 1: Home-based family caregiving at the end of life: A comprehensive review of published quantitative research (1998–2008). *Pall Medical* 25 (6): 573–593.
17. Aoun, S., Kristjanson, L.J., Currow, D.C., and Hudson, P.L. (2005). Caregiving for the terminally ill: At what cost? *Pall Medical* 19 (7): 551–555.
18. Shear, M.K. (2015). Complicated grief. *New England Journal of Medicine* 372: 153–160.
19. Shear, M.K., Boelen, P.A., and Neimeyer, R.A. (2011). Treating complicated grief: Converging approaches. In: *Grief and Bereavement in Contemporary Society* (ed. R.A. Neimeyer, D.L. Harris, H.R. Winokuer, and G.F. Thornton), 139–162. New York: Routledge.
20. Prigerson, H.G., Horowitz, M.J., Jacobs, S.C., Parkes, C.M., Aslan, M., Goodkin, K. et al. (2009). Prolonged grief disorder: Psychometric validation of criteria proposed for DSM-V and ICD-11. *PLoS Medicine* 6 (8): 1–12.
21. Bonanno, G.A. (2004). Loss, trauma and human resilience. *American Psychologist* 59 (1): 302–311.
22. Greene, R. (2002). Holocaust survivors: A study in resilience. *Journal of Gerontological Social Work* 37 (1): sourced from (PDF) Holocaust Survivors: A Study in Resilience | Roberta R Greene – https://Academia.edu.
23. Seligman, M.E.P. and Csikszentmihalyi, M. (2000). Positive psychology: An introduction. *American Psychologist* 55 (1): 5–14.
24. Stroebe, M. and Schut, H. (1999). The dual process model of coping with bereavement: Rationale and description. *Death Studies* 23 (3): 197–224.
25. Doka, K.J. (2016). *Grief Is a Journey. Finding Your Path through Loss*. New York: Atria.
26. Davis, C.G. (2008). Redefining goals and redefining self: A closer look at posttraumatic growth following loss. In: *Handbook of Bereavement Research and Practice* (ed. M.S. Stroebe, R.O. Hansson, H. Schut, and W. Stroebe), 309–327. Washington DC: American Psychological. Association.
27. Lobb, E.A., Kristjanson, L.J., Aoun, S.M. et al. (2010). Predictors of complicated grief: A systematic review of empirical studies. *Death Studies* 34 (8): 673–698.
28. White, C.A. (2018). Psychological symptoms and the promotion of psychological well-being. In: *Palliative Care Nursing: Principles and Evidence for Practice*, 3e (ed. C.

Walshe, N. Preston, and B. Johnston), 158–170. London: Open University Press.

29. Blackburn, P. and Dwyer, K. (2017). A bereavement common assessment framework in palliative care: Informing practice, transforming care. *Am J Hospice Pall Care* 34 (7): 677–684.

30. Sanders, C.M. (1993). Risk factors in bereavement outcome. In: *Handbook of Bereavement* (ed. M.S. Stroebe, W. Stroebe, and R.O. Hansson), 255–267. Cambridge: Cambridge University Press.

31. Neimeyer, R.A. (2000). Searching for the meaning of meaning: Grief therapy and the process of reconstruction. *Death Studies* 24 (6): 541–558.

32. Freud, S. (1917). *Mourning and Melancholia, Collected Papers*, Vol. 4. New York: Basic Books.

33. Kubler-Ross, E. (1969). *On Death and Dying*. New York: Macmillan.

34. Bowlby, J. (1984). *Attachment and Loss: Vol.1. Attachment*, 2e. Harmondsworth: Penguin.

35. Stroebe, M., Schut, H., and Boerner, K. (2017). Models of coping with bereavement an updated overview. *Studies In Psychology* 38 (3): 582–607.

36. Hall, C. (2010). Bereavement theory: Recent developments in our understanding of grief and bereavement. *Bereavement Care* 33 (1): 7–12.

37. Walter, T. (1999). *On Bereavement*. Buckingham: Open University Press.

38. Dodd, A., Guerin, S., Delaney, S., and Dodd, P. (2017). Complicated grief: Knowledge, attitudes, skills and training of mental health professionals. A systematic review. *Patient Education and Counselling* 100 (8): 1447–1458.

39. Payne, S. (2004). Overview. Loss and Bereavement. In: *Palliative Care Nursing. Principles and Evidence for Practice* (ed. S. Payne, J. Seymlour, and C. Ingleton), 435–462. Maidenhead: Open University Press.

40. Machin, L. (2001). *Exploring a framework for understanding the range of response to loss: a study of clients receiving bereavement counselling*. Unpublished PhD thesis. UK: Keele University.

41. Ainsworth, M.D.S., Blehar, M.C., Waters, E., and Wall, S. (1978). *Patterns of Attachment: A Psychological Study of the Strange Situation*. Hillsdale NJ: Erlbaum.

42. Sim, J., Machin, L., and Bartlam, B. (2014). Identifying vulnerability in grief: Psychometric properties of the adult attitude to grief scale. *Quality of Life Research* 23 (4): 1211–1215.

43. Lloyd- Williams, M. (2004). Emotions and cognitions. Psychological aspects of care. In: *Palliative Care Nursing. Principles and Evidence for Practice* (ed. S. Payne, J. Seymlour, and C. Ingleton), 299–312. Maidenhead: Open University Press.

44. Harding, S. (2021). *Hear Me Out. My Story, My Words, My Life*. London: Ebury Press.

45. Corr, C.A. (2007). Anticipatory grief and mourning. An overview. In: *Living with Grief before and after the Death* (ed.

K.J. Doka), 5–20. Washington DC: Hospice Foundation of America.

46. Nielsen, M.K., Neergaard, M.A., Jensen, A.B. et al. (2016). Do we need to change our understanding of anticipatory grief in caregivers? A systematic review of caregiver studies during end-of-life caregiving and bereavement. *Clinical Psychology Review* 44: 75–93.

47. Machin, L. (2018). Understanding and assessing grief and bereavement. In: *Palliative Care Nursing: Principles and Evidence for Practice*, 3e (ed. C. Walshe, N. Preston, and B. Johnston), 301–321. London: Open University Press.

48. Aujoulat, I., Luminet, O., and Decache, A. (2007). The perspectives of patients on their experience of powerlessness. *Qual Health Research* 17 (6): 772–785.

49. Kinghorn, S. and Duncan, F. (2005). Living with loss. In: *Palliative Care the Nursing Role* (ed. J. Lugton and R. McIntyre), 303–337. Edinburgh: Elsevier Churchill Livingstone.

50. Braine, M.E. and Wray, J. (2016). *Supporting Families and Carers: A Nursing Perspective*. Boca Raton, FL: CRC Press.

51. Didion, J. (2005). *The Year of Magical Thinking*. London: Fourth estate.

52. Witt Sherman, D. and Free, D. (2015). Culture and spirituality as domains of quality palliative care. In: *Palliative Care Nursing Quality Care to the End of Life*, 4e (ed. M. Matzo and D. Witt Sherman), 170–235. New York: Springer.

53. Papadatou, D. (2009). *In the Face of Death*. New York: Springer.

54. Soto-Rubio, A., Perez-Marin, M., Miguel, J.T., and Martin, P.B. (2018). Emotional distress of patients at end-of-life and their caregivers: Interrelation and predictors. *Frontiers in Psychology* 9: article 2199.

55. Kissane, D.W. and Parnes, F. (ed.) (2014). *Bereavement Care for Families*. New York: Routledge.

56. McLaughlin, D. and Nyatanga, B. (2018). Palliative care for those in disadvantaged groups. In: *Palliative Care Nursing: Principles and Evidence for Practice*, 3e (ed. C. Walshe, N. Preston, and B. Johnston), 221–239. London: Open University Press.

57. Payne, S., Horn, S., and Relf, M. (1999). *Loss and Bereavement*. Buckingham: Open University Press.

58. Monroe, B. and Oliviere, D. (2009). Communicating with family carers. In: *Family Carers in Palliative Care* (ed. P. Hudson and S. Payne), 1–20. Oxford: Oxford University Press.

59. Stevens, E. (2018). Communication and palliative care nursing. In: *Palliative Care Nursing: Principles and Evidence for Practice*, 3e (ed. C. Walshe, N. Preston, and B. Johnston), 117–33. London: Open University Press.

60. Walter, T. (2010). Grief and culture: A checklist. *Bereavement Care* 29 (2): 5–9.

61. National Institute for Clinical Excellence. (2004). *Guidance on Cancer Services: Improving Supportive and Palliative Care for Adults with Cancer. The Manual.* London: NICE.

62. Aoun, S.M., Breen, L.J., O'Connor, M. et al. (2012). A public health approach to bereavement support services in palliative care. *Australian and New Zealand Journal of Public Health* 36 (1): 14–16.

63. Schut, H.A.W., Stroebe, M.S., Van den Bout, J., and de Keijser, J. (1997). Intervention for the bereaved: Gender differences in the efficacy of two counselling programmes. *British Journal of Clinical Psychology* 36 (10): 63–72.

64. Harrop, E., Farnell, D., Longo, M. et al. (2020). *Supporting people bereaved during COVID-19: Study Report 1*, 27 November. Cardiff University and the University of Bristol.

9 Recognising Deterioration, Preparing and Planning for Dying

Jo Wilson and Sarah Russell

Death is inevitable, but the time before, is not.
– Sarah Russell, Handbook of Palliative Care

Introduction

In this chapter, we explore why it is important to recognise the possibility of deterioration and dying in an adult patient. We consider the concept of advance care planning, its terminology, and definitions. We go on to think about how we can recognise people who are approaching the end of their lives and the tools that can be used to aid this process. We cover the responsibility for advance care planning; how to start conversations and the importance of a relational approach by clinicians individually and as part of the wider health-care system in both updating care plans and acting on them at appropriate points of clinical deterioration. We discuss that advance care planning is a complex health intervention and the benefits and challenges with this intervention. We recommend advance care planning as a public health approach much earlier in the life course, where this is culturally acceptable, rather than at times of clinical deterioration, and the need for clinicians to hone their communication skills and comfort in this aspect of care. Throughout the chapter we use the term "family" to represent family and friends who matter to patients.

Why It Is Important to Recognise that People May Be in the Last Years of Their Lives

It is important to recognise when people are entering the latter stages of their life, in order to understand "what matters to the person" and that appropriate treatments are offered that bring benefits to the person's life and that the side effects are tolerable. This is illustrated by The National Confidential Enquiry into Patient Outcomes and Death undertaken in 2008, which recognised that patients were receiving systemic anti-cancer therapy in the last 30 days of life, when dying could have been recognised, and 43% died with grade 3 or 4 treatment toxicity and such things as needing blood transfusions [1]. These deaths were made more uncomfortable due to unrealistic active medical intervention. This is now recognised for patients with other diseases, for example those with dementia and an impaired swallow, where the introduction of an enteral feeding tube is rarely indicated, and risk feeding is a way forward that promotes quality of life for the time that is remaining, and care can more easily be provided outside of a hospital setting [2]. Another example is the importance of minimising polypharmacy as a person becomes frailer, for their health to be maintained and to lessen the patient and carer burden in terms of medication management [3].

It is relevant to think through the last years, months, and days in a planned manner wherever possible, as people are living longer, with multi-morbidity. This means that rather than a predictable "end-of-life" trajectory, many people suffer with acute exacerbations of illnesses such as heart failure, respiratory failure and renal disease. At any one of those moments' hospital clinicians cannot be certain patients will "pull through" despite offering optimal treatment. In the UK one of the aims of "good end-of-life care" is that patients experience less than three admissions to hospital in the last 90 days of life and spend more of the last 90 days outside of hospital [4].

Thinking ahead with patients and their families in a planned rather than a crisis-based manner means that their wishes, choices, and needs can be identified and accessed earlier to support them in receiving care in their preferred

Handbook of Palliative Care, Fourth Edition. Edited by Richard Kitchen, Christina Faull, Sarah Russell and Jo Wilson.
© 2024 John Wiley & Sons Ltd. Published 2024 by John Wiley & Sons Ltd.

place of death (e.g. home, hospice, or care home). This may include accessing fast track funding for care home or community support, financial assessment, equipment (e.g. hospital beds), community/district nursing and General Practitioner care, specialist palliative care, or hospice at home services, packages of care, referral for inpatient hospice care as well as supporting and preparing family members in their role as informal carers. This needs careful negotiation [5]. It is important for the patient and those around them to have a sense of emotional safety and security. It is key to the patient being able to remain at home [6] or their preferred place of care.

Recognising when a person may be entering the latter stages of their lives helps them and their families to plan and prepare for dying and bereavement. It is useful to think through such things as who can represent them, how to manage finances, write a will, consider the care of dependents such as pets, prepare young children in the family etc. and to consider all things held digitally such as photos and bitcoins (https://www.moneysavingexpert.com/family/death-plan and https://digitallegacyassociation.org/framework).

It is helpful for the bereaved if "dealing with the affairs" is as straightforward as it can be, as well as offering information to family members about what to do when their loved one has died. For example, if in hospital or care home, how long can they stay to say goodbye, what care is provided after death and what is the process to collect the death certificate. If death is at home, this may include offering advice about having a deceased person at home, and the process of care after death—verification, calling the funeral director, and calling the General Practitioner for Medical Certification of the Cause of Death.

Advance Care Planning

Advance care planning is a specific type of personalised care and support planning that focuses on preferences and decisions about future end-of-life care [7]. In 2017 an overarching international consensus definition of advance care planning was achieved [8]. The definition (Figure 1) has a focus on ongoing individualised support and communication for decision-making [8, 9].

The evolvement of the consensus statement, away from the narrow focus on decisions made in advance and appointment of surrogate decision makers, to wider social, emotional, and spiritual considerations including the quality of communication between the individual and people likely to be involved in health care decisions is welcomed as it enables a broader, relational consideration of

> *Advance care planning is a process that supports adults at any age or stage of health in understanding and sharing their personal values, life goals, and preferences regarding future medical care. The goal of advance care planning is to help ensure that people receive medical care that is consistent with their values, goals, and preferences during serious and chronic illness.*

Figure 1 Advance care planning consensus definition [8].

the complexity of advance care planning [7, 10]. This is further illustrated by recent reflections on high quality advance care planning who comment this includes past experiences and quality of life as well as individuals working with their families and proxy decision makers to reduce or prevent conflict [11].

The output of advance care planning is often described as an advance care plan which may include some or many of the aspects illustrated in Figure 2. The advance care plan can be a "live document" for a person when they have capacity, but it more helpfully comes into play if the person has lost the mental capacity to make decisions. The language around advance care planning needs clarifying at this point.

In 2022, NHS England published the Universal Principles of Advance Care Planning [12]. The purpose of this document is to set out six high-level principles for advance care planning in England. The principles are for the person, those important to them, practitioners, and notably also for organisations involved in supporting advance care planning conversations and honouring their outcomes. What is important to note is that people are supported to speak up if an individualised approach is not taken to advance care planning. The principles were written in response to the Care Quality report (2021) [13] that found that during COVID-19 advance decisions were not always personalised. The six principles are:

1. The person is central to developing and agreeing their advance care plan including deciding who else should be involved in the process.

2. The person has personalised conversations about their future care focused on what matters to them and their needs.

3. The person agrees the outcomes of their advance care planning conversation through a shared decision-making process in partnership with relevant professionals.

4. The person has a shareable advance care plan which records what matters to them, and their preferences and decisions about future care and treatment.

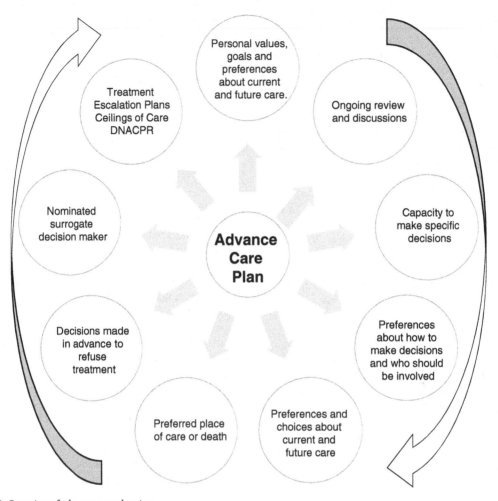

Figure 2 Overview of advance care planning.

5. The person has the opportunity, and is encouraged, to review and revise their advance care plan.

6. Anyone involved in advance care planning can speak up if they feel that these universal principles are not being followed.

Terminology and Definitions

Internationally, there are a variety of ways that advance care planning can be expressed. It is useful to be familiar with your own region or countries formats.

In England and Wales, advance care planning maybe expressed by, for example:

1. Advance Statements indicate an individual's preferences for care; they are not legally binding. In the United States, this may be known as a values history.

2. Advance Refusals of Future Treatment. In England and Wales, the advance decision to refuse treatment (ADRT) is a legally binding record of informed consent for withholding or withdrawal of certain treatments, including life-sustaining measures, under particular health scenarios. For the withholding or withdrawal of life-sustaining measures, the records must be in writing and signed by both the individual and a witness and include the term *even if my life is at risk*.

3. Proxies or Surrogate Decision Makers may be appointed. Surrogate decision makers in England and Wales are known as Lasting Powers of Attorney for Health and Welfare, and Lasting Power of Attorney for Property and Financial Affairs (see https://www.gov.uk/power-of-attorney). Elsewhere these may be known as Welfare Powers of Attorney (Scotland https://www.publicguardian-scotland.gov.uk/power-of-attorney); Durable Powers of Attorney for Health Care (Australia, Canada, and United States), or Representatives (Canada). These appointments may pertain to decision making for health and welfare and/or property/financial matters. Where appointments are made for health and welfare decisions, there will usually be a requirement to assign specific decision-making rights over life-sustaining measures.

Assessing mental capacity

England and Wales—Mental Capacity Act 2005
Northern Ireland—Mental Capacity Act 2016
Ireland—Assisted Decision Making (Capacity) Act 2015
Scotland—Adults with Incapacity Act 2000

In England and Wales there is a four-step process to assessing mental capacity. These steps are that the individual can understand the information given to them, retain that information, use and weigh the information to formulate a decision; and are able to communicate back that decision. All clinicians can contribute to an assessment of mental capacity, and it is helpful if it is a multidisciplinary decision. It is usual to have local policies and documentation in place. Considering capacity in advance care planning conversations, decisions, and documents is key to best practice regardless of diagnosis, prognosis, or the type of decision. The Mental Capacity Act (2005) emphasises that: *a person is not to be treated as unable to make a decision unless all practicable steps to help them do so have been taken without success.* (Principle 2, section 1(3), Mental Capacity Act 2005). In addition, enabling advocacy, supporting autonomy, and a framework to make decisions in the individuals' best interests are necessary.

It is vital that advance care planning considerations are considered early for patients whose mental functioning is likely to become increasingly impaired e.g. those with a new diagnosis of dementia, or who may have a neurological disease that will affect their expression of their capacious decisions e.g. those with a diagnosis of motor neurone disease. There are good examples and best practice recommendations of how this can be undertaken for patients with dementia [14] and by the motor neurone disease association:

https://www.mndassociation.org/professionals/management-of-mnd/management-by-symptoms/palliative-and-end-of-life-care.

It can also be challenging for patients who have no family or anyone who they can identify as able to represent them from their community. At times of crisis in the UK there is access to an Independent Mental Capacity Advocate (IMCA), although this is a Monday to Friday 9–5 service (https://www.scie.org.uk/mca/imca/do). It is important clinical work to help patients who are alone to think through their advance care plans prior to losing capacity.

The pre-emptive work undertaken by a person carrying out advance care planning for themselves, can be yielded by understanding the level of extreme diligence and attention in any best interest scenario. A best interest scenario is where the patient does not have mental capacity for a particular decision, and others known to the patient contribute to the decision-making process. The consultant or GP has responsibility for this. The complexities of this are beautifully documented in the article by Derek Wade [15].

A best interests meeting should consider for every decision the following:

The person's beliefs, wishes, feelings, values and any other factors they would consider if they were able to do so. Their current quality of life, best broken down into personal experiences; pain, distress, pleasure and happiness. Functional autonomy; the behaviours and goals within their capacity. Social interaction: roles, availability of others to interact with. Meaning in life; having future expectations and wishes. Their potential future quality of life (as they would see it) judged on same features, including the effect of any possible change in placement. The effect of any intervention, or stopping of any intervention, considered in probabilistic terms covering: Risks, pain, time taken, distress etc, set against the effect on one or more aspects of quality of life, broken down as above, and likely length of life.

In principle, each decision should be articulated as what the person would decide, were they able to, given the facts about their situation, prognosis and treatment considered at the meeting. At the end of the meeting, it is vital to: State explicitly what has been decided, checking that all agree and understand and if there was disagreement, then the reasons behind the decision must also be made explicit publicly. Either, if there is agreement confirm: What actions will follow, including: who will undertake them, and when by, and when the next meeting will be specifying either a date, time and place, or an event that will precipitate a meeting. In the case of disagreement, specify what the next steps will be, usually one or more of: Obtaining

further information and/or a further opinion, and/or involving a mediation expert, and/or starting the process of involving the Court of Protection. Confirm that a documented record will be written and distributed to all present and agree who else will get a copy.
[15, p. 1582]

The process for enacting an advance care plan for a person who has lost mental capacity for the relevant decision is helpfully described by NHS Cheshire and Merseyside Strategic Clinical Network [16]:

What is possible for these patients, however, is care planning as part of the best interest decision making process; this can be drawn from their previous wishes informally from their statement or formally from an Advance Decision to Refuse Treatment. An advance care plan is only a plan that helps inform decisions in future circumstances; it does not replace clinical decision making or the responsibility of the clinician when a decision is needed (except for a patient's advance decision to refuse a specified treatment (ADRT), if valid and applicable). It does not need to be used when patients still have capacity.
[16, p. 13]

Outcomes

Ahead of the discussions on the benefits and disadvantages of care planning, it is really important to note that there is lack of standardised outcomes for advance care planning. In a recent scoping review 170 outcomes were identified across a range of studies [7]. The authors of this scoping review argue for future research to consider the *Six Pillars of Advance Care Planning* which refer to key stakeholders or potential intervention targets: patients, surrogates, community, clinicians, health systems, and policy. They suggest each "pillar" may need its own tailored interventions and outcomes for which the intervention can reasonably be expected to affect.

Person-centred outcome measures (PCOMs) such as Palliative phase of illness, Australia-modified Karnofsky Performance Status and Integrated Palliative Care Outcome Scores are being variably used currently to identify, monitor, and direct clinical action to address the needs and symptoms of an individual and facilitate communication between patients and clinicians. These measures are based on what patients and their families prioritise as important in advanced illness and have been endorsed by NHS England and Public Health England. In

an outcome study, there is consideration as to how all of these PCOMs can be consistently delivered at individual/patient assessment level, team (e.g. focusing patient reviews and workload planning), service (e.g. service evaluation/development and making business cases) and population (e.g. benchmarking) levels of practice [17].

Benefits and Challenges of Advance Care Planning

Benefits of Advance Care Planning

There is evidence that advance care planning improves goals of care concordance because of ongoing discussion, review and documentation of preferences and decisions. This means wishes and choices can be implemented if or when an individual may not be able to express them themselves [9]. Other benefits include the production of advance directives (an international generic term representing decisions written in advance to refuse specific treatments), ceilings of medical treatment decisions, treatment escalation plans (TEP), and DNACPR decisions [12]. Commentators report that advance care planning increases satisfaction with care, reduces stress, anxiety, and depression in bereaved family members [18], as well reducing health care costs and the number of hospital admissions in the last year of life [19].

The COVID-19 pandemic emphasised the value of advance care planning conversations to provide clarity about a patient's choice, increase autonomy, and prevent crisis decision making [20]. This has been especially relevant with the absence of "in person" surrogate decision makers or family in hospital and residential care settings (due to social distancing restrictions) to articulate, contribute to, and support decision making [21]. Early advance care planning discussion is recommended between patients, families, and clinicians to minimise potential future misunderstandings or conflict at the time of clinical deterioration [22]. Although it is recognised that patients can change their mind at the point of clinical deterioration, which points to the importance of their relationship with their clinicians, and the clinician's ability to discuss this [23].

Challenges with Advance Care Planning

There are a number of challenges. In hospital settings where people are unwell, researchers have found that clinician's sensitivity and communication skills, time to have these conversations, support for any agreed plan, and the need to involve family as patients did not have capacity, which affected the ability to think meaningfully together about the future [24]. Also, because clinicians change rapidly it affected the handover of any agreed plans, which speaks to both the importance of individual relationship and to the need for consistent system relationship with the patient via accessible handover information. There are additional human factors which can negatively impact on patients being able to receive their own advance care plan e.g. staff confidence to trust previous advance care planning documentation, and clinicians' ability to act on previously recorded information [25].

There remains the challenge that a person continues to evolve in their life despite maybe losing their capacity for significant and specific decisions e.g. facilities, new pastimes can give new pleasures, and the person wishes and decisions may have changed since when they first expressed or documented them. This reinforces the need for the continued relationship and understanding with the clinical team and family.

Internationally there is low uptake of advance care planning. Much of the research is from high income countries with a focus on autonomy and individual decision-making, and discussions primarily on the refusal of health-care interventions—assuming that such interventions are available [26]. There is less attention paid to the

> **Box 1: Case study—"the consequences of no advance care planning"**
>
> Shaan was an 89-year-old gentleman, who lived in a Local Authority owned flat. His nephew lived with him and assisted with activities of daily living. Shaan had started haemodialysis fifteen years earlier due to advanced renal disease. He tolerated three times a week dialysis well, but over the previous five years had a progressive dementia. He and his nephew had a close relationship. Sadly, it was only as Shaan became too unwell to tolerate dialysis (he needed an ambulance to get him to and from dialysis, he was agitated on dialysis, and his oral intake was incredibly small) that conversations were started about the future. Shaan did not have mental capacity to take part in conversations about treatment options, which resulted in his nephew being involved in decisions in a best interests manner. Facing the loss of his uncle, plus his home and his source of financial support was incredibly stressful for the nephew and required much support. It was challenging to provide support in bereavement to accommodate the loss as Shaan's nephew was occupied in locating a new home, finding income, etc.

> **Box 2: Case study—"the consequences of advance care planning"**
>
> Michael was a 38 year old man with motor neurone disease. He lived at home with his wife and three children. He worked as a computer programmer until his disease process rendered him dependent on daily care. He arranged for his wife to have Lasting Power of Attorney for health and welfare, and finance. He applied for a personal health budget as he wanted to organise the meeting of his own care needs at the times of the day that suited him. He had completed an ADRT for Do Not Attempt Cardio-Pulmonary Resuscitation (DNACPR). He had a PEG tube for feeding. He was open to the treatment of Non-Invasive Ventilation if it was required. His wife, his children, and his regular carers, alongside his GP, respiratory consultants and palliative care team knew his wishes to be managed at home if possible. Ultimately, he died at home, with his symptoms managed and with his family with him. He lived as well as he was able, being in control, working and providing for his family until very late in the disease trajectory, the family were provided with bereavement support.

family or relational influence on how people make decisions about their future care [26, 27]. Researchers report numerous inconsistencies e.g. advance care planning document completion, behaviour change, health-care utilisation and care consistent with individual goals [8]. This means it is difficult to compare clinical initiatives, programmes, tools, or research findings across organisations, care settings, and regions. Furthermore, there are no widely accepted guidelines on how to implement advance care planning. More research is needed to set appropriate expectations of outcomes, standardize outcomes across studies, as well as tailor interventions and outcomes to local environmental resources and contexts [7, 28]. Two case studies are provided (Box 1 and Box 2) to illustrate the complexities of advance care planning.

Recognising People Who Are Approaching the Latter Stages of Their Lives

There are many screening tools and processes that if systematically applied help clinicians identify those people who may benefit from a conversation about the future However, many clinicians trust their "gut instinct" [29] before going onto systematically screen the patient with a recognised tool. Clinicians who have honed their skills in

---

Table 1 Examples of tools and processes to identify palliative and advance care planning needs and communicate uncertainty.

Integrated Palliative care Outcome Scale (IPOS) [31]

Holistic, well-validated, and global measure of symptom burden that uses 10 questions (scored on a 0–4 Likert-type scale) to assess the most important symptoms and concerns of patients affected by life-limiting illnesses across physical, psychological, social and existential domains of well-being.

Australia-modified Karnofsky Performance Scale (AKPS) [32]

Assessment of patient' overall performance/functional status across three dimensions: activity, work and self-care.

Palliative Phase of Illness (POI) [33]

Measure which describes the urgency of care needs for a person receiving palliative care.

Key Information Summaries (KIS) [34]

Anticipatory care plans written by general practitioners (GPs) could be routinely shared electronically and updated in real time, between GPs and providers of unscheduled and secondary care.

Amber Care Bundle: Patients whose recovery is uncertain [35]

To improve the quality of care for inpatients whose potential for recovery is uncertain and may be approaching the end of their lives despite treatment. It gives staff the opportunity to involve patients and their families in discussions about treatment and future care.

Supportive and Palliative Care Indicators Tool (SPICT) [36]

Helps identify people with deteriorating health due to one or more advanced conditions or a new serious illness so they benefit from holistic assessment and future care planning.

Gold Standards Framework Prognostic Indicator Guidance and the Surprise Question [37]

Predicting needs rather than exact prognostication including the Surprise Question: "Would you be surprised if this patient were to die in the next few months, weeks, days?"

The Multidimensional Prognostic Index (MPI), based on a Comprehensive Geriatric Assessment (CGA) [38]

The MPI assesses eight domains relating to functional, cognitive, and nutritional conditions, comorbidities, and pressure sore risk. It also considers clinical issues such as medication, and social aspects.

Palliative Care Needs Rounds [39]

Triage meetings with care home staff and specialist palliative care clinicians, focusing on residents at risk of dying without a plan in place.

Resident Assessment Instrument (RAI) [30]

Structured, standardised approach for care home staff to gather information on a resident's strengths and needs and identify problems.

Prognosis in Palliative care Study (PiPS) tools [40]

Models to predict survival probabilities in advanced cancer.

3D approach [41]

Developed to address the issues associated with managing patients with multi-morbidity in primary care in the UK.

---

particular specialties can all recognise the signs of deterioration in that specific area of care. Patients, those important to them, as well as the wider multi-disciplinary team (such as chaplains) all have access to this "gut instinct." It is important that all are listened to and then a considered approach taken to underpinning this gut instinct with a thorough review of the clinical history, a thought about available treatment options and an agreement from the wider MDT regarding the appropriateness of the future treatment plans before engaging with the patient and those important to them.

Tools and Processes to Identify and Act upon Palliative and Advance Care Planning Needs

There are a variety of person-centred tools, processes, and outcome measures to aid the identification of palliative and advance care planning needs, communicate uncertainty as well as demonstrate if an intervention has had benefit to an individual. Ellis-Smith et al.'s [30] systematic review of managing clinical uncertainty towards the end-of-life reported 63 tools in over 40 studies. Examples of beneficial tools and processes are illustrated in Table 1.

An example of how a tool can be used is demonstrated through the early assessment and intervention provided by the Scottish Palliative Care Directly Enhanced Service (DES) and the Key Information Summaries (KIS). The DES encourages general practitioners to identify more patients with non-malignant disease for palliative care by supporting them to use the Supportive and Palliative Care Indicators Tool to trigger a palliative care approach and to report specifically on numbers of non-malignant patients placed on their palliative care register. The KIS enabled shared medical records between healthcare professionals and results demonstrated that patients were more likely to die outside hospital if they had a KIS. Additionally anticipatory and palliative care was more equitable across different disease trajectories and earlier in the disease process [34].

More recently, the NHS England and Improvement EARLY Identification and Personalised Care Planning Toolkit for primary care [42] is promoted as offering an opportunity for individuals to discuss and develop a personalised care plan and supports the documentation of a personalised care plan on the local "Electronic Palliative Care Coordination System". All tools should be used alongside clinical judgement and as part of the multiprofessional, holistic assessment. This is relevant because the evidence for their use is still emerging and patient need, not prognosis, should be the driver for referral to palliative care [43].

Starting Conversations and Communicating Uncertainty

Starting conversations about the future of a patient can be challenging. The easiest starts are when patients give professionals verbal cues such as "I never feel well these days," "I am worried about the future" and "I just want to get home from hospital." When transitions occur in the patient's care e.g. discharge from hospital, or a move into a care home, or putting in an increased package of care at home, these can be helpful times to start a conversation. Sometimes a more bold and simultaneously gentle approach is required. This has been described by Eckberg as "framing illness projections and end-of-life in general terms" [44, p. 7]. When a patient or a family have not raised dying or end-of-life care then such an approach can be made in the following manner: "some patients when they have been critically ill and in hospital want to think about what will happen when they become unwell again." Ekberg says this "softens" the direct relevance of the topic being introduced to the patient and family and it means the patient can decline to talk about the topic if they wish. More information on communication can be found in Chapter 7: Conversations and Communication.

Prognosticating the future date of a patient's death is a challenging skill and individual clinicians are known to be inaccurate at prognostication no matter how experienced they are [45]. A multi-disciplinary approach rather than an individual approach is helpful to prognostication. The challenge with prognosticating is that it can leave patients and families feeling unhappy and mistrusting when either the patient dies sooner or later than the date range predicted. Cultural factors can affect the discussion and uptake of advance care planning. This may include religiosity, trust in the health-care system, patient and clinician comfort discussing death and patient attitudes regarding decision-making [46]. An individualised communication-based approach is likely to yield a stronger patient/family/clinician relationship even if the future cannot be discussed in detail.

Considering the setting of the conversation is important, and to allow time for discussions. The manner of the conversation needs to convey the respect for the seriousness of the conversation. Families find communication of uncertainty helpful, with evidence that "hoping for the best, whilst preparing for the worst" is helpful and they certainly value knowing that the patient is "sick enough to die" [47]. Even those patients and families who do not want to consider future health scenarios, and hope for cure, can still value having thought through the preparation for death such as wills, digital legacies etc.

Responsibility for Advance Care Planning

It is our belief that advance care planning is "everyone's business" because it is concerned with how someone prepares and plans for what is important to them in their dying and afterwards in terms of "care after death" and bereavement support. "Everyone's business" includes patients, families, health, and social care professionals as well as the wider community. A focus on only the medical or treatment decision making aspects of dying, while important, is only one part of advance care planning. Advance care planning therefore needs to balance the clinical and treatment choices about care with systems to communicate information about wishes and decisions as well as the lived experience of planning and preparing for dying. It tends to be clinically led as health and health decisions can seem to topple previously held "firm decisions" about homes, finances, faith, and relationships. While the medical aspects of the advance care plan from a clinical perspective is seen as the consultant/GP responsibility, the enactment of it requires the skills of the wider MDT as well as care for the patient and family. It is essential that there is a physical record available at the point of a clinical deterioration. This has led to the drive for electronic co-ordination records which are underpinned by national information standards [48].

Viewing Advance Care Planning Differently

Advance Care Planning as a Relational Approach

Advance care planning can be seen as an ongoing conversation, documentation, and sharing of a person's future choices and preferences. This puts the patient/ health and social care relationship at the heart of the process. It is holistic, collaborative, and individualised recognising that whilst home is often a preference for place of care that a person's preferences and priorities are complex and may change over time [23, 49]. The conversations can be had with families and friends, but it is vital that health and social care providers are part of the conversation and record conversations in a way that is accessible in the future, and especially in emergency situations [50].

Advance Care Planning as a Complex Health Intervention

Advance care planning is not only a complex intervention between patients, surrogates, communities, clinicians, health systems, and policy [24] but also an individual, relational, iterative process, and experience [7]. The embracing of the wider aspects of living with, preparing, and planning for the certainty of one's future death is illustrated by the growing guidelines and models not only for advance care planning decisions and documents but also communicating serious illness, prognostic uncertainty, and the context of a person's decision making [27]. The recent Lancet Commission on the Value of Death; bringing death back into life [26] reminds us that end-of-life conversations continue to be challenging for health-care practitioners but also points out how advance care planning has become part of how society understands, regulates, and manages death. The report argues that advance care planning has an over emphasis on individual autonomy and decision-making

and an overreliance on the refusal of treatments—something that is irrelevant in many societies as basic health care is still not present [26, p. 21]. Moreover, the report challenges the dominance of a medical hegemony on advance care planning with a call to arms for communities to reclaim death, dying, and grief as social concerns [40].

Advance Care Planning as a Public Health Approach

Along with others [26] we recommend advance care planning as a public health issue rather than as a prognostic, clinical need, or dying conversation. This is already seen elsewhere. For example, in 2015, the Institute of Medicine proposed a life-cycle model which was milestone specific (e.g. obtaining driver license, marriage, or buying a house), situation specific (e.g. high risk occupations such as military service), part of primary care (e.g. regular conversations when well), at the initial diagnosis of chronic disease (e.g. at the beginning of illness), as health worsens (e.g. at turning points in the disease) and in the final year of expected life with activity such as advance decisions and appointment of surrogate decision makers being seen as part of approaching death advance care planning activity [51]. The public health, life cycle, disease management, or prognosis approach to advance care planning conversations is of interest in terms of visualising preparing and planning for dying away from diagnosing dying towards conceptualising and recognising death as an inevitable part of living and dying.

Conclusion

While more work is undertaken on outcome measures, there is little doubt that the timely and sensitive introduction of the fact that life is uncertain, and preparation for the future via the concept of advance care planning is, on the most part, helpful for the patient, their families and for the health and social care system. The importance of communication and relationship skills cannot be underestimated. We would recommend that clinicians continue to hone their communication skills, and cultural competence to help with the ease of these conversations (see Chapter 7: Conversations and Communication), and to access clinical supervision to enable reflection and learning (see Chapter 23: Creating Space, Clarity and Containment: managing the emotional impact of palliative work by sustaining staff).

References

1. Mort, D., Lansdown, M., Protopapa, N.S., and Mason, M. (2008). For better, for worse? A review of the care of patients who died within 30 days of receiving anti-cancer therapy. https://www.ncepod.org.uk/2008report3/Downloads/SACT_summary.pdf (accessed 21 May 2022).

2. NICE. (2018). Decision aid Enteral (tube) feeding for people living with severe dementia. *Decision aid for Dementia: assessment, management and support for people living with dementia and their carers.* https://www.nice.org.uk/guidance/ng97/resources/enteral-tube-feeding-for-people-living-with-severe-dementia-patient-decision-aid-pdf-4852697007 (accessed 21 May 2022).

3. Francis, S.-A., Wilson, J., and Yardley, S. (2022). Good medicines management: from describing problems to a vision for change. *Palliative Medicine* [editorial]. https://doi.org/10.1177/2F02692163221076712

4. Makwana, A., Bowtell, A.P.N., Bowtell, N., and Verne, J. (2020) Emergency admissions in the 3 months before death. https://www.gov.uk/government/publications/emergency-admissions-in-the-3-months-before-death/emergency-admissions-in-the-3-months-before-death (accessed 21 May 2022).

5. Sathiananthan, M.K., Crawford, G.B., and Eliott, J. (2021). Healthcare professionals' perspectives of patient and family preferences of patient place of death: a qualitative study. *BMC Palliative Care* 20: 147.

6. Seipp, H. et al. (2021). How can we ensure the success of specialised palliative home-care? A qualitative study (ELSAH) identifying key issues from the perspective of patients, relatives and health professionals. *Palliative Medicine* 35 (10): 1844–1855.

7. McMahan, R.D., Tellez, I., and Sudore, R.L. (2021). Deconstructing the complexities of advance care planning outcomes: what do we know and where do we go? A scoping review. *Journal of the American Geriatrics Society* 69 (1): 234–244.

8. Sudore, R.L. et al. (2018). Outcomes that define successful advance care planning: a Delphi panel consensus. *Journal of Pain and Symptom Management* 55 (2): 245–255.e8.

9. Rietjens, J.A.C. et al. (2017 September). Definition and recommendations for advance care planning: An international consensus supported by the European Association for Palliative Care. *The Lancet Oncology* 18 (9): e543–e551.

10. Russell, S. and Detering, K. (2017). What are the benefits of advance care planning and how do we know? In: *Advance Care Planning in End of Life Care* (ed. K. Thomas, BenLobo, and K. Detering). Oxford University Press.

11. Bradshaw, A. et al. (2021). Understanding and addressing challenges for advance care planning in the COVID-19 pandemic: an analysis of the UK CovPall survey data from specialist palliative care services. *Palliative Medicine* 35: 1225–1237.

12. NHS England. (2022). Universal principles for advance care planning. https://www.england.nhs.uk/wp-content/uploads/2022/03/universal-principles-for-advance-care-planning.pdf (accessed 21 May 2022).

13. Care Quality Commission. (2021). Protect, respect, connect—decisions about living and dying well during COVID-19. https://www.cqc.org.uk/publications/themed-work/protect-respect-connect-decisions-about-living-dying-well-during-covid-19 (accessed 21 May 2022).

14. Harrison Dening, K., Sampson, E.L., and De Vries, K. (2019). Advance care planning in dementia: recommendations for healthcare professionals. *Palliative Care* 12: 1178224219826579.

15. Wade, D.T. and Kitzinger, C. (2019). Making healthcare decisions in a person's best interests when they lack capacity: clinical guidance based on a review of evidence. *Clinical Rehabilitation* 33: 1571–1585.

16. North Cheshire and Merseyside Strategic Clinical Network. (2015) Advance care planning framework. https://www.england.nhs.uk/north/wp-content/uploads/sites/5/2018/06/Advance_Care_Planning_Framework_2015-18_FINAL.pdf (accessed 21 May 2022).

17. Bradshaw, A., Santarelli, M., Khamis, A.M. et al. (2021). Implementing person-centred outcome measures (PCOMs) into routine palliative care: a protocol for a mixed-methods process evaluation of The RESOLVE PCOM implementation strategy. *BMJ Open* 2021, 11: e051904.

18. Weathers, E. et al. (2016). Advance care planning: a systematic review of randomised controlled trials conducted with older adults. *Maturitas* 91: 101–109. doi: 10.1016/j.maturitas.2016.06.016. Epub 2016 Jun 23. PMID: 27451328.

19. Zhang, B. et al. (2009). Health care costs in the last week of life: associations with end-of-life conversations. *Archives of Internal Medicine* 169: 480–488.

20. Ridgers, H. (2020). COVID-19: empowering patients with advance care. *Nursing Standard* 7: 42–44.

21. Block, B.L., Smith, A.K., and Sudore, R.L. (2020). During COVID-19, outpatient advance care planning is imperative: we need all hands on deck. *Journal of the American Geriatrics Society* 68: 1395–1397.

22. Abadir, P.M., Finucane, T.E., and McNabney, M.K. (2011). When doctors and daughters disagree: twenty-two days and two blinks of an eye. *Journal of the American Geriatrics Society* 59: 2337–2340.

23. Gray, N. (2022). Op-comic: my patients wrestle with end-of-life care, even if there's a living will. https://www.latimes.com/opinion/story/2022-04-25/living-will-end-of-life-care-die-hospital-home (accessed 21 May 2022).

24. Johnson, H. et al. (2020). Implementation of a complex intervention to improve care for patients whose situations are clinically uncertain in hospital settings: a multi-method study using normalisation process theory. *PLOS one* 15: e0239181–24.

25. Dinnen, T., Williams, H., Yardley, S. et al. (2019). Patient safety incidents in advance care planning for serious illness: a

mixed-methods analysis. *BMJ Supportive & Palliative Care* 0:1–8. doi:10.1136/bmjspcare-2019-001824

26. Sallnow, L. et al. (2022). Report of the Lancet Commission on the Value of Death: bringing death back into life. *Lancet* 399 (10327): 837–884.

27. Russell, S. (2016). Advance care planning and living with dying: the views of hospice patients. https://uhra.herts.ac.uk/handle/2299/17474 (accessed 21 May 2022).

28. Jimenez, G. et al. (2018). Overview of systematic reviews of advance care planning: summary of evidence and global lessons. *Journal of Pain and Symptom Management* 56: 436–459.e25.

29. Wilson, J. (2017). A mixed method, psychosocial analysis of how senior health care professionals recognise dying and engage patients and families in the negotiation of key decisions. https://researchportal.bath.ac.uk/en/studentTheses/a-mixed-method-psychosocial-analysis-how-senior-health-care-profe (accessed 21 May 2022).

30. Ellis-Smith, C. et al. (2021). Managing clinical uncertainty in older people towards the end of life: a systematic review of person-centred tools. *BMC Palliative Care* 20: 168.

31. Murtagh, F.E. et al. (2019). A brief, patient- and proxy-reported outcome measure in advanced illness: validity, reliability and responsiveness of the Integrated Palliative care Outcome Scale (IPOS). *Palliative Medicine* 33: 1045–1057.

32. Nicholson, C. et al. (2018). What are the main palliative care symptoms and concerns of older people with multimorbidity?—a comparative cross-sectional study using routinely collected Phase of Illness, Australia-modified Karnofsky Performance Status and Integrated Palliative Care Outcome Scale data. *Annals of Palliative Medicine* 7: S164–S175.

33. Masso, M. et al. (2015). Palliative Care Phase: inter-rater reliability and acceptability in a national study. *Palliative Medicine* 29: 22–30.

34. Tapsfield, J., Hall, C., Lunan, C. et al. (2019). Many people in Scotland now benefit from anticipatory care before they die: an after death analysis and interviews with general practitioners. *BMJ Supportive & Palliative Care* 9: e28.

35. Koffman, J. et al. (2019). The AMBER care bundle for hospital inpatients with uncertain recovery nearing the end of life: the improvecare feasibility cluster RCT. *Health Technology Assessment* 23: 1–150.

36. Highet, G., Crawford, D., Murray, S.A., and Boyd, K. (2014). Development and evaluation of the Supportive and Palliative Care Indicators Tool (SPICT): a mixed-methods study. *BMJ Supportive & Palliative Care* 4: 285.

37. Downar, J., Goldman, R., Pinto, R., Englesakis, M., and Adhikari, N.K.J. (2017). The "surprise question" for predicting death in seriously ill patients: a systematic review and meta-analysis. *Canadian Medical Association Journal* 189: E484–E493.

38. Pilotto, A. et al. (2021). The multidimensional prognostic index (MPI) for the prognostic stratification of older

inpatients with COVID-19: a multicenter prospective observational cohort study. *Archives of Gerontology and Geriatrics* 95: 104415.

39. Macgregor, A. et al. (2021). Palliative and end-of-life care in care homes: protocol for codesigning and implementing an appropriate scalable model of needs rounds in the UK. *BMJ Open* 11: e049486.

40. Stone, P.C. et al. (2021). The Prognosis in Palliative care Study II (PiPS2): a prospective observational validation study of a prognostic tool with an embedded qualitative evaluation. *PLOS One* 16: e0249297.

41. Smith, S.M., Wallace, E., Clyne, B. et al. (2021). Interventions for improving outcomes in patients with multimorbidity in primary care and community setting: a systematic review. *Systematic Reviews* 10 (271).

42. Stirling, C. (2020). End of life care clinical network NHS England and improvement (London region) EARLY identification and personalised care planning toolkit. https://www.england.nhs.uk/london/wp-content/uploads/sites/8/2022/01/London-EOLC-CN-London-Early-Identification-and-Personalised-Care-Planning-Toolkit-V2-24032021.pdf (accessed 21 May 2022).

43. Costantini, M., Higginson, I.J., Merlo, D.F., Leo, S.D., and Tanzi, S. (2017). About the "surprise question". *CMAJ* 12; 189 (23): E807.

44. Ekberg, S., Parry, R., Land, V. et al. (2021). Communicating with patients and families about illness progression and end of life: a review of studies using direct observation of clinical practice. *BMC Palliative Care* 20: 186.

45. White, N., Reid, F., Harris, A., Harries, P., and Stone, P. (2016). A systematic review of predictions of survival in palliative care: how accurate are clinicians and who are the experts? *PLOS one* 11: e0161407.

46. McDermott, E. and Selman, L.E. (2018). Cultural factors influencing Advance Care Planning in progressive, incurable disease: a systematic review with narrative synthesis. *Journal of Pain and Symptom Management* 56: 613–636.

47. Krawczyk, M. and Gallagher, R. (2016). Communicating prognostic uncertainty in potential end-of-life contexts: experiences of family members. *BMC Palliative Care* 15: 59.

48. NHS Digital. (2022). SCCI1580: palliative care co-ordination: core content. https://digital.nhs.uk/data-and-information/information-standards/information-standards-and-data-collections-including-extractions/publications-and-notifications/standards-and-collections/scci1580-palliative-care-co-ordination-core-content#:~:text=This%20information%20standard%20specifies%20the,manage%20their%20health%20and%20care (accessed 21 May 2022).

49. Gomes, B., Calanzani, N., Gysels, M., Hall, S., and Higginson, I.J. (2013). Heterogeneity and changes in preferences for dying at home: a systematic review. *BMC Palliative Care* 12: 7.

50. Millington-Sanders, C., Nadicksbernd, J.J., O'Sullivan, C., Morgan, T., Raleigh, A., Yeun, P., and Ormerod, G. (2012). Electronic palliative care co-ordination system: an electronic record that supports communication for end-of-life care—a pilot in Richmond, UK. *London Journal of Primary Care* 5 (1): 130–134.

51. Committee on Approaching Death: Addressing Key End of Life Issues; Institute of Medicine. (2015 March 19). *Dying in America: Improving Quality and Honoring Individual Preferences near the End of Life*. Washington, DC: National Academies Press (US). https://www.ncbi.nlm.nih.gov/books/NBK285681.

10 Pain and Its Management

Richard Kitchen

Introduction

Pain is a common symptom in the context of life-limiting illness, and one that is often feared by patients and those around them [1, 2]. The good news is that there are many strategies available to help manage pain. This chapter will initially look at the scale of the problem of pain in palliative care, and then consider what pain is, including the concept of total pain. The chapter will cover the neuroanatomy and physiology of pain and then consider some of the types of pain. Terminology of pain will be covered, and there will be a focus on pain assessment, including the real importance of this in providing best management. The management of pain will then be considered at length, with a particular focus on the importance of individualising management for every patient. Pain will be most commonly framed in the context of cancer pain, though the importance of pain related to other advanced illness will also be considered. Note that pain is also alluded to in the renal and neurological illness chapters of this book.

The Challenges Pain Presents in Palliative Care

Pain is a very common symptom in palliative care, for people with both malignant and non-malignant illness. Pain is the most common presenting symptom in people diagnosed with cancer [3]. In those with advanced cancer, 66% patients get pain, and 55% patients get pain with an intensity of 5/10 or more [4]. Such pain commonly has an impact on quality of life [5]. Furthermore at the end-of-life, 80% of people with AIDS and 67% of people with cardiovascular disease or chronic obstructive pulmonary disease experience moderate-severe pain [6].

Box 1: Case study

"Mr. Talbot is a 68-year-old man with colorectal cancer, which has metastasised to the liver and bones. Mr. Talbot is troubled by pain, particularly in the right upper quadrant of the abdomen, which is described as dull and constant. There is also pain radiating down the right leg that is "shooting" in nature. Mr. Talbot is already taking paracetamol and codeine. The codeine is stopped, and oral morphine is commenced. Despite three increases to the morphine dose by different healthcare professionals, Mr. Talbot's pain is partially improved at best. He last opened his bowels five days ago. Mr. Talbot says he is really struggling..."

Given this challenge, supporting patients with pain is of huge importance. We have many treatment options but despite this, pain is often poorly managed [7]. A study found that 32% patients were receiving analgesia that was too little for the pain they were experiencing [8]. Additionally, informal carers also perceive pain as a significant problem [9]. Supporting patients and those around them with an individualised and multi-modal approach is most likely to be helpful. In the case study of Mr. Talbot (Box 1), an individualised approach rather than a single analgesic strategy would have been more effective.

What Is Pain?

The International Association for the Study of Pain (IASP) defines pain as "An unpleasant sensory and emotional experience associated with actual or potential tissue damage, or described in terms of such damage" [10]. This definition was first released in 1979, but this more recent publication from the IASP defines six key notes alongside

Handbook of Palliative Care, Fourth Edition. Edited by Richard Kitchen, Christina Faull, Sarah Russell and Jo Wilson.
© 2024 John Wiley & Sons Ltd. Published 2024 by John Wiley & Sons Ltd.

the definition, particularly recognising the individual experience that people feel when they have pain [10]:

• Pain is always a personal experience that is influenced to varying degrees by biological, psychological, and social factors.

• Pain and nociception are different phenomena. Pain cannot be inferred solely from activity in sensory neurons.

• Through their life experiences, individuals learn the concept of pain.

• A person's report of an experience as pain should be respected.

• Although pain usually serves an adaptive role, it may have adverse effects on function and social and psychological well-being.

• Verbal description is only one of several behaviours to express pain; inability to communicate does not negate the possibility that a human or a nonhuman animal experiences pain.

The top point pays homage to the concept of "Total Pain," a term developed by Dame Cicely Saunders in the 1960s, and commonly used in palliative care since this time. Total pain considers pain to be a multi-faceted experience for the patient, with physical, psychological, social, and spiritual components [11]. A multi-dimensional assessment of all of these components is crucial to developing a coherent pain management plan, and neglecting elements will most likely lead to poorer outcomes. Figure 1 is a simple depiction of total pain. Table 1 outlines some of the problems a patient with pain may be experiencing, and groups them into the domains of total pain.

Neuroanatomy and Physiology of Pain

Pain is commonly classified as nociceptive and neuropathic pain. Though an oversimplification, this division is a good starting point and has lots of clinical relevance, which will be borne out in this chapter. The following discussion of pain pathways is focussed on nociceptive pain, as neuropathic pain is the result of abnormal activation of nociceptive pathways.

We already know that pain occurs due to tissue damage (from a "noxious stimulus"). There is a characteristic pathway that follows such an insult, involving four processes: transduction, transmission, perception, and modulation [12].

Transduction involves nociceptor stimulation. Pain is transmitted by nerve fibres of primary afferent neurones, namely A-δ ("fast") and C ("slow") fibres (Table 2). Nociceptors are the nerve endings of these fibres. In response to thermal, mechanical, or chemical noxious stimuli, damaged cells produce neurotransmitters such as substance P. These stimulate nociceptors and the pathway begins.

After nociceptor stimulation, transmission occurs. Afferent nerve fibres synapse in the dorsal horn of the spinal cord, and transmit via the spinothalamic tract on to

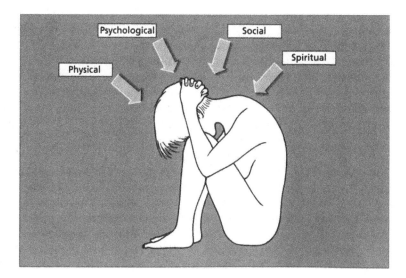

Figure 1 The four domains of total pain.

Table 1 Elements of pain, grouped into their total pain domain.

Physical	*Psychological*
"Traditional" pain	Anxiety/fear of worsening pain
Impact on mobility	Equating "pain" with "dying"
Requirement for analgesia	Equating pain relief (especially opioids) with dying
Other physical symptoms	Sense of inevitability of future severe pain
	Reminder of ill health/limitations/sick role
	Anger, despair, and hopelessness
Social	*Spiritual*
Inability to work	Loss of sense of purpose
Loss of role as earner, practical person, or carer for another person	Loss of role(s) and identity
Restricted social activities and contacts	Change to expected life narrative or journey
Loss of income	Feeling of being punished
Changes to housing to accommodate functional changes	Altered relationship with/feelings about a "higher authority" in whatever form

Table 2 Nerve fibres transmitting pain.

Nerve Fibre Type	A-delta	C
Myelin Sheath	Yes	No
Pain Characteristics	Sharp, well-localised	Dull, aching, poorly localised

the brainstem and thalamus, then to the cerebral cortex. Of note, A-beta nerve fibres, which are also sensory afferents, also terminate in the dorsal horn and can inhibit the transmission of the painful stimulus. This is known as "gate control" [13] and is the mechanism of action of a transcutaneous electrical nerve stimulator (TENS) machine.

Perception is the conscious awareness of pain [14]. Afferent input is interpreted by a number of systems within the brain: sensory-discriminative (somatosensory cortex), affective motivational (reticular and limbic systems) and cognitive-evaluative (cerebral cortex). These systems interact to produce the experience of pain for the patient. This is impacted upon by genetics and previous experiences among other factors, giving rise to the individual nature of pain [14].

Modulation is the body's impact on afferent input, with the periaqueductal grey area most important in this process. Modulation is most commonly recognised as descending inhibitory pathways, whereby neurotransmitters such as serotonin, noradrenaline, and GABA reduce pain perception (and also offer targets for adjuvant analgesics). In certain situations pain can be enhanced rather than inhibited, particularly in the case of neuropathic pain.

Understanding this pathway, and the sites of actions of analgesics within it (Figure 2), can help to individualise pain management options for a patient [15].

Opioid Receptors

Opioids are commonly used medications in palliative care and have effect at opioid receptors. Four opioid receptors have been identified: Mu (μ), Delta, (δ), Kappa (κ), and ORL-1 (opioid-receptor-like); these are also sometimes referred to as "MOP," "DOP," "KOP," and "NOP" [16]. These receptors appear throughout the body, most commonly in nervous tissue, but also in other areas such as the bowel. Endogenous opioid metabolism contributes to many physiological functions: pain, hormonal, and immune among others [17].

All clinically important opioid analgesics act at Mu receptors [17]. It is also Mu receptor activation that contributes to most opioid-related side effects.

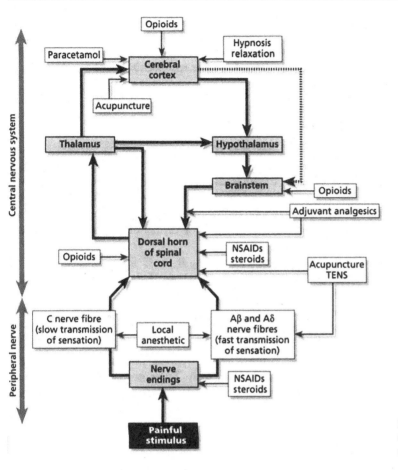

Figure 2 A schema of the neuroanatomy of pain and the sites of action of different analgesics.

Pain Types and Syndromes

Pain comes in many shapes and sizes. While pain is a personal experience it is useful to categorise it, for academic purposes, and particularly to guide clinical management. Though classifications can be more complex, pains can generally be classified according to their state (nociceptive/neuropathic), type (visceral/somatic) and temporality (constant/episodic). Table 3 displays the types of pain commonly seen in palliative care and also offers an overview of analgesics that are likely to be useful. Pains are sometimes seen as "opioid-responsive" and "non-opioid responsive." This split is not an absolute and it is common to see pains that are partially responsive to opioids; as always it is important to assess the effect in the individual taking the medication.

Nociceptive Pain

Nociceptive pain is very common in both cancer and non-cancer settings in palliative care. It appears in a variety of forms dependent upon the cause.

Visceral pain is that arising from pathology of an internal organ or tissue. It is commonly described as vague and poorly defined, though this is an oversimplification as the underlying cause can give rise to a number of presentations. Damage to solid organs such as the liver tend to cause pain that is "dull" in nature and difficult to localise. Pain may be referred due to underlying innervation (in the case of the liver, to the right shoulder tip). Some pains, related to more peripheral structures such as the peritoneum, will be more easily localised. Damage to a hollow viscus, such as the bowel, may present with colicky pain caused by muscular spasm of the bowel wall.

Table 3 Types of pain, possible opioid response, and other analgesic options.

Classification/Type of Pain	Temporal Characteristics	Example	Opioid Response	Co-analgesic or Other Modality
Nociceptive visceral	Constant	Liver capsule pain	Partial	Corticosteroid
Nociceptive visceral	Episodic	Partially obstructing bowel tumour	Partial response but may exacerbate constipation	Anticholinergic
		Radiation induced cystitis	Poor response	Anticholinergic
Nociceptive somatic	Constant	Bone metastasis	Partial	Nonsteroidal anti-inflammatory drug Paracetamol Radiotherapy Bisphosphonates
		Cutaneous metastasis	Partial	Topical anti-inflammatory Neuropathic agent
Nociceptive somatic	Episodic	Bone pain due to pathological fracture or vertebral collapse	Partial but may not cover movement-related pain Muscle spasm may also be involved	Surgical stabilization Nerve block Radiotherapy Muscle relaxant for muscle spasm
Neuropathic	Constant	Chemotherapy induced painful peripheral neuropathy OR Post-herpetic neuralgia	Partial response	Tricyclic antidepressant Antiepileptic
Neuropathic	Episodic	Lancinating pain due to brachial plexopathy	Poor response	Tricyclic or other antidepressant Antiepileptic Benzodiazepine

Somatic pain is that related to more peripheral structures such as bone. It is commonly described as "sharp" and is generally well-localised.

Classical nociceptive pain is caused by noxious stimuli activating nociceptors. An inflammatory pain state has been more recently recognised. In this instance, inflammatory mediators activate and sensitise nociceptors, due to causes such as inflammatory disorders or infection [18]. For this text it is reasonable to consider inflammatory pain a branch of nociceptive pain, though recognising this mechanism and the underlying cause is integral for best management.

Neuropathic Pain

Neuropathic pain arises from a disease or lesion affecting the somatosensory system – either the peripheral or central nervous system [19]. It is also common, affecting up to 40% patients with cancer [20]. In this setting it may be caused by direct invasion of the cancer (such as in brachial plexopathy), paraneoplastic syndromes, cancer treatment (systemic anti-cancer therapies such as platinum-based agents, and surgery) or non-cancer related causes. It is also prevalent in non-malignant life-limiting illnesses such as multiple sclerosis, peripheral vascular disease and chronic kidney disease (especially when due to diabetes mellitus).

Though neuropathic pain is a heterogeneous entity [20], with pain that can be constant or episodic, some classical findings are often seen. Words that patients commonly use include "burning," "stinging," and "shooting." There may be concomitant sensory and/or motor changes. Pain is usually seen in the distribution of the affected nerve(s). It is important to identify such features, to distinguish neuropathic pain and to identify the lesion or disease causing the pain, to allow a targeted plan to be developed [21].

Neuropathic pain is often considered harder to treat [22]. Although opioids may be useful, this is sometimes not the case. Neuropathic analgesics and interventional analgesia alongside non-pharmacological methods are often required to achieve significant improvements.

Pain Temporality

Background ("constant") pain is that present most or all of the time. It can be defined as occurring (or would be present without analgesia) at least 12 hours/day over the last week [23].

Breakthrough ("episodic") pain is that which "breaks through" controlled background pain. It can be specifically defined as "a transient exacerbation of pain that occurs either spontaneously, or in relation to a specific predictable or unpredictable trigger, despite relatively stable and adequately controlled background pain." [24] Within this definition, the authors describe two forms of breakthrough pain, spontaneous and incident [24]. Spontaneous ("idiopathic") pain occurs unexpectedly, whereas incident pain is related to specific events. Incident pain can be further divided into volitional (precipitated by a volitional act such as walking), non-volitional (precipitated by an act such as coughing) and procedural (related to a therapeutic intervention) [24]. Determining the type of pain is beneficial in developing a bespoke management plan. Bear in mind that patients can have more than one type of incident pain.

Terminology of Pain

Pain is complex, and often best managed with a multidisciplinary team approach. It is useful for clinicians to have a number of descriptors that can help classify pain, to allow accurate and succinct discussion. Some of the terms used are discussed below, and are often features of neuropathic pain. When in a consultation, it is usually safer (and simpler) to restrict the use of descriptors to those used by the patient to maintain a shared understanding of the patient's pain experience.

Allodynia

Pain due to a stimulus that does not usually provoke pain [25]. This could be due to a variety of modalities, including touch, heat, and pressure. The overlying skin may or may not be damaged.

Dysaesthesia

An unpleasant abnormal sensation that can be spontaneous or evoked [26]. Allodynia is a form of dysaesthesia, though the unpleasant sensation need not be painful.

Hyperaesthesia

Increased sensitivity to any stimulus, for example minor pressure being felt more severely.

Hyperalgesia

Increased pain from a stimulus that usually provokes pain [25]. For example, a minor insult causing severe pain.

Paraesthesia

An abnormal sensation that is not unpleasant. This may be experienced as "tingling," "prickling," or "itching" among other feelings.

Pain Assessment

Excellent pain assessment is the cornerstone of pain management. Getting this right will allow the clinician to best support the patient through their symptoms. Conversely, inadequate pain assessment and a lack of documentation are thought to be the greatest barriers to good pain relief [27]. A structured approach to assessment is advised, and some key points need to be remembered:

- Number: Patients often have more than one pain [28]. A rule of thumb is that a third of patients have one pain, 1/3 have two pains, and 1/3 have three or more pains.
- Causes: In those with cancer, also consider other causes of pain. A study found that in those with pain and cancer, 17% of pains were due to antineoplastic treatment, and 10% were due to aetiologies unrelated to cancer [29].
- Impact: The effect of pain on functionality is sometimes overlooked. It is important to establish this to allow development of a multidisciplinary plan.
- Re-assess: It is essential to re-assess pain, to ensure the correct pain mechanism has been identified, and the effect of management strategies is evaluated.

Assessment should begin as soon as the patient is seen, considering their appearance, behaviour, and gait. History taking is crucial, and using a systematic approach to define the pain such as the mnemonic SOCRATES (Box 2), adapted to the patient, is recommended [30].

Assessment tools can be used alongside history taking to form a picture of what the patient is experiencing.

Box 2: History taking in pain assessment – Using SOCRATES

- **Site** – Define where the pain is, checking on this for each different pain.
- **Onset** – When did the pain start, and when did it progress?
- **Character** – A description of what the pain feels like; this is particularly important in defining the type of pain.
- **Radiation** – Where the pain spreads to, which can be helpful in defining an anatomical cause.
- **Associated factors** – Are there co-existent symptoms or other features of note?
- **Timing** – Is the pain worse at a particular time of day?
- **Exacerbating/relieving factors** – Factors which make the pain better or worse; it is helpful to know these for defining a cause but also developing a management plan.
- **Severity** – A description of "how bad" the pain is. Tools such as a visual analogue scale (VAS) and numerical rating scale (NRS) can be useful to use.

Unfortunately no universally accepted tool exists [31]. The Expert Working Group of the European Association for Palliative Care have previously recommended using multidimensional tools like the Brief Pain Inventory (BPI-sf) and the Short Form McGill Pain Questionnaire for pain assessment in PC (SF-MPQ) [32]. However, clinical assessment is the gold standard [33], and it is often pragmatic to use history taking in the first instance, adding the use of a pain tool when pain assessment is more challenging. Tools can be useful in assessing pain in those with significant cognitive impairment, such as dementia. The PAINAD (Pain Assessment in Advanced Dementia scale) and DisDAT (Disability Distress Assessment Tool) have been shown to be effective in assessing nursing home residents with advanced dementia [34]. When using these it is important to try to distinguish distress and pain to ensure appropriate management. The LANSS (Leeds Assessment of Neuropathic Symptoms and Signs) can be used in suspected neuropathic pain [33].

Alongside pain characteristics, it is essential to ask about the effect of the pain on the patient's life and their goals for the future. Similarly, establish the patient's ideas about the cause of pain, their concerns and their expectations to further develop shared understanding. It is important to cover co-symptoms, such as bowel function if the patient is taking opioids. Physical examination, such as checking sensory function in suspected neuropathic pain, is valuable. Reviewing old investigations, to for example look

---

Box 3: Case study

"Mr. Talbot has come to the clinic. You have taken a full history as well as examined his abdomen and peripheral nerves. You have also reviewed his most recent scan results. You clearly explain that he likely has liver capsular pain as a result of liver metastases, and neuropathic pain in the leg due to spinal root compression from bone metastases. You consider referral for palliative radiotherapy to the spine as well as adjuvant analgesics, and help Mr. Talbot to start to develop some goals for the future."

---

for anatomical causes of pain, and considering new investigations is also vital.

The information gained through this process should be used to work out the type(s) of pain the patient is experiencing, and ultimately the mechanism(s) of the pain, which is important in developing a targeted management plan.

Finally, patients' underlying illnesses or co-morbidities need to be considered. Chronic pain in the context of no life-limiting illnesses (managed in primary care with referral to pain clinics rather than palliative care) requires a different approach to pain due to advanced cancer, though holistic assessment and a personalised management plan are needed in both cases. It is therefore important to consider prognosis alongside the potential long-term side effects of treatment when devising a plan.

Management of Pain

General Principles

Following assessment, a holistic management plan should be developed alongside the patient, using the approach in Box 4.

Box 4: Principles of pain management

- Complete the pain assessment and discuss this with the patient
- Consider managing the underlying cause of pain
- Support the patient to manage their pain and set realistic goals
- Utilise the multidisciplinary team
- Use pharmacological approaches to modify pain perception
- Consider interventional approaches to interrupt pain pathways
- Make a follow up plan

Complete Pain Assessment and Discuss This

A thorough assessment will have allowed the type of pain to be identified and a cause for the patient's pain(s) to be found. Talking this through will help to support the patient's understanding of the situation, which will in turn support discussion of pain management options, and subsequently compliance.

Consider Managing the Underlying Cause of Pain

If there is effective treatment available for the underlying cause of pain then this should be considered, weighing up the benefits and burdens with the patient. For example, this may include palliative radiotherapy in a patient with painful bone metastases such as in Mr. Talbot's case (Box 3), or surgical fixation where there is an impending fracture due to a lytic lesion in a bone.

Support the Patient

It is important to remember the concept of total pain, and the impacts each element can have. For example, if the patient is struggling with anxiety or depression, pain management is less likely to be effective, and so supporting this with pharmacological and non-pharmacological approaches will also help pain control.

As part of this element, it is also imperative to discuss reasonable expectations for management of the pain, and set realistic goals for the patient to work towards. For instance, removing a pain entirely may be very difficult, but improving it enough to allow a short car journey to the beach may be possible.

Utilise the Multidisciplinary Team

The multidisciplinary team brings many skills that can help a patient struggling with pain. If pain is exacerbated by movement, a physiotherapist may be able to support a patient's mobility, and an occupational therapist could modify the home environment to support this. If pain is impacted upon by spiritual challenges, a member of the pastoral care or chaplaincy team could support the patient to work through these.

Modify Pain Perception

Utilising medication is a cornerstone of pain management. Many types of analgesic are available and are discussed in the remainder of this chapter. Further approaches include complementary therapies (discussed in Chapter 24: Patient/Individual and Carer Wellbeing) and a TENS machine.

Interrupt Pain Pathways

Pain interventions can be neuraxial (epidural or intrathecal analgesia) or neurolytic (nerve blocks) and are usually carried out by anaesthetists. They are particularly useful for pain that has proved more resistant to analgesia, or where there are intolerable side effects to a number of medications. It is important to consider them early enough for the patient to derive good benefit.

Make a Follow-up Plan

Whatever management plan has been made with the patient, it is imperative to discuss how the benefit of this will be assessed and followed up, to ensure continuity of care.

Pharmacotherapeutic Intervention

The majority of this management section focusses on pharmacological options for pain management, and aims to provide the reader with a structured approach to this while also considering the patient as an individual.

There are many guidelines, local and national, available for pain management in palliative care, such as NICE guidance "CG140: Palliative care for adults: strong opioids for pain relief" [35]. This chapter is designed to work alongside rather than instead of these. Furthermore, certain texts such as the Palliative Care Formulary are referenced in this chapter and provide greater information on individual drugs. Product information on each specific drug should be noted. In clinical practice, advice can also be gained from specialists such as those working in specialist palliative care. As always, the reader is responsible for their own practice and should prescribe within the limits of their competence.

As an introduction to management, medications for pain can broadly be divided into three groups: non-opioids, opioids, and adjuvant drugs.

Non-opioid drugs are those with analgesic and antipyretic actions, with some having anti-inflammatory effects too. Principally this group includes Paracetamol (Acetaminophen) and non-steroidal anti-inflammatory drugs (NSAIDs).

Opioids are medications related in structure to the natural plant alkaloids found in opium, which is derived from the resin of the opium poppy, Papaver somniferum [36]. Opioids are grouped as "weak" (for "mild-moderate" pain) and "strong" (for "moderate-severe" pain), the key distinction being weak opioids having a ceiling dose and strong opioids not. Table 4 lists drugs in each class. The term "opiate" is sometimes used; this refers specifically to drugs derived directly from opium resin (morphine and codeine), whereas "opioids" are the wider group of analgesics of related structure.

Adjuvant analgesics are medications originally used for another indication (such as depression or epilepsy) that are now utilised for their analgesic effect.

Table 4 Opioids analgesics and their class.	
"Weak" Opioids	"Strong" Opioids
Codeine	Morphine
Dihydrocodeine	Diamorphine
Tramadol	Oxycodone
	Fentanyl
	Buprenorphine
	Methadone
	Hydromorphone
	Alfentanil

Box 5: Three steps in the WHO analgesic ladder

Step 1
Paracetamol and/or NSAID +/adjuvant
Step 2
Paracetamol and/or NSAID + weak opioid ± adjuvant.
Examples of weak opioids are codeine, dihydrocodeine, or tramadol.
For breakthrough analgesia, use low-dose normal release strong opioid, for example morphine NR 5 mg or equivalent.
Step 3
Paracetamol and/or NSAID + strong opioid ± adjuvant.
A normal release strong opioid should be prescribed for breakthrough analgesia alongside the regular strong opioid.

The WHO Analgesic Ladder

The ladder was originally developed in 1986 by a group of experts, brought together by the Cancer and Palliative Care Unit of the WHO. It comprises a three-step framework, designed for the management of cancer pain, based around pain intensity rather than aetiology [37].

Alongside the three pharmacological steps of non-opioids, weak opioids and strong opioids alongside adjuvant analgesics (see Figure 3 and Box 5), the ladder proposes two more principles. Firstly, that analgesia is given by mouth unless there is a compelling reason to utilise another route, and secondly, that analgesia is given regularly ("by the clock"), with breakthrough analgesia available alongside this. Conventional use of the ladder dictates starting at step 1 and assessing the effect of the analgesic for at least 48 hours (though a longer period of assessment may be required). If pain control is not significantly improved, a second step 1 analgesic could be added (if paracetamol has been commenced, a non-steroidal anti-inflammatory drug (NSAID) would be reasonable, considering contraindications), an adjuvant analgesic could be included, or analgesia can be changed to step 2 (addition of a weak opioid). A similar approach applies between steps 2 and 3, stepping up from weak opioids to strong opioids when appropriate.

Individualising Pain Management and Issues with the WHO Ladder

In Mr. Talbot's case, opioid analgesia was "stepped up" without adequate consideration of adjuvant analgesics and non-pharmacological options for pain. This led to poor pain control and side effects from opioids. This simple example demonstrates the need for a multi-dimensional pain assessment and an individualised management plan developed on the back of this.

The WHO analgesic ladder has been widely lauded, given the genuinely positive impact it has had on pain management in patients with advanced cancer [15,38]. However, more recently, challenges with the ladder have been identified. The first of these concerns the use of the ladder for chronic pain. It is accepted that chronic pain, while also multi-faceted and complex, is different from pain in advanced cancer in that it is present over a longer time course and is harder to predict [38]. Use of escalating opioids gives rise to the possibility of long term side effects, and a potentially unrealistic aim of resolving the pain, whereas the approach of managing the pain in the context of life as a whole is more likely to be effective.

The second limitation of the ladder is targeting analgesia to pain intensity rather than the underlying cause.

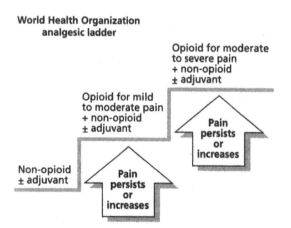

World Health Organization analgesic ladder

Opioid for moderate to severe pain + non-opioid ± adjuvant

Opioid for mild to moderate pain + non-opioid ± adjuvant

Non-opioid ± adjuvant

Pain persists or increases

Pain persists or increases

Figure 3 Visual depiction of the WHO analgesic ladder.

Opioids are very effective analgesics when used appropriately and pain intensity is an important part of assessment. However, the ladder has never been validated, and alternatives to opioids, including both alternative analgesics and non-pharmacological options, are preferable at times [15]. A multidimensional assessment will often find a number of contributors to the pain, and managing these as part of a whole person approach is much more likely to be effective.

Further work has looked at the role of weak opioids ('step 2'). Some have suggested that step 2 be eliminated, going straight from non-opioids to low doses of strong opioids [39]. This approach has already been adopted in paediatrics [40]. This approach is contingent on the availability of strong opioids, but is often reasonable where cancer pain is challenging.

The opinion of this author is to focus on pain assessment, and use this, working alongside the patient, to develop an individualised management plan. It can be useful to think about the hierarchy that the WHO analgesic ladder describes, particularly in pain due to advanced cancer, but this must be done in the context of the patient as a whole. With this in mind, the ladder will be referred to as a guide during the rest of this chapter, as part of an individualised approach.

Breakthrough Analgesia

Treating breakthrough pain is an important part of pain management, as such pains can be debilitating. As described earlier, characterising this into spontaneous or incident pain through assessment will allow an individualised approach. The analgesic prescribed for breakthrough pain will also partially rely on the analgesia used for background pain. For example, if a patient is using regular paracetamol, it is reasonable to prescribe a weak opioid as required if the breakthrough pain sounds visceral, whereas for breakthrough bone pain, an NSAID may be preferable.

Non-opioids
Paracetamol

Paracetamol is a synthetic analgesic and antipyretic. It works mainly in the central nervous system (CNS), through inhibition of cyclo-oxygenase (COX)-2 and also through a number of other pathways; opioid, cannabinoid, and serotoninergic descending pain inhibition [17]. Paracetamol can be given orally (tablets, soluble tablets, liquid), rectally or by intravenous infusion. It is well tolerated but toxic in overdose. The "usual dose" is 1gram PO QDS, though this should be reduced in those at risk of hepatotoxicity. Risks factors include weight <50kg, poor nutritional status, fasting/anorexia, older age and chronic alcohol use [17]; in a patient with at least one of these, the dose should be reduced to maximum 3 grams/24 hours. In those with severe renal impairment (glomerular filtration rate (GFR) < 30), the dose should also be reduced to maximum 3 grams/24 hours, It is a useful analgesic but in those where it is not effective it should be stopped, not least as this helps to reduce tablet burden.

NSAIDs

NSAIDs are anti-inflammatory, antipyretic, and analgesic in action. They act by inhibiting COX as part of the arachidonic acid cascade, ultimately reducing prostaglandin production which leads to their clinical effects.

NSAIDs are now categorised depending on their selectivity in inhibiting COX-2; those that are more selective for COX-2 have less detrimental effect on platelet function and therefore have less bleeding risk. This is important as one of the main risks of NSAIDs is gastrointestinal toxicity, which can commonly cause bleeding. See Table 5 for the relative impact of different NSAIDs on gastrointestinal toxicity.

These drugs are very useful for pain management in palliative care, though the benefits and risks need to be carefully weighed up. The risks can sometimes be mitigated, for example reducing gastrointestinal bleeding risk through picking a low risk NSAID, using "gastric-protection" (for example a PPI) and reducing other medications contributing to gastrointestinal bleeding (anticoagulants, aspirin, corticosteroids, selective serotonin reuptake inhibitors (SSRIs)). Cardiovascular risk cannot be removed but historically Naproxen has been thought to be the "safest" NSAID in this regard; more recent evidence suggests Celecoxib may also be preferable to others [17]. Renal toxicity is difficult to reduce other than by maintaining hydration. For more information on the adverse effects of NSAIDs see Table 6.

Table 5 Relative gastrointestinal toxicity of different NSAIDs.

Low Risk	Medium Risk	High Risk
Celecoxib	Naproxen	Piroxicam
Parecoxib	Diclofenac	Ketorolac
Ibuprofen		Ketoprofen
Nabumetone		

Table 6 Adverse effects of NSAIDs.

System Involved	Adverse Effects	Notes
Gastrointestinal tract	Gastro-duodenal inflammation, ulceration, bleeding, and perforation Pain, nausea, vomiting Lower GI bleeding	NSAIDs differ in their gastrointestinal toxicity (see Table 5)
Renal system	Water and sodium retention, oedema Hyperkalaemia Antagonism of diuretics and anti-hypertensives Acute renal failure especially if elderly, dehydrated, and renal artery stenosis present	Risk of renal toxicity greater in those with preceding renal impairment Contraindicated in myeloma and renal impairment
Cardiovascular system	Increased risk of thrombotic events (myocardial infarction and stroke) Fluid retention precipitating or exacerbating congestive cardiac failure	Contraindicated in severe heart failure Minimise risk by using lowest dose for shortest time
Respiratory system	Bronchospasm Exacerbation of known asthma Rhinitis	Contraindicated if known previous sensitivity Avoid if known severe asthma, chronic rhinitis, nasal polyps Use cautiously under close supervision in asthmatic patients aged > 40 years

Opioids
Weak Opioids
The medications in this class are Codeine, Dihydrocodeine, and Tramadol. Formulations and other information about each of these is shown in Table 7. Note that low dose compound preparations (such as co-codamol 8/500) are not recommenced in palliative care.

These drugs are designated as "weak" opioids as they have a ceiling dose; that is, when this dose is reached, there is no clinical indication to increase further. If this point is reached, and pain persists and is thought to be opioid-sensitive, the weak opioid should be stopped and a strong opioid commenced (see Figure 4 and strong opioids section).

In general, these drugs are thought to have a relative potency to morphine of 1/10th, hence the suggestions in Figure 4. Bear in mind that codeine is a pro-drug, with the vast majority of its effect being gained from conversion to morphine by the cytochrome enzyme CYP2D6. There is known variation in the activity of this enzyme due to genotypic variations, and those who are poor metabolisers of codeine will derive less analgesic effect [41]. This also means that when such individuals are switched to strong opioids, there is the risk that the initial opioid dose will be too potent and opioid toxicity will follow. A dose reduction of the strong opioid will be required in this situation to obtain the balance between clinical benefit and adverse effects.

Strong Opioids: Morphine
Morphine is usually the strong opioid of choice, given its familiarity, availability and cost [17, 42]. There is, however, no compelling evidence to suggest morphine is superior or inferior to other strong opioids. There are times when alternative strong opioids are useful, and these are discussed later. Morphine is an effective analgesic, with 70% of patients with cancer pain having a good therapeutic outcome [43].

Morphine mainly acts on μ-opioid receptors, both centrally and peripherally. It is readily absorbed by the gut and metabolised in the liver, mainly through the process of glucuronidation. Liver metabolism is maintained reasonably well in hepatic impairment, and morphine often remains the opioid of choice, though glucuronidation is reduced if the prothrombin time is prolonged (which obviates more cautious dosing) [17].

Table 7 Weak opioids.

Drug	Dose Range and Formulations	Potency Relative to Morphine	Notes
Codeine	30–60 mg QDS, maximum 240 mg/24 h Tablets, oral syrup, and solution (injection not used in palliative care) Compound preparations with paracetamol and aspirin exist	Codeine 30 mg ~ Morphine 3 mg (bear in mind potential issues with CYP2D6)	Also used to treat cough Metabolised to morphine Metabolites accumulate in renal impairment
Dihydro-codeine	30–60 mg QDS, maximum 240 mg/24 h Tablets and oral solution Modified release tablets exist Injection not recommended in palliative care Compound preparations with paracetamol exist	Dihydrocodeine 30 mg ~ Morphine 3 mg Similar potency to codeine when given orally but twice as potent as codeine when injected	Unlike codeine, dihydrocodeine is not a pro-drug; hence, its therapeutic effect is not limited by CYP2D6 inhibition Causes toxicity in renal impairment due to accumulation of metabolites
Tramadol	50–100 mg QDS (maximum 400 mg/24 h) Modified and normal release tablets and capsules Normal release oro-dispersible tablets Injection (not recommended in palliative care) Compound preparations with paracetamol exist	Trial evidence suggests 1/5th as potent as morphine by mouth (Tramadol 50 mg ~ Morphine 10 mg) but clinical experience suggests 1/10th A range of potencies have been found with injection, in practice used at 1/10th potency of morphine injection	Less constipating than codeine/dihydrocodeine but causes more nausea/vomiting Non-opioid properties (noradrenaline and serotonin) responsible for some efficacy and adverse effects Preferred weak opioid in renal impairment as converted by liver to inactive metabolites that are renally excreted, though caution still required Avoid in uncontrolled epilepsy Adds to risk of serotonin syndrome

The main metabolites of morphine are morphine-3-glucoronide (M3G) and morphine 6-glucoronide (M6G). Clinical effects, both analgesic but also adverse, can mainly be attributed to M6G. These metabolites are excreted by the kidney, and in renal impairment they can build up, precipitating opioid toxicity. For this reason, an alternative strong opioid to morphine is often chosen when there is significant renal impairment.

Initiating and Titrating Morphine

There are limited studies around the initiation of strong opioids. A systematic review found evidence for initiation with both immediate release (IR) and modified release (MR) morphine, with neither approach being superior [44].

The immediate release approach, with patients taking opioids every four hours, has historically been used. This was not based upon evidence, but upon pharmacological considerations given that immediate release morphine has a plasma half-life of 2–4 hours, and reaches a steady state within 4–5 half lives. Practically, however, the expectation of taking medication this regularly risks non-compliance, and a modified release approach may be preferable. Currently either approach is reasonable, and both are displayed in Figure 4. Further points to consider when starting strong opioids are found in Box 6, and considerations when titrating strong opioids are listed in Box 7.

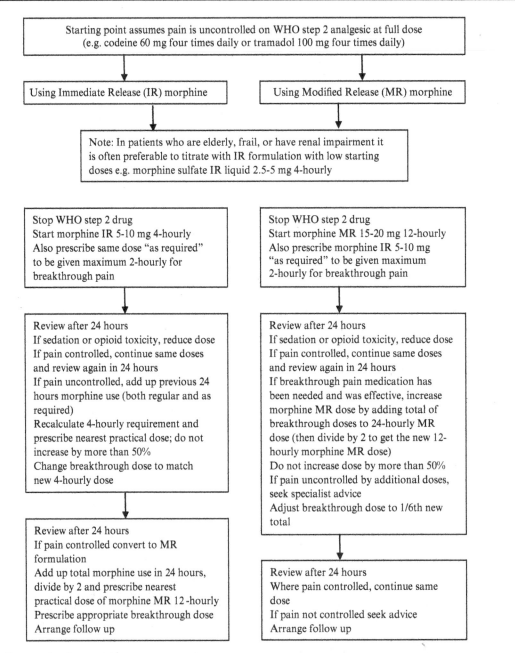

Figure 4 Commencing strong opioids.

Breakthrough Pain: Opioid Dose

It is crucial that all patient's taking regular opioids have a breakthrough opioid prescribed too. A task group of the Association for Palliative Medicine of Great Britain and Ireland reviewed this in 2009 [24] and the guidelines were more recently affirmed in an international review of practice [45].

Twelve recommendations about strategies for approaching the management of cancer-related breakthrough pain were devised based on low-grade evidence. These included assessing whether patients have breakthrough pain, that breakthrough pain should be assessed, and that an individual management strategy should be devised.

Box 6: Points to consider when starting strong opioids

- Ensure patients have been given clear oral and written instructions, and their understanding has been confirmed
- MR opioids should be instructed to be taken 12 hours apart (for example, 0800 and 2000) rather than the less precise instruction "twice daily"
- Clarify with the patient that regular opioids should still be taken even if a dose of breakthrough medication has just been used
- Ensure that a regular laxative has been prescribed and that bowel habit is monitored
- Ensure that patients have a supply of anti.emetic for regular or as required use for at least the first week on a strong opioid
- Monitor closely for efficacy, adverse effects, and opioid toxicity

Box 7: Considerations when titrating opioids

- When increasing the total regular daily dose of strong opioid, it is usual to do so by 30–50% (the equivalent of 2–3 "PRN" doses).
- It is not recommended to titrate with transdermal preparations when there is unstable pain.
- Always adjust the breakthrough dose if the regular dose is changed (up **or** down).
- Do not use two or more MR opioid formulations at the same time without specialist advice.
- If pain control deteriorates, a holistic pain assessment should be carried out.
- If an intervention takes place that may change the pain burden, such as a nerve block, the opioid dose may require reduction to avoid intolerance and adverse effects.

Classically using the same opioid for MR and IR use has been recommended where possible (this is not possible with opioid patches – see section on transdermal patches), with the IR dose at 1/6th of the total daily regular dose. However, effectiveness but also adverse effects related to breakthrough doses should be closely reviewed and then tailored to the patient.

More recently rapid-onset opioids (ROOs), namely transmucosal fentanyls, have been introduced. These come in a variety of formulations including sublingual tablets and nasal sprays. They may be particularly helpful for short duration pain (commonly incident pain) though more

evidence base is needed to fully understand their role. Their use should only be initiated under specialist care.

Pharmacogenomics and Opioid Analgesia

While response to opioids in terms of analgesia and side effects is quite predictable, individual response must be considered too. The prime example is the already discussed response to codeine and CYP2D6 expression, whereby a poor analgesic response to codeine suggests poor conversion of the codeine prodrug to morphine. Furthermore, a number of polymorphisms of the μ-opioid receptor have been described, impacting on the analgesic effects and adverse effects of opioids [46]. Such polymorphisms are very rarely characterised in a clinical setting, however, and when prescribing a strong opioid morphine remains first choice (when renal function is not grossly impaired).

Other Strong Opioids

While morphine is usually first choice, a number of strong opioids are available. In general they have no superiority in analgesic effect to morphine [43,47] but in some patients a change of opioid (an "opioid switch") is indicated because of intolerable side effects from morphine, by organ (mainly renal) impairment or sometimes, in the case of a switch to methadone, because of suboptimal analgesic effect.

There is evidence for this individualised therapeutic approach. Fewer patients report constipation for example when taking fentanyl as opposed to morphine [48]. Changing from morphine to oxycodone (or vice versa) can give analgesic benefit to the around 30% of people where the initial drug has been ineffective [43]. Since it seems people may respond differently to different opioids it is most important that if a switch is made, the patient is monitored closely to assess their individual effects.

Different opioids have different potencies, and these equivalences need to be used when calculating doses on changing opioids. It is usual practice to reduce the opioid dose by 25–50% when switching, though this reduction may be less for patients in severe pain, and more for those on very high doses [17]. Specialist advice is often needed in consideration of "switching."

Information about alternative opioids to morphine is found in Table 8, dose equivalence between morphine and other opioids is in Table 9, and equivalence between oral and subcutaneous opioids is found in Table 10.

Table 8 Alternative strong opioids to morphine.

Opioid	Formulations	Characteristics/Comments
Oxycodone	IR liquid and capsules, MR tablets, injection	Similar properties to morphine. MR formulation should not be used in severe renal impairment
Hydromorphone	IR and MR capsules, injection	Good oral option for patients with renal impairment (though dose reductions needed)
Fentanyl	Transdermal patches, transmucosal lozenges, buccal and sublingual tablets, nasal spray, injection	Potency often underestimated. Less constipating than morphine. Patches not suitable for unstable pain requiring rapid titration. Transmucosal formulations permit options for rapid absorption, but this requires close supervision in initial titration. Suitable in renal impairment
Buprenorphine	Transdermal patches, sublingual tablets, injection	Patches not suitable for unstable pain requiring rapid titration. Low strength transdermal formulations provide an option for less severe pain or for patients sensitive to other strong opioids. Suitable in renal impairment. Toxicity not reversed by standard doses of naloxone (higher doses needed)
Alfentanil	Injection	Only available as an injection. Better given in a syringe driver than on an as-required basis as short half-life. Suitable in renal impairment
Diamorphine	Injection	No analgesic advantage over parenteral morphine but more soluble and thus commonly used by infusion, especially when high doses are needed. Compatible with many drugs in SC infusion
Methadone	Tablets, oral solution, injection	Non.opioid receptor (NMDA) actions potentiate analgesic action. Highly variable pharmacokinetics and pharmacodynamics between individuals; hence, switching from other opioids and titration should be managed by specialists [48]

Table 9 Equivalence between morphine and other opioids. Note that these figures are a guide and this table follows recommendations from the Faculty of Pain Medicine [49] and PCF7 [17] rather than the manufacturers' stated ratios.

Opioid Dose Ratio	Example of Converted Prescriptions (with No Dose Reduction)
Switching between oral formulations	
Morphine: Oxycodone = 1.5: 1	Morphine 15 mg = Oxycodone 10 mg
Morphine: Hydromorphone = 5: 1	Morphine 30 mg = Hydromorphone 6 mg
Switching from oral to transdermal formulations	
Morphine PO: Fentanyl TD = 100: 1	Morphine MR 30 mg/24h = Fentanyl TD patch 12 mcg/h
	Morphine MR 60 mg/24 h = Fentanyl TD patch 25 mcg/h
	Morphine MR 120 mg/24 h = Fentanyl TD patch 50 mcg/h
Morphine PO: Buprenorphine TD = 100: 1	Morphine MR 12 mg/24h = Buprenorphine 5 mcg/h
	Morphine MR 24 mg/24h = Buprenorphine 10 mcg/h
	Morphine MR 48 mg/24h = Buprenorphine 20 mcg/h

Table 10 Equivalence between oral opioids. Note that these figures are a guide and this table follows the PCF7 clinical recommendations [17] rather than the manufacturers' stated ratios.

Opioid Dose Ratio	Example of Converted Prescription (with No Dose Reduction)
Morphine PO: Morphine SC = 2: 1	Morphine MR 30 mg PO 12 hourly = Morphine 30 mg/24 h through SC infusion
Morphine PO: Diamorphine SC = 3: 1	Morphine MR 30 mg PO 12 hourly = Diamorphine 20 mg/24 h through SC infusion
Morphine PO: Oxycodone SC = 2: 1	Morphine MR 30 mg PO 12 hourly = Oxycodone 30 mg/24 h through SC infusion
Morphine PO: Hydromorphone SC = 10: 1	Morphine MR 30 mg PO 12 hourly = Hydromorphone 4 mg/24 h through SC infusion
Morphine PO: Alfentanil SC = 30: 1	Morphine MR 30 mg PO 12 hourly = Alfentanil 2 mg/24 h through SC infusion
Oxycodone PO: Oxycodone SC = 1.5: 1	Oxycodone MR 20 mg PO 12 hourly = Oxycodone 25 mg/24 h through SC infusion
Hydromorphone PO: Hydromorphone SC = 2: 1	Hydromorphone MR 8 mg PO 12 hourly = Hydromorphone 8 mg/24 h through SC infusion

Transdermal Opioids

Currently the opioids fentanyl and buprenorphine are available as patches. This route of administration can offer specific advantages, though patches must be used in appropriate circumstances.

Opioid patches are indicated for opioid responsive pain that is stable; they are more difficult to titrate when analgesia requirements are escalating and so are not a good choice at this time. A switch to one of these opioids may be considered for the reasons previously discussed, to try to improve analgesia or to reduce adverse effects. A switch may also be considered to fentanyl and buprenorphine as both are well tolerated when kidney function is poor. Additionally, a patch can be considered when there are challenges with the oral route, such as impaired or painful swallowing due to cancer or treatment of this, or problems with drug absorption in the gut, such as malignant bowel obstruction or gastric outlet obstruction. A patient may be keen to switch to a patch to reduce their tablet burden; using a patch for this reason may also aid compliance. Finally, a patch can be considered where there are concerns about misuse or diversion of tablets (though patches can still be abused).

Practicalities

Transdermal patches need to be applied to a clean, dry, and flat and hairless area of skin. The back and upper outer arms are common sites. It is good practice to "rotate" the patch site, so that it is not recurrently applied to an identical area of skin. Ensure a good seal between the patch and the skin on application. Patients should avoid applying heat to the patch, such as in a hot bath, as this can increase the absorption rate (it is ok for patients to shower). When removed, patched should be folded over, sticky sides together, and disposed of safely such as in a sharps bin or returned to a pharmacist.

Fentanyl patches are available in a number of different strengths, but all patches are designed to be used for 72-hours. Occasionally a patient will experience an end of dose deterioration of pain, in which case changing patches 48-hourly can be helpful. Lower strength buprenorphine patches are changed every 7 days, with higher strength patches lasting 96-hours; in practice, it is best to change these twice weekly, on the same days of the week for clarity. Patches should not be cut to try to achieve alternative doses.

While it is ideal to use the same opioid for modified and normal release purposes, this is more challenging when using transdermal patches. It is usual to use IR morphine in the first instance as the as required opioid alongside transdermal patches, unless there are reasons to use alternatives (for example, severe renal impairment, when oxycodone may be used at low dose).

Initiating and Discontinuing Transdermal Patches

The practicalities of timings around changing opioids, including transdermal patches, can be challenging. See

Box 8: Guidance on timings of changing opioids. Guidance taken with permission from The North of England Cancer Network Palliative and End-of-Life Care Guidelines [50]

Oral to subcutaneous infusion
From IR opioid: start syringe driver immediately.
From 12-hourly MR opioid: start syringe driver 4 hours
    before next oral dose due.

Subcutaneous infusion to oral
Switching to either IR or MR opioid, stop the syringe driver
    and give first oral dose at the same time.

Oral to patch
From IR opioid: apply patch when convenient and use oral
    IR opioid as required.
From twice daily MR opioid: apply patch at same time as last
    dose of MR oral opioid.

Patch to oral
Remove patch 6 hours before giving first dose of oral MR
    opioid.
For first 24 hours (i.e. first two doses) give HALF the calcu-
    lated equivalent dose since the transdermal fentanyl will
    take time to be cleared from plasma and subcutaneous
    reservoir.
After 24 hours increase to the calculated equivalent dose if
    clinically indicated by pain.

Patch to subcutaneous infusion
For those likely in the last days-short weeks of life, it is
    reasonable to continue the patch and add a syringe driver
    in addition to this, being careful to calculate the correct IR
    opioid dose.
In other situations where a change from patch is required,
    remove patch and start syringe driver 6 hours later using
    HALF the calculated opioid equivalent dose for the first 24
    hours then adjust according to symptoms.

Subcutaneous infusion to patch
    Apply patch. Continue subcutaneous infusion for a fur-
    ther 6 hours then discontinue syringe driver.

Box 8 for guidance on this, remembering the importance of individual assessment in each case. Box 8 also contains guidance on the timings on switching opioids given by routes other than transdermal patches.

When changing from an alternative opioid to transdermal preparations, patients may experience an opioid withdrawal-like syndrome, with gastric upset a predominant feature. Utilising doses of IR opioid will help these symptoms [17].

Opioid Adverse Effects

It is important to counsel patients about the potential adverse effects of opioids on commencement, to aid understanding and so that patients know what to expect. Adverse effects occur with both weak and strong opioids.

Constipation is the commonest adverse effect of opioids, occurring in up to 95% of cases. All patients taking regular opioids should also take a stimulant laxative to counteract this.

Nausea and vomiting is also common in those taking opioids. This is much more likely during the first week of treatment, or when the opioid dose is increased. Metoclopramide or Haloperidol are appropriate antiemetics, and should be available for patients on an as required basis during these times, being stepped up to regular if nausea or vomiting occurs.

A dry mouth is also a common effect of opioids. It is worth reviewing the patient's medications as a whole as other offending medications may be discontinued. Local oral measures can also be useful.

Other well-recognised adverse effects include drowsiness, delirium, hallucinations and myoclonus. Sometimes these effects can settle down within a few days. If hallucinations are problematic they may improve with a small dose of haloperidol. If adverse effects remain problematic and opioids have been at least partially effective, an opioid switch should be considered.

Opioid toxicity occurs when opioids are escalated too quickly for the individual patient, or when opioids are not excreted as expected, such as in renal impairment. Earlier features include drowsiness, confusion, and myoclonus, later progressing onto respiratory depression. If opioid toxicity is diagnosed opioids should be reduced, or temporarily stopped in more severe cases. Naloxone is only indicated when the patient's respiratory rate is less than 8 breaths/minute and/or the patient's oxygen saturations are below baseline (due to opioids). Please refer to local guidelines when treating opioid toxicity with respiratory depression.

Fears and Concerns Related to Use of Morphine and Other Opioids

Guidelines on the use of and literature about opioids are freely available, though concerns remain relatively common among both healthcare professionals and patients (Box 9). Some fears may be related to the perception of opioids as "recreational drugs," while others are related to the use of opioids by professionals; though important to report on, events in the media such as the inquiry into

Box 9: Professional and patient concerns about opioids

Professional	Patient
Patient addiction/ dependence	Addiction/dependence
Diversion of patient supply to illegal use	Social stigma
Respiratory depression	Side effects
Excess sedation/confusion/ cognitive impairment	Morphine equated to imminent death
Fear of expediting death	Pain will become resistant to analgesia so "nothing left when pain severe later"
	Effect on functionality e.g. driving

Gosport War Memorial Hospital [51] are understandably concerning for patients and professionals alike.

Evidence and experience has shown that opioids, when used in an appropriate way, are excellent analgesics that are safe to prescribe. Fears around their use are unjustified [52] and often unfounded. However, it is of critical importance in discussing patients' fears about these medications, to address anxiety and to help secure concordance of pain management plans. Of particular importance is explaining that addiction (psychological dependence) does not occur when opioids are used for pain management in palliative care, and that if pain is reduced by other means (e.g. nerve blocks) then opioids can generally be reduced. Note, however, that opioids should be gradually reduced and not be stopped suddenly as withdrawal symptoms can occur.

It is important for patients in the UK taking opioids to know about driving legislation. Roadside drug tests were introduced in 2015, and those taking prescribed opioids should carry evidence of this (such as a prescription), which will prevent prosecution as long as their driving is not impaired [53].

Adjuvant Analgesics or Co-analgesics

Adjuvant analgesics are medications that were initially designed for another indication, but also have an analgesic benefit when given in the correct circumstances. Many adjuvant analgesics are particularly useful in the treatment of neuropathic pain. Note that the evidence base for many of these medications may be in a different setting, for example painful diabetic neuropathy rather than cancer-related nerve pain for neuropathic drugs. It is best practice to initially use one adjuvant analgesic and titrate up the dose, though it is common to then introduce a second analgesic that works synergistically. Medications are discussed below with a summary in Table 11.

Anti-convulsants

These medications have been used for neuropathic pain for a number of years, for example Carbamazepine for trigeminal neuralgia. For other causes of neuropathic pain, the gabapentinoids (gabapentin and pregabalin) should be used first line [54]. These medications work via voltage-gated calcium channels, helping reduce glutamate release. They are often well tolerated if titrated at an appropriate pace for the patient. The most common side effects are drowsiness and dizziness. The dose should be reduced in renal impairment [17]. Other anti-convulsants, such as sodium valproate, may also be effective but should be used under specialist supervision. Clonazepam is sometimes used by specialists but as yet has very limited evidence base for neuropathic pain.

Antidepressants

Medications in this group are the others recommend by NICE as first-line for neuropathic pain [54]. Tricyclic antidepressants, particularly amitriptyline, are commonly used, and have the lowest number needed to treat (NNT) value for medications in neuropathic pain [55]. They have a number of mechanisms of action, particularly through noradrenaline re-uptake [17]. Doses should be started low and titrated as required and tolerated. They are contra-indicated in heart disease and in those with arrhythmias. Adverse effects are commonly due to their anti-cholinergic properties, including dry mouth, urinary retention, constipation, and a risk of falls.

The other drug recommended by NICE is duloxetine, a serotonin and noradrenaline reuptake inhibitor (SNRI), for which most evidence is in diabetic neuropathy. The most common side effects are drowsiness and a dry mouth. Mirtazapine is also sometimes used for neuropathic pain but has a very limited evidence base; the risk of serotonin toxicity is lower with mirtazapine compared to other antidepressants.

Corticosteroids

Corticosteroids have multiple indications in palliative care, for which pain is one. They are most useful for liver capsular pain and neuropathic pain (see case study in Box 10). They have anti-inflammatory effects, but also work through reducing peri-tumoural oedema. Early side

Table 11 Adjuvant analgesics.

Group	Indication	Example(s) with Maximum Dose Range
Antiepileptics	Neuropathic pain	Gabapentin 100 mg TDS – 1.2 g TDS
		Pregabalin 25 mg BD – 300 mg BD
Antidepressants	Neuropathic pain	Amitriptyline 10–75 mg OD (nocte)
		Duloxetine 30 – 120 mg/day
Corticosteroids	Neuropathic pain	Dexamethasone 6 – 12 mg daily initially, reducing every few
	Liver capsular pain	days to stop (within 2–3 weeks)
Bisphosphonates	Bone pain (particularly in myeloma, breast cancer and prostate cancer)	Zoledronic acid 4 mg in 100 ml 0.9% saline infused over 30 min given every 4 weeks
Benzodiazepines	Muscle relaxant	Diazepam 2–10 mg daily
		Midazolam 2.5–5 mg SC per dose
	Neuropathic pain	Clonazepam 500 micrograms – 4 mg daily
Muscle relaxants	Muscle spasm	Baclofen 5 mg BD – 20 mg TDS
Anticholinergics	Bladder spasm	Tolterodine 2 mg BD
	Colic (in complete bowel obstruction) or rectal spasm	Hyoscine butylbromide 60–120 mg/24 h SC infusion
Ketamine (for use under specialist initiation and supervision only)	Neuropathic pain not responsive to other medications	Starting dose: 10–25 mg PO QDS or 50–100 mg/24 h by SC infusion
		Usual maximum dose: 50–100 mg PO QDS or 500 mg/24 h by SC infusion

Box 10: Case study

"Mr. Talbot's pain responded well to radiotherapy, corticosteroids, and neuropathic agents. His corticosteroids were down-titrated. He later developed visceral abdominal pain and morphine was appropriately titrated to allow adequate analgesia that was well tolerated. Discussions about his preferences for the future were supported and he was able to stay in his preferred place of care of home."

effects include gastric irritation and an increase in blood glucose, particularly in those with pre-existing diabetes mellitus, with later effects including proximal myopathy, a decrease in bone density, and other metabolic effects. It is best practice to review corticosteroids regularly, reducing them to their lowest effective dose, and ideally stopping after less than three weeks, to avoid the risk of Addisonian effects and late side effects. As they work quickly for nerve pain they are particularly useful to prescribe whilst other more standard neuropathic agents are being titrated.

Topical Analgesics

A number of agents are available as topical formulations. Levomenthol 1–2% (in Aqueous Cream) is helpful for itch through an effect on sensory nerve endings, but can also be useful for the "stretching" pain experienced from oedematous limbs. Capsaicin cream works by reducing substance P production and can be helpful for localised neuropathic pain, though it is an irritant and is best applied with a gloved hand. The local anaesthetic lidocaine is available in a medicated plaster, which is licensed for post-herpetic neuralgia. It can be useful for localised neuropathic pain though has a very limited evidence base. Plasters are used in a 12 hour on, 12 hour off pattern, and caution is advised in those with severe cardiac, renal, or hepatic impairment [17].

Interventional Analgesia

Procedures for pain are considered in those whose pain remains challenging despite specialist input and a trial of pharmacological and non-pharmacological options. This may be due to poorly responsive pain or intolerance to a number of analgesics. Such patients should always be referred to specialist palliative care services, who can liaise with interventional pain colleagues to consider neuraxial options (epidural or intrathecal inteventions) and/or neurolytic procedures (such as a coeliac plexus block or cervical cordotomy).

Non-pharmacological Interventions

In the early part of this chapter, the importance of a whole-person assessment was discussed. Pain is a complex symptom that is generally multi-dimensional in the setting of advanced illness. Management needs to reflect this. It is therefore important that the multi-disciplinary team (MDT) is involved in developing a management plan, and treatments are considered from different professionals within this group. This may include among other specialists:
• Physiotherapy and occupational therapy who may support the use of a TENS machine, acupuncture, rehabilitation, and goal setting
• Clinical psychology to explore psychological causes and impacts of pain
• A spiritual care team to support spiritual aspects of pain
• Complimentary therapies as reducing anxiety, increasing relaxation, and promoting self- efficacy such as through hypnosis are all valuable pain management strategies
Additionally, it is important to consider the underlying disease process and whether direct treatment for this will help pain, for example:
• The use of radiotherapy for painful bony metastases
• Surgical fixation of impending fractures from bony metastases
• Vertebroplasty for osteoporotic spinal fractures
Finally, the value of communicating to patients about their pain should not be underestimated, and there is evidence that patient-based educational interventions support pain management [56].

Conclusion

Pain is a complex, multi-dimensional symptom, particularly in the context of advanced illness. A whole person assessment and an individualised approach to management will allow the best outcome for the patient. Pharmacological approaches are very important, and clinicians should have a good grasp of a number of medications that are likely to be helpful in different circumstances. Clinicians should also recognise when referral on to specialist services is required for use of more complex analgesia, treatment of the underlying illness, and input from the wider MDT for non-pharmacological approaches.

Acknowledgement

Many thanks to Dr Alex Nicholson, previous author of this chapter, who allowed me to use the structure of and images from the previous edition in writing this chapter.

References

1. Abernethy, A.P., Kamal, A., and Currow, D.C. (2013). When should nonsteroidal antiinflammatory drugs be used to manage pain? *Evidence-Based Practice of Palliative Medicine* (N.E. Goldstein and R.D. Morrison), 49–53. Philadelphia: Saunders.
2. British Medical Association (2016). *End-of-life Care and Physician-assisted Dying (Volume 1)*. London: BMA.
3. Breivik, H., Cherny, N., Collett, B. et al. (2009). Cancer related pain: a pan-European survey of prevalence, treatment, and patient attitudes. *Annals of Oncology* 20 (8): 1420–1433.
4. van den Beuken-van Everdingen, M.H., Hochstenbach, L.M., Joosten, E.A. et al. (2016). Update on prevalence of pain in patients with cancer: systematic review and meta-analysis. *Journal of Pain and Symptom Management* 51 (6): 1070–1090.
5. Wiffen, P.J., Wee, B., Derry, S. et al. (2017 Jul). Opioids for cancer pain – an overview of Cochrane reviews. *Cochrane Database of Systematic Reviews* 2017 (7): CD012592.
6. World Health Organisation. *Palliative Care*. https://www. who.int/news-room/fact-sheets/detail/palliative-care (accessed 30 March 2021).
7. Natoli, S., Lazzari, M., and Dauri, M. (2015). Open questions in the treatment of cancer pain: time for a strong evidence-based approach? *Expert Opinion on Pharmacotherapy* 16: 1–4.
8. Greco, M.T., Roberto, A., Corli, O. et al. (2014). Quality of cancer pain management: an update of a systematic review of undertreatment of patients with cancer. *Journal of Clinical Oncology* 32 (36): 4149–4154.
9. Lynn, J., Teno, J.M., Phillips, R.S. et al. (1997). Perceptions by family members of the dying experience of older and seriously ill patients. SUPPORT investigators. Study to understand prognoses and preferences for outcomes and risks of treatments. *Annals of Internal Medicine* 126 (2): 97–106.
10. Raja, S.N., Carr, D.B., Cohen, M. et al. (2020). The revised International Association for the Study of Pain definition of pain: concepts, challenges, and compromises. *Pain* 161 (9): 1976–1982.

11. Saunders, C. (1998). The symptomatic treatment of incurable malignant disease. *Prescriber's* Journal. 1964; 4: 68-73. Cited in: Clark D. An annotated bibliography of the publications of Cicely Saunders – 1: 1958-1967. *Palliative Medicine* 12 (3): 181–193.

12. McCaffery, M. and Pasero, C. (1999). *Pain: A Clinical Manual.* St Louis, Missouri: Mosby.

13. Melzack, R. and Wall, P.D. (1965). Pain mechanisms: a new theory. *Science* 150 (3699): 971–979.

14. Ellison, D.L. (2017). Physiology of pain. *Critical Care Nursing Clinics of North America* 29: 397–406.

15. Raphael, J., Ahmedzai, S., Hester, J. et al. (2010). Cancer pain: Part 1: pathophysiology; oncological, pharmacological, and psychological treatments: a perspective from the British Pain Society endorsed by the UK Association of Palliative Medicine and the Royal College of General Practitioners. *Pain Medicine* 11 (5): 742–764.

16. McDonald, J. and Lambert, D.G. (2005). Opioid receptors. *Continuing Education in Anaesthesia, Critical Care and Pain* 5 (1): 22–25.

17. Wilcock, A., Howard, P., and Charlesworth, S. (2020). *Palliative Care Formulary*, 7th e. London: Pharmaceutical Press.

18. Vardeh, D., Mannion, R.J., and Woolf, C.J. (2016). Toward a mechanism-based approach to pain diagnosis. *The Journal of Pain* 17 (9 Suppl): T50–69.

19. Treede, R.D., Jensen, T.S., Campbell, J.N. et al. (2008). Neuropathic pain: redefinition and a grading system for clinical and research purposes. *Neurology* 70 (18): 1630–1635.

20. Bennett, M.I., Rayment, C., Hjermstad, M. et al. (2012). Prevalence and aetiology of neuropathic pain in cancer patients: a systematic review. *Pain* 153 (2): 359–365.

21. Haanpaa, M., Attal, N., Backonja, M. et al. (2011). NeuPSIG guidelines on neuropathic pain assessment. *Pain* 152 (1): 14–27.

22. Grond, S., Radbruch, L., Meuser, T. et al. (1999). Assessment and treatment of neuropathic cancer pain following WHO guidelines. *Pain* 79 (1): 15–20.

23. Davies, A.N. (2014). Breakthrough cancer pain. *Current Pain and Headache Reports* 18: 420.

24. Davies, A.N., Dickman, A., Reid, C. et al. (2009). The management of cancer-related breakthrough pain: recommendations of a task group of the Science Committee of the Association for Palliative Medicine of Great Britain and Ireland. *European Journal of Pain* 13: 331–338.

25. Jensen, T.S. and Finnerup, N.B. (2014). Allodynia and hyperalgesia in neuropathic pain: clinical manifestations and mechanisms. *Lancet Neurology* 13 (9): 924–935.

26. Martin, L.A. and Hagen, N.A. (1997). Neuropathic pain in cancer patients: mechanisms, syndromes, and clinical controversies. *Journal of Pain and Symptom Management* 14 (2): 99–117.

27. Herr, K., Titler, M.G., Schilling, M. et al. (2004). Evidence based assessment of acute pain in older adults: current nursing practices and perceived barriers. *The Clinical Journal of Pain* 20 (5): 331–340.

28. Greater Manchester Medicines Management Group. (2019). *Palliative Care Pain & Symptom Control Guidelines For Adults*, 5th e. Available from: http://gmmmg.nhs.uk/docs/guidance/GMMMG-Palliative-Care-Pain-and-Symptom-Control-Guidelines-for-Adults-v1-1.pdf (accessed 02 May 2021)

29. Grond, S., Zech, D., Diefenbach, C. et al. (1996). Assessment of cancer pain: a prospective evaluation in 2266 cancer patients referred to a pain service. *Pain* 64: 107–114.

30. Rayment, C. and Bennett, M.I. (2015). Definition and assessment of chronic pain in advanced disease. In: *Oxford Textbook of Palliative Medicine*, 5th e (ed. N. Cherny, M. Fallon, S. Kaasa et al.), 519–524. Oxford University Press.

31. Holen, J.C., Hjermstad, M.J., Loge, J.H. et al. (2006). Pain assessment tools: is the content appropriate for use in palliative care. *Journal of Pain and Symptom Management* 32: 567–580.

32. Caraceni, A., Cherny, N., Fainsinger, R. et al. (2002). Pain measurement tools and methods in clinical research in palliative care: recommendations of an Expert Working Group of the European Association of palliative care. *Journal of Pain and Symptom Management* 23: 239–255.

33. Callin, S. and Bennett, M.I. (2008). Diagnosis and management of neuropathic pain in palliative care. *International Journal of Palliative Nursing* 14 (1): 16–21.

34. Jordan, A., Regnard, C., O'Brien, J.T. et al. (2012). Pain and distress in advanced dementia: choosing the right tools for the job. *Palliative Medicine* 26 (7): 873–878.

35. National Institute for Clinical Excellence. (2016). *Palliative care for adults: Strong opioids for pain relief.* Available from: https://www.nice.org.uk/guidance/CG140 (accessed 20 May 2021).

36. Trang, T., Al-Hasani, R., Salvemini, D. et al. (2015). Pain and poppies: the good, the bad, and the ugly of opioid analgesics. *The Journal of Neuroscience* 35 (41): 13879–13888.

37. World Health Organisation. (1996). *Cancer Pain Relief; with a guide to opioid availability*, 2nd e. Available from: http://apps.who.int/iris/bitstream/handle/10665/37896/9241544821.pdf; jsessionid=EE2B5F851E110017444AAD7167C89D79?sequence=1 (accessed 30 May 2021).

38. Ballantyne, J.C., Kalso, E., and Stannard, C. (2016). WHO analgesic ladder: a good concept gone astray. *BMJ* 352: i20.

39. Vadalouca, A., Moka, E., Argyra, E. et al. (2008). Opioid rotation in patients with cancer: a review of the current literature. *Journal of Opioid Management* 4 (4): 213–250.

40. Glare, P. (2011). Choice of opioids and the WHO Ladder. *Journal of Pediatric Hematology/oncology* 33 (Suppl 1): S6–S11.

41. Carranza-Leon, D., Dickson, A.L., Gaedigk, A. et al. (2021). CYP2D6 genotype and reduced codeine analgesic effect in

real-world clinical practice. *The Pharmacogenomics Journal.* https://doi.org/10.1038/s41397-021-00226-8.

42. Hanks, G.W., Conno, F., Cherny, N. et al. (2001). Morphine and alternative opioids in cancer pain: the EAPC recommendations. *British Journal of Cancer* 84 (5): 587–593.

43. Riley, J., Branford, R., Droney, J. et al. (2015). Morphine or oxycodone for cancer-related pain? A randomized, open-label, controlled trial. *Journal of Pain and Symptom Management* 49 (2): 161–172.

44. Klepstad, P., Kaasa, S., and Borchgrevink, P.C. (2011). Starting step III opioids for moderate to severe pain in cancer patients: dose titration: a systematic review. *Palliative Medicine* 25 (5): 424–430.

45. Davies, A.N., Elsner, F., Filbet, M.J. et al. (2018 September). Breakthrough cancer pain (BTcP) management: a review of international and national guidelines. *BMJ Supportive & Palliative Care* 8 (3): 241–249.

46. Nicholson, A.B., Watson, G.R., Derry, S. et al. (2017). Methadone for cancer pain. *Cochrane Database of Systematic Reviews* 2 (2): CD003971.

47. Tassinari, D., Sartori, S., Tamburini, E. et al. (2008). Adverse effects of transdermal opiates treating moderate-severe cancer pain in comparison to long-acting morphine: a meta-analysis and systematic review of the literature. *Journal of Palliative Medicine* 11 (3): 492–501.

48. Faculty of Pain Medicine. (2020). *Dose equivalents and changing opioids.* Available from: https://fpm.ac.uk/opioids-aware-structured-approach-opioid-prescribing/dose-equivalents-and-changing-opioids (accessed 14 September 2021).

49. The North of England Cancer Network. (2012). *Palliative and end of life care guidelines for cancer and non-cancer patients.* Available from: https://www.nth.nhs.uk/content/uploads/2015/06/necn-palliative-care-guidelines-booklet-2012.pdf (accessed 14 June 2021).

50. Gosport Independent Panel. (2018). *Gosport War memorial hospital: the report of the Gosport Independent Panel.* Available from: https://www.gosportpanel.independent.gov.uk/media/documents/070618_CCS207_CCS03183220761_Gosport_Inquiry_Whole_Document.pdf (accessed 02 June 2021).

51. McQuay, H. (1999). Opioids in pain management. *Lancet* 353 (9171): 2229–2232.

52. National Institute for Clinical Excellence. (2020). *Strong opioids.* Available from: https://cks.nice.org.uk/topics/palliative-cancer-care-pain/prescribing-information/strong-opioids (accessed 02 June 2021).

53. National Institute for Clinical Excellence. (2020). *Neuropathic pain in adults: Pharmacological management in non-specialist settings.* Available from: https://www.nice.org.uk/Guidance/CG173 (accessed 15 June 2021).

54. Finnerup, N.B., Attal, N., Haroutounian, S. et al. (2015). Pharmacotherapy for neuropathic pain in adults: systematic review, meta-analysis and updated NeuPSIG recommendations. *Lancet Neurology* 14 (2): 162–173.

55. Bennett, M.I., Bagnall, A. and Closs, J.S. (2009). How effective are patient-based educational interventions in the management of cancer pain? Systematic review and meta-analysis. *Pain* 143 (3): 192–199.

56. Vieira, C.M.P., Fragoso, R.M., Pereira, D. et al. (2019). Pain polymorphisms and opioids: an evidence based review. *Molecular Medicine Reports* 19 (3): 1423–1434.

11 The Management of Gastrointestinal Symptoms and Advanced Liver Disease

Andrew Chilton, Christina Faull, Wendy Prentice and Monica Compton

With thanks to Dr Laura Clipsham for reviewing the chapter for the 4th edition of The Handbook of Palliative Care

Introduction

Patients with advanced disease, of whatever nature, commonly have symptoms related to the gastrointestinal (GI) tract. All such patients should be specifically asked about dry and sore mouth problems, eating, nausea, and constipation. Unrelenting nausea can be more disabling than pain, and effective management requires a logical, systematic, and persistent approach. Constipation is often neglected and can be prevented for most patients. Cancer may obstruct the GI tract causing well-defined syndromes and the options for palliation of these symptoms are described in detail in this chapter.

Eating and defecating can be a major point of reference for patients and their carers about their health, and their dysfunction may carry enormous significance about sustaining life and the approach of death. The importance of this in caring for patients should never be underestimated.

The palliative care needs of patients with advanced liver disease are now more recognised [1, 2]. Given the dramatic and often highly symptomatic complications of end-stage liver disease, many of these patients spend the last months of their lives in acute hospitals where many of them will also die. A small number of patients have access to specialist palliative care services, and further work is needed to support this increasing number of patients to receive appropriate palliative care delivered according to need and if possible in a place of their choosing.

Cachexia, Anorexia, and Nutrition

Cachexia and anorexia are commonly experienced symptoms of advanced malignant and non-malignant diseases, and up to 10% of patients with cancer in the community will have a body mass index of less than 20 m²/kg. The associated distress can be marked, especially in terms of body image and quality of life. Cachexia has been found to be associated with a shorter prognosis for many diseases including cancer [3], chronic obstructive airways disease [4], heart failure (HF) [5], liver disease [6], and acquired immunodeficiency syndrome (AIDS) [7].

Detailed discussion of pathophysiology is beyond the scope of this book but might include the following:
- Unresolved nausea.
- Mechanical effects of tumours and ascites.
- Cytokines (e.g. tumour necrosis factor) causing increased basal metabolic rate; increased hepatogluconogenesis, using protein as substrate; increased glucose intolerance; altered lipid metabolism; and anorexia.
- Adverse effect of medications.
- Jaundice and obstructed biliary system.
- Poor oral hygiene.
- Psychological factors including low mood and anxiety.
- Unresolved pain.

Management requires active involvement of the multidisciplinary team (MDT), and best outcomes are gained by using a range of approaches that aim to ameliorate the

Handbook of Palliative Care, Fourth Edition. Edited by Richard Kitchen, Christina Faull, Sarah Russell and Jo Wilson.
© 2024 John Wiley & Sons Ltd. Published 2024 by John Wiley & Sons Ltd.

underlying cause and address symptoms directly. Patients and carers need to be fully involved in decision-making and goal-setting. It is often the carer's job to prepare meals, and this sustaining role is of vital importance to them.

Before embarking on enteral nutritional support, clear goals and plans need to be thought through and discussed with the patient. Enteral tube feeding is considered to be a medical treatment in UK law. Its initiation, stopping, and withdrawal are medical decisions; however, these need to be made in concert with the patient [8]. If the patient is not competent to make decisions, then it is incumbent on the doctor to make these decisions in the "best interests" of the patient in consultation with those who know the patient best, the wider multi-professional team and taking into consideration any previously expressed wishes. In some countries, there is legal provision for an individual to nominate another individual to be involved in health-care decisions for them, if they are to lose the capacity in the future [9].

Drugs to Increase Appetite and Weight Gain

The following drugs have been shown to have some effect on the symptoms in cancer patients [10]. They should initially be used on a trial basis, with treatment being continued only if benefit is confirmed.

Steroids

Dexamethasone 2–4 mg (or equivalent dose of an alternative steroid) is useful for increasing appetite and energy but not weight gain. The side effects of these drugs can limit their use (e.g., diabetes, psychological effects, immunosuppression, fluid retention, and proximal muscle weakness).

Progesterones

Megestrol acetate 160 mg daily (increased up to 800 mg if required), and medroxyprogesterone acetate 480–960 mg daily, can improve appetite and weight in cancer and perhaps also AIDS patients. These drugs are usually well tolerated but can cause mild oedema, impotence, and vaginal bleeding. Unlike steroids their effect is not immediate but may occur within 2 weeks and is generally more sustained [11].

In cardiac cachexia, both angiotensin-converting enzyme (ACE) inhibitor and beta blockers can reduce weight loss.

Nutritional Support

Nutritional support has benefits for nonterminal patients in terms of quality of life and other outcomes. For example,

it increases patient tolerance of chemotherapy; in alcoholic cirrhosis may influence prognosis; and nutritional supplements benefit people during acute exacerbations of illness [12]. In advanced disease previously advised dietary restrictions, such as reducing salt to assist in managing ascites, should be regularly reviewed as they can exacerbate a reduced intake and outweigh the benefits.

The causes of insufficient nutritional intake in advanced disease are multifactorial and can place emotional strain on both the patient and the carer. In most situations, patients are unable to meet requirements in both the macro and the micronutrients. Improvements can be made concentrating on energy and protein sources in the diet with a multivitamin mineral tablet to provide micronutrients. The key message to the patient is to think differently about his/her diet, there is no such thing as "bad" food. Cream and chocolate provide a beneficial source of energy. Additionally, the following advice can be helpful:

- Eat when and what is enjoyable. Little and often can assist in reducing nausea.
- Make foods interesting and if possible plan ahead.
- Have snacks freely available around the house, or when going out, to maximise when the patient has an appetite and/or nausea is reduced.
- Use a small plate (it gives the impression of finishing a complete meal. Some patients feel defeated when seeing large portions, reducing intake further).
- Softer foods that reduce chewing can sometimes be better tolerated.
- Readymade meals reduce energy expenditure for fatigued patients.
- Encourage the family and carer to create a rota system for supplying hot meals (can be frozen and used later).
- Provide emotional support to the patient and carer to ensure meal/food related tension and anxiety are reduced.
- Make use of aperitifs.

When attempts at diet manipulation do not improve, commercially prepared supplements may be helpful in some situations [13]. Patients undergoing treatments or having episodic illness seem to benefit the most with supplements. There are many types of supplements varying in composition and presentation, such as milk and juice-based drinks (sweet and savoury flavour), puddings, pre-thickened drinks, and powders made into drinks. They are available on prescription in the United Kingdom and are therefore free to most patients. Nutritional companies are continually introducing new products with varying nutrient formulations.

The most appropriate type and quantity of supplement should be determined based on the patient's food preferences, medical condition, nutritional requirements, and nutrient deficit [14]. If there is not a clear understanding of the specific composition when selecting the supplement, the patient's diet will be further imbalanced negating any potential improvement. Regular reviews are essential to ensure tolerance and effectiveness. Nutritional supplements can leave an unpleasant after-taste, are rich in texture and can lead to a monotonous diet; therefore, it is unlikely the patient is able to sustain this as an effective long-term option. Supplements should be used for short periods of time transitioning back to food as the patient's intake improves. Dietitians provide more detailed advice on nutritional needs of patients and are an excellent source of information on dietary supplementation. The Royal College of Physicians and the British Society of Gastroenterology have published an excellent resource to guide decision-making for patients with oral feeding difficulties towards the end-of-life and is recommended to the reader [15].

As the patient deteriorates further, the main aim of nutritional intervention shifts to the emotional support since there is little clinical benefit from nutritional supplements, and supplements can have a deleterious effect on the GI system and mouth care. The carer may feel they are providing the best for the patient by offering nutritional supplements; however, they should be reassured that sips of soup and favourite drinks are equally beneficial, if not superior, to the quality of the patient's death.

For some patients, the inability to meet nutrition and hydration requirements or ability to administer medications orally will severely impact on the quality of life, necessitating the decision to proceed with enteral nutrition. If the patient has a functional GI tract, the patient should be referred to the Nutrition Team or Gastroenterologist in secondary care to conduct an assessment, present the most appropriate plan of care and to assist in coordinating community support with the Community Home Enteral Nutrition Team. Enteral feeding tube options available to the patient are nasogastric (NG) tube or gastrostomy tube.

Nasogastric Tube

An NG feeding tube is generally 5–8 French gauge, placed in the nostril and fed down into the stomach. Professionals, who have competency to pass NG tubes, typically insert them at the bedside. They are generally indicated for short term and dependent on the material of the tube can be left in-situ up to six weeks before requiring replacement. Indications are:

- Patients undergoing chemotherapy/radiotherapy.

- Preparation for surgery in severely malnourished patients [14].
- Post-surgery complications impeding oral nutrition.
- As a trial to assess effectiveness and tolerability (e.g., patients with motor neurone disease) before commencing more permanent feeding options if appropriate.

There are many practical difficulties in using the NG tube in the community; most importantly is the risk of tube displacement into the lungs. The risk is minimised by checking the pH of aspirated tube contents (should be less than 5.5 unless taking a proton pump inhibitor [PPI]) before each administration of feed, water, and medication. In secondary care an X-ray is conducted if the pH cannot confirm position; however, this is not practical in primary care. The safest option for the patient without confirmation is to withhold the feed and consider having a new tube placed [14]. There may be limited professionals in the community with competency to pass NG tubes, requiring the patient to have it passed in secondary care. The arduous process limits the feasibility of this option.

Percutaneous Endoscopic Gastrostomy (PEG) Tube

Fixed placement of a tube through the abdominal wall into the stomach is useful for patients who require long-term interventional nutrition (months to years) or those undergoing treatment for head and neck cancer. The procedure is well tolerated even by quite sick patients and is generally done under benzodiazepine sedation (Figure 1). It may be placed endoscopically (the majority), radiologically, or by a mini laparotomy. It is a day case procedure endoscopically, but patients may remain in hospital while learning about the enteral feeding apparatus and techniques. Around 6% of people will die within 30 days (around 40% of endoscopic deaths), and robust consideration of risks by the MDT is needed to assure selection of appropriate patients [16].

Box 1 outlines the indications and contraindications and Box 2 describes the possible complications of PEG.

Jejunal Tube Feeding

Some patients have considerable problems with enteral feeding into the stomach with symptoms of reflux, hiccup, aspiration, nausea, and vomiting. If prokinetic agents (e.g., metoclopramide) do not resolve this, then jejunal placement of the NG or PEG tube (usually endoscopically) may alleviate symptoms. However, patients with jejunal feeding tubes will be unlikely to tolerate bolus feeds since there is no longer the gastric reservoir and therefore will be more practically constrained by the time required for feed to be given.

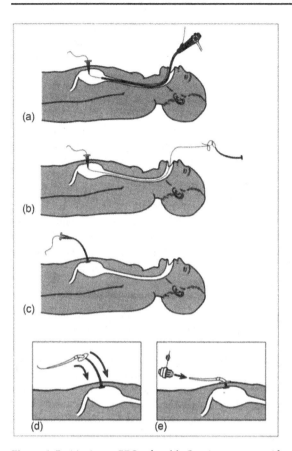

Figure 1 Positioning a PEG tube. (a) Gastric puncture with a sheathed needle and introduction of a string or metal wire through the sheath after the removal of the needle. While grasping the string or the metal wire, the endoscope is removed. (b) The loop of the gastrostomy tube is knotted at the string projecting from the mouth and by pulling at the abdominal end of the string the gastrostomy tube passes through the oesophagus and stomach and finally pierces the abdominal wall. (c) The retention disc of the gastrostomy tube is apposed against the gastric wall. (d) The outer retention disc, and (e) the feeding adaptor are put in place. (Reproduced from Reference 16)

Daily Care for Patients Requiring Enteral Feeding

Risk can be minimised with good daily care and the Community Home Enteral Nutrition team can be a valuable resource for the patient and carer providing training and support.

Flushing before and after each administration with either freshly drawn tap water or cooled boiled water will reduce the risk of the tube becoming blocked with feed and/or medication residue. Any medicine administered through the enteral feeding tube must be in the liquid form or a dissolvable preparation. The community pharmacist

Box 1: Factors to assess before PEG insertion

Indications	Contraindications
	Ileus
Oropharyngeal disease	Blood coagulation disorder
Oesophageal obstruction-but may be technically problematic	Poor wound healing Ascites
Neurogenic dysphagia with risk of aspiration	Sepsis
Neurological injury and neurodegenerative disease	Tumour infiltration of stomach
	Respiratory insufficiency on lying flat (radiologically inserted gastrostomy [RIG] may be possible)
Major oral surgery	
Preradiotherapy	
If it is impossible to site a gastrostomy endoscopically, it may be possible radiologically with ultrasound guidance (RIG)	

or prescribing advisors supporting the general practitioner (GP) can provide advice. If the tube does become blocked, the Home Enteral Nutrition team may be contacted to provide support. Techniques available are:

- Inspect the tube to see if the blockage is visible. Wrap a warm flannel around the tube and once cooler massage the tube at the blockage. With a 50-ml syringe **gently** attempt to aspirate alternating with flushing warm water. If this is

Box 2: Complications of PEG

Major	Minor
Perforation with peritonitis	Wound infection/stomal leak
Haemorrhage Haematoma	Regurgitation and aspiration (consider jejunal placement)
Death	Ileus, abdominal bloating, diarrhoea
	Tube migration/extubation
	Anorexia

not successful, rest and repeat in 30 min. Do not force flush the tube.

- Pancreatic enzymes such as Pancreatin only help if the blockage is due to feed [18].
- If all attempts fail, seek specialist advice or replacement.

Many patients do not feel it is necessary to continue with mouth care if not eating and drinking orally. However, daily oral, dental, and pharyngeal hygiene will help to minimize incidence of oral thrush, tooth decay, and halitosis. Evidence also suggests oropharyngeal microorganisms can migrate into the respiratory tract causing infections [19, 20].

PEG Care

To minimise the risk of infections the puncture site (stoma) requires daily cleaning with warm soapy water. Discharge can be common and is not always indicative of an infection. Dressings may assist in managing the discharge however should be balanced with the risk of infections caused from ideal breeding conditions. The Home Enteral Nutrition team and/or District Nurse can support the patient and provide advice.

Trouble Shooting

The tube can be displaced regardless of the type of fixation device used. In the United Kingdom, National Patient Safety Agency (NPSA) put out a Rapid Response Alert in 2010, recommending that in the first 72 h.

> If there is pain on feeding, prolonged or severe pain post-procedure, or fresh bleeding, or external leakage of gastric contents, stop feed/medication delivery immediately, obtain senior advice urgently and consider CT scan, contrast study, or surgical review [21].

If late displacement occurs (i.e., once the tract is mature), the stoma tract can potentially close within hours. Some Home Enteral Nutrition teams have staff competent in changing balloon gastrostomies and may be available for immediate support, or the patient should be instructed to go to hospital as soon as possible bringing spare tubes if available. If indicated a urinary Foley catheter can be inserted to maintain the integrity of the tract.

Gastroesophageal reflux is common and can be treated with a PPI. Positional change and avoidance of overnight continuous feeding is also helpful. Aspiration occurs frequently in both NG and PEG feeding and may present with pneumonia. Patient position, type of feed and prokinetic medication may be useful. Jejunal feeding may benefit patients with persistent problems.

Nausea, bloating, and cramps occur frequently. Diarrhoea occurs in approximately 30% of patients and can present a significant challenge. These problems can be addressed by alteration of feed type and mode of feeding. Close liaison with the Community Home Enteral Nutrition team is essential.

Parenteral Nutrition

If the gut is functional use it! Parenteral nutrition (PN) is not physiological and is fraught with pitfalls. PN is never an emergency. Electrolytes and micronutrients must be corrected to prevent the re-feeding syndrome in malnourished patients.

In the United Kingdom, most home PN is given for intestinal failure due to the short bowel syndrome. In parts of Europe and the United States however, the bulk of home PN is provided for malignant disease. There is, however, no convincing evidence that PN enhances either quality of life or survival in patients with advanced malignancy. Patients with advanced cancer who currently receive PN in the United Kingdom have usually either been commenced on it before diagnosis or before potentially curative treatment and have continued on it. PN may occasionally be used in cancer patients who have intestinal failure (complete bowel obstruction) with no other disease spread; further guidance can be taken from the ESPEN guidelines for clinical nutrition in cancer [22]. For patients with cachexia due to advanced nonmalignant disease, the place of PN is equally uncertain. This is an area of practice that is likely to continue to challenge us all in the coming years.

Care for patients with oral feeding difficulties should have their needs carefully assessed by the MDT. As far as possible the oral route should be preserved by detailed assessment and modification of food and liquid to facilitate maintenance of oral nutrition.

Mouth Care

Mouth care is very important. Studies have shown that in the elderly aspiration pneumonia is related to poor oral hygiene [19, 20]. The aim of oral hygiene is to keep the lips and oral mucosa clean, soft, and intact and the basis for this is daily tooth brushing, dental flossing, and consideration of a mouth wash (one teaspoonful of sodium bicarbonate per large cup of water). Commercial mouthwashes may cause pain in patients with stomatitis since they contain alcohol, lemon, and glycerine.

Oral complications including a dry mouth (xerostomia) are common and a major problem for many patients with advanced disease [22]. Saliva helps us to chew, talk, and swallow. It protects against infection and begins digestion of food. Normally about 1–1.5 L of saliva containing amylase and bicarbonate are produced daily. A reduction in this is most commonly a side effect of drugs (e.g., opioids, antihistamines, anticholinergics, diuretics, beta blockers, and anticonvulsants) but dehydration, anxiety, and mouth breathing also result in a dry mouth. Patients who have had radiotherapy to the head and neck may have considerable problems with dry mouth, altered anatomy, and function leading to debris accumulation and pain. Dentures in patients who have lost weight can become ill-fitting and cause soreness and abrasions.

As well as keeping the lips and mucosa moist, clean and intact patients may need extra mouth care in order to:
- prevent infection;
- alleviate pain and discomfort thus enabling greater oral intake;
- prevent halitosis;
- enhance taste and appetite;
- facilitate speech; and
- minimise psychological distress.

Key Point in Mouth Care

The *frequency* of mouth care is of greater importance than what is used to clean it.

Painful Mouth

Mouth ulcers can be helped by choline salicylate gel (Bonjela) or, if persistent, corticosteroid in the form of a hydrocortisone buccal tablet (2.5 mg), dissolving slowly in contact with the ulcer up to four times a day. The bioadherent gel, *Gelclair*, can also sooth and promote healing.

A sore mouth, from whatever cause, may be helped by sucking anaesthetic lozenges or using local anaesthetic mouthwashes or sprays. Severe pain may require opioid analgesia often by subcutaneous (SC) rather than oral administration.

Management of Xerostomia

Table 1 outlines the measures that may help patients with dry mouths. Sialogogues increase the production of saliva, and chewing gum (sugar free) has been shown to be helpful and liked by patients with advanced cancer who are able to produce some saliva [23]. Most salivary substitutes provide relief for only a short time, and those that contain mucin improve symptoms more than those that don't. However, the mucin is derived from pigs and may therefore not be suitable for some patients. Salivary substitutes that have a low pH may cause demineralisation of teeth.

A few additional tips: Salivary substitutes should be applied or sprayed beneath the tongue and between the buccal mucosa and the teeth (i.e., mimic the pooling of saliva) and not in the back of the throat, the mouth should be moistened with water before spraying; lemon and glycerine swabs and mouthwashes containing glycol should not be used due to adverse effects of irritation and rebound drying effects; moist cotton swabs (e.g., Moistir) or sponge swabs on sticks dipped in water may help very frail patients.

Cholinergic agonist agents such as pilocarpine have been shown to increase saliva production post-irradiation. It is very useful in patients with post-radiotherapy xerostomia in head and neck cancer (start with 5 mg TDS with meals). However, it is often poorly tolerated, usually because of sweating or GI side effects. It is contraindicated in obstructive airways disease and asthma.

Prevention and Management of Oral Infections

Thrush

Attention to the care of the oral cavity, teeth, and dentures will help minimise infection. Patients on steroids, antibiotics, or those who have diabetes are at particular risk. Thrush is the commonest infection. Candida prefers an acid environment and sodium bicarbonate mouthwashes repeated regularly (2 hourly), coupled with gentle

Table 1 A summary of approaches to the management of a dry mouth.

General measures	Cleanliness/tongue coating	Salivary substitutes	Increased salivary secretion
Sips of water	Pineapple	Carboxymethycellulose	Chewing gum Pilocarpine 5 mg TDS with or after food
Ice poles Brushing with soft toothbrush Moistened sponges on stick Mild bicarbonate mouth wash	Effervescent vitamin C	Mucin	

brushing of the teeth (or cleaning dentures) twice per day is effective prevention [23].

Established thrush is treated with nystatin or miconazole topically. Patients should be instructed to keep the gel or suspension in contact with as much of the oral mucosa as possible, for as long as possible. Ice lollipops made with diluted nystatin are soothing and engender a long duration of mucosal contact. Miconazole acts both topically and systemically. If the patient is severely affected, has symptoms suggestive of oesophageal infection, or is taking antibiotics and/or steroids a systemic antifungal is indicated; for example, fluconazole 50 mg OD for 7–14 days, or itraconazole 100 mg OD for 10–15 days. To avoid reinfection, dentures must be cleaned in Sterident or Milton with or without nystatin. If oral thrush persists then mouth swabs should be taken to evaluate further.

Herpes Simplex

Herpes simplex infections present as very painful, vesicular, and ulcerating lesions. Oral acyclovir 200 mg five times daily, or valacyclovir 500 mg BD for 5 days is indicated.

Oesophageal Problems

Swallowing may be difficult for patients with oesophageal cancer for several common reasons:

- Oesophageal compressive and/or obstructive lesions
- Functional dysphagia
- Odynophagia (painful swallowing)
- Oro-Oesophageal thrush.

In addition, patients may experience copious thick, tenacious mucus, which may also cause coughing.

Treatment options include surgery (not for disease with metastatic spread), external beam and endoluminal radiotherapy, chemotherapy, endoscopic recanalisation, and expanding metal stents. Endoscopic interventions are discussed below. General symptom control is vital whatever the cause of obstruction or possibility of intervention.

Pain should be managed by the standard titration of analgesics as per the World Health Organisation (WHO) analgesic ladder. Strong (non-oral) opioids, such as SC diamorphine/morphine or transdermal fentanyl, may be required to control background pain. Sucralfate will coat ulcerated tumour and may reduce bleeding and pain.

In total obstruction of the oesophagus, coping with saliva and secretions can be distressing for the patient. The following may be helpful:

- Hyoscine hydrobromide (Kwells), 1–2, tablets sublingually QDS.
- Hyoscine hydrobromide SC 1.2–2.4 mg/24 h.
- Hyoscine butylbromide SC 40–120 mg/24 h (less sedating than hydrobromide).
- Glycopyrronium bromide SC 0.6–1.2 mg/24 h (less sedating than hyoscine hydrobromide).

Nebulized water or saline may help reduce the tenacity of mucus secreted by the cancer, and nebulised local anaesthetic (5 ml of 0.25% bupivacaine) may be helpful in very advanced disease if the pharynx is dysfunctional and swallowing of saliva or mucus results in aspiration with distressing bouts of coughing.

Endoluminal Recanalisation

Exophytic growth of tumours into a lumen will lead to obstruction. Endoscopic procedures that recanalise the oesophagus may offer alternatives or additional options to endoluminal stenting (see following section) for dysphagia:

- *Argon plasma coagulator (APC)*: This is a safe and effective method. APC provides predictable penetration of normal and abnormal mucosa. The equipment is relatively cheap and has multiple other applications. The main drawback is that it may take a number of sessions to achieve the desired outcome.
- *Laser (YAG)*: Not widely available and has statutory restriction on its use. Very "powerful" with limited room for error.
- *Injection of absolute alcohol*: Cheap with good results if injected into exophytic tumour. It usually requires multiple sessions and can give rise to mediastinal discomfort at the time of injection. Will cause ulceration of the normal mucosa if injected into it.
- *Dilatation*: Useful for constrictive rather than exophytic tumours. Dilatation can be done with bougies over a guide wire or balloons under direct vision. Balloon dilation of the oesophagus, pylorus, duodenum, and colon can be undertaken. The perforation rate is 1–5%.

A combination of the above modalities focused on the nature of the individual clinical problem should be employed.

Nausea and Vomiting

Nausea and/or vomiting are common in advanced disease and can be a major cause of poor quality of life. The prevalence in patients with advanced cancer is up to 70% and up to 50% in those with advanced non-malignant disease [24]. The symptoms may be more distressing than pain.

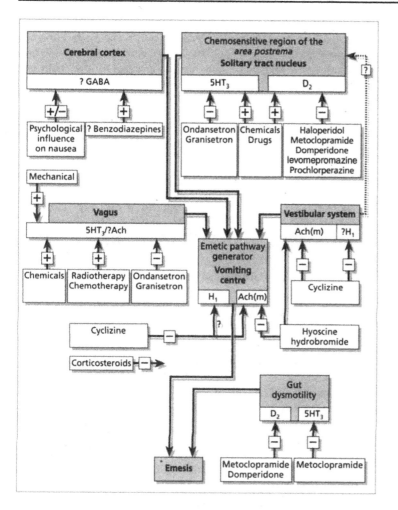

Figure 2 A schema of the pathways of emesis (nausea and vomiting), important neurotransmitters, and site of action of antiemetics. The neurokinin receptor and antagonist is not shown as this is an area of specialist only prescription in oncology. Receptor types – GABA; H, histamine; D, dopamine; Ach(m), acetylcholine muscarinic; 5HT, serotonin (5-hydroxytryptophan). Subscript denotes receptor subtype: + denotes agonist or enhancing stimulus; – denotes antagonist or blocking stimulus; ? denotes limited evidence for effect through this mechanism.

Five components are the key to management:

1. Careful assessment of the patient to try and identify possible avoidable and reversible aetiologies.
2. Knowledge of common syndromes.
3. Reversal of the reversible (where appropriate).
4. An understanding of the mechanism of action of antiemetic drugs (Figure 2).
5. Consideration of the route of administration of antiemetic and other drugs. Since nausea can cause gastric stasis, the SC or rectal routes may be needed even when there is no vomiting.

Figure 3 outlines the management. An aetiological based approach to management generally underpins most guidelines although an empirical-based approach may be as effective [24, 25]. Generally the first-line choice of antiemetic is one of metoclopramide, haloperidol, or cyclizine.

Control of symptoms using one antiemetic is possible in 60% of patients. However, about one-third of patients require concurrent administration of a second antiemetic. In these patients antiemetics of different mechanisms of action should be combined (e.g. cyclizine and haloperidol). A third-line choice would be a broader spectrum antiemetic, which has risks of more side effects. This is discussed further below under the section "Persistent nausea and vomiting."

Acupuncture and ginger are two commonly used complementary techniques. Other approaches such as relaxation therapy, hypnosis, or neurolinguistic programming (NLP) are invaluable for patients with a high degree of anxiety or to combat the anticipatory nausea induced by chemotherapy treatments.

Table 2 provides a quick view of the range of antiemetics and gives prescription guidance.

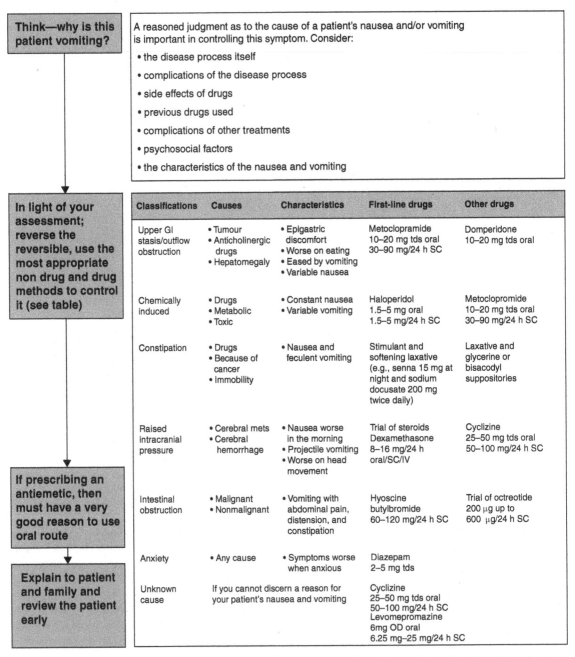

Think—why is this patient vomiting?	A reasoned judgment as to the cause of a patient's nausea and/or vomiting is important in controlling this symptom. Consider: • the disease process itself • complications of the disease process • side effects of drugs • previous drugs used • complications of other treatments • psychosocial factors • the characteristics of the nausea and vomiting

	Classifications	Causes	Characteristics	First-line drugs	Other drugs
In light of your assessment; reverse the reversible, use the most appropriate non drug and drug methods to control it (see table)	Upper GI stasis/outflow obstruction	• Tumour • Anticholinergic drugs • Hepatomegaly	• Epigastric discomfort • Worse on eating • Eased by vomiting • Variable nausea	Metoclopramide 10–20 mg tds oral 30–90 mg/24 h SC	Domperidone 10–20 mg tds oral
	Chemically induced	• Drugs • Metabolic • Toxic	• Constant nausea • Variable vomiting	Haloperidol 1.5–5 mg oral 1.5–5 mg/24 h SC	Metoclopromide 10–20 mg tds oral 30–90 mg/24 h SC
	Constipation	• Drugs • Because of cancer • Immobility	• Nausea and feculent vomiting	Stimulant and softening laxative (e.g., senna 15 mg at night and sodium docusate 200 mg twice daily)	Laxative and glycerine or bisacodyl suppositories
	Raised intracranial pressure	• Cerebral mets • Cerebral hemorrhage	• Nausea worse in the morning • Projectile vomiting • Worse on head movement	Trial of steroids Dexamethasone 8–16 mg/24 h oral/SC/IV	Cyclizine 25–50 mg tds oral 50–100 mg/24 h SC
If prescribing an antiemetic, then must have a very good reason to use oral route	Intestinal obstruction	• Malignant • Nonmalignant	• Vomiting with abdominal pain, distension, and constipation	Hyoscine butylbromide 60–120 mg/24 h SC	Trial of octreotide 200 μg up to 600 μg/24 h SC
	Anxiety	• Any cause	• Symptoms worse when anxious	Diazepam 2–5 mg tds	
Explain to patient and family and review the patient early	Unknown cause	If you cannot discern a reason for your patient's nausea and vomiting		Cyclizine 25–50 mg tds oral 50–100 mg/24 h SC Levomepromazine 6mg OD oral 6.25 mg–25 mg/24 h SC	

Figure 3 Summary of the approach to the management of nausea and vomiting.(Adapted from Faull C and Woof R. 2002. *Palliative Care: An Oxford Core Text* with permission from the publishers Oxford University Press.)

Common Syndromes of Nausea and Vomiting and Their Management

Gastric Stasis and Outflow Obstruction

This is common in patients with GI malignancy because of ascites, liver enlargement, and direct effects of tumour on the stomach. It is also common in patients with advanced congestive cardiac failure because of ascites and in patients with diabetics because of autonomic neuropathy. It is a component of the nausea induced by opiates. Nausea is of varying intensity. It may be very transient, just before vomiting and is often relieved by vomiting. The vomitus can be

Table 2 Antiemetic prescription.

Drug	Oral dose	Subcutaneous dose	Rectal dose
Metoclopramide	10–20 mg TDS	30–90 mg/24 h	
Domperidone	10–20 mg TDS	–	
Levomepromazine	5–25 mg OD	6.25–25 mg/24 h, may be given once daily	
Haloperidol	1–5 mg OD	1.5–5 mg/24 h, may be given once daily	
Ondansetron	8 mg BD	8–16 mg/24 h	16 mg OD
Granisetron	1–2 mg OD	1–2 mg/24 h	
Cyclizine	50 mg TDS	50–100 mg/24 h	
Prochloperazine	3–10 mg TDS	Not suitable	
Hyoscine hydrobromide	300 µg QDS		

of considerable volume and may contain undigested food. Vomiting may be provoked by movement of the torso. A succussion splash and other features of autonomic failure may be present.

Metoclopramide or Domperidone are the drug treatments of choice. Erythromycin may be helpful in a few patients but needs to be given intravenously. Flatulence may be relieved with dimethicone.

In complete obstruction prokinetic drugs should be stopped. PPIs may be helpful in reducing acidity and volume of secretions. A NG tube (for aspiration or free drainage) may help to relieve symptoms and is tolerated well by some patients but many prefer to have intermittent vomiting and no NG tube, especially if nausea is controlled. Insertion of a gastrostomy tube (see previous section) for venting purposes has been found to be effective and acceptable but is not commonly used in the United Kingdom [26].

Chemically Induced Nausea

A vast array of drugs cause nausea. The initiation of opioids causes nausea in up to 30% of patients but usually settles within 3–4 days although it can reappear with an escalation of dose, and it persists in a small percentage of patients. Metabolic causes of nausea are common in advanced disease: renal failure, liver failure, hypercalcaemia, hyponatraemia, and ketoacidosis. Anti-dopaminergic are the drugs of choice, for example, haloperidol. 5HT3 antagonists are useful for highly emetogenic chemotherapy and perhaps in cases of intractable vomiting of metabolic cause, but their cost-effectiveness in other circumstances is

not yet established. These drugs are also used in the postoperative period.

Raised Intracranial Pressure

Nausea may be worse in the morning, and the vomiting can be projectile in nature. Nausea and vomiting provoked by head movement is associated with vestibular pathway aetiology. There is usually headache, which may be worse in the morning. Neurological signs may be absent. Steroids and cyclizine are the treatments of first choice. If there are signs of vestibular pathway aetiology, hyoscine hydrobromide may be useful.

Persistent Nausea and Vomiting

Thirty percent of patients require the concurrent use of two antiemetics. These should be selected for different mechanisms of action that are compatible in effects. Haloperidol with cyclizine is a good choice. Both cyclizine and hyoscine hydrobromide will counteract the prokinetic effect of metoclopramide and domperidone but will not counteract the central antiemetic effect of metoclopramide.

Alternatively, low-dose levomepromazine can also be useful. It is a "broad-spectrum" antiemetic (antihistamine, anticholinergic, anti-dopaminergic, and serotonin antagonist activity) and in low doses does not generally cause troublesome sedation or hypotension.

Corticosteroids are potent antiemetics although their mechanism of action is not fully understood. They are thought to potentiate the effects of other antiemetics but also have an antiemetic effect in their own right. Dexamethasone at 2–6 mg OD is useful to add to an antiemetic regimen for patients with resistant problems.

Malignant Bowel Obstruction

Malignant GI obstruction occurs most commonly in patients with advanced abdominal or pelvic cancers: in 25% of patients with a primary bowel cancer; in 6% of patients with a primary ovarian cancer; and in about 40% of advanced ovarian cancer patients.

Where surgery is technically not possible, is inappropriate, or is not acceptable to the patient, medical management of malignant GI obstruction can offer good symptom control. Patients may live for surprisingly long periods of time (sometimes months) and be able to take small quantities of food and fluids as desired, usually without the need for an NG tube or parenteral fluids. Most patients can be cared for at home.

The clinical scenario may only have some of the classic features of complete bowel obstruction outlined in Box 3. Malignant obstruction may present acutely but more commonly is gradual in onset, intermittent, and variable in severity. Gross distension is often absent, even in lower bowel obstruction since the bowel may be constricted at several points. Patients with lower bowel obstruction will often have infrequent, faeculent vomiting, while those with high bowel obstruction may vomit undigested food. It is always useful to determine whether colic is present or absent since this will affect the management strategy (see following paragraphs).

Box 3:   Classical features of complete intestinal obstruction

- Large-volume vomits.
- Nausea worse before vomiting.
- Nausea relieved by vomiting.
- Nil per rectum or per stoma.
- Abdominal distension.
- Visible peristalsis.
- Increased bowel sounds, classically tinkling, but may be absent.
- Background abdominal pain.
- Colicky abdominal pain.

Nonmalignant causes of obstruction or gut paresis must be considered, which may be amenable to surgical or other appropriate intervention. These include adhesions, constipation, drugs, unrelated benign conditions, and metabolic abnormalities.

Investigations can be helpful and may include a biochemical profile (hypokalaemia may cause ileus; hypercalcaemia may cause pseudo-obstruction due to constipation). A plain abdominal X-ray will demonstrate constipation, but can be misleading when multiple levels of obstruction are present. A CT/MRI scan can be indicated if surgery is to be considered.

Chemotherapy may offer a palliative option for some patients with chemosensitive tumours, for example, ovarian carcinoma. Any surgical or oncological intervention should run in parallel with more immediate symptomatic treatment. Expanding stents placed endoscopically or radiologically are occasionally helpful and are discussed shortly.

Surgical Intervention

Surgery should always be considered in malignant GI obstruction. However, it will often be inappropriate or technically impossible. Surgical intervention is unlikely to be successful in the following situations:

- Radiological or previous surgical evidence indicating that a surgical procedure will not be technically possible.
- A stiff, doughy abdomen with little abdominal distension [27].
- Diffuse intra-abdominal carcinomatosis.
- Massive ascites that re-accumulates rapidly after paracentesis.
- Poor general physical status [28].
- Previous radiotherapy to the abdomen or pelvis, in combination with any of the above.

Medical Management

A NG tube and intravenous (IV) fluids are rarely necessary if the following strategy is used.

Pain

Analgesia for background pain is obtained by using a continuous SC infusion of an opioid, for example, morphine (dose: 1/2 total daily oral morphine equivalent dose ± 30–50% increment as dictated by the pain). If opioid naive, start on a morphine dose of 10 mg/24 h. Not all patients require opioid analgesia if no background pain is present and colic can be relieved by more appropriate drugs (see following paragraphs).

Colic and Gut Motility

If colic is present avoid all drugs that could worsen this (i.e., metoclopramide, bulk-forming, osmotic, and stimulant laxatives). If colic persists, add hyoscine butylbromide SC, starting at 60 mg/24 h (up to 200 mg/24 h as needed).

If colic is absent, a trial of metoclopramide SC 30–90 mg/24 h should be cautiously instigated with close monitoring for development of colic. In the absence of colic, incomplete obstruction in the large bowel may be helped by a stool-softening laxative, such as docusate sodium 200 mg BD-QDS. Corticosteroids may reduce bowel obstruction in those with advanced malignancy, particularly GI and ovarian cancer. A 5-day trial of dexamethasone 6–16 mg SC/IV should be given [29].

Nausea

The choice of antiemetic depends on whether the patient is experiencing colic. If colic is not a feature, metoclopramide is administered SC 30–90 mg/24 h (see earlier paragraph). If colic is present, give haloperidol (SC 3–5 mg/24 h) or cyclizine (SC 50–100 mg/24 h). A combination of haloperidol and cyclizine is sometimes necessary.

5HT 3 antagonist antiemetics may have a role in relief of the nausea induced by bowel distension and stimulation of the vomiting centre through vagal afferents (see above), but this is unclear. They can be given rectally or subcutaneously.

Vomiting

Reduction in the volume of GI secretions will reduce colic, nausea, pain, and the need to vomit. This can usually be adequately achieved with hyoscine butylbromide (SC 60–200 mg/24 h [30]) with or without an H^2 antagonist or PPI.

If large-volume vomiting persists despite hyoscine butylbromide, the somatostatin analogue, octreotide, will further decrease the volume of intestinal secretions in the gut lumen [31]. A trial of octreotide, given at a rate of 300 µg/24 h by SC infusion, should be performed. The dose can be titrated over 2–3 days to 600 µg/24 h; If there is no benefit at 600 µg/24 h it should be stopped. The dose should be reduced daily by 100 µg/24 h to the lowest effective dose (mean dose 300 µg/24 h) [32].

In some cases, particularly in high obstructions such as gastric outlet obstruction, these strategies are not effective. It may then be helpful to use a NG tube or consider a venting gastrostomy to allow the patient to continue to drink and eat as desired without the fear of provoking immediate vomiting. Venting gastrostomy can be performed under local anaesthetic either endoscopically or radiologically and may facilitate discharge and dying at home. In one

series of 51 patients median survival was 17 days with a range of 1–190 days; 92% of patients gaining symptomatic improvement of nausea and vomiting with some restoration of diet [26].

Contraindications to the use of a venting gastrostomy are:

- The presence of significant ascites as it would precipitate peritonitis.
- Tumour infiltration of the stomach.

In an obstructed abdomen with malignant infiltration, the risk of perforating the bowel with resultant peritonitis is significant and the patient should be clear about this risk.

It is important that at least a 16–20 F bore gastrostomy tube should be used to facilitate adequate decompression.

Subcutaneous Drug Delivery

Patients may require the use of more than two drugs to obtain symptom control and not infrequently two SC infusions are required. Studies of the compatibility of multiple drug combinations are often not available (see Chapter 22), but clinical observation suggests the following drugs mixed in water for injection are compatible and maintain efficacy:

- Morphine/diamorphine, haloperidol, and cyclizine.
- Morphine/diamorphine, haloperidol, and hyoscine butylbromide (compatibility may depend on order of mixing).
- Morphine/diamorphine and octreotide.
- Morphine/diamorphine, haloperidol, and octreotide.

Diet and Hydration

Sensitive, pre-emptive discussion of the situation is a vital part of care for the patient and family. Many patients with obstruction can eat and drink in modest amounts when symptoms are controlled. A liquid, low-residue diet may be the least problematic.

Hydration should be considered on an individual basis. Oral discomfort and dryness can largely be relieved by frequent, attentive mouth care, ice to suck, and drinks as desired and tolerated. Profound thirst is not common but some patients may benefit from parenteral fluids, for example, SC infusion of 1–2 litres 0.9% saline/24 h or IV fluids. The use of parenteral fluids can impact on choices regarding place of care.

Hiccup

This is an abnormal respiratory reflex characterised by spasm of one or both sides of the diaphragm, causing sudden inspiration with associated closure of the vocal cords. The phrenic nerve, vagus nerve, thoracic sympathetic fibres, brainstem, and hypothalamus are all involved in the reflex arc. An inhibitory pathway through the pharyngeal and glossopharyngeal nerves is present. Disturbance of any of these components may cause hiccup. Identification of cause may sometimes enable a logical and successful approach to treatment.

Management

Stimulation of the pharynx may be successful in reducing hiccup. This can be achieved in various ways, including holding iced water in the oropharynx, soft palate massage, oropharyngeal, or nasopharyngeal catheter placement.

Common empirical treatments are:
• A defoaming antiflatulent before and after meals and at bedtime (e.g. Simeticone).
• Domperidone 10–20 mg TDS; or metoclopramide 10 mg TDS half an hour before meals if delayed gastric emptying.
• Nifedipine 10–20 mg BD-TDS (assess effect on blood pressure).
• Midazolam 5–10 mg SC/24 h (this option is for those in the last days of life; the dose can be titrated to a maximum of 60 mg/24 h).
• Baclofen 5–10 mg BD-TDS (higher doses can be used with caution).
• Chlorpromazine – use with care and only if simpler measures fail: 10–25 mg PO TDS (it has a diffuse depressant effect on the reticular formation).
• Sodium valproate – for hiccup of central origin.

In general, the drugs should be started at low dose and gradually increased to avoid side effects.

Phrenic nerve stimulation or ablation is only occasionally an appropriate treatment in patients with advanced disease.

Endoluminal Stents

Stenting is a widely used therapeutic intervention for palliation of GI and hepatobiliary malignant obstruction. Stents are available as expandable metal systems (covered or uncovered) or in plastic (for biliary obstruction). Stents are usually placed through a guidewire under endoscopic and fluoroscopic guidance, although radiologists do place them under fluoroscopic guidance alone. Uncovered stents embed well in luminal tissues but may become occluded by further tumour growth. Covered stents prevent the ingress of tumour but are more prone to migration and displacement. Stenting is usually a day case procedure but depends on patient performance status and complications.

Oesophageal Stents

Expandable metal stents (EMS) provide relief or improvement of dysphagia in 90% of cases and result in shorter hospital stays and fewer procedures than non-stenting options. Covered stents are particularly effective in tracheoesophageal fistula. Stents are most useful in mid to low oesophageal tumours. Tumours of the gastroesophageal junction respond well, but stent migration is more common and the function of the lower oesophageal sphincter is lost and can result in problematic gastroesophageal reflux (patients will need PPIs). Stenting of high oesophageal tumours can cause significant and persistent discomfort.

Complications:
• 0.5–2% mortality as a result of stent insertion. [33].
• Pain/mediastinal discomfort (NB: surgical emphysema may indicate perforation).
• Bleeding.
• 3% perforation rate.
• Stent migration (more common following chemotherapy and tumour regression).
• Tumour overgrowth.
• Food blockage.

After stenting patients need to modify their diet: more liquidised/sloppy food, avoid leafy vegetables and chunks of steak, etc. Possible acute food blockage may be relieved by carbonated drinks. Total dysphagia with drooling and aspiration requires emergency review.

Tumour overgrowth can be dealt with by laser, alcohol injection, or argon (see recanalisation earlier).

Gastroduodenal Stents

Pancreatic, duodenal, and gastric cancers frequently precipitate gastric outflow obstruction, and EMS are as effective in relieving this as palliative bypass surgery. Most patients gain significant clinical improvement. Where there is functional gastric-outlet obstruction due to tumour invasion of neural supply or diffuse peritoneal infiltration with bowel encasement and gut failure, improvement will not be seen.

The EMS are best placed using the combined modalities of endoscopic and fluoroscopic guidance; however, this can be achieved fluroscopically alone. Gastroduodenal stents can be inserted as an outpatient procedure. Patients with duodenal involvement frequently develop biliary obstruction, and it is advisable that the biliary obstruction is treated first. Complications are similar to those mentioned earlier.

Biliary Stents

Patients with biliary obstruction experience nausea, anorexia, weight loss, fat malabsorption with steatorrhoea, itch, and occasionally cholangitis, although the severity of these symptoms varies between individual patients.

Jaundice can also be a significant visual reinforcement affirming the disease process. The obstructed biliary tree is decompressed by endoscopic retrograde cholangiopancreatography (ERCP) or percutaneous transhepatic cholangiography (PTC). Plastic stents are subject to bacterial and biliary encrustation resulting in occlusion and usually last between three and four months. The more expensive EMS have larger diameters and longer patency than plastic stents. If patient survival is greater than four to six months, then metal stents appear more cost-effective with fewer endoscopic interventions and hospital admissions required.

Patients may benefit from re-stenting and recurrence of jaundice should not be assumed to be due to tumour progression.

Complications of biliary stenting (ERCP and PTC):
- Pancreatitis
- Bleeding
- Perforation
- Biliary leak and peritonitis
- Malposition
- Cholangitis.

Colorectal Stents

Colorectal stents can be used as a bridge to surgery or in patients with extensive disease who are poor surgical candidates. Covered stents are also useful in assisting closure of colo-vesical and colo-vaginal fistulas. Right-sided colonic stents require endoscopic placement. Left-sided stents can be placed radiologically.

Complications:
- Perforation (devastating as it will cause a florid faecal peritonitis)
- Stent migration
- Stool occlusion
- Bleeding
- Tenesmus1
- Faecal incontinence.[1]

Patients should be advised to consume a low residue diet and take faecal softeners.

Liver Disease

Liver disease is the only major cause of death that is continuing to rise year on year, and it is now the fifth "big killer" in England and Wales after heart disease, cancer, stroke, and respiratory disease [34]. Therefore, cirrhosis and

advanced chronic end-stage liver disease represent a major public health and potential palliative burden. Worldwide hepatitis B and C are the most common causes of cirrhosis. In the developed world, alcohol is the most common cause, but viral infections and liver disease associated with obesity (non-alcoholic steatohepatitis) are both increasing.

The UK incidence of cirrhosis is approximately 17 per 100,000 (prevalence 76 per 100,000) in adults over 25 years. More than 80% of liver-related deaths in the United Kingdom are due to cirrhosis secondary to alcohol [35].

Prognosis is related to the severity of the underlying disease (see Figure 4) and the development of disease-related complications. In stable compensated cirrhosis (Childs A) the five-year survival is excellent; however, in decompensated cirrhosis (development of portal hypertension, ascites, portal hypertensive bleeding, encephalopathy), the five-year survival is 50%. The model for end-stage liver disease (MELD) is a validated scoring system used to predict the survival of patients with end-stage liver disease in America and Europe [36]. The UK equivalent is UKELD, and a UKELD score of greater than 49 is the minimum criteria for entry onto the transplant waiting list.

Complications of Cirrhosis

The development of complications (see Figure 5) associated with decompensated cirrhosis have a marked impact on survival:
- Refractory Ascites (RA).
- Spontaneous Bacterial Peritonitis (SBP).
- Hepatorenal Syndrome (HRS).
- Variceal Bleeding (VB).
- Hepatocellular Carcinoma (HCC).
- Portosystemic Encephalopathy (PSE).

Ascites and Refractory Ascites

While response to the use of diuretics in malignant ascites is variable and unpredictable, they are highly effective in ascites of decompensated liver disease. Response may be seen using spironolactone up to 400 mg/day and furosemide up to 160 mg/day. Diuretics should be titrated to effect while monitoring electrolyte balance and renal function.

RA is associated with a high frequency of complications (PSE and infections). The 1-year survival is approximately 50%. Patients should have the patency of the portal vein checked (ultrasound) and development of a HCC excluded (serum alpha feto protein and imaging if appropriate).

---

[1]In stents placed in the lower rectum.

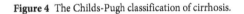

	1 point	2 points	3 points
Bilirubin (μmol/L)	<34	34–51	>51
Albumin (g/L)	>35	28–35	<28
Prothrombin time (s)	1–4	4–6	>6
Ascites	Absent	Mild (easily controlled)	Moderate to severe (poorly controlled)
Encephalopathy	None	1–2 (slight)	3–4 (moderate to severe)

Figure 4 The Childs-Pugh classification of cirrhosis.

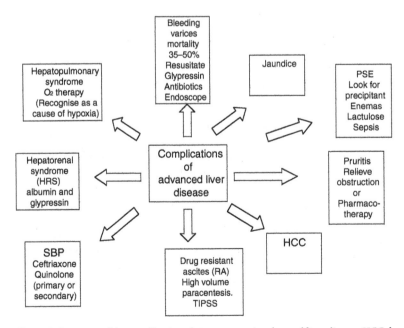

Figure 5 Summary of the complications that may occur in advanced liver disease. HCC, hepatocellular carcinoma; TIPSS, transjugular intrahepatic portosystemic shunt; SBP, spontaneous bacterial peritonitis; PSE, portosystemic encephalopathy.

Treatment of RA includes the following:

- *Transplantation*: By far the best treatment but not all patients will be suitable.
- *Transjugular intrahepatic portosytemic shunt (TIPSS)*: Reduces the rate of ascites recurrence and the development of HRS, has no effect on survival and is associated with a 20% incidence of encephalopathy. The ongoing management of patients with TIPSS is hospital intensive, and it is not recommended for those with severe liver failure, concomitant active infection, progressive renal failure, or severe cardiopulmonary disease.
- *Paracentesis* (see Box 4) [37]: The treatment of choice for most patients. Large volume paracentesis (>5 L) requires hospitalisation and concurrent administration of IV albumin; however, smaller volume paracentesis (<5 L) can be done as an outpatient, and the need for volume expansion is less clear and needs to be considered within the overall goals of care for a patient*. A palliative procedure out of the hospital setting may be appropriate, but the risks and benefits for the patient need to be considered carefully. Palliative long-term abdominal drains (LTADs) are routinely used in refractory malignant ascites but are not standard of care in cirrhosis, pending results of a national definitive trial. Currently, outside of a research setting, LTADs should only be considered in cirrhosis on a case by case basis after careful patient selection.

Spontaneous Bacterial Peritonitis (SBP)

SBP carries a 10–30% mortality with a 1-year survival of 38% after the first episode. It may lead to circulatory dysfunction and HRS that has a very poor survival rate. Administration of albumin with antibiotic therapy prevents HRS and improves prognosis.

There is good evidence for the administration of prophylactic quinolone antibiotics in patients with ascites due to cirrhosis for the prevention of SBP however concerns exist over the emergence of quinolone-resistant species of bacteria and antibiotic-induced complications. The suggested schedule is ciprofloxacin 250 mg OD.

Hepatorenal Syndrome (HRS)

In patients whose renal function deteriorates, HRS should be considered and urgent specialist advice sought. HRS occurs in 5–10% of cirrhotic patients with ascites and is a very sinister development with greater than 90% mortality.

Portosystemic Encephalopathy

This is common and if mild is easily controlled. There are multiple causes; however, the most common are sepsis, dehydration, GI bleed, and the co-administration of sedating drugs. It is a marker of decompensation and therefore potentially reversible.

---

*Note that for malignant ascites in patients without cirrhosis, IV albumin is not required.

> ### Box 4:   Large volume paracentesis (>5 L)
>
> - If patient on diuretics, withhold.
> - Under local anaesthetic insert paracentesis catheter into peritoneal cavity.
> - Give albumin 8 g/L of ascitic fluid drained.
> - Drain to dryness.
> - Remove catheter after 24 h to reduce chances of infection and peritonitis.
> - Place stoma bag over site if ascites leakage. Start albumin infusion before or at same time as starting paracentesis.

Treatment includes the following:

- Correction of the reversible (sepsis, SBP, dehydration, hypokalaemia, underlying bleeding, constipation).
- Enemas to achieve bowel clearance.
- *Laxatives*: lactulose has traditionally been used as it reduces colonic pH and nitrogen load in the gut. However, in practice it is acceptable to use alternatives that may be better tolerated.

Variceal Bleeding

Varices are related to elevated portal pressure and the development of a portosystemic shunt through collateral vessels, allowing portal blood to be diverted to the systemic circulation. The size of the varix and the severity of the underlying liver disease are risk factors for bleeding. Propanolol (40 mg BD) reduces the incidence of first variceal bleeds by 50%. Alcohol causes marked increase in portal hypertension, and every effort should be made to get patients to cease drinking. Banding of varices has a role in preventing further bleeds, and if practical, should be carried out on a regular basis until the varices are obliterated.

The average mortality of a first variceal bleed is approximately 50%; however, this is closely related to the underlying severity of liver disease. Bleeding may result in severe decompensation and fatal liver injury. Variceal bleeding is always a frightening and dramatic occurrence.

Prescribing in Liver Disease

Patients with advanced liver disease are symptomatic and therefore need their symptoms to be appropriately assessed and treated. Concern exists in prescribing for patients with liver disease as there is little evidence to guide practice. The liver has a huge reserve and has to be damaged significantly before it starts to have an effect; however, this is unpredictable and each patient should therefore be assessed as an individual and closely monitored after any medication is prescribed.

Pain Management in Advanced Liver Disease

The dose of paracetamol should be reduced to a maximum of 3g/24h for those with liver disease. Further dose reduction is required if the patient's weight is less than 50 kg. Nonsteroidal anti-inflammatory drugs (NSAIDs) should be avoided since their salt retention and other renal effects may lead to decompensation in patients with cirrhosis.

All opioids require liver metabolism and may accumulate in liver impairment. There are also many other factors that impact on the effects of opioids, for example, underlying diagnosis and speed of deterioration, presence of ascites. There is no evidence base to inform prescribing advice and we therefore suggest:

- Use reduced doses and consider increasing the dosing interval.
- Avoid drugs with long half-lives.
- Titrate slowly against effect.
- Re-evaluate daily.

Liver Transplantation Issues

Liver transplant is the gold standard treatment for advanced chronic liver disease and fulminant hepatic failure with a one-year survival of 80–90% and 5-year survival of 60–80%. However, for various reasons not all patients will be eligible for transplantation, and there is a limited pool of donor grafts available. Four people will die for every one transplanted.

For those who are not suitable for transplantation (e.g. those with alcoholic cirrhosis who cannot cease drinking or those whose performance status precludes transplantation) palliative care is the key focus of care. Even for those who are suitable for transplantation and on the waiting list, one in five will die. Appropriate symptom management and assessment of quality of life needs therefore to be considered for all those with advanced disease whether they are listed or not. This will include support for patients and their families often at a time of uncertainty and consideration of place of death when patients are removed from the transplant list because of deterioration.

Cholestatic Liver Disease

The key symptoms resulting from stasis of bile are pruritus and jaundice.

Pruritus

The pruritic effect is mediated through a central mechanism, a response to a rise in endogenous opioid levels. Large variations in individual response are seen and there is no correlation between plasma bilirubin concentration and intensity of pruritus. Approximately 20–25% of jaundiced patients complain of itch. There is no standard or generally accepted regimen for treatment and many different medications, with a limited evidence base, have been tried. The most effective treatment is to achieve biliary drainage, although this is not always possible and not without complications.

Drugs for pruritis include the following:

- *Antihistamine*: Sedating antihistamine has no effect on the itch but may assist in promoting sleep through their sedating effect, best avoided during the daytime.
- *Exchange resins*: Colestyramine is a bile salt binder, give 4 g bd. Best taken on an empty stomach first thing in the morning and before the evening meal (can add to orange juice to improve palatability).
- *Choleuretic agents*: Ursodeoxcholic acid 250 mg TDS.
- *Enzyme inducers*: Rifampicin 150 mg daily or phenobarbital. Moderate to low efficacy with variable response.
- *5HT3 antagonists*: Anecdotal reports of therapeutic response to ondansetron.
- *Selective serotonin reuptake inhibitor (SSRI) antidepressants*: Sertraline 25 mg OD and titrating to effect.
- *Opioid antagonists*: specialist guidance is required as opioid withdrawal may be provoked.

Jaundice

In cholestatic or obstructive jaundice, patients frequently feel unwell, anorexic, and nauseated. Bile is essential for digestion and absorption of fat, an essential fuel source.

They may develop symptoms of malabsorption. Active palliation through decompression of the biliary system (see endoluminal stents mentioned in the earlier section) is the only effective treatment, if at all practical. The approach can be through an ERCP or PTC, either as a day case or a short stay in hospital. However, on many occasions, decompression is not practically possible and therefore active palliation of the resulting symptoms with medication needs to be aimed for.

Constipation

Constipation is a big problem for patients with advanced disease. For instance more than 50% of patients admitted to hospices in the United Kingdom complain of constipation [38]. Physical illness, immobility, poor oral intake, opioids, and many other drugs are risk factors for constipation. Constipation can be prevented in the majority of patients by prescription of appropriate laxatives and careful review.

All patients prescribed a weak or strong opioid should be advised to also take a stimulant laxative unless a contraindication exists. The dose of laxative will usually need to be increased as the dose of opioid is increased. It is not appropriate to wait until (predictable) constipation occurs before commencing laxative treatment. The vicious cycle of inappropriately treated abdominal pain and constipation should be anticipated in all patients with cancer, or others taking opioid analgesics.

Management

Management will involve removing any underlying causes if possible, prescribing an appropriate oral laxative and considering the use of per rectal/stomal measures (see Table 3). It should be remembered that one of the commonest reasons for failure of therapy is prescription of a laxative that the patient dislikes.

Table 4 shows the various types of laxative that are available. Macrogols and sodium picosulfate are probably best used as second-line laxatives for patients with established constipation resistant to other laxatives. Lactulose may cause substantial gaseous distension, especially in resistant constipation.

Rectal laxatives may be needed and include:
- *Suppositories*: glycerine (softening and mild stimulant); bisacodyl (stimulant).
- *Enemas*: arachis (peanut) oil (130 ml) (softening); phosphate, sodium citrate (stimulant).

Table 3 Treatment of constipation.

Examination finding	Treatment
Rectum full of hard faeces	Soften with glycerin suppositories +/ – arachis oil enema. Commence combined stimulant and softening oral laxative
Rectum full of soft faeces	Stimulate evacuation with bisacodyl suppository +/ – stimulant enema. Commence stimulant oral laxative
Empty distended rectum	Exclude obstruction. Stimulant suppository or enema will enhance colonic contraction. Commence oral laxative

If the rectum is empty and stool is high in the colon, enemas should be administered through a rubber Foley catheter. Oil enemas should be warmed before use.

Bulk-forming laxatives have a very limited place in the management of constipation in patients with advanced disease, since they are generally troublesome to take, rely on a high oral fluid intake, and are not appropriate for the management of opioid-induced constipation. All laxative doses should be titrated according to response.

In 2008 methylnaltrexone (an opioid antagonist) was licensed for use in the United States and Europe. This is given subcutaneously and may be appropriate to consider using when standard management of constipation has failed in those patients with opioid-induced constipation. Oral opioid antagonists such as naloxegol are now available for opioid-induced constipation too. Specialist advice should be sought when considering the use of opioid antagonists for constipation [39].

Rectal Problems of Advanced Cancer

The presence of tumour in the rectum may lead to bleeding, faecal incontinence, and offensive discharge, in addition to pain. The quality of life may be severely impaired. Such problems occur not only in patients with primary rectal cancers but also in patients with other pelvic cancers: cervix, vagina, uterus, and bladder. Treatment options include:
- radiotherapy;
- palliative surgery with stoma formation;
- endoscopic injection of absolute alcohol;
- laser therapy and diathermy;
- metal stent alone or in combination with laser or alcohol; and
- pharmacological palliation.

The stool should be kept very soft to pass through the obstructive lesion. Docusate sodium is given at a dose of 200 mg at least TDS but titrated to stool consistency; it can be combined with a stimulant laxative. Careful insertion of softening enemas may be useful.

Pain and Tenesmus

Pain from rectal cancer may be troublesome in a number of ways; constant nociceptive, visceral and bone, which may be worsened by movement. In some cases, sitting may be impossible. The pain may be present only on, or worsened by, either standing or defecation. Neuropathic pains can result from infiltration of the lumbosacral plexus. Some patients experience tenesmus: a painful sensation of rectal fullness and an urge to defecate.

Table 4 Laxatives and their characteristics.

Laxative type	Drugs	Starting dose	Latency of action
Stimulant	Bisacodyl	10 mg nocte	6–12 h
	Senna	15 mg nocte	
	Sodium picosulfate	5 ml nocte	
Softening	Docusate sodium	200 mg BD-TDS	1–2 days
	Lactulose	15 ml BD	
	Macrogol	1 sachet daily in 125 ml water	

The WHO ladder (see Chapter 9) will be helpful for all of these pain syndromes. Pain will be additionally helped by keeping the faeces soft. For some patients, a palliative colostomy will be the best form of pain relief.

Neuropathic pain, of which tenesmus is one type, may be helped by opioids but will probably require adjuvant analgesics such as amitriptyline 10–75 mg nocte. Tenesmus may also be helped by:

• steroids – dexamethasone 4–16 mg daily;

• calcium channel antagonists – nifedipine 10–20 mg BD-TDS (smooth muscle relaxant);

• radiotherapy;

• bupivacaine enema;

• sacral epidural injection of steroid and local anaesthetic, and

• intrathecal 5% phenol to posterior sacral nerve roots.

Occasionally epidural infusion of opioids and local anaesthetic may be appropriate for relief of pain at rest and on defecation, particularly if the obstructive lesion is very low in the bowel.

Rectal Bleeding and Discharge

While radiotherapy, alcohol injection, diathermy, or laser therapy is being planned, or if these are not possible or helpful, other measures may be needed to reduce the distress and discomfort from rectal bleeding. Enemas may be performed using various active ingredients, including: tranexamic acid (2–4 g/day made up in KY jelly) [40]; and aluminium coating through an enema (1% alum or sucralfate in KY jelly) [41]. Distress or discomfort due to rectal discharge may be alleviated by steroid enemas and metronidazole suppositories.

Stoma Care

Patients with stomas require both physical and psychological support. Good preparation before stoma formation and adequate time spent with the patient after stoma formation by a specialist (stoma care) nurse help in the transition and continued successful management. Patients vary in the time needed to adapt to and manage their stoma.

The most common physical difficulties are:

• when a bowel stoma becomes overactive, often with a more fluid faecal output;

• when constipation occurs; and

• when patients are less able to manage their own stoma care because of the effects of their treatment or their disease.

Evaluation and management of these problems will involve examination of the stoma and effluent, including a digital examination of the stoma. There must also be a review of skin protectives/adhesives and bag size, together with a review of laxatives and antidiarrhoeal agents along with all other drugs.

If a stoma is impacted, suppositories and enemas can be given as for rectal impaction; however, a stoma has no sphincter. Suppositories should be gently pushed through the stoma as far as possible and gauze held over the stoma for a few minutes. If an enema, either oil or phosphate, is used it should be administered through a medium-sized Foley catheter. This should be passed well into the stoma (identify direction of the bowel by digital examination beforehand). Inflate the balloon to 5 ml for 10 min while instilling the enema.

Control of fluid loss from an overactive ileostomy can be troublesome and specialist advice may need to be sought.

Various treatments are available. The administration of opioids can reduce bowel motility; for example, loperamide 4–8 mg BD or codeine phosphate 30–60 mg QDS If the patient is already taking morphine for pain relief, an increase in this may reduce bowel motility further but will also increase sedation and other central effects, and is not the preferred option unless it is also useful to improve pain control. A reduction of bowel motility and secretions may be achieved by use of anticholinergics, for example, hyoscine butylbromide SC 60–200 mg/24 h, while H^2 antagonists or PPIs can reduce gastric secretions.

Ispaghula (1–2 sachets TDS) aids thickening of the motions, as does the use of isotonic and avoidance of hypotonic oral fluids. Marshmallows may also help increase stool consistency. An SC infusion of octreotide can reduce small bowel secretions (see previous section). However, doses required can be much greater than in treating obstruction.

The principles of management of a stoma and stomacare equipment can also be used to contain the output from faecal fistulae and protect the skin. SC octreotide has been used to decrease the volume of fistula effluent and in some cases has aided healing.

References

1. Roth, K., Lynn, J., Zhong, Z. et al. (2000). Dying with end stage liver disease with cirrhosis: Insights from SUPPORT. Study to understand prognoses and preferences for outcomes and risks of treatment. *Journal of the American Geriatrics Society* 48 (5 Suppl): S122–S130.
2. Hansen, L., Saaski, A., and Zucker, B. (2010). End-stage liver disease: Challenges and practice implications. *Nursing Clinics of North America* 45: 411–426.
3. Dewys, W.D., Begg, D., Lavin, P.T. et al. (1980). Prognostic effect of weight loss prior to chemotherapy in cancer patients. *American Journal of Medicine* 69: 491–496.
4. Wagner, P.D. (2008). Possible mechanisms underlying the development of cachexia in COPD. *European Respiratory Journal* 31: 492–501.
5. Anker, S.D., Negassa, A., Coats, A.J. et al. (2003). Prognostic importance of weight loss in chronic heart failure and the effect of treatment with angiotensin-converting-enzyme inhibitors: An observational study. *Lancet* 361: 1077–1083.
6. Plauth, M. and Schutz, E.T. (2002). Cachexia in liver cirrhosis. *International Journal of Cardiology* 85: 83–87.
7. Grunfield, C. (1995). What causes wasting in AIDS? *NEJM* 333: 123–124.
8. General medical Council (2010). *Treatment and Care Towards the End of Life: Good Practice in Decision Making*. London: GMC.
9. HM Government UK (2005). *Mental Capacity Act*. London: The Stationary Office.
10. Bruera, E. and Sweeney, C. (2003). Pharmacological interventions in cachexia and anorexia. In: *Oxford Textbook of Palliative Medicine*, 3e (ed. D. Doyle, G.W.C. Hanks, N. Cherney, and K. Calman), 552–560. Oxford: Oxford University Press.
11. Ruiz Garcia, V., Lopez-Briz, E., Carbonell Sanchis, R., Gonzalvez Perales, J.L., Bort-Marti, S. (2013). Bort-Marti S. Megestrol acetate for treatment of anorexia-cachexia syndrome. *Cochrane Database of Systematic Reviews*, Issue 3. CD004310. https://www.cochranelibrary.com/cdsr/doi/10.1002/14651858.CD004310.pub3/full
12. Stratton, R.J. and Elia, M. (2007). A review of reviews: A new look at the evidence for oral nutritional supplements in clinical practice. *Clinical Nutrition Supplements* 2: 5–23.
13. Elia, M. (Chairman and ed.) (2000). Guidelines for detection and management of malnutrition. Maidenhead: Malnutrition Advisory Group (MAG), Standing committee of British Association of Parenteral and Enteral Nutrition (BAPEN).
14. National Institute for Clinical Excellence (2006). CG32 guidance for nutrition support in adults.
15. Royal College of Physicians (2010). Oral feeding difficulties and dilemmas. A guide to practical care, particularly towards the end of life. Report of a working party. Royal College of Physicians.
16. Mathus-Vliegen, E.M.H. (2000). Feeding tubes and gastrostomy. In: *Practice of Therapeutic Endoscopy* (ed. G.N.J. Tygat, M. Classen, J.D. Waye, and S. Nkazawa), Philadelphia, PA: Saunders.
17. NCEPOD (2004). Scoping our practice. The 2004 report of the national confidential enquiry into patient outcome and death. London: NCEPOD.
18. Wilcock, A., Howard, P., and Charlesworth, S. (ed.). (2020). Drug administration to patients with swallowing difficulties or enteral feeding tubes. In: *Palliative Care Formulary*, 7e, 837–867. Nottingham: Pharmaceutical Press.
19. Scannapieco, F.A. (2010). Pneumonia in nonambulatory patients: The role of oral bacteria and oral hygiene. *The Journal of the American Dental Association* 137: 21s–25s.
20. Bassim, C.W., Gibson, G., Ward, T. et al. Modification of the risk of mortality from pneumonia with oral hygiene care. *Journal of the American Geriatrics Society* 2008 56: 1601–1607.
21. National Patient Safety Agency. (2010). Rapid response alert– Early detection of complications after gastrostomy No.1214 NPSA/2010/RRR010.
22. Petrina Sweeney, M. and Bagg, J. (2000). The mouth and palliative care. *American Journal of Hospice and Palliative Medicine* 17: 118–124.
23. Muscaritoli, M., Arends, J., Bachmann, P. et al. (2021). ESPEN practical guideline: Clinical Nutrition in cancer. *Clin Nutr* 40(5): 2898–2913.
24. Davies, A. and Finlay, I. (eds.) (2005). *Oral Care in Advanced Disease*, 97–114. Oxford: Oxford University Press.
25. Harris, D.G. (2010). Nausea and vomiting in advanced cancer. *British Medical Bulletin* 96: 175–185.

26. Ang, S.K., Shoemaker, L.K. and Davis, M.P. (2010). Nausea and vomiting in advanced cancer. *American Journal of Hospice and Palliative Medicine* 27 (3): 219–225.

27. Brooksbank, M.A., Game, P.A., and Ashby, M.A. (2002). Palliative venting gastrostomy in malignant intestinal obstruction. *Palliative Medicine* 16: 520–526.

28. Taylor, R.H. (1985). Laparotomy for obstruction with recurrent tumour. *British Journal of Surgery* 72: 327.

29. Krebs, H. and Goplerud, D.R. (1983). Surgical management of bowel obstruction in advanced ovarian cancer. *Obstetricians and Gynecologists* 61: 327–330.

30. Feuer, D.D.J. and Broadley, K.E. (2000). Corticosteroids for the resolution of malignant bowel obstruction in advanced gynaecological and gastrointestinal cancer. *Cochrane Database of Systematic Reviews* 1: CD001219. doi: 10.1002/14651858.CD001219.

31. DeConno, F., Caraceni, A., Zecca, E. et al. (1991). Continuous subcutaneous infusion of hyoscine butylbromide reduces secretions in patients with gastrointestinal obstruction. *Journal of Pain and Symptom Management* 6: 484–486.

32. Ripamonti, C.I. Easson, A.M. and Gerdes, H. (2008). Management of malignant bowel obstruction. *European Journal of Cancer* 44: 1105–1115.

33. Riley, J. and Fallon, M.T. (1994). Octreotide in terminal malignant obstruction of the gastrointestinal tract. *European Journal of Palliative Care* 1: 23–25.

34. Ramirez, F.C., Dennert, B., Zierer, S.T. et al. (1997). Esophageal self-expandable metallic stents-Indications, practice, techniques and complications, results of a national survey. *Gastrointestinal Endoscopy* 45: 360–364.

35. Office for national statistics (2008). Health service quarterly. *Winter* 40: 59–60.

36. Macnaughtan, J. and Thomas, H. (2010). Liver failure at the front door. *Clinical Medicine* 10 (1): 73–78.

37. Medici, V., Rossaro, L., Wegelin, J.A. et al. (2008). The utility of the model for end-stage liver disease score: A reliable guide for liver transplant candidacy and, for select patients, simultaneous hospice referral. *Liver Transplantation* 14: 1100–1106.

38. European Association for the Study of the Liver. (2010). EASL clinical practice guidelines on the management of ascites, spontaneous bacterial peritonitis, and hepatorenal syndrome in cirrhosis. *Journal of Hepatology* 53: 397–417.

39. Sykes, N.P. (2010). Constipation and diarrhoea. In: *The Oxford Textbook of Palliative Medicine*, 4e (ed. G. Hanks, N.I. Cherny, N.A. Christakis, M. Fallon, S. Kaasa, K. Russell, and R.K. Portenoy), Oxford: Oxford University Press.

40. Larkin, P.J., Sykes, N.P., Centeno, C. et al. (2008). The management of constipation in palliative care: Clinical practice recommendations. *Palliative Medicine* 22: 796–807.

41. McElligot, E., Quigley, C. and Hanks, G.W. (1991). Tranexamic acid and rectal bleeding. *Lancet* 29: 37–39.

42. Regnard, C.F.B. (1991). Control of bleeding in advanced cancer. *Lancet* 337: 974.

Further Reading

Nutrition, tube feeding, and PEG

Stroud, M., Duncan, H., and Nightingale, J. (2003). Guidelines for enteral feeding in adult hospital patients. *Gut* 52 (Suppl VII): vii1–vii12.

Cirrhosis and its complications

Menon, K.V. and Kamath, P.S. (2000). Managing the complications of cirrhosis. *Mayo Clinic Proceedings* 75 (5): 501–509.

12 The Management of Respiratory Symptoms and Advanced Chronic Obstructive Pulmonary Disease

Frances Hakkak

When you're actually gasping, you think this is the last breath, you really do. I can only put it down to feeling someone's choking you and then just at the last second, as you're about to die, they loosen their hands off and you get a grasp of air and you start again and it is bloody frightening it really is.

Patient with COPD [1]

Introduction

In this chapter, we will look at the causes of breathlessness and other respiratory symptoms in both malignancy and advanced non-malignant disease. We will start by considering specific symptoms related to malignancy and their management; we will then discuss the assessment and management (both non-pharmacological and pharmacological) of breathlessness and cough, regardless of the cause. Finally, we will look at some particular issues associated with managing patients with non-malignant lung diseases such as chronic obstructive pulmonary disease (COPD) and interstitial lung disease (ILD).

Respiratory disease affects one in five people in the UK and is the third most common cause of death. Hospital admissions for respiratory-related diseases are rising at three times the rate of admissions for other conditions [2] and 20% of all ambulance arrivals to hospital are due to acute-on-chronic breathlessness [3].

Breathlessness and other respiratory symptoms are frequently experienced in advanced disease and can be extremely distressing and debilitating. Yet, in comparison to pain, they are poorly recognised, understood, researched, assessed and managed. Dyspnoea is a better predictor of five-year survival than airway obstruction in patients with COPD [4]. In almost any condition, breathlessness worsens in the last few months of life [5] and has a significant impact on quality of life [6]. These are important symptoms that when paid attention to, can often be improved by relatively simple interventions.

Causes of Respiratory Symptoms in Advanced Disease

As with pain, it is important to make a detailed assessment in order to ascertain the likely cause of breathlessness or cough. Some causes may be reversible or have specific treatments (see Table 1).

Managing Specific Problems Associated with Malignancy

Lung Cancer and Lung Metastases
Systemic treatment (chemotherapy, immunotherapy, and targeted therapy), radiation therapy, surgery, and steroids may be used palliatively to help control symptoms including breathlessness.

Pleural Effusions
Malignant pleural effusions can be a complication of various primary cancers including lung, breast, lymphoma, gynaecological, and mesothelioma [7]. Effusions are

Handbook of Palliative Care, Fourth Edition. Edited by Richard Kitchen, Christina Faull, Sarah Russell and Jo Wilson.
© 2024 John Wiley & Sons Ltd. Published 2024 by John Wiley & Sons Ltd.

Table 1 Causes of breathlessness.

Causes of Breathlessness
Related to malignant disease
Lung cancer
Mesothelioma
Lung metastases
Malignant pleural effusion
Pulmonary embolism
Superior vena cava obstruction
Lymphangitis carcinomatosis
Anaemia
Ascites
Drug-related pneumonitis
Large airway obstruction and problems with tracheostomy/laryngectomy in head and neck cancer
Related to non-malignant disease
Chronic obstructive pulmonary disease
Interstitial lung disease (ILD)
Heart failure
Atrial fibrillation and other arrhythmias
Pericardial effusion
Respiratory muscle weakness for example, in Motor Neurone Disease (MND)
Respiratory tract infection (bacterial, viral – including COVID-19)
Obesity/physical deconditioning

Many of the causes of breathlessness listed here can also cause cough.

usually a sign of advanced disease. They are commonly associated with progressive breathlessness although patients can be asymptomatic. Chest pain, cough, and haemoptysis can also be experienced.

The drainage of pleural effusions is usually done in the hospital setting because of the requirement to use ultrasound guidance and the small risk of causing a pneumothorax. A one-off drain can be followed by talc pleurodesis to reduce the risk of effusion recurrence; however this usually requires a short inpatient stay. Increasingly, indwelling pleural catheters (PleurX™, Rocket®) are inserted which enable more regular drainage of small amounts of fluid by patients themselves, family members, or district nurses in a community setting. Drainage can be guided by symptoms, offering a sense of

control to most patients. Ultimately, the optimal management will be influenced by patient preference, with some choosing to avoid any form of drainage.

Pulmonary Embolism (PE)

Cancer and chemotherapy are both risk factors for developing a PE, which can cause acute and chronic breathlessness as well as cough and haemoptysis. As patients with cancer can also have an increased bleeding risk, the diagnosis should be confirmed on computed tomography pulmonary angiogram (CTPA) before committing to an extended period of anticoagulation. Treatment is usually with low-molecular-weight heparin (LMWH) injections initially and then a switch to a direct-acting oral anticoagulant (DOAC) can be considered depending on individual factors including renal function and bleeding risk. Treatment is usually for 3–6 months although ongoing active cancer remains a risk factor and some advocate near life-long treatment or prophylaxis in these circumstances. In practice for each individual the risks, burdens and benefits should be considered and regularly reassessed and it is often appropriate to discontinue long-term anticoagulation in a person entering the last weeks of life, and certainly in the last days. In addition to chronic breathlessness, some patients experience "post-thrombotic panic" [8]. The interplay between breathlessness, anxiety and panic attacks and how to best manage this, will be discussed later.

Lymphangitis Carcinomatosis

Lymphangitis carcinomatosis is uncommon and is due to the diffuse infiltration and obstruction of the pulmonary parenchymal lymphatic system by tumour cells. It causes progressive dyspnoea and a dry cough and is associated with a poor prognosis [9]. It most commonly occurs in people with breast, lung, gastric, and pancreatic cancer [10] but can also occur with many other primaries. Systemic corticosteroids can be helpful [11] for example, dexamethasone 8 mg OD PO.

Superior Vena Cava (SVC) Obstruction

The SVC can be compressed directly by lung tumours or by lymph nodes in the chest from breast, oesophageal, bowel, testicular primaries, or lymphoma. Breathlessness and other features (oedema and redness of face/neck/upper limbs, headaches, dizziness, altered vision, dysphagia, and prominent distended upper chest wall veins) can develop rapidly over a period of days to weeks. Urgent radiotherapy, stenting, or in some circumstances chemotherapy may be indicated. Supportive measures include diuretics, oxygen, steroids, and maintaining an upright position. Dexamethasone 16mg[1] daily PO/SC/IV is an appropriate steroid dose in this situation [12]. As with all causes of breathlessness, opioids, and benzodiazepines can be helpful in alleviating symptoms.

Drug Related Pneumonitis

Pneumonitis is an uncommon but serious side effect of the immunotherapy checkpoint inhibitors (a subclass of monoclonal antibodies – MABs) sometimes used to treat melanoma, Hodgkin's lymphoma, urinary tract, breast and lung cancers. The timing of onset can be variable [13]. Pneumonitis can also be a side effect of radiotherapy or chemotherapy. Symptoms include breathlessness and a dry cough. Fever and chest pain can also occur. The clinical and radiological picture can be difficult to distinguish from other causes of lung disease for example lymphangitis carcinomatosis or infection. Treatment is with steroids e.g. 8–16 mg dexamethasone daily, tapering over 6–12 weeks, plus supportive measures as needed, and the causative drug should usually be discontinued.

Anaemia

Cancer-related anaemia can be due to bleeding, chronic disease, bone marrow infiltration, or cancer treatment (chemotherapy or radiotherapy). Some patients, with a haemoglobin level of less than 70–80 g/L may benefit symptomatically from a blood transfusion [14], although the benefits can be short-lived that is, for just up to 2–4 weeks [15, 16] and therefore the potential risks, benefits and burdens need to be considered for each individual's circumstances. Those with a sufficient prognosis may benefit from investigating and treating iron/B12/folate deficiency. Treatment with B12/folate can result in a haemoglobin rise in just 7–10 days [17]. Some centres treat iron deficiency in people with heart failure with intravenous iron which can significantly increase quality of life, exercise capacity, and symptoms of heart failure [18]. Tranexamic acid can be used to reduce blood loss without increasing the risk of thrombosis [19] and this can be particularly useful for patients who are distressed by their bleeding. However, it is not recommended in those with urinary bleeding because of the risk of clot retention.

Stridor (Large Airway Obstruction)

Stridor is a harsh, high pitched noise on inspiration due to upper airway obstruction. Generally, stridor results from a narrowing of a central airway or the larynx caused by intrinsic or extrinsic tumour compression for example, in head and neck, oesophageal and lung cancers. It can be associated with SVCO. For those at risk, it is important to establish and plan ahead regarding how it should be managed. It is rarely a hyperacute problem but in some circumstances needs to be treated as an emergency. Dexamethasone 16 mg IV/SC/PO can be given and oxygen, with urgent ENT assistance sought for consideration of surgical airway if appropriate. More often it is an anticipated problem associated with advancing disease. Radiotherapy, chemotherapy, or stenting may be appropriate. Otherwise, symptoms can be managed with dexamethasone 8–16 mg daily, nebulised salbutamol, opioids, and benzodiazepines. Advanced airway obstruction at the very end-of-life can be distressing for patients and is best managed with reassurance and midazolam 10 mg IM/SC.

Nebulised adrenaline 1 ml of 1:1000 diluted to 5 ml with 0.9% saline QDS can be beneficial [20]. Heliox 80:20 (80% helium, 20% oxygen) can be considered if available. Heliox is less dense and viscous than air and can help reduce the respiratory work needed to overcome upper airway obstruction.

Neck Breathers

Patients with head and neck cancer and tracheostomy or laryngectomy can also be at risk of airway obstruction when there is recurrent/advanced disease.

Secretion management can be problematic in this group. Strategies to manage this include suctioning, use of carbocisteine and/or nebulised saline to reduce secretion viscosity, and antimuscarinics for example, glycopyrronium/ hyoscine butylbromide (via injection) or hyoscine hydrobromide (via a patch) to dry secretions. It may also be helpful to seek advice from your local team specialising in tracheostomies and laryngectomies.

Haemoptysis

Haemoptysis is blood coughed up from a pulmonary source. It can be distressing for patients and, when extensive, can be a pre-terminal event. It most commonly occurs in patients with lung cancer or lung metastases; however, it can also be associated with infection or PE. Palliative radiotherapy can be effective if due to tumour and the prognosis is long enough for the patient to benefit. If infection is the cause, treatment with antibiotics can help. Suspected PE

---

[1] Note that parenteral dexamethasone is prescribed differently in some units through considering the dexamethasone base only (e.g. 3.3mg parenteral dexamethasone could be considered equivalent to 4mg oral dexamethasone for dexamethasone 3.3mg/ml solution).

should be investigated and diagnosed if low-molecular-weight heparin is to be considered. After excluding potentially reversible causes, review and consider stopping any drugs that might increase bleeding. Tranexamic acid 1 g TDS can be considered for tumour related haemoptysis which is frequent and distressing. Massive terminal haemoptysis is rare but, as with those at risk of airway obstruction, it is wise to discuss and plan ahead just in case. Use of dark towels/sheets/blankets/tissues can lessen distress by reducing the visibility of the bleeding. Have benzodiazepines to hand including midazolam 10 mg IM/SC in case of a catastrophic bleed. A calming environment and reassurance however is often more important than any medications given when death is imminent.

A Note on Steroids

Steroids can be considered to manage several of the above scenarios. In a palliative care context, dexamethasone is often the steroid of choice as it can be given subcutaneously, as well as in soluble tablets and oral solution if necessary. Steroids should generally be prescribed at the lowest effective dose for the shortest time necessary to prevent side effects and physical dependence. Prescribe early in the day where possible (with or after food) to reduce insomnia, and consider night sedation for example, low dose zopiclone, especially if the steroid dose used is high. Always consider gastroprotection for example, with a proton pump inhibitor (PPI). Screen for steroid induced diabetes within 48 h of commencing or increasing the dose. Initially this can be done with urinalysis or with a late afternoon/early evening capillary blood glucose check.

Assessing and Managing Dyspnoea

Dyspnoea is the subjective sensation of breathlessness, of difficult or uncomfortable breathing. As with pain, breathlessness is what the person feeling it says it is. As with pain, the concept of "total breathlessness" should be considered, with emotional, psychological, and social components contributing to the overall experience.

Assessing Symptoms

As with assessing any symptom in palliative care, taking a detailed history is key. It is important to ascertain any precipitating and alleviating factors. Look for associated symptoms of cough, sputum, wheeze, pain, fevers, palpitations, fatigue, oedema, orthopnoea, and paroxysmal nocturnal dyspnoea. Ask about associated anxiety, depression and panic attacks. Which starts first? Does breathlessness lead to anxiety or the other way round?

Table 2 The MRC dyspnoea scale.

1959 MRC Breathlessness Scale
Grade 1: Are you ever troubled by breathlessness except on strenuous exertion?
Grade 2: (If yes) Are you short of breath when hurrying on the level or walking up a slight hill?
Grade 3: (If yes) Do you have to walk slower than most people on the level? Do you have to stop after a mile or so (or after ¼ hour) on the level at your own pace?
Grade 4: (If yes to either) Do you have to stop for breath after walking about 100 yds. (or after a few minutes) on the level?
Grade 5: (If yes) Are you too breathless to leave the house, or breathless after undressing?

Used with the permission of the Medical Research Council [21]

Severity can be assessed using dyspnoea scores such as the Medical Research Council (MRC) Dyspnoea Scale (see Table 2).

The MRC dyspnoea scale has been in use for many years for grading the effect of breathlessness on daily activities. This scale measures perceived respiratory disability and is simple to administer as it allows the patients to indicate the extent to which their breathlessness affects their mobility.

The impact of breathlessness can be significant and is important to acknowledge. Consider the following: What impact does it have on activities of daily living (ADLs) such as washing, dressing, walking, eating, drinking, and sleeping? What have their family members or carers noticed? What can they still do or no longer do? What do they struggle or need help with? Taking a shower can be particularly difficult because of the enclosed space and the steam that is generated. What is the impact of their breathlessness on them and those that matter to them? There can be many losses experienced – loss of occupation, status, role, identity. The social, financial, psychological, and emotional impact can be huge and this can influence how the symptoms are experienced for an individual.

The meaning of the breathlessness for an individual patient is also important to assess. In addition to the associated losses, there may be fear. Fear of what the breathlessness means in terms of diagnosis, prognosis, of what dying might be like. It is common for patients to be fearful of dying gasping for breath, but it is uncommon that this actually happens. Understanding and acknowledging someone's fears or concerns is the first step in being able to address them and perhaps reassure. Even the most severe states of breathlessness can be helped pharmacologically and with support to bring comfort and relief. It is important for patients and their families to understand this to enable them to regain some quality of life and to consider their options for example, regarding preferred place of care and death.

The impact can go beyond the individual patient, with symptoms significantly impacting on family and carers. People can feel very helpless when looking after someone experiencing significant breathlessness and panic attacks. Night times can be particularly difficult with fewer healthcare professionals to call upon, often resulting in unwanted ambulance calls and trips to hospital emergency departments.

When assessing breathlessness and its severity, it is important to remember that, for the reasons already discussed, the severity of symptoms do not necessarily reflect the disease status or severity overall. Symptoms can cause distress but are often intermittent and short-lived.

Chronic Breathlessness Syndrome

Chronic breathlessness syndrome has recently been recognised and defined as "the experience of breathlessness that persists despite optimal treatment of the underlying pathophysiology and results in disability for the patient" [22].

Despite optimal treatment of the underlying cause, breathlessness often persists at rest or on minimal exertion, worsening over time as the underlying cause progresses. Chronic breathlessness is under-reported by patients and under-recognised by clinicians who focus on the underlying disease or only see patients when acutely unwell. It is therefore a silent and invisible problem [23], a neglected symptom, with patients often wrongly assuming there is nothing that can be done.

The Breathing Thinking Functioning (BTF) Clinical Model [24]

The inconsistent relationship between pathology and breathlessness perception explains why optimising disease management alone does not guarantee good symptom control [24].

The neurophysiology of breathlessness is complex with thoughts and emotions contributing to breathlessness perception. As already alluded to, the human reaction to the perception of breathlessness can worsen the symptom. There is no quick fix, or one-size fits-all simple interventions. Complex symptoms require complex interventions and there is good evidence emerging for the effectiveness of multi-faceted non-pharmacological interventions such as pulmonary rehabilitation and dedicated breathlessness services [25–29].

The Cambridge Breathlessness Intervention Service (CBIS), a multidisciplinary home-based intervention of proven cost-effectiveness, developed the BTF model. The model advocates careful assessment in order to ascertain the main drivers involved, enabling a more targeted approach to developing an individualised evidence-based management plan. The model is based on three predominant cognitive and behavioural reactions to breathlessness

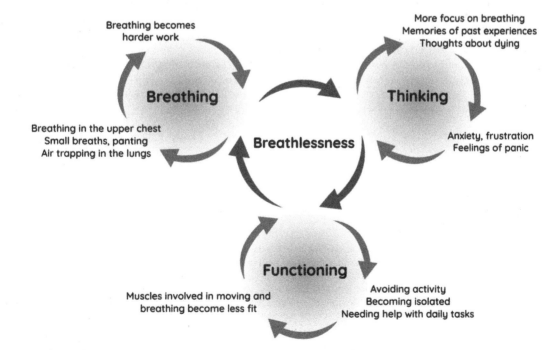

Figure 1 The Breathing, Thinking, Functioning clinical model [24]. Reproduced with permission of the Cambridge Breathlessness Intervention Service.

Table 3 The Breathing, Thinking, Functioning clinical model – three domains [24].

Breathing domain	Dysfunctional breathing patterns are common. Breathless patients experience a sense of "needing more air" and so increase their respiratory rate, using predominantly the upper chest and accessory muscles, further increasing the work of breathing and intensifying breathlessness.
Thinking domain	Breathlessness can cause fear and anxiety which in turn can worsen the perception of breathlessness. This can easily lead to panic attacks which in turn can increase the respiratory rate and cause muscle tension, further increasing the work of breathing and the feeling of breathlessness.
Functioning domain	Breathlessness leads to inactivity which leads to muscle deconditioning which increases the demand on the respiratory system, and worsens breathlessness further.

Table 4 The Breathing, Thinking, Functioning clinical model – interventions [24].

Domain	Interventions
Breathing	Breathing techniques
	Handheld fan
	Airway clearance techniques
	Inspiratory muscle training
	Chest wall vibration
	Non-invasive ventilation
Thinking	Cognitive behavioural therapy (CBT)
	Relaxation techniques
	Mindfulness
	Acupuncture
Functioning	Pulmonary rehabilitation
	Activity promotion
	Walking aids
	Pacing
	Neuromuscular electrical stimulation

that, by causing vicious cycles, worsen and maintain the symptom (see Figure 1 and Table 3).

These three vicious cycles combine to make a "vicious daisy". Patients and their families can often easily understand aspects of the model. Vicious cycles can be broken and there are evidence-based interventions that can be helpful for each of these. Even just challenging the misconceptions driving a vicious cycle can be highly effective. Although all three vicious cycles occur to a degree in each breathless patient, in practice, one or two tend to predominate. Focusing on those interventions which affect the

predominant cycle is recommended and can increase adherence (see Table 4).

Managing Breathlessness

As for pain, a stepwise ladder approach should be used when managing breathlessness (see Figure 2).

Non-Pharmacological Interventions

There are numerous non-pharmacological interventions available for breathlessness, many of which are unknown about or poorly understood by most healthcare professionals.

Step 3
Palliative pharmacological interventions e.g. opioids

Step 2
Non-pharmacological interventions

Step 1
Optimise disease treatment & treat reversible causes

Figure 2 Dyspnoea Ladder (adapted from Rocker et al.) [30]. **Step 1** Some of the specific scenarios related to malignancy and targeted interventions for these have already been discussed. Similarly, there are well evidenced disease specific interventions for chronic respiratory diseases such as COPD and ILD which will be discussed here. For patients with advanced disease and debilitating symptoms the risks/burdens versus benefits need to be carefully considered for significant step one options, which can always be revisited if a patient's situation is stabilised by interventions in steps 2 and 3. **Step 2** Non-pharmacological interventions should always be considered ahead of introducing medications such as opioids. Some of these have been listed in the BTF section earlier and will be discussed in more detail next. In addition to patient interventions it is important to consider education and support for family and carers in this step. Planning for how a breathlessness crisis/exacerbation will be managed is an extremely helpful intervention that is best done with patient and family/carers together. **Step 3** Opioids are safe and effective. How to best use these and other medications to manage breathlessness is discussed next.

The BTF model can help clinicians identify which interventions are most suitable for an individual patient. Dedicated Breathlessness Intervention Services deliver some interventions, often predominantly by physiotherapists and occupational therapists but others will be available elsewhere. Take the time to identify what services are available to you locally. Some interventions are simple and can be delivered by anyone. Non-pharmacological measures can help to empower patients at a time when the majority of their symptom management is prescriptive [31].

Breathing Techniques

A very simple technique that anyone can advise patients on is to focus on the exhale or "out breath". Breathless patients experience a sense of "needing more air" and so tend to focus on the inhale or "in breath", taking small fast breaths from the upper chest which actually tends to make the situation worse. Ask patients to forget about the in-breath and instead focus on long slow breaths out. Reassure them that in doing this an adequate in breath will follow automatically. Some people find it helpful to visualise or focus on a rectangle when doing this (see Figure 3) [32].

A physiotherapist can teach additional techniques and include breathing control, pursed lips breathing, exhalation on effort (blow as you go!), relaxed slower deeper breathing, and paced breathing. Energy conservation strategies and walking aids can support activities of daily living. Inspiratory muscle training may help some patients. Airway clearance techniques can also be used for those that need them. Positioning techniques include fixing the shoulder girdle passively and forward lean postures for example, elbows resting on knees or a table when seated, or simply sitting more upright in bed. A physiotherapist will be able to select and tailor these techniques to an individual, taking into account the cause of their breathlessness [33].

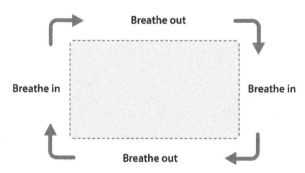

Figure 3 Breathe a rectangle. Reproduced with permission of the British Lung Foundation.

Fan Therapy

A cool breeze across the face can help reduce the sensation of breathlessness. Patients often recognise this themselves when they seek to open windows and doors. The beneficial effects of oxygen therapy may be in part due to this cool breeze. A cool breeze acts on sensory neuron receptors (Transient Receptor Potential Melastatin 8 – TRPM8 – channels) on/in the nose, mouth, and facial skin and can lead to reduced breathlessness. In terms of effective positioning, portability and control, a handheld fan is recommended and there is evidence for its effectiveness [34–39].

A handheld fan can improve recovery time from exertion-induced breathlessness [40], which can then enable people to be more active.

If you are not in a position to give patients a handheld fan then keep one to hand in order to demonstrate its use (see Table 5). Direct patients to on line resources (e.g. Cambridge Breathlessness Intervention Service) [41] or give written information, and let them know where they can purchase a fan. All of these measures will increase uptake of use.

Use of a cool moist flannel is a suitable alternative for those who don't tolerate fan therapy or where it is contraindicated.

Cognitive Behavioural Therapy (CBT)

CBT is an evidence-based, patient-centred, individualised, structured psychological intervention, which aims to understand a patient's current difficulties by exploring the links between their situation, physical symptoms, thoughts, emotions, and behaviour. Patients are encouraged to identify unhelpful thinking or behaviour driving vicious cycles and to find ways to break these and improve their quality of life. It is a very practical form of talking therapy, where a self-management plan is developed and progress monitored. Common misconceptions can be challenged for example, "When I am breathless I need oxygen", "When I feel breathless it means my disease is getting worse and I am going to die soon", "Physical exertion makes me feel breathless and is therefore dangerous".

Table 5 Advice for patients using a handheld fan.

Advice for patients using a handheld fan
• Hold the fan about six inches (15cm) from your face or the distance you find most helpful.
• Aim the cool air at your cheeks, nose, and mouth.
• Either hold the fan still or move it around slightly, whatever you find most helpful.

From Bringing Breathlessness into View – a guide to living well with breathlessness (hyms.ac.uk) [42]

Evidence suggests that healthcare professionals can learn and deliver CBT techniques as brief interventions, which can improve symptoms of anxiety and breathlessness and reduce Emergency Department (ED) attendances and hospital admissions [43–45].

Relaxation and Mindfulness

Breathlessness can often cause anxiety and feelings of panic which in turn make the breathlessness worse. Relaxation is a skill that can be taught, learnt, practiced, and improved, and there are numerous techniques available. Patients can be guided through a relaxation exercise in person or via a Compact Disc or app. Family members can read from scripts. Some people find more specific interventions such as complementary therapy (massage, aromatherapy, reflexology, reiki), hypnotherapy [46], acupuncture [47], or autogenic therapy helpful and these can sometimes be available through hospice services. Mindfulness meditation is now very popular and easily accessed via apps such as *Headspace* and *Calm*. All of these interventions help people focus on the present moment rather than the past/future and on the body or a visualisation rather than on thoughts and feelings. While some techniques encourage a focus on the breath, this is not essential and indeed an alternative focus for example, on various parts of the body via a "body scan" may be preferable for those affected by breathlessness.

Pulmonary Rehabilitation (PR)

PR is an exercise and education programme for people with lung disease who experience symptoms of breathlessness. A course usually lasts six to eight weeks, with two sessions of around two hours each week. Courses are delivered in small groups by a multidisciplinary team and may be held in local hospitals, community halls, leisure centres, and health centres. Evidence shows that accessing PR improves people's ability to walk further and helps them feel less tired and breathless when carrying out day-to-day activities. 90% of patients who complete a PR programme have higher activity and exercise levels, and report an improved quality of life. PR can improve a patient's ability to self-manage and can reduce unplanned hospital admissions [48]. Some services are able to deliver lower intensity programmes in a patient's own home. While many patients may initially appear too unwell to benefit from pulmonary rehabilitation, if deconditioning and "functioning" is their main vicious cycle then PR could make a big difference. Needing oxygen therapy isn't a contraindication – patients can take part using portable oxygen. PR is usually for those with chronic lung conditions rather than malignancy.

Support and Activity Groups

For those unable to manage PR or who find peer support particularly beneficial there are a range of options available. The British Lung Foundation run local Breath Easy support groups and many localities offer similar via NHS or hospice services for example, the FAB (Fatigue, anxiety and breathlessness) Programme [49] and Singing for Health [50].

Pharmacological Management

Several palliative pharmacological interventions are available to help with breathlessness, and associated anxiety/panic, regardless of the underlying cause. They are best reserved for use in advanced disease where symptoms have not been optimally managed by disease specific treatments and non-pharmacological interventions, and when breathlessness occurs at rest or on minimal exertion (e.g. talking, eating).

Opioids

With evidence available to support their use, opioids are the drug of choice in this context. Opioids are safe and effective in the palliation of breathlessness due to a variety of malignant and non-malignant causes and can improve overall quality of life [51–55]. Their mechanism of action is not fully understood however they appear to reduce respiratory rate by acting on brainstem respiratory control, and depress anticipatory activity in the amygdala and hippocampus reducing "breathlessness unpleasantness" [56].

The best evidence is for morphine (oral or parenteral) and a variety of opioids appear to be effective in practice. The dose required tends to be lower than used for pain with doses as low as 5 mg oral morphine per day conferring some benefit, and doses greater than 20–30 mg oral morphine per day rarely needed [51, 55]. Opioids are well tolerated when used appropriately, and anticipated side effects explained and addressed proactively. Nebulised opioids are not recommended.

Opioids for breathlessness, as for pain, are best given regularly in order to achieve a steady state. The simplest way of doing this is to use a modified release (MR) preparation but in some circumstances an immediate release (IR) preparation prescribed regularly may be preferable (see Table 6).

It is possible that opioids can, in addition to improving breathlessness and quality of life, improve exercise capacity. Certainly when assessing if the introduction of regular opioids has been successful it is helpful to include

Table 6 A practical guide to using oral morphine for breathlessness.

Option 1	Option 2	For All Patients
Start with 10 mg modified release morphine PO per day. **e.g. MST Continus 5 mg BD** Use of MST allows for a low start dose and further titration. Review effectiveness weekly and titrate as needed to a maximum of 15 mg BD (30 mg/24 h). Some localities use Zomorph in preference to MST however this offers less flexible dosing as a 5 mg preparation is unavailable. Zomorph 10 mg BD can be considered however the start dose may be too much for some patients so if MST is unavailable it may be best to start with option 2.	Consider this option if there is significant renal/hepatic impairment, risk of renal function changing unpredictably/rapidly, or in any other situation where lower/more easily adjustable doses and slower titration may be desirable. Start with **liquid morphine IR** (2 mg/ml strength) **1 mg (0.5 ml) BD PO.** Increase after 48 h to 1 mg QDS PO (e.g. 8 am, 12 pm, 4 pm, 8 pm). Then increase as needed weekly to 2 mg QDS, then 3 mg qds, then 4 mg QDS, then 5 mg QDS PO etc. (max 28 mg/24 h) Issue 1 ml oral syringes to measure doses and show the patient/carer how to do this. Consider switching to a MR preparation once an effective dose is reached.	Give written information about opioids and the dosing schedule. Explain that the potential initial side effects of drowsiness and nausea are generally short-lived (a few days max). Prescribe an antiemetic in case of need if there is concern e.g. haloperidol 500 mcg or metoclopramide 10 mg PRN. Explain that opioids can cause constipation and prescribe a laxative e.g. senna 15 mg OD to be titrated as needed.

this as a measure in very practical terms for example, ability to walk upstairs, do housework etc. Using as required (PRN) opioids pre activity is an option but is not yet well researched. In practice, exertional breathlessness in patients requiring opioids is likely to occur many times per day and so regular dosing is likely to be more practical and effective. Using prn opioids for exertional breathlessness is controversial. Most episodes of acute-on-chronic breathlessness take less than half an hour to recover and so are more amenable to non-pharmacological than drug interventions followed by titration of regular opioids if occurring frequently.

Equivalent doses can be used in a syringe pump to deliver a continuous subcutaneous infusion (CSCI) over 24 hours. Parenteral morphine is two times stronger than oral so a suitable start dose might be 5 mg/24 h.

Morphine is the gold standard opioid however a switch to an alternative opioid can be considered if morphine is poorly tolerated for example, to oxycodone.

Some people with breathlessness don't respond to opioids in which case they should be discontinued. Opioids can also be reduced/discontinued if someone responds very well and you are able to step down the treatment ladder and gain more benefit from non-pharmacological approaches for example, exercise to tackle deconditioning.

Breathlessness in the last days of life can be very distressing. Larger doses of morphine may be required in this situation for example, 2.5–5 mg SC injection PRN and 5–10 mg by CSCI over 24 hours, titrated to effect.

Benzodiazepines

Although there is still a lack of evidence to support their use, in practice benzodiazepines are used widely and appear to offer some benefit in certain circumstances. They are particularly helpful for managing the anxiety and panic often associated with breathlessness, especially in a crisis situation which can lead to unnecessary ambulance call outs/emergency hospital visits.

Shorter acting benzodiazepines (midazolam, lorazepam) are recommended over longer acting options (diazepam).

For example, Lorazepam 500 mcg sublingual PRN

Midazolam 2.5 mg SC injection PRN

In order to administer lorazepam sublingually (for quicker onset of action) prescribe the Genus brand (half a 1 mg tablet).

Midazolam can be used in a syringe driver for example, 5–10 mg/24h.

For breathlessness in the last days of life it can be particularly beneficial to use a combination of morphine and midazolam [57].

Antidepressants

Antidepressants are not a treatment for breathlessness per se however; many people experiencing breathlessness do experience associated anxiety and panic (and depression). If prognosis is sufficient (months), these symptoms can be best managed with antidepressants (rather than benzodiazepines) if non-pharmacological interventions alone are insufficient. Underlying anxiety and depression can amplify the perception of breathlessness. It is also worth noting that the response to opioids can be reduced by anxiety and depression [58, 59].

Suitable antidepressants to use in this situation are selective serotonin reuptake inhibitors for example, Sertraline 25–50 mg OD or Citalopram 10 mg OD. Mirtazapine 15 mg nocte is an alternative option which may also help with insomnia. Doses can be titrated to effect.

Oxygen

Palliative oxygen (O_2) (e.g. 2–4 L/min) can be considered for symptom management if the O_2 saturations are less than 90–92% on air and other measures have not helped. Benefit is not necessarily related to the degree of hypoxia, and other interventions for example, opioids are likely to be more beneficial in most cases [60]. If someone is not hypoxic then O_2 is no more helpful than air and a cool breeze may be as beneficial (see fan therapy). Be careful about introducing oxygen therapy unnecessarily as psychological dependence can be an issue and home oxygen can be very limiting in terms of someone's mobility and ability to go outdoors. When oxygen is used for the palliation of breathlessness, it's effectiveness should be assessed in terms of an improvement in breathlessness, rather than an improvement in O_2 sats, and if it is unhelpful should be discontinued. Oxygen therapy can often be withdrawn in the last days of life without problems [61].

Long-term oxygen therapy (LTOT), used for 16 h + per day, plus or minus ambulatory oxygen is used in specific circumstances and generally improves survival rather than offering symptomatic benefit. It should be prescribed and monitored by a respiratory specialist. Some patients who desaturate only on exertion (e.g. those with ILD) may be prescribed ambulatory oxygen alone.

Home oxygen should not be prescribed when anyone in the household still smokes because of the risk of fire. Oil-based emollients, petroleum jelly, and paraffin-containing products should be avoided. Oxygen use does not in itself prevent someone from being able to drive. Nasal cannulae (prongs) are often better tolerated than a mask. Humidification can help prevent dryness and advice on mouth and skin care should be provided.

Managing Cough

As with breathlessness, the first step in managing cough where possible is to identify and treat the underlying cause. When assessing and managing cough it is important to distinguish between a dry cough and one where sputum management is the main issue.

Productive Cough

It is common for patients with lung cancer and chronic respiratory disease for example, COPD, bronchiectasis to experience a chronic productive cough. Patients with tracheostomies and those with MND may experience similar problems with secretions. Infective exacerbations can be treated with appropriate antibiotics. Chronic sputum which is thick and viscous and difficult for patients to expectorate can be helped by mucolytics such as carbocisteine 750 mg TDS which can be reduced to a maintenance dose of 375 mg TDS or 750 mg BD in time. Nebulised sodium chloride 0.9% (normal saline) qds + prn can also be effective. Nebulised hypertonic saline (3–7%) is sometimes recommended in bronchiectasis. Some patients find that simple measures can help such as keeping well hydrated, drinking hot drinks, and steam inhalation. For those with more problematic sputum, physiotherapists can recommend specific techniques and equipment such as a flutter device or cough assist machine in certain circumstances.

For those not responding fully to the above protussive measures, antitussives can be used in addition (see dry cough). For patients nearing the end-of-life, suctioning may be appropriate and/or the use of antimuscarinic medication for example, glycopyrronium or hyoscine butylbromide as well as careful patient positioning, mouth, and skin care.

Dry Cough

First of all, consider if the cough is unrelated to any lung condition for example, secondary to medication (e.g. ACE inhibitor) or due to gastro-oesophageal reflux disease (GORD) or post-nasal drip (PND). Consider a two-month trial of a proton pump inhibitor (PPI) BD for GORD [62, 63], or intranasal therapy (steroid, antihistamine, ipratropium bromide) for PND [64].

For some people simple linctus (5 ml TDS-QDS) or menthol lozenges can help.

Opioids for Dry Cough

A dry cough can be managed by cough suppression. Opioids are effective antitussives (see Table 7 for options).

For those most bothered by cough overnight, a dose of opioid can just be given OD at bedtime.

Table 7　Opioids for cough.
Codeine phosphate linctus (15 mg/5 ml strength) 15–30 mg PO PRN, then regularly TDS-QDS if beneficial
Morphine liquid IR 2–5 mg PO PRN, then regularly QDS if beneficial (or MR preparation 5–10 mg BD PO)

Table 8 Alternative antitussives.

Gabapentin 100–300 mg OD and titrate dose/frequency every few days to effect.

Diazepam 5 mg nocte.

Amitriptyline 10 mg nocte.

Baclofen 10 mg TDS or 20 mg OD.

Alternative Antitussives for Dry Cough

Some alternative antitussive options, if opioids are unsatisfactory are listed in Table 8.

Each have neuro-inhibitory effects and may act by interfering with the cough reflex and/or central sensitisation which leads to cough hypersensitivity present in most patients with chronic cough.

Thalidomide can be considered for intractable cough due to Idiopathic Pulmonary Fibrosis (IPF) not helped by other measures. This should be under the guidance of an ILD specialist [65].

COPD

In the UK alone there are 1.2 million people living with COPD and 30,000 deaths per year. Patients are often highly symptomatic for many years but, due to the invisibility of chronic breathlessness already discussed, symptoms are often ignored or poorly managed. Patients with COPD have a very different illness trajectory to those with cancer. They experience exacerbations (infective or non-infective) which often lead to hospitalisation and any one of these can potentially lead to death. Despite an overall gradual decline in condition, death can be difficult to predict and can appear unexpected (see Figure 4).

This can lead to "prognostic paralysis" [67] where clinicians avoid talking about the future and people's wishes because they cannot predict when a significant deterioration will happen. Actually, this lack of a crystal ball shouldn't stop important conversations taking place. A helpful mantra is to "hope for the best but prepare for the worst" [68]. The Gold Standards Framework (GSF) Proactive Identification Guidance (PIG) is a useful tool for identifying people with COPD who could benefit from a palliative care approach, conversations about the future, and possibly a referral to specialist palliative care services/hospice (see Table 9) [69].

Usual therapy for patients with COPD includes inhaled/nebulised beta-2 agonists, muscarinic antagonists, and inhaled corticosteroids. Long-acting and combination preparations are available. Spacers can be helpful. For nebulised medications, some patients find a mouthpiece less claustrophobic than using a mask. Long-term use of oral corticosteroids should be avoided. Oral theophylline is occasionally recommended. Prophylactic antibiotics (e.g. azithromycin 250 mg 3 times a week) are sometimes used for those who have frequent/prolonged/severe infective exacerbations. Diuretics can be helpful for those with oedema due to cor pulmonale. A small selection of patents are suitable for lung reduction surgery or transplantation [70].

The stepwise approach to breathlessness management described above should be used for people with COPD. If symptoms persist despite optimisation of usual COPD therapy (step 1) then non-pharmacological (step 2) measures should be considered using the BTF model to assess which would be most effective, followed by palliative pharmacological interventions if needed.

People with COPD often experience frequent exacerbations. Patients should have a clear and regularly reviewed

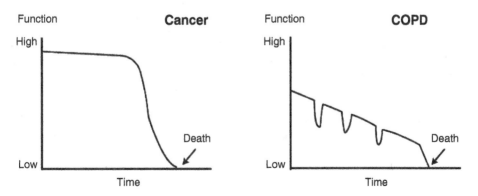

Figure 4 Illness trajectories in cancer and COPD. Adapted from Lunney, J.R., Lynn, J. and Hogan, C. (2002) [66].

Table 9 Gold Standards Framework (GSF) Proactive Identification Guidance (PIG) for COPD [69].

GSF PIG for COPD – at least two of the following indicators:

- Severe disease (e.g. FEV1 < 30% predicted), persistent symptoms for example, breathlessness despite optimal therapy, causing distress
- Recurrent hospital admissions (at least three in last year due to COPD)
- Hypoxia/fulfilling long term oxygen therapy criteria (PaO2 < 7.3kPa)
- Too unwell for surgery or pulmonary rehabilitation
- MRC grade 4/5 – shortness of breath after 100 metres on level surface
- Required ITU/NIV during admission or ventilation contraindicated
- Other factors for example, right heart failure, anorexia, cachexia, >six weeks steroids in preceding six months, despite specialist review/treatment optimisation, requires palliative medication for breathlessness.

Reproduced with permission of the National GSF Centre in End-of-Life Care UK.

plan for how to manage these when they occur in order to avoid unnecessary hospital admissions. Patients are taught how to recognise signs of infection and often have rescue packs (antibiotics and steroids) at home to treat these without delay. Non-infective exacerbations are best managed with step 2 and 3 measures tailored to the individual. It can be useful to have a written plan for patients and their carers to follow in a crisis.

Acute exacerbations sometimes require hospitalisation for intravenous antibiotics (although sometimes these can be given at home), closer monitoring, and invasive or non-invasive ventilation (NIV). Patients with chronic hypercapnic respiratory failure can be considered for long-term home NIV. NIV can be quite a distressing intervention for patients. Those who have experienced it and those who are at risk should have the opportunity to discuss their preferences regarding future treatment escalation. Some people choose to refuse this treatment in advance. Some choose to have it withdrawn when they are unwell and gaining no overall benefit from it. NIV withdrawal in either an acute or chronic situation is a complex intervention and should be done jointly by respiratory and palliative care specialists.

Interstitial Lung Disease (ILD)

There are numerous types of ILD. One of the most common is Idiopathic Pulmonary Fibrosis (IPF). IPF has a poor prognosis and patients should be offered a palliative care approach at diagnosis. A few patients will be suitable for lung transplantation and some will meet the strict criteria for antifibrotics (pirfenidone or nintedanib). Most patients with ILD are very symptomatic at diagnosis and will benefit from step 2 and 3 interventions for breathlessness management as well as interventions for cough. Patients are often hypoxic requiring increasing levels of home oxygen therapy. Exertional desaturation is common and so patients often have one oxygen prescription for at rest and a second higher flow rate prescribed for when mobilising. Although patients with ILD can experience infective exacerbations, this is not so much a feature as it is for those with COPD and patients tend to have a slightly more predictable illness trajectory, more similar to those with malignancy. Patients with both COPD and ILD have a particularly poor prognosis.

COVID-19

On 12 March 2020, COVID-19 was declared a pandemic by the World Health Organisation. In severe cases symptoms can escalate rapidly therefore an anticipatory approach to symptom management is key [71]. Symptoms can include breathlessness, cough, fatigue, anxiety, agitation, drowsiness, and delirium. As with all causes of breathlessness, opioids and the non-pharmacological measures described above can be helpful. However, the use of a handheld fan is not recommended in COVID-19 because of the theoretical risk of increasing droplet and aerosol spread. Patients who are able to adopt a prone position themselves should be encouraged to try it for relief of breathlessness. Benzodiazepines and/or antipsychotic medication can be used to manage anxiety, agitation, and delirium. Communication with patients and family can be challenging due to noisy NIV machines, the use of personal protective equipment (PPE), social distancing and restricted visiting in hospitals. Technology can be helpful here, for example, for remote consultations and to support at the bedside communication. Simple bedside tools include transparent face masks and handheld whiteboards.

Hospitalised patients deteriorating despite non-invasive ventilation (NIV), usually Continuous Positive Airway Pressure (CPAP), may choose to have this withdrawn, or a decision to withdraw treatment may be made in best interests when the patient lacks capacity. Parenteral opioids and benzodiazepines are usually required to enable a patient to be comfortable enough to tolerate this. This is a complex intervention which usually requires both respiratory and specialist palliative care team input.

A Joint Specialty Multidisciplinary Team (MDT) Approach

In some localities, there is joint specialty working between respiratory and palliative care teams. Patients can be referred for an MDT discussion and some services offer joint consultations in outpatient clinics or other settings. These services tend to focus on patients with non-malignant conditions who experience chronic symptoms, exacerbations, crises, and frequent hospital admissions. This approach enables a greater proportion of patients to live and die in their preferred place while improving their physical, emotional, and social wellbeing [72].

Summary

In this chapter, we have reviewed the causes of breathlessness and other respiratory symptoms in advanced malignant and non-malignant disease and how to best manage these. Careful assessment and the use of a stepwise approach to management is important. Non-pharmacological interventions should always be considered ahead of palliative pharmacological measures. Understanding illness trajectories in non-malignant disease helps clinicians communicate more effectively about prognosis and treatment options. As with all areas of palliative care, a holistic approach and good use of the full multidisciplinary team is key.

> *To leave the world a bit better; to know that one life has breathed easier because of you. This is to have succeeded.*
> Ralph Waldo Emerson

References

1. Hakkak, F., Forbes, K., and Dowson, L. (2014). Living with COPD and facing death: information and communication needs about end-of-life issues. *BMJ Supportive & Palliative Care* 4: A9–A10.
2. NHS England > Respiratory Disease. https://www.england.nhs.uk/ourwork/clinical-policy/respiratory-disease (accessed 14 March 2021).
3. Hutchinson, A., Pickering, A., Williams, P. et al. (2017). Breathlessness and presentation to the emergency department: a survey and clinical record review. *BMC Pulmonary Medicine* 17: 53.
4. Nishimura, K. et al. (2002). Dyspnea is a better predictor of 5-year survival than airway obstruction in patients with COPD. *Chest* 121 (5): 1434–1440.
5. Johnson, M.J., Bland, J.M., Gahbauer, E.A. et al. (2016). Breathlessness in elderly adults during the last year of life sufficient to restrict activity: prevalence, pattern, and associated factors. *Journal of the American Geriatrics Society* 64: 73–80.
6. Currow, D.C., Dal Grande, E., Ferreira, D. et al. (2017). Chronic breathlessness associated with poorer physical and mental health-related quality of life (SF-12) across all adult age groups. *Thorax* 72: 1151–1153.
7. Penz, E., Watt, K.N., Hergott, C.A. et al. (2017). Management of malignant pleural effusion: challenges and solutions. *Cancer Management and Research* 9: 229–241.
8. Duffett, L., Castellucci, L.A., and Forgie, M.A. (2020). Pulmonary embolism: update on management and controversies. *BMJ* 370: m2177.
9. Klimek, M. (2019). Pulmonary lymphangitis carcinomatosis: systematic review and meta-analysis of case reports, 1970-2018. *Postgraduate Medicine* 131 (5): 309–318.
10. Johkoh, T., Lee, K.S., Nishino, M. et al. (2021). Chest CT diagnosis and clinical management of drug-related pneumonitis in patients receiving molecular targeting agents and immune checkpoint inhibitors: a position paper from the fleischner society. *Radiology* 298 (3): 550–566.
11. Lin, R.J., Adelman, R.D., and Mehta, S.S. (2012). Dyspnea in palliative care: expanding the role of corticosteroids. *Journal of Palliative Medicine* 15 (7): 834–837.
12. Superior Vena Cava Obstruction (2019). Scottish palliative care guidelines. NHS Scotland. https://www.palliativecareguidelines.scot.nhs.uk/guidelines/palliative-emergencies/superior-vena-cava-obstruction.aspx (accessed 27 March 2021).
13. Wang, H., Guo, X., Zhou, J. et al. (2020). Clinical diagnosis and treatment of immune checkpoint inhibitor-associated pneumonitis. *Thorac Cancer* 11: 191–197.

14. Aapro, M. et al. (2018). Management of anaemia and iron deficiency in patients with cancer: ESMO clinical practice guidelines. *Annals of Oncology* 29: iv96–iv110. doi: 10.1093/annonc/mdx758.

15. Preston, N.J., Hurlow, A., Brine, J., and Bennett, M.I. (2012 15). Blood transfusions for anaemia in patients with advanced cancer. *Cochrane Database of Systematic Reviews* 2012 (2): CD009007.

16. Neoh, K., Gray, R., Grant-Casey, J. et al. (2019). National comparative audit of red blood cell transfusion practice in hospices: recommendations for palliative care practice. *Palliative Medicine* 33 (1): 102–108.

17. Devalia, V., Hamilton, M.S., and Molloy, A.M. (2014). Guidelines for the diagnosis and treatment of cobalamin and folate disorders. *British Journal of Haematology* 166: 496–513.

18. Ponikowski, P., van Veldhuisen, D.J., Comin-Colet, J. et al; CONFIRM-HF Investigators. (14 March 2015). Beneficial effects of long-term intravenous iron therapy with ferric carboxymaltose in patients with symptomatic heart failure and iron deficiency. *European Heart Journal* 36 (11): 657–668.

19. Roberts, I., Perel, P., Prieto-Merino, D. et al; CRASH-2 Collaborators. (2012 September 11). Effect of tranexamic acid on mortality in patients with traumatic bleeding: prespecified analysis of data from randomised controlled trial. *BMJ* 345: e5839.

20. Flockton, R.J., Dickman, A., and Ellershaw, J.E. (2007). Letter to the editor: use of nebulised adrenaline in the management of steroid-resistant stridor. *Palliative Medicine* 21 (8): 723–724.

21. Medical Research Council, MRC Breathlessness Scale (1959). https://mrc.ukri.org/research/facilities-and-resources-for-researchers/mrc-scales/mrc-dyspnoea-scale-mrc-breathlessness-scale (accessed 21 March 2021).

22. Johnson, M.J., Yorke, J., Hansen-Flaschen, J. et al. (2017). Towards an expert consensus to delineate a clinical syndrome of chronic breathlessness. *The European Respiratory Journal* 49: 1602277.

23. Gysels, M. and Higginson, I.J. (2008). Access to services for patients with chronic obstructive pulmonary disease: the invisibility of breathlessness. *Journal of Pain and Symptom Management* 36 (5): 451–460. doi: 10.1016/j.jpainsymman.2007.11.008.

24. Spathis, A., Booth, S., Moffat, C. et al. (2017). The Breathing, Thinking, Functioning clinical model: a proposal to facilitate evidence-based breathlessness management in chronic respiratory disease. *NPJ Primary Care Respiratory Medicine* 27: 27.

25. McCarthy, B., Casey, D., Devane, D., Murphy, K., Murphy, E., and Lacasse, Y. (2015). Pulmonary rehabilitation for chronic obstructive pulmonary disease. *Cochrane Database of Systematic Reviews* 23 (2): CD003793.

26. Farquhar, M.C., Prevost, A.T., McCrone, P., Brafman-Price, B., Bentley, A., Higginson, I.J., Todd, C., and Booth, S. (31 October 2014). Is a specialist breathlessness service more effective and cost-effective for patients with advanced cancer and their carers than standard care? findings of a mixed-method randomised controlled trial. *BMC Medicine* 12: 194.

27. Higginson, I., Bausewein, C., Reilly, C., Gao, W., Gysels, M., Dzingina, M. et al. (2014). An integrated palliative and respiratory care service for patients with advanced disease and refractory breathlessness: a randomised controlled trial. *The Lancet Respiratory Medicine* 2: 979–987.

28. Johnson, M.J., Kanaan, M., Richardson, G. et al. (2015). A randomised controlled trial of three or one breathing technique training sessions for breathlessness in people with malignant lung disease. *BMC Medicine* 13: 213.

29. Bausewein, C., Schunk, M., Schumacher, P., Dittmer, J., Bolzani, A., and Booth, S. (2018 February). Breathlessness services as a new model of support for patients with respiratory disease. *Chronic Respiratory Disease* 15 (1): 48–59.

30. Rocker, G.M., Sinuff, T., Horton, R., and Hernandez, P. (2007). Advanced chronic obstructive pulmonary disease: innovative approaches to palliation. *Journal of Palliative Medicine* 10 (3): 783–797.

31. Taylor, J. (2007). The non-pharmacological management of breathlessness. *End of Life Care* 1 (1).

32. British Lung Foundation (2020). How to manage breathlessness. https://www.blf.org.uk/support-for-you/breathlessness/how-to-manage-breathlessness (accessed 26 March 2021).

33. Bott, J., Blumenthal, S., Buxton, M. et al. (2009). Guidelines for the physiotherapy management of the adult, medical, spontaneously breathing patient. *Thorax* 64: i1–i52.

34. Kako, J., Kobayashi, M., Oosono, Y. et al. (2020). Immediate effect of fan therapy in terminal cancer with dyspnea at rest: a meta-analysis. *American Journal of Hospice and Palliative Medicine* 37 (4): 294–299.

35. Schwartzstein, R.M., Lahive, K., Pope, A. et al. (1987 July). Cold facial stimulation reduces breathlessness induced in normal subjects. *The American Review of Respiratory Disease* 136 (1): 58–61. doi: 10.1164/ajrccm/136.1.58.

36. Galbraith, S., Perkins, P., Lynch, A.G., and Booth, S. (2008). Does the use of a handheld fan improve intractable breathlessness? *Palliative Medicine* 22: 597–598.

37. Swan, F., Newey, A., Bland, M. et al. (2019 June). Airflow relieves chronic breathlessness in people with advanced disease: an exploratory systematic review and meta-analyses. *Palliative Medicine* 33 (6): 618–633.

38. Luckett, T., Phillips, J., Johnson, M.J. et al. (2017). Contributions of a hand-held fan to self-management of chronic breathlessness. *European Respiratory Journal* 50 (2): 1700262. doi: 10.1183/13993003.00262-2017.

39. Morélot-Panzini, C. (2017 August). *European Respiratory Journal* 50 (2): 1701383. doi: 10.1183/13993003.01383-2017.

40. Swan, F., English, A., Allgar, V. et al. (2019). The hand-held fan and the calming hand for people with chronic breathlessness: a feasibility trial. *Journal of Pain and Symptom Management* 57 (6): 1051–1061.

41. Cambridge university hospitals breathlessness intervention service: video and audio to help manage breathlessness. https://www.cuh.nhs.uk/our-services/breathlessness-intervention-service/video-and-audio-help-manage-breathlessness (accessed 26 March 2021).

42. Bringing Breathlessness Into View. Hull York Medical School. https://www.hyms.ac.uk/assets/docs/research/bringing-breathlessness-into-view.pdf (accessed 26 March 2021).

43. Livermore, N., Dimitri, A., Sharpe, L. et al. (2015). Cognitive behaviour therapy reduces dyspnoea ratings in patients with chronic obstructive pulmonary disease (COPD). *Respiratory Physiology & Neurobiology* 216: 35–42.

44. Heslop-Marshall, K., Baker, C., Carrick-Sen, D. et al. (2018 October). Randomised controlled trial of cognitive behavioural therapy in COPD. *ERJ Open Research* 4 (4).

45. Howard, C. and Dupont, S. (2014). 'The COPD breathlessness manual': a randomised controlled trial to test a cognitive-behavioural manual versus information booklets on health service use, mood and health status, in patients with chronic obstructive pulmonary disease. *NPJ Primary Care Respiratory Medicine* 24: 14076.

46. Plaskota, M., Lucas, C., Pizzoferro, K. et al. (2011). The effectiveness of hypnotherapy in the treatment of anxiety in patients with cancer receiving palliative care. *BMJ Supportive & Palliative Care* 1: 235.

47. von Trott, P. et al. (2020). Acupuncture for breathlessness in advanced diseases: a systematic review and meta-analysis. *Journal of Pain and Symptom Management* 59 (2): 327–338. e3. doi: 10.1016/j.jpainsymman.2019.09.007.

48. NHS England. Pulmonary rehabilitation. https://www.england.nhs.uk/ourwork/clinical-policy/respiratory-disease/pulmonary-rehabilitation (accessed 26 March 2021).

49. Pollock, K. A service evaluation of the Fatigue, Anxiety and Breathlessness (FAB) programme. Marie Curie Hospice Edinburgh. https://www.palliativecarescotland.org.uk/content/publications/02-FAB-evaluation-poste.pdf (accessed 26 March 2021).

50. Singing for Lung Health. British Lung Foundation. https://www.blf.org.uk/support-for-you/singing-for-lung-health (accessed 26 March 2021).

51. Barnes, H., McDonald, J., Smallwood, N., and Manser, R. (2016 March 31). Opioids for the palliation of refractory breathlessness in adults with advanced disease and terminal illness. *Cochrane Database of Systematic Reviews* 3 (3):CD011008. (accessed 31 March 2016).

52. Ekström, M., Nilsson, F., Abernethy, A.A., and Currow, D.C. (2015 July). Effects of opioids on breathlessness and exercise capacity in chronic obstructive pulmonary disease. A systematic review. *Annals of the American Thoracic Society* 12 (7): 1079–1092.

53. Verberkt, C.A., van den Beuken-van Everdingen, M.H.J., Schols, J.M.G.A. et al. (2017). Respiratory adverse effects of opioids for breathlessness: a systematic review and meta-analysis. *European Respiratory Journal* 50 (5).

54. Verberkt, C.A., van den Beuken-van Everdingen, M.H.J., Schols, J.M.G.A. et al. (2020 October 1). Effect of sustained-release morphine for refractory breathlessness in chronic obstructive pulmonary disease on health status: a randomized clinical trial. *JAMA Internal Medicine* 180 (10): 1306–1314.

55. Currow, D.C., McDonald, C., Oaten, S. et al. (2011 September). Once-daily opioids for chronic dyspnea: a dose increment and pharmacovigilance study. *Journal of Pain and Symptom Management* 42 (3): 388–399. doi: 10.1016/j.jpainsymman.2010.11.021.

56. Hayen, A., Wanigasekera, V., Faull, O.K. et al. (2017). Opioid suppression of conditioned anticipatory brain responses to breathlessness. *NeuroImage* 150: 383–394.

57. Navigante, A.H., Cerchietti, L.C., Castro, M.A. et al. (2006 January). Midazolam as adjunct therapy to morphine in the alleviation of severe dyspnea perception in patients with advanced cancer. *Journal of Pain and Symptom Management* 31 (1): 38–47.

58. Edwards, R.R., Dolman, A.J., Michna, E. et al. (2016 October). Changes in pain sensitivity and pain modulation during oral opioid treatment: the impact of negative affect. *Pain Medicine* 17 (10): 1882–1891.

59. Abdallah, S.J., Faull, O.K., Wanigasekera, V. et al. (2019). Opioids for breathlessness: psychological and neural factors influencing response variability. *The European Respiratory Journal* 54: 1900275.

60. Clemens, K.E., Quednau, I., and Klaschik, E. (2009 April). Use of oxygen and opioids in the palliation of dyspnoea in hypoxic and non-hypoxic palliative care patients: a prospective study. *Support Care Cancer* 17(4): 367–77.

61. Campbell, M.L., Yarandi, H., and Dove-Medows, E. (2012 March). Oxygen is nonbeneficial for most patients who are near death. *Journal of Pain and Symptom Management* 45 (3): 517–523.

62. Kahrilas, P.J. et al. (2013). Response of chronic cough to acid-suppressive therapy in patients with gastroesophageal reflux disease. *CHEST* 143 (3): 605–612.

63. Ojoo, J.C., Everett, C.F., Mulrennan, S.A. et al. (2013). Management of patients with chronic cough using a clinical protocol: A prospective observational study. *Cough* 9: 2.

64. Macedo, P., Saleh, H., Torrego, A. et al. (2009 November). Postnasal drip and chronic cough: an open interventional study. *Respiratory Medicine* 103 (11): 1700–1705.

65. Idiopathic pulmonary fibrosis in adults: Diagnosis and management. NICE Clinical guideline [CG163] Published 2013, updated 2017. https://www.nice.org.uk/guidance/cg163 (accessed 26 March 2021).

66. Lunney, J.R., Lynn, J., and Hogan, C. (2002). Profiles of older medicare decedents. *Journal of the American Geriatrics Society* 50: 1108–1112.

67. Murray, S.A., Boyd, K., and Sheikh, A. (2005). Palliative care in chronic illness. *BMJ* 330: 611.

68. Mori, M., Fujimori, M., and Ishiki, H. (2019). Adding a wider range and "Hope for the Best, and Prepare for the Worst"

statement: preferences of patients with cancer for prognostic communication. *Oncologist ep* 24 (9): e943–e952.

69. Thomas, K. et al. (2022). GSF proactive identification guidance. National GSF Centre in End of Life Care UK. https://goldstandardsframework.org.uk/pig (accessed 05 September 2022).

70. Chronic obstructive pulmonary disease in over 16s: diagnosis and management. NICE guideline [NG115] Published 2018, updated 2019. https://www.nice.org.uk/guidance/NG115 (accessed 26 March 2021).

71. Ting, R., Edmonds, P., Higginson, I.J., and Sleeman, K.E. (2020). Palliative care for patients with severe COVID-19. *BMJ* 370.

72. Huntley, C., Hakkak, F., and Ward, H. (2020 March 2). Palliative care for chronic respiratory disease: integrated care in outpatient settings. *British Journal of Community Nursing* 25 (3):132–138.

13 Managing Complications of Cancer

Lesley Charman, Rachael Barton and Katie Spencer

Introduction

Patients with advanced or metastatic cancer often experience complications caused by their disease or its treatment. These may have a profound effect on their functional ability and quality of life. Although such complications are commonly seen in oncology, they may be rare outside the specialty. It is important to identify early those who may benefit from specific treatment, since a prompt referral allows the rapid palliation of symptoms minimising their impact on quality of life. It is equally important to identify those patients who are in the terminal stage of their illness who may be helped more by symptomatic measures than by referral for investigation and treatment. Advance care planning and understanding of patients' priorities in the context of their expected disease trajectory can help ensure that the care delivered aligns with patient preferences. This chapter outlines the clinical problems most frequently encountered and suggests management guidelines, so that non-specialists may have confidence in dealing with what is often a distressing situation for both patient and carer.

Malignant Spinal Cord Compression (MSCC)

MSCC is an oncological emergency requiring urgent recognition, diagnosis, and management. Where function has been lost at the point of treatment, it is rarely regained. It is therefore essential to have a high level of suspicion in patients with known cancer, particularly where bony metastatic disease has been previously demonstrated.

Post-mortem evidence suggests MSCC may be present in 5–10% of patients with advanced cancer and an estimated 2.5% will present clinically in their final five years of life [1]. Approximately a quarter of those presenting with MSCC have no known cancer diagnosis [2]. The risk of MSCC differs widely between cancer diagnoses; over half of patients have a diagnosis of breast, lung, or prostate cancer with haematological, gastro-intestinal and renal cell cancers much less frequent [3].

Early Suspicion and Clinical Diagnosis

Patients with known bone or spinal metastases and those at high risk of developing spinal metastases, should be given written information explaining the symptoms to look out for [4].

In patients with MSCC, 94% experience back pain, with pain often developing over a median of 3 months before further symptoms and signs occur, giving a "window of opportunity" for diagnosis [3]. Localised pain in the vertebral column may be associated with bony tenderness and radicular pain, sometimes radiating in a dermatomal distribution. Pain is severe and unremitting, often preventing sleep and worsening with activities that raise intra-abdominal pressure, involve movement, lying supine, percussion over the vertebrae or neck and hip flexion.

Myelopathy manifests as weakness, variable sensory disturbance, and loss of bowel and bladder function. Weakness is often symmetrical although unilateral presentation can occur early on. Sphincter dysfunction occurs late in spinal cord compression but is an earlier feature of cauda equina compression, resulting in urinary retention, constipation, faecal incontinence, and loss of anal tone [5]. The clinical picture varies and the frequency of symptoms is shown in Table 1 [6]. Infrequently, myelopathy due to MSCC can manifest with neurological impairment in the absence of pain.

Handbook of Palliative Care, Fourth Edition. Edited by Richard Kitchen, Christina Faull, Sarah Russell, and Jo Wilson.
© 2024 John Wiley & Sons Ltd. Published 2024 by John Wiley & Sons Ltd.

Table 1   The frequency of symptoms in MSCC. Source: Levack et al. [6].

Symptom	% with symptom
Pain	94
Weakness or difficulty walking	82
Changes in sensation	68
Difficulty passing urine	56
Constipation	66
Faecal incontinence	5

Investigations

Patients with new or unremitting spinal pain on a background of known malignancy, or a suspicious history in patients not known to have cancer, with or without clinical signs, require urgent clinical assessment. If clinically suspicious for MSCC, urgent discussion with the local MSCC co-ordinator is required, and an MRI of the whole spine should be performed within 24 hours unless there is a specific contraindication [4]. Occasionally MRI will be required sooner than 24 hours if there is a pressing clinical need for emergency surgery.

Treatment

Immediate Management

All patients with suspected or confirmed MSCC should be prescribed dexamethasone 16 mg immediately. This should only be given parenterally if there is concern about oral absorption [7]. This should be followed by dexamethasone 16 mg daily (in 1–2 divided doses, the latest given before 2p.m. to avoid night-time wakefulness, although this should not preclude emergency administration of the first day's dose). Patients who remain on steroids for more than a week should be issued with a steroid alert card and advice regarding the necessity of gradual weaning to avoid adrenal crisis [8]. Concurrent prescribing of gastric protection is required. Strong opioids and nonsteroidal anti-inflammatories (NSAIDs) (where appropriate) are often required for pain, and potentially also antispasmodics and neuropathic agents if appropriate.

Patients with severe mechanical pain suggestive of spinal instability or symptoms/signs suggestive of MSCC should be nursed flat with neutral spinal alignment until bony and neurological stability are established and

cautious mobilisation can begin [7]. In the absence of surgical stabilisation, or brace support, following initial assessment, the need to maintain neutral alignment requires careful consideration. In all cases the risks and benefits of potentially permanent immobilisation versus the risks of mobilisation as pain allows should be discussed with the patient and decisions made in line with their preferences.

Subsequent Treatment Options

Despite the development of MSCC being a poor prognostic sign, active management is indicated in the majority of patients. Definitive treatment is arranged via the MSCC coordinator and needs to begin before further neurological deterioration, ideally within 24 hours of diagnosis.

The potential benefit of treatment is extremely limited in patients very near the end-of-life or where paraplegia is established in the absence of pain. For these patients multidisciplinary assessment and sensitive discussion can guide a more appropriate management plan focussing on the medical management of symptoms.

Surgery

Surgery is considered when there is structural spinal instability with or without pain, particularly if neurological compromise can be prevented. Spinal decompression and stabilisation followed by radiotherapy improves the outcome in terms of maintenance of mobility and continence compared with radiotherapy alone [9]. Other relative indications for surgery include malignancy of unknown primary (to support histological diagnosis) or disease that is radio-resistant. Patients most likely to benefit from surgery are those with a good prognosis and limited sites of metastatic disease. Patients with a prognosis of less than three months should not be managed surgically given the time required for recovery. A recognised prognostic scoring system such as that described by Tokuhashi is recommended to aid decision making (see Box 2) [7, 10].

Radiotherapy

Radiotherapy is the mainstay of treatment, and pain improvement is seen in approximately 50–60% of patients [11]. In general, radiotherapy is more effective when cord compression occurs without bony collapse and instability [12]. A single fraction is as effective as two or five fractions in patients with limited prognosis while for those with a better prognosis limited evidence supports consideration of a longer course [7, 13, 14]. Where a patient with poor prognosis has complete paraplegia and no pain, a holistic approach to symptom control may be more appropriate than radiotherapy [11].

Table 2 Tokuhashi prognostic scoring system in spinal cord compression [10].

Predictive Factor	Score (Points)
Performance status (KPS)	
Poor (KPS 10–40%)	0
Moderate (KPS 50–70%)	1
Good (KPS 80–100%)	2
Number of extraspinal bone metastases	
≥3	0
1–2	1
0	2
Number of metastases in vertebral bodies	
≥3	0
2	1
1	2
Metastases to visceral organs	
Unresectable	0
Resectable	1
No metastases	2
Primary cancer diagnosis	
Lung, Pancreas, Oesophageal, Gastric, Bladder, Osteosarcoma	0
Liver, Gallbladder, Unidentified	1
Others	2
Uterus, Kidney	3
Rectum	4
Thyroid, Prostate, Breast, Carcinoid	5
Paralysis	
Complete	0
Incomplete	1
None	2

Using this system, patients scoring 0–8: Prognosis <6 months; 9–11: Prognosis 6–12 months; ≥12: Prognosis >12 months. KPS = Karnofsky Performance Status, a measure of a patient's functional ability and activity levels which deteriorate near the end-of-life.

Chemotherapy

Chemotherapy may be indicated for chemosensitive tumours such as lymphoma, small-cell lung cancer, and germ cell tumours, and is usually followed by radiotherapy.

Outcomes

Function

Most patients who are ambulant at the point of treatment will maintain ambulation subsequently. Where ambulatory function is lost this is regained in less than a third of patients undergoing radiotherapy and less than 10% of patients presenting with paraplegia [15]. Of those not requiring a urinary catheter before treatment, 80% will remain catheter-free compared to 20% of those who require a catheter at diagnosis.

Survival and Prognostic Factors

In patients diagnosed with MSCC, 18–30% survive for one year. Prognosis, however, may vary from short days to a number of years. Factors influencing survival are summarized in the Tokuhashi score (see Table 2) [10].

Rehabilitation and Discharge Planning

The physiotherapist and occupational therapist play a key role in supporting adjustment and, where appropriate, rehabilitation in patients presenting with MSCC. Patients and carers may need support to adapt to a limited prognosis, loss of mobility and bladder/bowel function but also to the distress associated with loss of social status and change in body image.

Immediate needs may include:

- Special equipment or adaptations at home.
- An alternative place of care such as a care home or palliative care unit.
- A "package" of social and health care.
- Psychosocial support.

Follow-up

More than 70% of patients will have other vertebral sites affected by metastatic disease giving a risk of further MSCC at both the treated site and beyond. Radiotherapy is often given where other lesions are painful although there is no evidence to support prophylactic treatment. To continue to optimise function, pain control, and quality of life, regular follow-up is vital and this may be community rather than hospital led.

Superior Vena Cava Obstruction (SVCO)

SVCO describes a syndrome characterised by obstruction to blood flow through the superior vena cava (SVC). Malignancy is the major cause of SVCO (in excess of 90% of cases) with a majority of cases being due to lung cancer (75%) **or** lymphoma (15%) [16]. Where malignancy is present SVCO is frequently the initial clinical presentation.

Symptoms and Clinical Diagnosis

Patients with lung cancer, especially right-sided, are at particular risk of SVCO. Symptom onset is often insidious, over weeks, allowing collateral blood vessels to develop, resulting in visibly engorged subcutaneous veins on the chest, neck and upper abdomen. Two-thirds of patients complain of breathlessness and half of facial swelling or a feeling of fullness in the head. The symptoms (see Table 3) may be exacerbated by bending forwards or lying down. Occasionally symptoms of SVCO may develop acutely due to sudden occlusion. In these cases, the patient may become acutely unwell.

Investigations and Initial Management

Although symptoms are often uncomfortable, SVCO is rarely life-threatening unless oxygenation is severely compromised. For patients without a known cancer diagnosis, urgent referral to the respiratory or acute oncology team is required. For those with a known cancer, urgent contact should be made with their existing oncology team. A contrast-enhanced CT thorax confirms the diagnosis.

The role of steroids is unproven although they are often given; dexamethasone 16 mg daily (with gastric protection) may help. Steroids should not be given "blind" without specialist guidance if the underlying diagnosis is not known. Rarely, high-grade mediastinal lymphoma may present as SVCO, in which case steroids may induce tumour lysis syndrome, threatening renal function, and obscuring a histological diagnosis. Anticoagulants are only indicated where associated thrombosis is demonstrated.

Table 3 Symptoms and signs of SVCO.

Symptoms	Physical Signs
• Breathlessness	• Neck vein distension
• Head fullness	• Facial/arm swelling
• Headache	• Dyspnoea
• Nasal congestion	• Distension of superficial veins (chest/abdominal wall)
• Epistaxis	
• Cough	• Plethora
• Chest pain	• Facial or conjunctival oedema
• Dizziness	
• Dysphagia	• Central or peripheral cyanosis
• Hoarse voice	

Active treatment of SVCO may provide relief from distressing symptoms and is indicated in all but the frailest, terminally ill patients who may be helped more by palliative symptomatic measures alone.

If the patient is breathless, bed rest and elevation of the bed head may be helpful. Oxygen should be used only if it gives symptomatic relief or when the patient is hypoxic. Analgesia and antitussives may help patients who have headache and cough.

Subsequent Treatment

The aim of treatment is to relieve symptoms and, if possible, reverse the underlying process. Treatment decisions are based upon an understanding of the underlying malignant diagnosis, prognosis and likely sensitivity to chemotherapy and radiotherapy.

Where response to chemotherapy or radiotherapy may be delayed or insufficient, insertion of a stent under radiological control gives rapid and often immediate relief of symptoms, most resolving within 72 hours [17]. Urgent referral for stenting should be considered for severe symptoms or for relapse following treatment with other modalities. Caution must be exercised however, with the placement of stents in patients with a good prognosis, especially those with curable disease, as fibrosis and narrowing occurring some months after stenting may require further intervention with the risk of intractable symptoms. Following stenting, treatment with chemotherapy or radiotherapy can be considered for patients who remain fit enough.

Outcome

The average survival of patients diagnosed with a malignant cause of SVCO is eight months, but the prognosis depends heavily on the underlying histology and stage of disease at presentation. In lung cancer, relapse occurs following radiotherapy and/or chemotherapy in approximately 17% of patients over a period of 1–16 months following treatment [16].

Follow-up

Where anti-cancer treatment is undertaken, care should be centred at the specialist unit providing the treatment until toxicity has settled. Following treatment, patients with incurable disease should be cared for in a home setting with GP and palliative care support, with oncology available as an "SOS" option.

Bone Metastases

Bone metastases are common, especially in cancers of the breast, prostate, lung, and kidney. Widespread bone lesions are also a feature of multiple myeloma. Up to 70% of women dying of breast cancer have been found to have radiological evidence of bone metastases while these are present in almost all men dying of prostate cancer [18, 19]. Although many patients will be asymptomatic, around a third present with pain [20]. Other complications of bone metastases include pathological fracture, nerve compression, and hypercalcaemia.

Symptoms and Clinical Diagnosis

Pain due to bone metastases is commonly unrelenting, nagging and progressive. It may be present at rest, is often exacerbated by movement (functional pain) and can be associated with referred pain, restriction of movement, and neurological impairment.

Investigations

Initial investigation with plain X-rays of the affected area is required to confirm the diagnosis and rule out pathological fracture ahead of specialist review. Orthogonal (i.e. perpendicular) views of long bones are required as some metastases may be visible only on one view. Lesions may be sclerotic (with areas of increased bone density due to bone deposition) or lytic (with areas of increased bone lucency due to bone destruction). Prostate cancer classically results in sclerotic metastases although lytic disease may occur, whereas myeloma causes marked lysis of the bone. Breast and lung cancer often give a mixed picture of sclerotic and lytic metastases. Renal cancer metastases are often large and vascular.

An isotope bone scan is more sensitive than a plain radiograph for the investigation of bone metastases and can be considered where suspicion remains despite an unremarkable plain radiograph. In cases of difficulty, or if surgery is contemplated, an MRI scan of the affected area may be helpful.

Pathological Fracture

Approximately 20–50% of patients with bone metastases will experience a pathological fracture [21]. These are usually associated with lytic bone metastases, particularly in weight-bearing bones, including both spinal and long bones. Sudden loss of function or mobility, especially with a sudden increase in pain, makes a pathological fracture likely. Spinal cord compression should also be considered and urgent specialist referral for investigation is indicated (see MSCC section).

Management

The management of bone metastases depends upon the symptoms arising, disease trajectory, patient condition and wishes, and, importantly, the presence/risk of pathological fracture.

The Mirel's score is a well-established scoring system to estimate the probability of a given metastatic lesion resulting in fracture [22] (Table 4). A score of eight or more indicates a high risk of fracture and orthopaedic review should be sought to consider prophylactic fixation with weight-bearing minimized through the affected region until definitive treatment is complete. Good results are anticipated in all but the frailest patient. Where surgical stabilisation is not possible the risks and benefits of weight-bearing should be discussed with the patient.

Treatment of Uncomplicated Bone Metastases

General Measures

The initial priority is analgesia. While nonsteroidal anti-inflammatory drugs (NSAIDs) are routinely used in practice, the evidence supporting their role was found to be weak in a systematic review of the available literature [23]. Steroids, for example dexamethasone 4–6 mg daily, can be helpful as a short-term adjunct to other analgesics but, if not helpful after a week's trial, should be discontinued. If NSAIDs or steroids are continued, gastric protection should be prescribed. The mainstay of managing severe pain from bony metastases is, however, strong

Table 4   Mirels' score for impending pathological fracture [22].

	Score		
	1	2	3
Site	Upper limb	Lower limb	Peritrochanteric
Pain	Mild	Moderate	Functional
Lesion	Blastic	Mixed	Lytic
Size	<1/3	1/3–2/3	>2/3

opioids [20]. Pre-emptive analgesia is helpful for incident pain (pain on movement). Pain may also be reduced by resting the affected area. Consultation with physiotherapists and occupational therapists may be helpful, particularly if aids and adaptations are required.

Radiotherapy

For uncomplicated, painful bony metastases requiring strong opioids, local radiotherapy is the treatment of choice [24]. In bone metastases, approximately 60% of patients will experience pain relief with a complete response in 24%, a median of 2-4 weeks after a single dose of radiotherapy [25]. Palliative radiotherapy given in this way can be repeated if the pain recurs with a good chance of a second response and little added toxicity [26].

A flare of pain is experienced by approximately one third of patients during the first week following radiotherapy. This can be reduced from one in three to one in four patients by dexamethasone, 8 mg OD, taken at least one hour prior to radiotherapy and for the following four days [27]. Concurrent gastric protection should be considered.

"Hemibody radiotherapy" in which a single dose is delivered either to the upper or to the lower half of the skeleton [28] is rarely used in current practice due to the availability of systemic therapy options.

Systemic Anticancer Treatments

Systemic anti-cancer treatments, including hormones for breast and prostate cancer, chemotherapy, targeted agents, and immunotherapy may be beneficial in appropriately selected patients.

Bone-targeted Agents

Bone-targeted agents such as bisphosphonates and denosumab inhibit bone resorption and have been shown to reduce skeletal-related events (SREs) across a range of cancer diagnoses [29]. SREs include pathologic long bone fracture, spinal cord compression, radiotherapy for pain relief, requirement for surgery and episodes of malignancy associated hypercalcaemia. Bisphosphonates can be delivered intravenously or orally and although oral preparations improve the convenience of treatment they are less well-tolerated. Denosumab is delivered subcutaneously under specialist guidance. In both cases specific side-effects include flu-like symptoms, hypocalcaemia (the risk of which is reduced by checking for and correcting vitamin D deficiency prior to commencement) and osteonecrosis of the jaw (a rare but painful event, minimized by undertaking dental checks and completing preventative dentistry prior to commencement).

Bisphosphonates can also be used to manage malignant bone pain for patients with myeloma, breast, lung, and prostate cancer [30]. This approach is particularly valuable for patients with multi-focal bone pain and those with relapse beyond radiotherapy. In this situation they are usually delivered as an intravenous (IV) infusion. In bone metastases from prostate cancer, a single trial has demonstrated the non-inferiority of intravenous ibandronate to a single fraction of palliative radiotherapy [31].

Percutaneous Ablation

Where conventional treatments are unsuccessful, radiofrequency ablation (RFA) or cryotherapy can be used to destroy bone metastases, with or without the subsequent injection of cement into the bone to consolidate bone structure. This is particularly useful for lytic lesions of the pelvis that are not amenable to prophylactic surgical fixation. These techniques require operator expertise, are not available in all centres and are supported by very limited randomized data.

Outcome

For bony metastases not complicated by nerve compression, fracture, or hypercalcaemia, treatment outcomes are relatively good. Many patients will be able to reduce their analgesic requirement and/or improve their mobility following treatment. Prognosis is strongly influenced by primary diagnosis, performance status, and the presence of visceral metastases.

Follow-up

Patients with bony metastases often have several sites of pain and more will usually reveal themselves with time. Close follow-up is therefore required in the community to ensure adequate analgesia and appropriate, prompt referral back to specialist services when needed. Social services, occupational and physiotherapy services may also be needed to allow patients with reduced mobility to return safely and comfortably to their own homes.

Treatment of Impending or Completed Pathological Fracture

Surgical Fixation

An established pathological fracture in a weight-bearing long bone is treated surgically in all but the frailest patient. Those of the upper limb may be fixed surgically but in unfit patients immobilisation will usually provide improved pain control and radiotherapy can be considered. The decision to pursue surgery in those near the end-of-life requires careful multi-disciplinary consideration of the risks and benefits of intervention and discussion with the patient. Functional outcome after surgical fixation of an impending pathological fracture is usually excellent although overall outcome will depend on the patient's general state of health and performance status.

Vertebroplasty

For spinal lesions, vertebroplasty is frequently used in the treatment of osteoporotic vertebral fractures and can be considered for the treatment of painful spinal metastases not responsive to conservative approaches [32, 33]. A vertebra that contains a painful metastasis is injected with bone cement under sedation and radiological screening. If there is loss of bony height, there is also an option to restore some of the lost height by the use of a balloon, termed a kyphoplasty [34]. A randomized study demonstrates this approach offers superior pain control to non-surgical treatment [35].

Radiotherapy

Following surgery for either an impending or established fracture, postoperative radiotherapy is usually offered 4–6 weeks after the surgery to allow for soft-tissue healing. This aims to prevent local progression and reduce the need for further surgical intervention although the evidence supporting this is extremely limited [36]. The role of post-operative radiotherapy should be considered in the context of expected prognosis; local progression and implant failure take time to occur. A pathological fracture can be managed with radiotherapy alone, although reduction in functional pain is very uncertain and significant risk of fracture non-union exists.

Rehabilitation and Discharge Planning

The chances of a patient rehabilitating successfully will depend on many factors, particularly their general health and performance status. Other painful bony metastases may slow progress, especially if they occur in a limb that is required to take more weight following surgery. As for spinal cord compression, discharge planning may require the coordinated action of several teams.

Brain Metastases

Metastases to the brain affect 5–20% of patients with cancer [37, 38]. They are common in lung cancer (affecting approximately 20% of patients), with markedly lower rates in other diagnoses; renal cancer (6–10%), melanoma (7%), breast cancer (5%) and colorectal carcinoma (<2%). In most patients, the diagnosis of cerebral metastases carries a poor prognosis.

Diagnosis and Early Suspicion

Brain metastases frequently present with headaches, although approximately 18% present with seizures [39, 40]. Brain metastases should be considered in all those known to have cancer presenting with any of the symptoms listed in Table 5. Initial investigation is usually with neurological examination and CT scan.

Management

In many patients, the presence of cerebral metastases is a component of widely disseminated disease. The focus of management for this group is symptomatic care and consideration of psychosocial needs. For a selected group of patients with a better prognosis, anti-cancer treatments may be appropriate.

General Symptomatic Measures

Cerebral Oedema and Raised Intracranial Pressure

Acute treatment with steroids is guided by symptom severity and associated oedema on imaging. An initial dose of 8 mg dexamethasone is reasonable and should be given parenterally only when absorption is uncertain (e.g. in the presence of vomiting). Concurrent gastric protection is required. This should be followed by regular dexamethasone (up to 16 mg daily in one or two doses, the later dose given before 2 p.m. to avoid night-time wakefulness (though this should not preclude emergency administration of the first day's dose)). The steroid dose can be swiftly decreased, over days to weeks, to the minimum dose necessary to manage symptoms. IV mannitol is rarely needed to reduce intracranial pressure in patients whose condition is worsening rapidly.

Table 5   Common symptoms and signs of brain metastases.

Common Symptoms and Signs of Brain Metastases	%
Headache	49
Nausea/vomiting	30
Focal weakness/hemiparesis	32
Confusion	21
Unsteadiness	18
Seizures	12
Dysphasia	6
Visual disturbance	6

Source Tsao *et al.* [40].

Headache

Headache usually responds to steroids. Regular paracetamol with the addition of a weak or strong opioid (with concurrent laxatives) may be required.

Seizures

Once intracranial pressure is reduced, seizures may subside, however some patients require regular anticonvulsant medication (e.g. levetiracetam). Advice can be sought from the patient's oncology team or local neurology services. For terminally ill patients with cerebral metastases and uncontrolled fitting parenteral benzodiazepines may be required, for example, midazolam by continuous subcutaneous infusion (CSCI) (see Chapter 20: Care in the Last Days of Life and after Death). This can cause drowsiness, and levetiracetam via CSCI is an option where avoidance of sedation is preferred.

For patients whose seizures have previously been well controlled, consideration should be given to the role of concurrent medications which can lower the seizure threshold. Prophylactic use of anti-epileptic medications (before seizures have occurred) has not been shown to reduce seizure incidence [41].

Nausea and Vomiting

This usually responds to measures which reduce intracranial pressure, but anti-emetics, such as cyclizine, may be required and may need to be given parenterally at first.

Confusion, Agitation, or Psychosis

The introduction of steroids may reverse acute problems but occasionally sedation may be required until the steroids take effect or as part of the management of terminal agitation.

Specific Anti-cancer Treatment Options

Limited Brain Metastases

Surgical resection or stereotactic radiosurgery (SRS) are both used widely for the treatment of patients with a limited volume and small number of brain metastases, diagnosis of which requires MRI confirmation. Patients also need to have controlled/controllable extra-cranial disease and a good performance status and prognosis. Decision-making is guided by the local neuro-oncology multi-disciplinary team.

SRS uses finely focused beams of radiation, very restrictive immobilisation, and image guidance to precisely treat metastases and limit toxicity. This is available in the United Kingdom in several larger radiotherapy centres. Limited data are available to inform the comparison between surgery and SRS. The choice depends on local expertise, fitness for surgery, the size and site of the metastasis, and patient choice [42]. Surgery may be considered more appropriate where there is no known primary cancer, when the metastasis is too large for SRS, and when raised intracranial pressure causes severe symptoms, especially with hydrocephalus due to posterior fossa lesions.

The addition of whole brain radiotherapy to either of these local treatments reduces the risk of relapse in the brain but does not impact on overall survival and is associated with more side-effects [40, 43].

Extensive Brain Metastases

Whole Brain Radiotherapy (WBRT)

WBRT has previously been a common treatment for brain metastases. With the increasing availability of SRS, WBRT use has declined dramatically to only those who would be eligible for SRS but whose cerebral disease is too extensive. It is usually delivered over 1 to 2 weeks. Steroids are continued throughout and reduced once treatment is complete as determined by symptoms. Cessation is not possible for many patients.

Recent studies using patient-rated scales suggest that symptomatic benefit following WBRT is the exception (approximately 20% at 1 month), with benefit often outweighed by side-effects (Table 6) [44, 45]. Indeed, the practice-changing QUARTZ randomised trial in non-small cell lung cancer demonstrated radiotherapy offered no benefit over steroids alone, in terms of survival, quality of life or steroid sparing effect [46]. For patients with a poor performance status and poor prognosis, treatment with steroids, concentrating on end-of-life care, symptom control, and supportive measures may be the best option.

Table 6   Side effects of whole brain radiotherapy.

Acute	Late (>6 Months after Completion of Treatment)
Temporary alopecia	Difficulties with memory and concentration
Headache	Deterioration on neurocognitive testing
Nausea	Persistent alopecia
Redness and soreness of the skin	
Tiredness and sleepiness	

Chemotherapy

Systemic chemotherapy is useful for some chemo-sensitive tumours, such as small-cell lung cancer, germ cell tumours and cerebral lymphoma. It may also be valuable in patients with breast cancer. This is often part of multi-modality care (including radiotherapy) and the benefits and side-effects of its addition need careful consideration in the context of the patient's expected prognosis and other disease.

Rehabilitation and Discharge Planning

Many patients with brain metastases have a dramatic change in their functional ability, independence and, sometimes, personality. Their rehabilitation needs are similar to those outlined for patients with MSCC. In addition, some patients may need speech and language therapy. Where swallowing is compromised, route of nutrition should be considered and discussed with the patient with input from dietetics team. For many patients, remaining at home may be challenging due to loss of independence, cognitive decline, and need for nursing care. Changes in cognitive function can make the safe delivery of care at home problematic while often causing distress for relatives. There is a need for psychological support for both the patient and their carers.

Outcome

The survival of patients with cerebral metastases is usually limited. Performance status is the strongest predictor of survival although patients with non-small-cell lung cancer have a particularly poor prognosis with a median survival of 2–3 months. Table 7 summarises the factors influencing survival [47].

Follow-up

Symptomatic progression of brain metastases is common and is often accompanied by progressive extra-cranial disease. Close follow-up should be arranged in the community where care is usually centred for those without further anti-cancer treatment options.

Hypercalcaemia of Malignancy (HCM)

HCM is a usually reversible, potentially life threatening condition with a significant symptom burden. Around 20% of patients with cancer develop hypercalcaemia [48], making it a differential diagnosis for patients presenting with symptoms of unknown origin. A mean survival of 2–3 months identifies HCM as a condition of advanced disease [49].

HCM is most associated with: myeloma, breast, lung, renal, and bladder cancers and squamous cell carcinomas (SCC) – including head and neck, and cervix cancers. "Red flags" for HCM are a diagnosis of SCC and the presence of bone metastases (particularly in breast cancer and myeloma) [49, 50]. Alternative causes of hypercalcemia should be considered, including endocrine and pharmaceutical causes.

Hypercalcaemia is defined as a raised level of corrected calcium [51]. As calcium binds to albumin, frail, cachexic patients with low albumin level will present with artificially low calcium levels, hence the use of corrected calcium levels. Severity of hypercalcaemia is defined in Table 8 [51].

HCM is life threatening if untreated and, for a proportion of presenting patients, this will be a "terminal event." In this situation, patients presenting with "refractory HCM" (recurrent episodes of increasing frequency on a background of extensive disease) may choose to remain at home rather than seek hospital admission and treatment. Open, honest discussions with patients and families about the clinical picture, prognosis, treatment burden, and wishes about place of care and death will guide shared decision-making. Patients unable

Table 7   Factors affecting survival in patients with brain metastases.

Factors that Improve Survival	Factors that Reduce Survival
Solitary metastasis	Poor performance status
Long disease-free interval before relapse	Uncontrolled extra-cranial disease
Primary site breast	Meningeal disease
Younger age	

Table 8   Severity of hypercalcaemia.

	Corrected Serum Concentration
Mild Hypercalcaemia	2.60 – 3.00 mmol/l
Moderate Hypercalcaemia	3.01 – 3.40 mmol/l
Severe Hypercalcaemia	Greater than 3.40 mmol/l

to make their wishes known because of a loss of capacity may have an Advance Care Plan that can guide decision making alongside discussion with family or significant others.

Symptoms and Clinical Diagnosis

Clinical manifestations of hypercalcaemia are detailed in Box 1. Symptoms may be subtle and slow to manifest or present acutely with a rapid physical and cognitive decline related to rising calcium levels. The more quickly levels have risen the greater the severity of symptoms [52].

Box 1: Clinical Manifestations of Hypercalcaemia	
Clinical Manifestations	
Neurological	Fatigue and drowsiness; cognitive changes ranging from poor concentration, forgetfulness, mood changes to delirium, stupor and coma
Gastrointestinal	Nausea, vomiting, anorexia, constipation, and with more insidious onset, gastric ulcers, and pancreatitis
Renal	Polyuria (excessive diuresis), polydipsia (thirst), dehydration, renal function impairment. Less commonly in HCM – nephrolithiasis (stone formation)
Cardiac	Arrythmias, shortened QT, Prolonged PR, wide T, bradycardia and potentially, cardiac arrest
Other	Bone pain, hypotension, dry mouth, itch

Management of Associated Symptoms

Until normocalcaemia is established it may be necessary to palliate associated symptoms. Anti-emetics and laxatives administered via an appropriate route may be required. Local management guidelines for delirium should be followed with support from the palliative care team or psychiatry colleagues as necessary. Monitoring fluid balance, serial blood tests, and ECGs can add to the clinical picture.

Treatment

First line treatment is rehydration with intravenous normal saline (rate dictated by clinical condition and comorbidities). Nephrotoxic medications (e.g. NSAIDs) and drugs that inhibit urinary calcium secretion, for example, thiazide diuretics should be discontinued.

Intravenous bisphosphonates (e.g. zoledronic acid, pamidronate, and ibandronate) are the mainstay of treatment as they inhibit the action of osteoclasts and reduce bone resorption and calcium release. Side-effects are discussed earlier in the section on Bone Metastases and locally agreed guidelines on dosing and treatment regimens should be consulted with dose modifications for patients with renal impairment. Denosumab (a human monoclonal antibody that inactivates RANK-L) and cinacalcet are available but not widely used for management of HCM [53, 54].

An episode of hypercalcaemia may precipitate a change in anti-cancer treatment, reducing the risk of subsequent recurrence.

Follow Up

A robust management plan incorporating regular monitoring of calcium levels and early identification of symptoms should be agreed [51]. This may be coordinated by the GP, community palliative care team, or oncology team. Advance Care Plans should be regularly reviewed in the context of the individual's clinical situation. While for many, regular bisphosphonate treatment is appropriate, for some the increasing burden of hospital admission or regular out-patient visits in the face of increasing frailty and symptom burden from advanced cancer becomes unacceptable, and a plan for end-of-life care will be made.

Urinary Tract Obstruction

Obstruction of either the upper or lower urinary tract can occur. The level of obstruction dictates management. Severe obstruction can result in obstructive nephropathy (ON) with subsequent deterioration in renal function leading to acute kidney injury (AKI) and, potentially, death if both kidneys are affected [55].

Lower urinary tract obstruction is precipitated by bladder outflow obstruction, detrusor muscle dysfunction or urethral obstruction (Table 9) [55, 56]. Symptoms include urinary retention, supra-pubic, or abdominal pain.

Upper urinary tract obstruction involves obstruction of the renal collecting system, usually at the level of the

Table 9   Causes of Lower Urinary Tract Obstruction [55, 56].

Bladder outlet obstruction	Tumour mass – pelvic, abdominal, or retroperitoneal mass/es; lymphadenopathy
	Calculi
	Blood clot – "clot retention"
	Benign Prostatic Hypertrophy
	Prostate Cancer
	Constipation
	Drug induced (commonly caused by drugs with anti-cholinergic activity)
	Indwelling or supra-pubic catheter blockage
Bladder dysfunction	Neurogenic bladder dysfunction
	Detrusor muscle dysfunction
	Drug induced dysfunction – opioids; calcium channel antagonists; "anticholinergics" and others
Urethral obstruction	Obstructing tumour or lesions
	Fibrosis (secondary to radiotherapy)
	Urethral stricture
	Paraphimosis

ureter (see Table 10). Symptoms include abdominal or flank pain, nausea, and vomiting.

Investigations

Initial management is guided by the severity of obstruction, degree of urinary retention, and renal impairment. Assessment may include urinalysis, abdominal examination, neurological assessment, medication review, serial blood tests – particularly urea and electrolytes to gauge the degree, and progression of renal impairment. A urinary tract Ultra Sound Scan (USS) will confirm urinary retention, megaureter, and hydronephrosis. Abdominal/pelvic CT can identify underlying causes of obstruction. Malignant Spinal Cord Compression should be considered as a cause of urinary retention.

Table 10   Causes of Upper Urinary Tract Obstruction.

Intraluminal sources	Obstructing tumour or lesions
	Calculi
	Ureteric stricture
	Blood clot
Extraluminal source	Tumour mass- pelvic, abdominal, or retroperitoneal mass/es; lymphadenopathy
	Fibrosis

Management

The primary aim of any intervention is to relieve the obstruction [55]. Prompt discussion with urology colleagues is advised as management options, including surgery, stenting, or bladder irrigation, may be considered before anti-cancer treatments. Where renal function deterioration is life threatening, discussion with renal physicians should be considered to assess the role of temporary renal replacement therapy.

Early management of lower urinary tract obstruction can include urethral or supra-pubic catheterization, which also ensures accurate fluid balance measurement, particularly important in the management of AKI.

The two commonest management options for upper tract ON are placement of percutaneous nephrostomy or insertion of internal ureteric stents [55, 57]. Percutaneous nephrostomy placement is radiologically guided: a tube is placed through the skin into the kidney. Urine then drains into a bag placed on the skin. Sedation is required and patients may experience discomfort and pain during and after the procedure.

Insertion of ureteric stents requires general anaesthesia but avoids the requirement for external drains. Post-procedure discomfort is possible.

There is little consensus on which approach is best. Both bring risks of bleeding, infection/sepsis, tube, or stent blockage and pain. Tube/stent replacement every 3–4 months is required to reduce complications and necessitates hospital attendance.

Decision-Making and Outcomes

For patients with extensive or rapidly progressive disease and no anti-cancer treatment options, it is essential to discuss the implications of interventions. Evidence of the benefits of an interventional approach for patients with advanced cancer and metastases is mixed. Some studies demonstrate no significant difference in outcomes between observation and intervention; others demonstrate poor survival outcomes alongside complications affecting quality of life if the interventional approach is adopted [57, 58].

In the palliative phase, quality of life concerns must be balanced against the inherent risks of invasive interventions. Reversing an AKI/ON may prolong life in the short term, however, the patient may continue to deteriorate from widespread cancer, or develop further distressing symptoms. A purely palliative approach to symptom management and emotional/spiritual support may be more appropriate.

Follow Up

An interventional approach requires patients to be followed up by urologists alongside their oncologist. Community nursing and palliative care support may be required, particularly for those electing for a conservative management approach.

For information on the management of renal impairment please see Chapter 18: Palliative Care in Advanced Renal Disease.

Haemorrhage

Patients with cancer may develop bleeding for several reasons:

- bleeding directly from a tumour or metastasis, including malignant wounds (see the following section)
- invasion of tumour into blood vessels
- bleeding tendency due to thrombocytopenia, disseminated intravascular coagulopathy (DIC), uraemia, or anticoagulants
- post radiotherapy telangiectasia (especially bladder and GI tract)
- non-cancer causes, for example gastric ulceration due to steroids or NSAIDs.

Where tumour invades a major vessel, a risk of life-threatening "catastrophic" bleeding exists. Given the anxiety associated with bleeding, this risk should be identified and discussed calmly and sensitively with the patient and those important to them. Patients should be prepared that a small bleed may herald a subsequent larger event. Dark coloured towels should be available and anticipatory prescribing completed (acknowledging that, during the event, this may not be used and staying with the patient may be best) [59]. Management can be detailed in a bleeding crisis plan. After such an event occurs all involved may require an opportunity to de-brief.

The management of massive, terminal haemorrhage is discussed separately in Chapter 20: Care in the Last Days of Life and after Death.

Initial Assessment and Management

Initial assessment includes identification of bleeding source and systemic impact by review of observations, Full Blood Count (FBC), and clotting. Acute intervention decisions are taken in the context of the patient's prognosis and advance care plan. Intravenous fluid, blood and platelet transfusions maybe necessary.

Early medication review is required to identify the prescription of drugs that increase risk of bleeding such as NSAIDS, SSRIs, corticosteroids, and anticoagulant therapy. A risk versus benefit approach to their use may be required, necessitating discussion with the patient about their choices. For example, balancing the risk of further bleeding against that of thromboembolic events. Patients with gastric bleeding should be commenced on a proton pump inhibitor if this is not already in place.

Where bleeding is persistent and accessible, packing may aid haemostasis in the short-term. In the case of epistaxis this is best carried out by an ENT surgeon. Similarly, packing to reduce bleeding due to locally advanced cervical cancer should be carried out by a gynaecologist or appropriately trained clinical oncologist. Topical therapies are detailed in Table 11.

Drugs that reduce bleeding tendency may be helpful, for example, tranexamic acid. Given as a dose of 500 mg-1 g three times daily (orally or intravenously), this reduces bleeding due to cancer without increasing the risk of venous-thrombosis [60]. It should be continued for one week after cessation of bleeding but can be re-trialled subsequently if necessary. The risk of clot retention where tranexamic acid is used for the treatment of haematuria requires careful monitoring. DIC is a contraindication to use of tranexamic acid.

Subsequent management is determined following discussion with the patient, recognising their preference for further intervention, expected prognosis, prior treatments, and extent of persistent bleeding.

Radiotherapy

Palliative radiotherapy is used to control bleeding from both primary and metastatic cancers. Reduction in bleeding is reported in 80–100% of patients depending upon diagnosis [61–65]. Treatment is usually restricted to a short course; typically 1–5 days. Previous radiotherapy to the area does not necessarily preclude further treatment – this is an oncological decision.

Endoscopic Procedures

Endoscopic procedures, including bronchoscopy, oesophago-gastroscopy, cystoscopy, and colonoscopy offer visualisation and treatment of a range of bleeding sites. Improvement is frequently observed but rebleeding remains a problem [65]. These invasive procedures require careful consideration and discussion with the patient in the context of prognosis.

Vascular Embolisation

Occasionally, bleeding from a vascular tumour can be reduced by embolisation of its blood supply. The type of bleeding and vasculature of the tumour and surrounding normal tissues are critical to the decision to proceed. Patients must be able to lie flat throughout the procedure.

An interventional radiologist can advise on the suitability of the procedure, including further investigations to define this. Post-procedure rebleeding can occur early (due to incomplete embolization) and late (due to re-vascularisation). Tumour necrosis may occur, leading to pain and flu-like symptoms [65].

Symptomatic Measures

Where initial management, radiotherapy, endoscopy, and embolization are unsuccessful bleeding from a range of sites can be managed as detailed in Table 11 in the malignant wounds section.

Malignant Wounds

Primarily arising from skin neoplasms, malignant wounds are also caused by localised or metastatic infiltration of tissue and vasculature from other primary cancer sites [66]. Prevalence may be up to 14.5% in patients with advanced cancer, with malignant wounds most seen in patients with breast, head and neck, and primary skin cancers [67]. Classification of the wound dictates management.

Distinct from pressure sores or ulcers, malignant wounds may be classified as:

- Sub-cutaneous nodules (including metastatic deposits, primary tumours, and sub/cutaneous lymphoma)
- Malignant ulcers (Marjolin's ulcers)

Table 11 Management of symptoms related to malignant wounds [72–74, 77].

Symptom	Management
Bleeding (including from sub-cutaneous, rectal, bladder, gynaecological, or oral cancers)	Topical dressings soaked in adrenaline (epinephrine) 1/1000 – short term use for superficial wounds
	Haemostatic alginate dressings (with caution)
	Intravesical (bladder instillation) of tranexamic acid
	Topical administration of tranexamic acid or sucralfate as soaks, pastes/gels, mouthwash
	Wound dressings / packs (+/- haemostatic medication as above)
	Silver nitrate sticks to cauterise bleeding points
	Radiotherapy
Wound pain	Regular analgesia
	Appropriate non-adherent dressings
	Morphine 0.1%: Mix 1 mL of Morphine Sulfate 10mg/mL with 8g of Intrasite gel

(Continued)

Table 11 *(Continued)*

Symptom	Management
Pain associated with dressing changes	Pre-emptive "short acting" opioids Non-adherent dressings Entonox (caution required in longer term use)
Exudate	Appropriate dressings (seek advice from tissue viability team) Exemplary skin hygiene to prevent surrounding skin breakdown Use of barrier products
Malodour	Activated charcoal dressings Silver dressings (caution if undergoing radiotherapy treatment) Systemic metronidazole 400 mg PO TDS initially, reducing to 200 mg OD Topical metronidazole – 0.75% gel or 200 mg tablet crushed in water soluble gel – changed 1–2 times daily Environmental management strategies – de-odourisers, essential oils etc. Psychological support

- Eroding Malignant Wounds
- Fungating Malignant Wounds

Other presentations such as pressure damage and non-cancer wounds are not discussed. See Chapter 20 (Care in the Last Days of Life and after Death).

Anorexia-cachexia, immune-suppression, and other medical comorbidities can contribute to accelerating wound breakdown. Optimising nutrition and managing other conditions such as diabetes may help maintain skin integrity but not progression of the disease process. Early discussion with the treating oncologist and plastic surgeons will ensure management options such as radiotherapy, systemic treatments, or surgical debridement are considered.

Eroding Malignant Wounds

As eroding wounds develop and ulcerate, superficial capillaries or large blood vessels may be exposed. Superficial eroding wounds in highly vascular areas such as the scalp may bleed freely. The management of eroding malignant wounds aligns with that of bleeding from other malignant sources, as detailed earlier and in Table 11.

Malignant Fungating Wounds

Malignant fungating wounds develop secondary to tissue hypoxia, the associated tissue necrosis, and subsequent skin breakdown. Colonisation by anaerobic and aerobic bacteria leads to the characteristic malodour and exudate associated with a fungating wound.

Often thought of as "unhealable," these wounds present a significant physical and emotional burden for patients and their families (See Box 2) [68]. Psychological distress, depression, embarrassment, reduced self-esteem, reduced mobility, and social isolation are all issues associated with malignant fungating wounds [69, 70].

The priority of care for most patients presenting with a malignant wound is management of associated symptoms and distress with the aim of improvement of quality of life. The psychological burden of living with a malodorous, exuding wound and complexity of wound care demands a holistic approach and individualised management plan.

Box 2: Symptoms associated with malignant wounds [67, 68, 69, 70]

Pain (nociceptive and neuropathic)

Malodour – caused by release of volatile agents from action of aerobic and anaerobic bacteria

Exudate (sometimes excessive)

Bleeding

Itch

Perceived wound status (impact on body image)

Perceived bulk effect of dressings or underlying masses

Impact on functional status

Psychological impact

Management of Symptoms Associated with Malignant Wounds

Advice from a local tissue viability nurse (TVN) team is advised as wounds may require frequent dressing changes or dressings unfamiliar to generalist teams in order to reduce symptom burden by containing odour and exudate. Gentle wound cleansing with warmed saline may be more tolerable for patients. Oropharyngeal wounds may require mouth-washes to help manage infection or bleeding. Warming saline mouthwashes/gargles may make these more tolerable. A limited evidence base for malignant wound management means that any suggestions are based on small-scale studies, anecdotal evidence or case studies. Table 11 summarises treatment options for symptoms related to malignant wounds. Novel treatments such as electro-chemotherapy may reduce symptom burden and can be considered [71].

Itch

Itch (pruritis) is "an unpleasant sensation that triggers the need for a mechanical response such as scratching, rubbing or pressure" [75]. Itch negatively impacts on quality of life, affecting function, mood, and sleep [76]. The reflexive response of scratching may cause excoriation, pain, or secondary infection. Patients with advanced cancer experience a significant symptom and emotional burden and the additional impact of itch on quality of life cannot be underestimated.

Conditions associated with itch are detailed in Box 3.

Box 3: Conditions associated with itch

- Cholestasis (Cholestatic pruritis)
- Uraemia (Uraemic pruritis)
- Haematological – including leukaemia, lymphoma, poycythaemia rubra vera
- Thyroid function disorders
- Skin infections/infestations
- Skin conditions – dermatitis/eczema/psoriasis
- Allergies – urticaria/rashes
- Iron deficiency anaemia
- Cancer (paraneoplastic presentation or skin metastases)
- Multiple sclerosis
- AIDS
- Psychogenic causes e.g. psychosis (acknowledged but not explored in this chapter)

Management

Understanding the cause of an individual's itch guides management. Relief is best achieved by removal of stimuli/exacerbating factors and interruption of the neural pathway through medication. Clinical examination and blood tests add to the clinical picture, for example, full blood count, liver, and renal function tests.

Reversible and underlying causes should be explored:

- obstructive cholestasis may be managed by stenting or use of steroids to reduce localised obstruction secondary to tumour bulk
- medication review may identify drugs with the side effect of itch, for example, ACE inhibitors or morphine, which can be deprescribed or switched to an alternative
- skin infections or infestations can be treated
- systemic anti-cancer treatment can be considered for paraneoplastic itch
- radiotherapy may help for some presentations of metastatic infiltration of the skin.

Early discussion with colleagues is advisable to identify possible interventions in a timely manner.

Non-pharmacological and pharmacological interventions to manage itch, according to its cause, are detailed in Box 4 and Table 12. Management must take account of medication or treatment burden in the context of prognosis and the patients' quality of life priorities. As patients at the very end-of-life become too weak to manage oral medication, management shifts from direct management of the itch towards management of the distress or agitation caused by itch.

Fever

Fever is an elevation of core body temperature above normal (generally accepted as above 38°C) and is often the hallmark of immune system activation. Temperature regulation is directed by the hypothalamus in response to

---

Box 4: Non-drug measures to manage itch

- Regular use of emollients
- Use of topical preparations: menthol and aqueous cream, capsaicin cream
- Light loose clothing
- Avoid spicy foods and alcohol
- Reduce sweating

Table 12   Drug Treatment of itch changes to table content as below:

Aetiology	Drug and dose Ranked by Quality of evidence (77–79)	Mechanism
Uraemic pruritis in advanced chronic kidney disease	See Chapter 18: Palliative Care in Advanced Renal Disease	
Cholestatic pruritis (irreversible)	**Rifampacin** 150–600 mg OD	Unclear – possible effect on bile acid detoxification
	Naltrexone 50 mg OD	Opioid preceptor pathway (Risk of precipitating pain because of loss of analgesia)
Non-specific itch in palliative care patients	**Paroxetine** 5–20 mg OD	Selective serotonin reuptake inhibition
	Chlorpheniramine 4 mg – 12 mg TDS	Anti-histamine
	Cetrizine 10 mg OD	

a complex feedback system mediated by neurotransmitters such as cytokines and prostaglandins. The causes of fever in patients with advanced cancer are presented in Box 5.

Box 5: Causes of fever in patients with cancer [80, 81]

- Infection, particularly in neutropenic patients and patients with in-dwelling catheters: central venous lines, urethral, or percutaneous catheters
- Blood Transfusion
- Radiation Pneumonitis
- Thrombosis
- Chemotherapeutic agents including bleomycin, cisplatin, interferons
- Immunotherapy/targeted treatments including dabrafinib, rituximab, nivolumab
- CNS metastases
- Paraneoplastic fever – can be associated with lymphoma (Hodgkins and non-Hodgkins); renal cell carcinoma; bone sarcoma; adrenal cancer; neuro-endocrine tumours; solid tumours with liver metastases
- Rarely – Sweet syndrome, adult Still's disease

Management

Unless a decision has been made not to pursue further intervention, a temperature of 38°C or more, in a patient on systemic anti-cancer therapy must prompt urgent review and discussion with the treating oncology team (see management of treatment side-effects section below).

For other patients receiving palliative care, it is appropriate to discuss investigation and treatment of any reversible causes of fever, such as infection, if this aligns with their wishes and does not limit other choices regarding preferred place of care or death. For example, treating infection with IV antibiotics in the last days of life may be appropriate to reduce symptom burden, but if this requires patients to remain in hospital, continued treatment may limit their choices about their preferred place of death.

A comprehensive clinical history and investigations such as full blood count, urea and electrolytes, and septic screen will aid identification of the cause of fever and subsequent management. Alongside appropriate treatment of the underlying cause (see Table 13), antipyretic medication such as paracetamol and NSAIDs should be given; limited evidence suggests Naproxen over other NSAIDs [80]. Paraneoplastic fever is often a diagnosis of exclusion, precipitating management of symptoms to ensure patient comfort.

Table 13 Treatment of reversible causes of fever in cancer patients [80].

Cause	Treatment
Infection	Antibiotic Therapy
Radiation pneumonitis	Corticosteroids and appropriate gastric protection
Thrombosis	Anti-coagulation
Chemotherapeutic agents	Anti-pyretics and discussion with treating oncologist
Immunotherapy/targeted treatments	Anti-pyretics and discussion with treating oncologist
CNS metastases	Anti-pyretics and discussion with treating oncologist
Paraneoplastic fever (including lymphoma)	Anti-pyretic agents. Corticosteroids and appropriate gastric protection
Sweet Syndrome, Adult Still's disease	Consult Rheumatologist

Sweating

Sweating is a normal response to regulate core body temperature and prevent hyperthermia. It may be associated with fever. Patients with advanced cancer identify sweating as a symptom that causes discomfort, insomnia, and affects body image [81]. Causes of excess sweating (hyperhidrosis) are identified in Box 6.

Management

Once infection associated fever is excluded, other causes and management options may be considered. A comprehensive drug history may identify medication as a cause; if opioids are identified, a dose reduction or opioid switch may be required. Hormone therapy is contra-indicated in patients with breast and endometrial cancer experiencing hot flashes; early discussion with the treating oncologist is advised. Evidence-based alternative options include SSRIs, venlafaxine, and gabapentin for

hot flashes [77, 82]. A trial of corticosteroids may reduce sweats associated with lymphoma.

Maintaining comfort is essential. Consider light bed clothing and clothes, damp cloths to forehead and wrists, adequate hydration, and rigorous skin care.

Side-effects of Palliative Oncology Treatments

The side effects of oncological interventions weigh heavily in the cost–benefit analysis of anti-cancer treatments. It is important for patients, health-care teams, and carers to know what effects are expected and how these can be alleviated.

While radiotherapy side-effects are localised to the treated area, the side-effects of systemic therapies are generally more widespread. Symptom management is discussed below.

Immunotherapy side-effects fall into a distinct class to those resulting from chemotherapy and radiotherapy. These side-effects are predominantly immune-mediated, and their management reflects this. These are considered separately.

Radiotherapy and Chemotherapy Related Side-effects

Gastrointestinal System

Oral Mucositis

Oral mucositis can occur following chemotherapy or radiotherapy to the head and neck area. Evidence for the efficacy of many commonly used treatments for mucositis is poor. The mainstay continues to be exemplary assessment and oral hygiene measures [83]. This should include:

Box 6: Causes of abnormal/excess sweating in patients with cancer

- Induced menopause (secondary to treatment) – hot flashes
- Medical or surgical castration for prostate cancer – hot flashes
- Endocrine disorders
- Lymphoma (particularly at night)
- Drug induced sweating – opioids
- Fever

- frequent brushing of teeth/dentures with a soft toothbrush;
- moisturising lips;
- rinsing after each meal with saline;
- treatment of secondary infections, for example, candida.

Patients with mucositis require analgesia, often with strong opioids. Topical measures include Gelclair™; this forms a protective barrier and can be particularly helpful if used before attempts to eat. Mouthwashes often cause stinging, but the recently introduced mouthwash, Caphosol™ shows superiority over a standard regime in reducing the duration and severity of mucositis in patients undergoing bone marrow transplantation or head and neck radiotherapy [84].

Nausea and Vomiting

Nausea and vomiting are worsened by anxiety about cancer, the treatment, and its side-effects; hence, psychological support is vital throughout treatment. For some patients this anxiety can result in anticipatory vomiting which may benefit from an anxiolytic or benzodiazepine ahead of chemotherapy [85].

Highly Emetogenic Chemotherapy

Nausea and vomiting usually occur in the first 24–72 hours post-chemotherapy. It is managed by administering a $5-HT_3$ antagonist (e.g. ondansetron) plus dexamethasone intravenously pre-chemotherapy. This is followed by domperidone 10 mg tds or metoclopramide 10 mg tds PO TDS plus dexamethasone 4–6 mg PO daily for 3 days afterwards. Use of steroids may lead to gastritis and gastric protection can be considered if symptoms develop. Increasingly, neurokinin-1 receptor antagonists (e.g. aprepitant) are administered with highly emetogenic chemotherapy based on randomized data demonstrating superior control of chemotherapy induced emesis [85].

Less Emetogenic Chemotherapy

Where chemotherapy is less emetogenic, oral anti-emetics usually suffice, for example, cyclizine 50 mg TDS or domperidone 10 mg TDS.

Radiotherapy

Nausea and vomiting can occur within hours of radiotherapy, especially if the stomach, small bowel, or liver are in the treatment field. While oral anti-emetics (such as cyclizine) often suffice, $5-HT_3$ antagonists have been shown to be more effective in a single randomized study [86]. Dexamethasone is also frequently used and has the advantage of reducing pain flare following treatment for painful bone metastases [27]. Vomiting may be a side-effect of radiotherapy to the brain, in which case it will usually respond to an increase in the dose of oral steroids with the addition of cyclizine.

Diarrhoea

Diarrhoea is common with pelvic or abdominal radiotherapy. It often begins in the second week of radiotherapy and lasts 1–2 weeks after completion.
Management includes:

- dietary assessment and reduced fibre diet for the duration of the radiotherapy;
- loperamide titrated to effect +/ – codeine phosphate 30–60 mg 6 or 12 hourly (if the patient is not already receiving a strong opioid);
- attention to oral hydration;
- barrier creams to perianal skin.

If patients develop abdominal pain during radiotherapy, review by the treating oncologist should be sought before continuation.

Proctitis

Proctitis is common following pelvic radiotherapy. The timing of its occurrence is the same as for diarrhoea (see previous paragraphs). It may be associated with mucous discharge and rectal bleeding. In the acute setting steroid enemas are routinely used, although evidence supporting this is limited. Warm baths may help to alleviate symptoms. Late radiation proctitis may result in rectal bleeding more than six months after radiotherapy due to telangiectasia but has fallen in frequency with increasingly conformal radiotherapy techniques. Sigmoidoscopy is used to diagnose the cause of bleeding although biopsies and surgery should be undertaken with caution due to poor tissue healing. Management involves the use of sucralfate enemas and appropriate analgesia [87].

Skin

The skin is not usually severely affected by chemotherapy although mild rashes are common. Discoloration, erythema, and peeling of the palms and soles are sometimes seen, particularly with drugs such as capecitabine and 5-FU.

Skin reactions are common with high-dose radiotherapy, although uncommon in most palliative treatments where the total dose is generally low. Reactions develop in the second to third week of radiotherapy and start to improve two weeks after completion. Table 14 details the types of skin reactions.

Table 14   Skin reactions to radiotherapy.

Category of Skin Reaction	Detail of Signs and Symptoms
Erythema	The area in the radiotherapy field becomes slightly inflamed and may tingle, usually occurring after 1–2 weeks of treatment
Dry desquamation	The skin becomes hot, flaky, very itchy, and uncomfortable usually occurring at least 2–3 weeks into treatment
Moist desquamation	Blisters form on the epidermis that slough leaving a denuded, painful area of dermis that may exude serum. Moist regions with opposed skin surfaces, such as the perineum or inframammary fold, are particularly affected

Several steps can be taken to improve the comfort of the skin and prevent further damage:

- Protect from friction, by avoiding tight clothing, elastic straps, and underwired bras, etc.
- Avoid strong sunlight, hot baths, wet shaving, cosmetics, deodorants, adhesive plasters, and perfumed creams.
- Wash with warm water and usual soap. Pat dry with a soft towel and air-dry if possible.
- For erythema, apply moisturising cream, for example, aqueous cream twice daily.
- For dry desquamation, increase frequency of moisturising to 4–5 times daily.
- Occasionally hydrocortisone cream 1% is used, if the treated skin is particularly itchy.
- Intrasite gel® can be soothing for dry desquamation.
- For very itchy dry desquamation, a glycerine-based hydrogel sheet is very cooling.
- Moist desquamation heals best in a warm, moist environment. Conformable, non-adherent dressings are used. Intrasite gel® absorbs exudate and helps lift debris and can be used with Mepilex® dressings, which are a low adherent silicone dressing.

For patients who are undergoing or have recently completed radiotherapy and have significant skin toxicity, discussion with the treating radiotherapy centre is valuable to guide the use of appropriate dressings. Both the treating oncologist and radiotherapy department nurses or radiographers will be able to offer advice.

Hair Loss

Temporary hair loss is a variable feature of many chemotherapy regimens. Radiotherapy will also cause temporary alopecia limited to the irradiated area. The psychological impact should not be underestimated, and wigs and camouflage should be discussed before treatment.

Marrow Suppression

Patients with advanced cancer may have reduced bone marrow reserve and symptomatic anaemia is common. Thrombocytopenia is less common in the absence of chemotherapy, wide field radiotherapy, or bone seeking isotopes (particularly in prostate cancer). Anaemia and thrombocytopenia may require transfusion.

Clinically significant neutropenia is uncommon in the absence of cytotoxic chemotherapy. It predisposes to overwhelming bacterial sepsis, particularly when the absolute neutrophil count is less than $1 \times 10^9/l$. Neutropenic sepsis requires urgent specialist inpatient treatment with fluid resuscitation and IV antibiotics. Urgent admission to the treating oncology unit should be arranged for assessment of any patient having chemotherapy who develops symptoms or signs of sepsis, infection or fever > 38° C [88]. In advanced leukaemia, and rarely solid organ cancers with extensive bone metastases, neutropenic sepsis may result from bone marrow infiltration. In this situation, in discussion with the patient and those around them, a decision not to admit to hospital in the event of sepsis may be considered.

Immunotherapy Related Side-effects

Immunotherapy is increasingly used for a range of cancer diagnoses including melanoma, renal, lung, urothelial, and head and neck cancers and relapsed Hodgkin's lymphoma. It is showing promising results in an ever-increasing number of solid organ malignancies [89]. These treatments aim to enhance the body's natural immune response to target tumour cells. As a consequence, side-effects result from inflammation due to excessive immune activation; causing "itis" of the affected tissue. These side-effects can affect a wide range of tissues and are quite distinct, in terms of their presentation and management, from those of more traditional cytotoxic therapies.

Immunotherapy toxicity generally occurs in the first few months of treatment, however it has been reported up to a year after discontinuation of treatment. Consequently, vigilance is required when managing patients who have previously received immunotherapy and who present with unexplained inflammatory syndromes [90]. Where immunotherapy toxicity is suspected discussion with the treating oncologist is recommended.

Side-effects of immunotherapy include:

Rash

Rashes affect 30–50% of patients receiving immunotherapy. These are generally mild, requiring topical emollients, oral anti-histamines and sometimes a mild topical steroid. Where skin toxicity is affecting daily life, oncology review should be sought and a pause in treatment ± oral steroids [90].

Endocrinopathies

Depending upon the specific regimen, thyroid dysfunction is seen in 5–50% of patients undergoing immunotherapy and is frequently identified on routine blood tests, although patients may present with symptoms of under or over active thyroid. Hypothyroidism requires thyroid replacement therapy, usually long-term. For those with hyperthyroidism, a beta-blocker may suffice although a few patients will go on to require carbimazole or steroids [90].

Immunotherapy related underactivity of the pituitary gland (hypophysitis) is less frequent, however, it should be borne in mind in patients who have received immunotherapy and present with new onset of headache and visual disturbance or symptoms in keeping with pituitary dysfunction. MRI based imaging can help to distinguish hypophysitis from other intra-cranial disease and hormone tests are necessary to determine the need for replacement therapy [90]. Steroids are used for headache and visual disturbance, the treating oncologist should be contacted and endocrinology review sought.

Rarely type 1 diabetes can develop as a result of immunotherapy toxicity.

Colitis

The frequency of immune-colitis is heavily dependent upon the regimen used, ranging from less than 5% to approximately 20%. It is one of the most frequently observed and severe toxicities. Most patients present with diarrhoea although abdominal pain, weight loss, fever, nausea, and vomiting and rectal bleeding are also seen [91].

Patients who are well and passing less than four liquid stools a day can be managed symptomatically, although routine blood tests (including CRP) and stool cultures should be carried out to rule out infective causes. Severe symptoms or those that persist for more than 14 days require review by the treating oncology team. Further investigations include imaging and colonoscopy. Oral steroids are often commenced, and these may be escalated to intravenous steroids, and indeed Infliximab, if symptoms fail to resolve. While uncommon, bowel perforation can occur with a risk of mortality [90].

Hepatitis

Immune hepatitis is reported in 5–10% of patients receiving single agent immunotherapy [90]. Patients are frequently asymptomatic initially with hepatitis identified on routine blood test monitoring. As with colitis, alternative causes of hepatitis should be excluded. Early discussion with the treating oncology team is required. In mild cases a pause from treatment may deliver resolution, however, for many patients steroids will be needed and, rarely, further immunosuppression. Hepatology review may be necessary with failure to resolve.

Pneumonitis

Pneumonitis is relatively rare, with more serious symptoms occurring in 1–2% of patients. Many patients undergoing treatment, and particularly those with lung cancer, have pre-existing lung disease and may be unable to tolerate even relatively mild pneumonitis. Patients present with cough and shortness of breath, on average, a few months into treatment but cases are reported almost two years after commencement. As with other presentations, exclusion of alternative causes should be carried out. Cross-sectional CT imaging will often confirm the diagnosis although in some cases bronchoscopy is required to rule out atypical infection. Treatment is with steroids and should be led by the treating oncologist.

Other rare immune-toxicities include renal, cardiac, neurological, ocular, rheumatological and haematological toxicity. Where there is doubt about the cause of a patient's symptoms, in the context of immunotherapy, oncological review should be sought.

Lymphoedema

Introduction

Lymphoedema is a progressive, chronic, inflammatory condition that results in the accumulation of protein-rich fluid within the interstitial tissue space. Often affecting the limbs, it also manifests in other body areas, for example trunk, genital area, head, and neck. The associated symptoms of swelling, "heaviness" and discomfort impact on quality of life, function, independence, and body image [92, 93].

Management of chronic lymphoedema requires specialist advice as tissue changes over time require a long-term management plan. A more rapid onset is seen in patients with secondary lymphoedema in advanced cancer and may require a different approach to management with simple measures to maintain comfort often most appropriate.

Benefits and burdens of treatments should be weighed up carefully with patients, alongside advice from lymphoedema specialist teams and allied health professionals. It is important to consider other causes of swelling/fluid retention such as thrombosis or heart failure and treat accordingly. Alongside the clinical features noted in Table 15, stasis and accumulation of fluid increases the risk of cellulitis in the affected body part requiring monitoring and potentially treatment with antibiotics.

Management

Early holistic assessment and management of lymphoedema minimises both the physical and psychological effects of this chronic condition. Assessment should include:

- consideration of all possible aetiologies
- identification of any treatable precipitating factors
- physical effects including functional impairment
- recognition of acute complications
- identification of the psychological and social effects on patient and carers [93].

Current best practice guidance is published and updated on the International Lymphoedema Framework Website [94]. Early discussion or referral to lymphoedema services can ensure an appropriate management plan is identified and agreed with patients. The emphasis for palliative care patients, however, must be promotion of comfort and realistic goal setting.

Frail, fatigued palliative care patients may be less able to tolerate prolonged or invasive treatments. Management is then aimed at reducing discomfort, minimising risk of complications (cellulitis) and maintaining dignity. Simple measures such as analgesia and careful positioning for bed or chair bound patients may help. Support garments can aid comfort, for example, scrotal supports [95].

Table 16 outlines the four main pillars of lymphoedema treatment [96]. These can be adapted according to patient wishes and ability.

Table 15   Clinical Features of Lymphoedema.

Short Term	Long Term
• Swelling	• Reduced mobility
• Decreased skin mobility	• Discomfort and pain
• Skin tightness	• Skin folds
• Changes to skin texture and tone	• Hyperkeratosis
• Changes to skin integrity	• Papilomatosis
• Discomfort and pain	• Lymphorrhea (leakage of lymph through skin surface)

Table 16   The four main pillars of lymphoedema treatment [96].

Movement	Remaining active in a safe way assists the lymphatic system in collecting, transporting and excretion of lymph. Moving large and small muscles in the body and deep breathing helps move fluid through the system. Movement can mean simple activities like walking, stretching and heel-raises
Skin care	Keep the skin moisturised and clean to prevent dryness, cracking, and cellulitis
Compression	The use of garments and bandages to compress the affected areas will aid draining of lymphatic fluid and reduce swelling. There are many options and it is important to determine what will work best for the individual
Lymphatic drainage	The use of massage techniques to move fluid through the lymphatic system. This may be done by a practitioner or by the patient once a personalised plan is outlined.

Management of Cellulitis

To prevent systemic illness, early diagnosis and treatment of cellulitis is essential. Features include: acute onset of red, painful, hot, swollen, and tender skin that spreads rapidly and can be associated with fever, malaise, nausea, shivering, and rigors [97]. Treatment with antibiotics as per local protocols is recommended alongside evaluation of other contributory factors.

Follow Up

Input from community nursing services, allied health professionals (to promote and maintain independence and mobility), local tissue viability and lymphoedema specialists will ensure patients feel supported and that comfort and dignity is maintained. Management plans must be flexible and adaptable to changing patient needs and condition.

Airway Patency and Care of the Patient with a Tracheostomy or Laryngectomy

There are two ways of ensuring a patent airway where the larynx/upper airway is either obstructed or removed surgically: tracheostomy and laryngectomy.

A tracheostomy is an artificial opening from the anterior neck into the trachea [98, 99]. Tracheostomies are always kept patent using a plastic/metal tube. A tracheostomy is indicated for:

- bypassing an obstructed upper airway;
- long-term ventilation;
- facilitating suction

A laryngectomy is the surgical removal of the larynx to form an end stoma of the trachea on the anterior neck. The stoma does not usually require a tube to maintain the opening unless it has a tendency to shrink or distort. In an oncology setting a laryngectomy is most commonly used for locally advanced laryngeal cancer or dysfunctional larynx following non-surgical treatments [100].

In all cases, the tracheostomy/laryngectomy replaces the patient's upper airway. As a result, **where oxygen is required, this must be via the tracheostomy/laryngectomy not via mouth/nose.**

Communication

With removal of the larynx or placement of a tracheostomy, speech is initially lost or changed dramatically. Communication can be challenging causing frustration and fatigue for patients and carers. The identification of communication aids and strategies is vital to relieving associated stress and anxiety.

Where a patent airway remains above the tracheostomy/laryngectomy, phonation can be achieved by some patients using finger occlusion of the airway to force air upwards into the mouth. In patients with a tracheostomy, the air will pass around the outside of the tube or through fenestrations if these are present. Speaking valves can be incorporated in either airway type to aid speech. In a tracheostomy this is incorporated into the tube itself, while for patients with a laryngectomy a valve is positioned surgically in the posterior-superior trachea to allow air into the upper airways on occlusion of the stoma. Occasionally a hand-held electronic voice box or electrolarynx can be used. Speech via the upper airways requires significant coordination and can be challenging for those who are particularly frail.

Non-verbal communication is frequently used by patients. Resources include: paper and pen; magnet or digital writing boards; text to speech phone applications; and tablet applications which can be accessed via local speech and language therapy teams. For patients unable to read or write, picture boards displaying a key selection of issues, lip reading and bespoke single word solutions can be used. Body language is almost universal including pointing, thumbs up, eyebrows lifted, etc.

Types of Tracheostomy Tube in Use

Multiple different types of tracheostomy tube exist. All tubes have an outer and an inner tube. The latter facilitating cleaning of the tube and removal of secretions to prevent the tube becoming crusted and obstructing. In all cases the most important element of care is ensuring the tube remains patent and that the inner tube is cleaned regularly (see following paragraphs) [98, 99].

Tubes can be cuffed or uncuffed. The cuff is inflated within the trachea to provide a seal where there is a risk of aspiration (of own saliva or secretions) or bleeding from the tumour. Cuffed tubes require regular monitoring so patients are rarely discharged from hospital and guidance sought from the local hospital team if they remain in situ.

Patients who maintain speech via the upper airways will commonly use a fenestrated tube. Small holes allow air to pass out of the tube and into the upper airways to facilitate speech. The inner tube is used to open and close the fenestrations. A fenestrated tube should be exchanged for a non-fenestrated one overnight and replaced again in the morning. It should also be removed when performing deep suction; if the suction catheter were to escape through one of the fenestrations this could result in trauma [98].

Routine Care for Patients with a Tracheostomy

For all tube types, it is essential that a spare tube of the same size as the patient's and one of a size smaller should be kept at the patient's bedside in case the tube is accidentally dislodged. Accompanying these should be a pair of tracheal dilators for use in emergencies. This equipment is routinely provided for the patient when they are discharged from hospital and should be taken with the patient if admitted elsewhere. If the tube is dislodged it should be reinserted swiftly to ensure airway patency.

Inner Tubes Cleaning

The inner tracheostomy tube should be removed, cleaned, and replaced at least every four hours or more frequently if the patient produces copious secretions. Inner tubes should be cleaned under running water or using appropriate equipment/sterile water. A disposable cleaning swab should be used to dislodge any tenacious secretions. The tube should be dried after cleaning. Ideally the patient should have two inner tubes used in rotation and should not be left without an inner tube for more than very limited periods.

Tracheostomy Replacement

Routine guidance suggests that the whole tracheostomy tube should be changed every 28 days. In the palliative setting, delaying a tube change to ensure comfort (avoiding trauma, bleeding, or pain) is entirely reasonable if there is no concern about the condition of the tube.

Cleaning the Tracheostomy Site

The tracheostomy site should be cleaned using a clean or, where possible, aseptic technique, twice a day, removing all secretions from under and around the flange.

Dressings and Tapes

Tracheostomy tube tapes should be changed daily. One person must hold the tube in place while another changes the tapes. In the palliative setting it is appropriate to leave the tapes for longer periods if these remain clean and changing them would result in discomfort for the patient. If a dressing is indicated (due to large amounts of secretions,

tumour fungation, etc.) this should be changed at least daily but more if required. Pre-cut dressings should be used to prevent lint being introduced into the tract. Barrier creams can be applied to the skin around the tube if this looks sore.

Humidification

When intact, the upper airways warm and moisten incoming air. A heat and moisture exchange (HME) device or a bib should be used to replace this function and prevent the airway becoming dry between nebulisers. Any oxygen administered must be warmed and humidified. Good systemic hydration and, where necessary, regular saline nebulisers help to prevent secretions crusting.

Suction

Where possible patients should be encouraged to cough up secretions and the inner tube cleaned regularly. Suction should be carried out following assessment of the patient rather than at set intervals. The patient will need suction if:

- secretions are audible, the patient is distressed/agitated and secretions are not cleared by cleaning the inner tube
- the patient is desaturating or the work of breathing is increasing
- there is any indication that the patient may have aspirated

The technique for suction should follow local guidelines and advice can be sought from local hospital teams where necessary.

Routine Care for Laryngectomy Patients

Cleaning

The skin surrounding the stoma is cleaned regularly with tap water and a cloth (sterile water should be used in the inpatient setting). Liquid secretions can be removed from the stoma by the patient coughing and wiping them away or by suction. Crusted secretions should be removed gently from the stoma with round-ended forceps.

Tubes, Studs, and Tapes

If the patient is using a laryngectomy tube or a stoma stud to maintain the shape of the stoma, it should be removed and cleaned at least twice a day under running/sterile water and dried before re-insertion. It is usually necessary to use lubricating gel to re-insert laryngectomy tubes. Silicone laryngectomy tubes do not have inner tubes as it is safe to remove the whole tube to clean it. Tube tapes, if used, are replaced daily, or for patients near the end-of-life, only when soiled.

Speaking Valves

There may be a speaking valve visible at the back of the stoma. Care should be taken to prevent it being dislodged during cleaning. The valve can be carefully cleaned in situ, with a special brush. If there are any problems with the speaking valve, or worries about a possible leak or aspiration, the local hospital team should be contacted if appropriate considering the patient's prognosis. Transfer to hospital is required if a valve change is needed [101].

Humidification

A heat moisture exchange (HME) device should be used to replace the function served normally by the upper airways. This can be a bib, a disposable foam cover, a base-plate, or a base-plate/laryngectomy tube with a HME filter. Bibs can be washed and re-used three times. Base-plates can be worn until they start to come away from the skin. The HME filter or foam cover is changed at least daily, and frequently more often, depending upon secretions/soiling. This is a non-invasive intervention and should not result in discomfort.

Nebulisers should be used regularly, and any oxygen used should be warmed and humidified.

Suction

Suction is discouraged for patients with a laryngectomy and infrequently required. Patients should be encouraged to cough and wipe away expectorated secretions. Superficial suction around the stoma may be used where patients are particularly weak and struggle to expectorate. Humidification is important to ensure secretions can be cleared easily. Regular carbocisteine can be used to help loosen secretions where necessary. For patients with significant secretions suction may be required, although near the end-of-life hyoscine butylbromide can be considered to reduce secretions.

Where any concerns or questions about the care of a patient with a tracheostomy or laryngectomy exist, the local ENT ward or head and neck cancer clinical nurse specialist team should be contacted.

Summary

Advanced incurable cancer and its treatment can result in a wide range of symptoms that reduce quality of life. The key message of this chapter is that a melded approach, understanding, and respecting each individual's preferences to balance palliation and intervention, is key to achieving the best possible quality of life for each patient. Clarity of decision-making and regular review of advance care plans will ensure best outcomes for patients and their families.

References

1. Loblaw, D.A., Laperriere, N.J., and Mackillop, W.J. (2003 June). A population-based study of malignant spinal cord compression in Ontario. *Clinical Oncology* 15 (4): 211–217.
2. Levack, P. *et al.* (2002 December) Don't wait for a sensory level – listen to the symptoms: A prospective audit of the delays in diagnosis of malignant cord compression. *Clinical Oncology* 14 (6): 472–480.
3. National Collaborating Centre for Cancer (Great Britain). (2008). *Metastatic Spinal Cord Compression: Diagnosis and Management of Patients at Risk of or with Metastatic Spinal Cord Compression.* Cardiff: National Collaborating Centre for Cancer. (accessed 21 April 2021). [Online]. Available:. http://www.ncbi.nlm.nih.gov/books/NBK55007.
4. Metastatic spinal cord compression in adults | Guidance and guidelines | NICE. https://www.nice.org.uk/guidance/qs56 (accessed 23 October 2017).
5. "Scottish Palliative Care Guidelines – Malignant spinal cord compression," *Scottish Palliative Care Guidelines.* http://www.palliativecareguidelines.scot.nhs.uk (accessed 27 April 2021).
6. Levack, P., Graham, J., and Kidd, J. (2004 October). Listen to the patient: Quality of life of patients with recently diagnosed malignant cord compression in relation to their disability. *Palliative Medicine* 18 (7): 594–601.
7. NICE, "Treating metastatic spinal cord compression." 11 April 2020.
8. MHRA, "Medicines and Healthcare products Regulatory Agency – National patient safety alert for Steroid Emergency Card to support early reognition of adrenal crisis in adults." https://www.cas.mhra.gov.uk/ViewandAcknowledgment/ViewAlert.aspx?AlertID=103082 (accessed 07 January 2022).
9. Patchell, R.A. *et al.* (2005 August) Direct decompressive surgical resection in the treatment of spinal cord compression caused by metastatic cancer: A randomised trial. *The Lancet* 366 (9486): 643–648.
10. Tokuhashi, Y., Matsuzaki, H., Oda, H., Oshima, M., and Ryu, J. (2005). A revised scoring system for preoperative evaluation of metastatic spine tumor prognosis. *Spine* 30 (19): 2186–2191.
11. Spencer, K., Parrish, R., Barton, R., and Henry, A. (2018 March). Palliative radiotherapy. *BMJ* 360 k821.
12. Loblaw, D.A. and Laperriere, N.J. (1998). Emergency treatment of malignant extradural spinal cord compression: An

evidence-based guideline. *Journal of Clinical Oncology* 16 (4): 1613–1624.

13. Hoskin, P.J. *et al.* (2019 December) Effect of single-fraction vs multifraction radiotherapy on ambulatory status among patients with spinal canal compression from metastatic cancer: The SCORAD randomized clinical trial. *JAMA* 322 (21): 2084.

14. Maranzano, E. *et al.* (2009 November) 8Gy single-dose radiotherapy is effective in metastatic spinal cord compression: Results of a phase III randomized multicentre Italian trial. *Radiotherapy and Oncology* 93 (2): 174–179.

15. Rades, D. *et al.* (2008 November) A score predicting posttreatment ambulatory status in patients irradiated for metastatic spinal cord compression. *International Journal of Radiation Oncology*Biology*Physics* 72 (3): 905–908.

16. Rowell, N.P. and Gleeson, F.V. (2002 October). Steroids, radiotherapy, chemotherapy, and stents for superior vena caval obstruction in carcinoma of the bronchus: A systematic review. *Clinical Oncology* 14 (5): 338–351.

17. Ganeshan, A., Hon, L.Q., Warakaulle, D.R., Morgan, R., and Uberoi, R. (2009 August). Superior vena caval stenting for SVC obstruction: Current status. *European Journal of Radiology* 71 (2): 343–349.

18. Coleman, R.E. and Rubens, R.D. (1985 December). Bone metastases and breast cancer. *Cancer Treatment Reviews* 12 (4): 251–270.

19. Coleman, R.E. (2006 October). Clinical features of metastatic bone disease and risk of skeletal morbidity. *Clinical Cancer Research* 12 (20): 6243s–6249s.

20. Kane, C.M., Hoskin, P., and Bennett, M.I. (2015 January). Cancer induced bone pain. *BMJ* 350 (jan29 7): h315–h315.

21. Coleman, R.E. (2004). Bisphosphonates: Clinical experience. *The Oncologist* 9 (S4): 14–27.

22. Mirels, H. (1989 December). Metastatic disease in long bones. A proposed scoring system for diagnosing impending pathologic fractures. *Clinical Orthopaedics and Related Research* (249): 256–264. https://journals.lww.com/corr/Abstract/1989/12000/Metastatic_Disease_in_Long_Bones_A_Proposed.27.aspx.

23. Derry, S. *et al.* (2017). Oral nonsteroidal anti-inflammatory drugs (NSAIDs) for cancer pain in adults. *Cochrane Database of Systematic Reviews* (4) Art. No.: CD012638. DOI: 10.1002/14651858.CD012638.

24. Lutz, S. *et al.* (2011 March) Palliative radiotherapy for bone metastases: An ASTRO evidence-based guideline. *International Journal of Radiation Oncology*Biology*Physics* 79 (4): 965–976.

25. Rich, S.E. *et al.* (2018 March) Update of the systematic review of palliative radiation therapy fractionation for bone metastases. *Radiotherapy and Oncology* 126 (3): 547–557.

26. Chow, E. *et al.* (2006 March) A phase III international randomised trial comparing single with multiple fractions for re-irradiation of painful bone metastases: National Cancer Institute of Canada Clinical Trials Group (NCIC CTG) SC 20. *Clinical Oncology* 18 (2): 125–128.

27. Chow, E. *et al.* (2015 November) Dexamethasone in the prophylaxis of radiation-induced pain flare after palliative radiotherapy for bone metastases: A double-blind, randomised placebo-controlled, phase 3 trial. *Lancet Oncology* 16 (15): 1463–1472.

28. Dearnaley, D.P., Bayly, R.J., A'Hern, R.P., Gadd, J., Zivanovic, M.M., and Lewington, V.J. (1992 January). Palliation of bone metastases in prostate cancer. Hemibody irradiation or strontium-89? *Clinical Oncology* 4 (2): 101–107.

29. Coleman, R., Body, J.J., Aapro, M., Hadji, P., and Herrstedt, J. (2014 September). Bone health in cancer patients: ESMO clinical practice guidelines. *Annals of Oncology* 25 (suppl_3): iii124–iii137.

30. Wong, R.K.S. and Wiffen, P.J. (2002). Bisphosphonates for the relief of pain secondary to bone metastases. *Cochrane Database of Systematic Reviews* (2): Art. No.: CD002068. doi: 10.1002/14651858.CD002068. (accessed 23 September 2022).

31. Hoskin, P. *et al.* (2015 October) A multicenter randomized trial of ibandronate compared with single-dose radiotherapy for localized metastatic bone pain in prostate cancer. *Journal of the National Cancer Institute* 107 (10): djv197.

32. "Overview | Percutaneous vertebroplasty | Guidance | NICE." https://www.nice.org.uk/guidance/ipg12 (accessed 12 November 2021).

33. Buchbinder, R., Johnston, R.V., Rischin, K.J., Homik, J., Jones, C.A., Golmohammadi, K., and Kallmes, D.F. (2018). Percutaneous vertebroplasty for osteoporotic vertebral compression fracture. *Cochrane Database of Systematic Reviews* (11): Art. No.: CD006349. doi: 10.1002/14651858.CD006349.pub4. (accessed 23 September 2022).

34. "Overview | Balloon kyphoplasty for vertebral compression fractures | Guidance | NICE." https://www.nice.org.uk/guidance/ipg166 (accessed 12 November 2021).

35. Berenson, J. *et al.* (2011 March) Balloon kyphoplasty versus non-surgical fracture management for treatment of painful vertebral body compression fractures in patients with cancer: A multicentre, randomised controlled trial. *The Lancet Oncology* 12 (3): 225–235.

36. Willeumier, J.J. (2016). Lack of clinical evidence for postoperative radiotherapy after surgical fixation of impending or actual pathologic fractures in the long bones in patients with cancer; a systematic review. *Radiotherapy and Oncology* 5.

37. Barnholtz-Sloan, J.S., Sloan, A.E., Davis, F.G., Vigneau, F.D., Lai, P., and Sawaya, R.E. (2016 September). Incidence proportions of brain metastases in patients diagnosed (1973 to 2001) in the Metropolitan Detroit cancer surveillance system. *Journal of Clinical Oncology* 22 (14).

38. Schouten, L.J., Rutten, J., Huveneers, H.A.M., and Twijnstra, A. (2002). Incidence of brain metastases in a cohort of patients with carcinoma of the breast, colon, kidney, and lung and melanoma. *Cancer* 94 (10): 2698–2705.

39. Achrol, A.S. *et al.* (2019 December) Brain metastases. *Nature Reviews Disease Primers* 5 (1): 5.

40. Tsao, M.N. *et al.* (2018). Whole brain radiotherapy for the treatment of newly diagnosed multiple brain metastases. *Cochrane Database of Systematic Reviews* 1.

41. Kong, X., Guan, J., Yang, Y., Li, Y., Ma, W., and Wang, R. (2015 July). A meta-analysis: Do prophylactic antiepileptic drugs in patients with brain tumors decrease the incidence of seizures? *Clinical Neurology and Neurosurgery* 134: 98–103.

42. Fuentes, R., Osorio, D., Hernandez, J.E., Simancas-Racines, D., Martinez-Zapata, M.J., and Cosp, X.B. (2018). Surgery versus stereotactic radiotherapy for people with single or solitary brain metastasis. *Cochrane Database of Systematic Reviews* 8.

43. Kocher, M. *et al.* (2011 January) Adjuvant whole-brain radiotherapy versus observation after radiosurgery or surgical resection of one to three cerebral metastases: Results of the EORTC 22952-26001 study. *Journal of Clinical Oncology* 29 (2): 134–141.

44. Bezjak, A. *et al.* (2002). Symptom response after palliative radiotherapy for patients with brain metastases. *European Journal of Cancer* 38 (4): 487–496.

45. Gerrard, G.E. *et al.* (2003 October) Investigating the palliative efficacy of whole-brain radiotherapy for patients with multiple-brain metastases and poor prognostic features. *Clinical Oncology (Royal College of Radiologists)* 15 (7): 422–428.

46. Mulvenna, P. *et al.* (2016 October) Dexamethasone and supportive care with or without whole brain radiotherapy in treating patients with non-small cell lung cancer with brain metastases unsuitable for resection or stereotactic radiotherapy (QUARTZ): Results from a phase 3, non-inferiority, randomised trial. *The Lancet* 388 (10055): 2004–2014.

47. Sperduto, P.W., Berkey, B., Gaspar, L.E., Mehta, M., and Curran, W. (2008 February). A new prognostic index and comparison to three other indices for patients with brain metastases: An analysis of 1,960 patients in the RTOG database. *International Journal of Radiation Oncology*Biology*Physics* 70 (2): 510–514.

48. Gastanaga, V.M. *et al.* (2016 June) Prevalence of hypercalcemia among cancer patients in the United States. *Cancer Medicine* 5 (8): 2091–2100.

49. Zagzag, J., Hu, M.I., Fisher, S.B., and Perrier, N.D. (2018). Hypercalcemia and cancer: Differential diagnosis and treatment. *CA: A Cancer Journal for Clinicians* 68 (5): 377–386.

50. Minisola, S., Pepe, J., Piemonte, S., and Cipriani, C. (2015 June). The diagnosis and management of hypercalcaemia. *BMJ* 350 (jun02 15): h2723–h2723.

51. "Hypercalcaemia | Health topics A to Z | CKS | NICE." https://cks.nice.org.uk/topics/hypercalcaemia (accessed 28 oct 2021).

52. Stewart, A.F. (2005 January). Clinical practice. Hypercalcemia associated with cancer. *New England Journal of Medicine* 352 (4): 373–379.

53. Bower, M., Robinson, L., and Cox, S. *Endocrine and Metabolic Complications of Advanced Cancer.* Oxford University Press. (accessed 16 June 2021). [Online]. Available. https://oxfordmedicine.com/view/10.1093/med/9780199656097.001.0001/med-9780199656097-chapter-142.

54. Beland, P. (2018). Malignant hypercalcaemia: Definition, symptoms and treatment. *Nursing Times* 114 (11): 39–43.

55. Chávez-Iñiguez, J.S., Navarro-Gallardo, G.J., Medina-González, R., Alcantar-Vallin, L., and García-García, G. (2020 November). Acute Kidney injury caused by obstructive nephropathy. *International Journal of Nephrology* 2020: e8846622.

56. Verhamme, K.M.C., Sturkenboom, M.C.J.M., Stricker, B.H.C., and Bosch, R. (2008). Drug-induced urinary retention: Incidence, management and prevention. *Drug Safety* 31 (5): 373–388.

57. Wong, L.-M., Cleeve, L.K., Milner, A.D., and Pitman, A.G. (2007 July). Malignant ureteral obstruction: Outcomes after intervention. Have things changed? *Journal of Urology* 178 (1): 178–183. discussion 183.

58. Tatenuma, T., Tsutsumi, S., Yasui, M., Noguchi, G., Umemoto, S., and Kishida, T. (2020 February). Outcome of Palliative urinary diversion and observation for malignant extrinsic ureteral obstruction. *Journal of Palliative Medicine* 23 (2): 254–258.

59. Harris, D., Finlay, I., Flowers, S., and Noble, S. (2011 October). The use of crisis medication in the management of terminal haemorrhage due to incurable cancer: A qualitative study. *Palliative Medicine* 25 (7): 691–700.

60. Montroy, J. *et al.* (2017 July) The safety and efficacy of lysine analogues in cancer patients: A systematic review and meta-analysis. *Transfusion Medicine Reviews* 31 (3): 141–148.

61. Fairchild, A. *et al.* (2008 August) Palliative thoracic radiotherapy for lung cancer: A systematic review. *Journal of Clinical Oncology : Official Journal of the American Society of Clinical Oncology* 26 (24): 4001–4011.

62. Duchesne, G.M. *et al.* (2000). A randomized trial of hypofractionated schedules of palliative radiotherapy in the management of bladder carcinoma: Results of medical research council trial BA09. *International Journal of Radiation Oncology* Biology* Physics* 47 (2): 379–388.

63. Cameron, M.G., Kersten, C., Guren, M.G., Fosså, S.D., and Vistad, I. (2014 January). Palliative pelvic radiotherapy of symptomatic incurable prostate cancer – A systematic review. *Radiotherapy and Oncology* 110 (1): 55–60.

64. Cameron, M.G. *et al.* (2016 December) Palliative pelvic radiotherapy for symptomatic rectal cancer – A prospective multicenter study. *Acta Oncologica* 55 (12): 1400–1407.

65. Johnstone, C. and Rich, S.E. (2018 April). Bleeding in cancer patients and its treatment: A review. *Annals of Palliative Medicine* 7 (2): Art. no. 2.

66. Grocott, P., Gethin, G., and Probst, S. Common symptoms and disorders: Skin problems. In: *Oxford Textbook of Palliative Medicine*, 5th, 715–723. (accessed 23 April 2021). [Online]. Available. https://oxfordmedicine.com/view/10.1093/med/9780199656097.001.0001/med-9780199656097-part-11.

67. Maida, V., Corbo, M., Dolzhykov, M., Ennis, M., Irani, S., and Trozzolo, L. (2008 June). Wounds in advanced illness: A prevalence and incidence study based on a prospective case series. *International Wound Journal* 5 (2): 305–314.

68. Tilley, C.P., Fu, M.R., Van Cleeve, J., Crocilla, B.L., and Comfort, C.P. (2020 June). Symptoms of malignant fungating wounds and functional performance among patients with advanced cancer: An integrative review from 2000 to 2019. *Journal of Palliative Medicine* 23 (6): 848–862.

69. Alexander, S. (2009 August). Malignant fungating wounds: Key symptoms and psychosocial issues. *Journal of Wound Care* 18 (8): 325–329.

70. Lund-Nielsen, B., Müller, K., and Adamsen, L. (2005 January). Malignant wounds in women with breast cancer: Feminine and sexual perspectives. *Journal of Clinical Nursing* 14 (1): 56–64.

71. Morley, J., Grocott, P., Purssell, E., and Murrells, T. (2019 December). Electrochemotherapy for the palliative management of cutaneous metastases: A systematic review and meta-analysis. *European Journal of Surgical Oncology* 45 (12): 2257–2267.

72. Alexander, S. (2009 September). Malignant fungating wounds: Managing malodour and exudate. *Journal of Wound Care* 18 (9): 374–382.

73. Alexander, S. (2009 October). Malignant fungating wounds: Managing pain, bleeding and psychosocial issues. *Journal of Wound Care* 18 (10): 418–425.

74. Scottish Palliative care guidelines – Bleeding. Scottish Palliative Care Guidelines. http://www.palliativecareguidelines. scot.nhs.uk (accessed 24 January 2022).

75. Smothers, A. *Pruritus, Fever, and Sweats*, 285–290. Oxford University Press. (accessed 05 July 2021). [Online]. Available. https://oxfordmedicine.com/view/10.1093/med/9780190862374.001.0001/med-9780190862374-chapter-20.

76. Silverberg, J.I. *et al.* (2018 October) A comprehensive conceptual model of the experience of chronic itch in adults. *American Journal of Clinical Dermatology* 19 (5): 759–769.

77. Wilcock, A., Howard, P., and Charlesworth, S. (2022) Palliative Care Formulary PCF8 Pharmaceutical Press. https://www.pharmpress.com/product/9780857113689/pcf (accessed 23 April 2021).

78. Siemens, W. *et al.* (2016 November). Pharmacological interventions for pruritus in adult palliative care patients. *Cochrane Database of Systematic Reviews* 2016 (11).

79. Hercz, D., Jiang, S.H., and Webster, A.C. (2020). Interventions for itch in people with advanced chronic kidney disease. *Cochrane Database of Systematic Reviews* 12.

80. Zell, J.A. and Chang, J.C. (2005 November). Neoplastic fever: A neglected paraneoplastic syndrome. *Support Care Cancer* 13 (11): 870–877.

81. Rojas-Concha, L., Hansen, M.B., Petersen, M.A., and Groenvold, M. (2020 April). Which symptoms and problems do advanced cancer patients admitted to specialized palliative care report in addition to those included in the EORTC QLQ-C15-PAL? A register-based national study. *Support Care Cancer* 28 (4): 1725–1735 (accessed 1 November 2023).

82. Boehlke, C., Joos, L., Coune, B., Becker, C., Meerpohl, J.J., Buroh, S., Hercz, D., Schwarzer, G., Becker, G. (2023). Pharmacological interventions for pruritus in adult palliative care patients. *Cochrane Database of Systematic Reviews* 4: CD008320. doi: 10.1002/14651858.CD008320.pub4. PMID: 37314034. (accessed 14 April 2023).

83. Lalla, R.V. *et al.* (2014 May) MASCC/ISOO clinical practice guidelines for the management of mucositis secondary to cancer therapy. *Cancer* 120 (10): 1453–1461.

84. Papas, A.S., Clark, R.E., Martuscelli, G., O'Loughlin, K.T., Johansen, E., and Miller, K.B. (2003 April). A prospective, randomized trial for the prevention of mucositis in patients undergoing hematopoietic stem cell transplantation. *Bone Marrow Transplant* 31 (8): 705–712.

85. Navari, R.M. and Aapro, M. (2016 April). Antiemetic prophylaxis for chemotherapy-induced nausea and vomiting. *New England Journal of Medicine* 374 (14): 1356–1367.

86. Priestman, T.J. *et al.* (1990). Results of a randomized, double-blind comparative study of ondansetron and metoclopramide in the prevention of nausea and vomiting following high-dose upper abdominal irradiation. *Clinical Oncology* 2 (2): 71–75.

87. Andreyev, H.J.N., Davidson, S.E., Gillespie, C., Allum, W.H., and Swarbrick, E. (2012 February). Practice guidance on the management of acute and chronic gastrointestinal problems arising as a result of treatment for cancer. *Gut* 61 (2): 179–192.

88. "Introduction | Neutropenic sepsis: Prevention and management in people with cancer | Guidance | NICE." https://www.nice.org.uk/guidance/cg151/chapter/Introduction#when-to-refer-patients-in-the-community-for-suspected-neutropenic-sepsis (accessed 24 June 2021).

89. "Immunotherapy and its side effects," Cancer Research UK, 21 April 2020. https://www.cancerresearchuk.org/health-professional/treatment-and-other-post-diagnosis-issues/immunotherapy-and-its-side-effects (accessed 24 June 2021).

90. Haanen, J.B.A.G. *et al.* (2017). Management of toxicities from immunotherapy: ESMO Clinical Practice Guidelines for diagnosis, treatment and follow-up. *Annals of Oncology* 28: 24.

91. Marthey, L. *et al.* (2016 April) Cancer immunotherapy with anti-CTLA-4 monoclonal antibodies induces an inflammatory bowel disease. *Journal of Crohn's and Colitis* 10 (4): 395–401.

92. Frid, M., Strang, P., Friedrichsen, M.J., and Johansson, K. (2006). Lower limb lymphedema: Experiences and

perceptions of cancer patients in the late palliative stage. *Journal of Palliative Care* 22 (1): 5–11.

93. Fu, M.R., Ridner, S.H., Hu, S.H., Stewart, B.R., Cormier, J.N., and Armer, J.M. (2013 July). Psychosocial impact of lymphedema: A systematic review of literature from 2004 to 2011. *Psychooncology* 22 (7): 1466–1484.

94. Lymphoma United. International Lymphoedema Framework. https://lymphoedemaunited.com/international-lymphoedema-framework/ (accessed 26 Oct 2023).

95. Fu, M.R., Lasinski, B.B., Cleave, J.H.V., and Tilley, C.P., Lymphedema Management. Oxford University Press, pp. 238–250. (accessed 05 July 2021). [Online]. Available: https://oxfordmedicine.com/view/10.1093/med/9780190862374.001.0001/med-9780190862374-chapter-18

96. Sneddon, M. (2021 February). British Lymphology Society's EveryBodyCan campaign: 2021 relaunch. *British Journal of Community Nursing* 26 (2): 81–82.

97. "Cellulitis – acute | Health topics A to Z | CKS | NICE." https://cks.nice.org.uk/topics/cellulitis-acute (accessed 26 Oct 2023).

98. "Temporary tracheostomy." https://www.macmillan.org.uk/cancer-information-and-support/impacts-of-cancer/temporary-tracheostomy-for-head-and-neck-cancer (accessed 05 July 2021).

99. NICE, "Tracheostomy using a breathing tube passed from within the windpipe to the outside of the neck." August 2013. (accessed 05 July 2021). [Online]. Available: https://www.nice.org.uk/guidance/ipg462/resources/tracheostomy-using-a-breathing-tube-passed-from-within-the-windpipe-to-the-outside-of-the-neck-pdf-366162733

100. "What is a laryngectomy?" https://www.macmillan.org.uk/cancer-information-and-support/treatments-and-drugs/laryngectomy (accessed 05 July 2021).

101. "Laryngectomy stoma care and changes after laryngectomy." https://www.macmillan.org.uk/cancer-information-and-support/impacts-of-cancer/living-with-a-laryngectomy-stoma (accessed 05 July 2021).

14 Palliative Care for People with Progressive Neurological Disorders

David Oliver and Idris Baker

Introduction

The needs of people with progressive neurological disease may vary greatly due to the variation between diseases and individual variation within a disease. However, palliative care is often appropriate to support quality of life since these patients face continual loss – of mobility, speech, swallowing, breathing, and cognition as well as experiencing a range of burdensome symptoms. This has been emphasised in the UK, for instance in England in the National Service Framework for Long Term Conditions [1], and the End-of-Life Care Programme document "End-of-life care in long term neurological conditions" [2]. Palliative care is now included within several National Institute for Health and Care Excellence (NICE) guidelines [3, 4].

Neurological disease is a major cause of death worldwide (when stroke and dementia are included) with 9 million deaths worldwide, which was 16.5% of all deaths in 2016 –an increase by 39% from 1990 [5]. Palliative care aims to minimise the problems faced by patients and their families, and maximise their quality of life, despite disability and disease progression. Although new treatments are being developed, the care provided by a wide variety of disciplines will remain essential to enable patients and families to live as fully as possible, and to die with minimal symptoms and distress.

Background

There are many different progressive neurological diseases – see Table 1. They have very different trajectories, rates of progression, and prognosis, and there is also great individual variation within a disease group. Additionally, disease modifying treatments (DMT) will modify the disease patterns. In multiple sclerosis (MS) for example such treatments have changed the disease profile, with many patients experiencing stable disease, with no progression.

The Role of Palliative Care

Palliative care has been involved in the care of people with progressive neurological disease for over 50 years. When St. Christopher's Hospice in London was first opened in 1967 people with motor neurone disease (MND) and multiple sclerosis (MS) were admitted in the first few months. There has been a gradual increase in palliative care in neurology. In 2000, the End-of-Life Care Programme in England published a report "End-of-life care in long term neurological conditions: a framework for implementation" [2] to stimulate discussion.

In 2016 the European Association for Palliative Care (EAPC) and the European Academy of Neurology (EAN) produced a Consensus Statement which recommended that palliative care should be considered early in the disease trajectory, depending on the underlying diagnosis [6]. The paper also recommended the multidisciplinary approach to care, with palliative care included within the team. This has been seen now in the NICE Guideline on MND where palliative care expertise is recommended within the multidisciplinary team (MDT) and discussion about deterioration and end-of-life should be considered at any time during disease progression, depending on the

Handbook of Palliative Care, Fourth Edition. Edited by Richard Kitchen, Christina Faull, Sarah Russell and Jo Wilson.
© 2024 John Wiley & Sons Ltd. Published 2024 by John Wiley & Sons Ltd.

Table 1 Progressive Neurological Disorders.

	Prevalence	Number of people in UK	Prognosis	Causation	Symptoms	Variations	Treatment
Motor Neurone Disease (MND) Also known as Amyotrophic Lateral Sclerosis (ALS)	6/100,000	6000	Average 3–5 years 10% live more than 10 years	Most unknown 5–10% Family history (60% genetic mutation found)	Upper and lower motor neurone damage Frontal lobe and other parts of the brain may be affected Weakness Flaccidity/spasticity Respiratory muscle weakness Speech and swallowing problems Cognitive change 10–15% Frontotemporal dementia	Amyotrophic lateral sclerosis 66% of patients Upper and lower motor neurone loss Weakness, Spasticity, and flaccidity; Muscle wasting and fasciculations Progressive bulbar palsy – 26% of patients; involvement of the brain stem motor nuclei; presenting with swallowing and/or speech problems Progressive muscular atrophy (PMA) – lower motor neurones Weakness of legs or arms initially; prognosis of up to 10–15 years Primary lateral sclerosis – rare form; predominantly upper motor neurone involvement; spasticity and stiffness; longer prognosis, often over 10 years	Riluzole may slow the rate of progression Many treatments on clinical trials
Multiple Sclerosis (MS)	190–250/100,000	130,000	5–10 years lower than average	Autoimmune disease Aetiology not known	Demyelination in the nervous system Variable presentation, according to the area affected Hemiparesis Hemisensory loss Ophthalmoplegia Optic neuritis Ataxia Tremor Progressive disability	Primary progressive MS Gradual worsening – rate of deterioration is variable Starts under 40s Relapsing, remitting MS 85% of patients Relapse or flare up of symptoms with remissions in between Secondary progressive MS 65% of people with relapsing, remitting MS develop into this in 15 years Continued deterioration, with or without relapses	There are many Disease Modifying Treatments for relapsing, remitting MS Alemtuzumab Cladribine Glatiramer acetate Ocrelizumab Natalizumab Teriflunomide Early primary progressive MS Ocrelizumab

Table 1 (*Continued*)

	Prevalence	Number of people in UK	Prognosis	Causation	Symptoms	Variations	Treatment
Parkinson's disease (PD)	220/100,000	145,000	Variable Can be normal life expectancy	Not known	Neuronal loss in the substantia nigra, with inclusion bodies (Lewy bodies) Lewy body dementia in about 20%	Bradykinesia, cogwheel rigidity, rest tremor Dementia common later Autonomic dysfunction Cognitive change and dementia	Dopaminergic medication Levodopa – with dopa-decarboxylase inhibitors Dopamine agonist Apomorphine Cabergoline Pramipexole Ropinirole Catechol-O-methyltransferase inhibitors Entacapone Tolcapone
Multiple system atrophy (MSA)	7/100,000	3000	6-9 years	Not known	Alpha-synuclein deposits in Olivopontine area Cerebellum Nigrostriatal area	Parkinsonism (muscle rigidity with or without tremor and bradykinesia) Ataxia Later Speech and swallowing problems Breathing problems and stridor MSA-C – primarily cerebellar symptoms – gait ataxia, limb kinetic ataxia, scanning dysarthria, cerebellar ocular disturbances MSA-P – primarily parkinsonian symptoms – progressive akinesia and rigidity Autonomic changes Incontinence Postural hypotension Temperature control Sexual problems	Symptomatic treatment only

(*continued*)

Table 1 (*Continued*)

	Prevalence	Number of people in UK	Prognosis	Causation	Symptoms	Variations	Treatment
Progressive supranuclear palsy (PSP)	7/100,000	4000	6-7 years		Tau is deposited in neurofibrillary tangles in the brain	Unsteadiness, falls Slowing down Quietening of voice Emotional/behavioural changes – apathy Depression and anxiety Visual problems Fatigue Deterioration with: Dementia Swallowing and speech problems Immobility Muscle stiffness	Symptomatic treatment only
Huntington's disease (HD)	6/100,000	6500	10-30 years	Autosomal dominant inheritance		Usually presents after 30 years old Personality change Irritability Aggression Choreiform movements Bradykinesia Slowness of speech Depression Suicide increased Cognitive change and dementia	Symptomatic treatment Tetrabenazine for chorea Families may ask for genetic counselling
Corticobasal syndrome (CBS) Also known as Corticobasal degeneration (CBD)	5/100,000	3500	6-8 years	Not known	Tauopathy – with accumulation of tau in the cortex and basal ganglia	Similar to PSP Tremor Dystonia Balance and co-ordination problems Difficulty in moving one limb Slow/slurred speech Swallowing problems Dementia	Symptomatic treatment
Muscular dystrophies (MD)	80/100,000 Duchenne MD (DMD) 4/100,000	68,000 Duchenne MD 2500	Variable Duchenne MD 30 years	Group of disorders Duchenne MD is an X-linked recessive	Muscle degeneration	Proximal weakness Difficulty in walking and standing Progresses to wheelchair Respiratory muscle weakness may require ventilatory support Heart and respiratory muscle damage	Symptomatic Families may ask for genetic counselling

patient's request and particularly when new interventions are discussed [3]. The NICE Guideline on Parkinson's disease (PD) also stresses the importance of offering opportunities to discuss the prognosis and planning ahead [4].

How palliative care is provided may depend on the disease and the services involved. There is evidence in MND that the MDT is effective in maintaining quality of life and may extend life by several months [7, 8]. This multidisciplinary approach is essential to provide the overall holistic care of the patient and family and has been widely recommended [3, 6] and the EAPC/EAN Consensus Statement has stressed the need for education of those involved – neurologists in palliative care and palliative care specialists in neurology – to enable the collaborative approach to develop [6]. In the USA the concept of Neuro-palliative care has developed, with neurologists undertaking palliative care training and experience and then providing both neurology and palliative care support [9].

There will be patients and families with more complex needs – symptom or psychosocial issues – at any stage of their illness who would benefit from more input from specialist palliative care services. For instance, a person with MND may have distressing concerns about the diagnosis when they are first told the diagnosis, symptom management issues at any time, the need for careful discussion and consideration of interventions, such as gastrostomy or ventilatory support, and increased needs as they come nearer to the end-of-life. In MND this heightened need may be intermittently during a period of 2 to 3 years, whereas there may be similar varying needs for someone with MS over a period of 20 years. There may also be the need for the assessment of complex ethical decisions, such as whether to use and when to stop some treatments

and interventions, which may benefit from a collaborative approach and from the involvement of palliative care specialists. Specialist palliative care may be more closely involved in the care of the patients and family at certain periods of time, helping with specific issues, and in between these occasions the neurological MDT may provide the ongoing support [10]. This is illustrated in Figure 1.

The recognition of the needs of patients and families could be facilitated by the regular use of a patient outcome measure, which can highlight new areas of need or distress to the caring team, such as the Integrated Palliative care Outcome Scale for neurological conditions (IPOS Neuro) (https://pos-pal.org/maix/ipos_neuro.php) which has been found to be acceptable and helpful [11].

Studies of such short-term specialist palliative care intervention have shown benefits. For people with MS there was an improvement in symptoms, reduced caregiver burden and cost effectiveness [12, 13]; a short-term palliative care intervention for people with MS by an MS team, who had received extra training, did reduce symptom burden but did not influence quality of life [14]. A randomised controlled trial of a multidisciplinary approach of palliative care did show a reduction in symptoms – pain, breathlessness, sleep disorders, and bowel symptoms – and there was an improvement in quality of life [15]. A large study of short-term palliative care involvement in the UK has again shown that there was improvement in pain, sleep, nausea, and bowel issues, with no change in mortality, and reduced health and social care costs. Patients and caregivers appreciated the services and felt that the care helped to increase their resilience, attended to deficits and needs, and enabled the carer to continue with care at home [16].

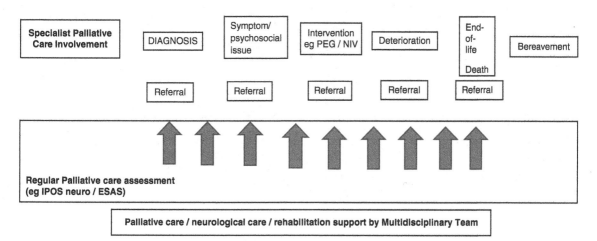

Figure 1   The involvement of palliative care for people with neurological disease.

Symptom Management

As there are no curative treatments for these progressive neurological diseases the primary aims of management should be quality of life, longevity for some, symptom management, and addressing other issues – physical, psychological, social, and spiritual. As outlined in Chapter 1, good symptom management requires:
• Impeccable assessment of the problem (to identify, where possible, causes and mechanisms and to inform prioritisation)
  ○ Careful history of the symptom
  ○ Careful physical examination
  ○ Relevant investigation
• Discussion with the patient, and those close to them, about possible options – including the advantages and disadvantages of treatments that might be offered.

Pain

Pain is common in people with progressive neurological diseases and may be due to the disease process itself, or be caused by the changes imposed by the disease, such as immobility. It is important to be aware that there may be coincidental pains, from other causes that may be worsened by the progression of neurological dysfunction, such as immobility increasing arthritic pain.

Pain is common in all neurological disease groups (Box 1):

> **Box 1: Prevalence of Pain in people with neurological disorders**
>
> | | |
> |---|---|
> | Motor neurone disease | 73% [17] |
> | Parkinson's disease | 85% [18] |
> | Multiple sclerosis | 77% [19] |
> | Multiple systems atrophy | 73% [20] |
> | MSA C | 41% |
> | MSA P | 63% |
> | Corticobasal syndrome | 25% [20] |
> | Progressive supranuclear palsy | 52% [20] |
> | Huntingdon's disease | 41% [21] |
> | Duchenne muscular dystrophy | 69% [22] |

The careful assessment of pain is essential, and later in the disease progression specific scales may be necessary. The DisDaT scale is used if the patient has limited communication or severe cognitive change [23]. It compares the cues that the patient is content and the cues of distress, as described by close carers, so that the presence of distress can be identified and then assessment undertaken of possible causes of pain, followed by appropriate reassessment to ascertain if the distress has lessened [23]. The PAINAD scale allows carers to assess various aspects of the patient [24]. It is important to involve carers in these assessments and where possible to differentiate pain from non-pain distress, which may be due to many different causes. Close assessment, examination, and re-evaluation are necessary. See Chapter 10: Pain and Its Management for more detail.

Common causes of pain are:

Musculoskeletal Pain
This may occur due to altered muscle tone around joints – particularly the shoulder and spine – or to restricted movement. Management includes:
• Careful positioning
• Physiotherapy, including passive movements, to maintain joint mobility, splints, and support aids
• Non-pharmacological strategies such as heat pads, massage, and acupuncture
• Non-steroidal anti-inflammatory drugs – although the risks of gastrointestinal, renal, and cardiovascular toxicity may limit their use in some patients
• Intra-articular injections of steroid and local anaesthetic may be helpful.

Muscle Cramps
If muscles are spastic – due to upper motor neurone damage in MND or MS – cramp and spasm may be troublesome. Careful positioning and physiotherapy are helpful and muscle relaxant drugs may be tried (see Box 2).

All these drugs may cause drowsiness and may reduce mobility (as lower limb spasticity may allow some mobility and if this is reduced walking may be more difficult).

> **Box 2: Treatment of muscle cramps**
>
> Baclofen 5 mg–20 mg TDS/QDS
> Tizanidine 2 mg–24 mg/day
> Dantrolene 25 mg–100 mg QDS
> Diazepam 5 mg nocte increasing slowly

Botulinum toxin injections can be helpful if spasticity is localised to one muscle group.

Tissue Pressure Pain

If a patient is immobile and remains in one position for some time they may experience discomfort and the insidious onset of pain developing slowly over time. Good positioning and regular help in movement is essential but analgesics are often also required. The WHO analgesic ladder, developed for cancer pain, is a good guide to their use in neurological disease – see Chapter 10. Opioids are often helpful and experience, particularly in MND, has shown that they can be used effectively and safely [25].

Neuropathic Pain

Some neurological disorders affect the sensory nervous system causing a number of pain syndromes, including allodynia and hyperalgesia. For instance, in MS paroxysmal pains, similar to trigeminal neuralgia, are common and may require treatment with anticonvulsant drugs used as analgesic adjuvants (see Chapter 10 (Pain and Its Management) for more information).

Breathlessness and Respiratory Issues

Patients with neurological disease may develop problems with respiration for several reasons see Box 3.

Box 3: Causes of breathlessness

- Swallowing problems – may lead to aspiration pneumonia.
- Posture – a person who is wheelchair or bed-bound may have restricted chest movement and hypoventilation and develop stasis pneumonia.
- Weakness of respiratory muscles – the diaphragm and intercostal muscles, particularly in MND and Duchenne muscular dystrophy (DMD). This may cause breathlessness but may present as respiratory failure without much breathlessness, with symptoms of orthopnoea, poor sleep due to arousals caused by hypoxia, dreams, morning headache due to carbon dioxide retention, non-refreshing sleep, anorexia and feeling unwell or other sleep issues, such as nocturia as an arousal at night may be misconstrued as the need to go to pass urine.
- Coexistent cardiac or lung pathology. Common co-morbidities may be present such as chronic obstructive pulmonary disease and cardiac failure. Additionally, patients with DMD have an associated cardiomyopathy, and are at risk of arrhythmias and muscle weakness if given diuretics which reduce potassium levels.

Management

- Infection – appropriate antibiotics and physiotherapy. If there is evidence of aspiration a full assessment of swallowing and consideration of alternative feeding methods should be considered, including gastrostomy.
- Respiratory muscle weakness – careful positioning: if the diaphragm is affected, patients may find lying flat distressing and raising the head of the bed may be helpful. The NICE Guideline on MND suggests early discussion of the issues when monitoring of ventilatory capacity is started, so that discussions are not rushed in an emergency situation when there is increasing respiratory failure [3]. Respiratory support, using non-invasive ventilation (NIV), may be appropriate in MND and DMD and has been shown to reduce symptoms, at least initially, and to improve quality of life in MND [26]. The discussion of the risks and benefits may be complex. Many people find the mask difficult to tolerate, and dependence and increasing disability are likely. It should be made clear that the NIV does not alter the progression of the disease. Life may be prolonged but with increasing disability, and although the patient's quality of life may be maintained this continued treatment during disease progression may cause distress and strain on the family. Discussion of future steps (see Box 4) should therefore be encouraged before starting NIV and in ongoing care [27, 28] as part of the wider consideration of advance care planning. This may at any stage lead to an Advance Decision to Refuse Treatment (ADRT) (see Chapter 9), perhaps covering circumstances in which the person would want the NIV to be withdrawn, or to a statement of wishes and values that will serve to inform future decisions if cognitive or communication failure or progressive fatigue compromise their ability to participate in decision-making.

Box 4: Areas to cover when considering starting non-invasive ventilation

- Continued disease progression in spite of NIV and that while it may prolong life it will not prevent death
- Likelihood of increasing ventilator dependence in the future
- Ceilings of care and escalation to tracheostomy ventilation, if it is available or if it is raised by patient or family
- Consideration of future withdrawal of ventilation if it is no longer wanted, no longer tolerated, or no longer working, or if it becomes incompatible with other goals

These may be hard topics to raise and require good communication skills, but patients and families often find it reassuring and helps them plan

---

Some patients may have invasive ventilation (IV), with a tracheostomy. People with MND may receive a tracheostomy when they present as an emergency with respiratory failure, before the diagnosis has been made. Some people may request elective IV, although this is rare in the UK, whereas internationally the prevalence of IV is higher – in Japan it is up to 38% [29]. Similar discussions should be undertaken, particularly as IV leads to increased burden and distress for the caregivers [30]. Withdrawal should also be discussed.

Discussions about cessation of ventilatory support are complex and the process of withdrawal is difficult for all concerned. Although the withdrawal of a treatment that a person no longer wishes, at their direct request or in a clear advance care plan, is both ethical and legal, the procedure may feel like assisting dying [31, 32]. Moreover, to prevent distress at withdrawal, medication may be necessary beforehand, or available at the time of withdrawal, to ensure that the person does not become distressed. The professionals involved may need support and there are guidelines available [33] and the need for support of everyone is important [31, 32].

• Medication is helpful in alleviating the subjective experience and possible distress of breathlessness:
  o Benzodiazepines, such as Diazepam 2–5 mg TDS or sublingual Lorazepam 500 micrograms to 1 mg for acute situations
  o Opioids, such as regular Morphine elixir 2.5–5 mg up to every 4 hours

Careful titration of medication is necessary to ensure the symptoms are effectively managed, without over-sedation. Depending on the pattern of symptoms and the response, administration may be either regularly or as required.

• Cough may be troublesome for patients with respiratory muscle weakness, or where posture reduces the ability to produce a good cough. Careful physiotherapy assessment will help in ensuring the cough is as effective as possible. The use of breath stacking or mechanical cough assist devices may be considered [3].

Mucolytics (such as Carbocisteine 500mg TDS) and nebulised saline may be helpful if the secretions are thick. Small doses of opioids, such as morphine elixir 2.5–5 mg every 4 hours, may be considered. Anticholinergic drugs used to reduce the volume of secretions (see below) may make them more tenacious and harder to clear.

• Inspiratory stridor develops in about 30% of people with MSA and can be distressing. Continuous positive airways pressure (CPAP) can be helpful. Quick acting benzodiazepines, such as sublingual Lorazepam, can be helpful in reliving the distress. Tracheostomy may also be considered. Sleep apnoea may also be seen in this patient group, and again CPAP may be helpful.

Nutrition and Dysphagia

Swallowing difficulties are very common. There may be involvement of muscles in the chewing, handling of the bolus of food in the mouth, moving the bolus to the pharynx or in swallowing itself. Other problems may contribute to nutritional failure, such as upper limb weakness and respiratory failure, and assessment by the occupational therapist may help to overcome these problems. Careful assessment by a speech and language therapist and dietitian is essential and videofluoroscopic examination of swallowing may be helpful.

Management

Other causes of dysphagia, such as oral and oesophageal candidiasis, should be excluded and treated appropriately. Following assessment, dietary advice from the speech and language therapist and dietitian is helpful – often a custard-consistency is easiest to swallow and high calorific value foods should be encouraged. As dysphagia worsens, education of carers – both family and professional – is helpful to ensure food with the best consistency for the person is presented in the most appropriate way.

If there is increasing difficulty, weight loss, and significant risk of aspiration, alternative methods of nutrition may be considered. Nasogastric feeding is rarely used, except for short-term use in a crisis situation. Percutaneous endoscopic gastrostomy (PEG) or percutaneous radiological gastrostomy (PRG) or per-oral image guided gastrostomy (PIG) may be considered – see Chapter 11. This can be a very difficult decision for patients and their families and should be discussed early in the disease progression, rather than in an emergency situation. Moreover, the practicalities of a gastrostomy may be more pronounced as the disease progresses, due to immobility or, in MND, respiratory muscle weakness, making the procedure more hazardous. A period of discussion, over several weeks, may allow the patient to discuss the issues and it should always be stressed that the gastrostomy does not, of itself, preclude oral feeding, which may continue, at risk, allowing the taste and pleasure of eating.

Early discussion about the possible cessation of feeding at the end-of-life, or if it is no longer tolerated, is important. Discussion about treatment choices and burdens and benefits should begin before a gastrostomy is formed and feeding started. Continued feeding close to the end-of-life can lead to an increased risk of reflux and aspiration.

However, the gastrostomy may allow hydration and the continuation of medication which may, in turn, allow a family to care for the person at home. As with ventilatory support an ADRT may be considered, specifying future circumstances under which continued feeding would be refused – see Chapter 9.

Drooling

Drooling of saliva may occur if there is reduced swallowing and weakness of facial muscles, causing poor lip control, and neck weakness leading to the head falling forwards. Drooling is usually due to reduced swallowing of the normal production of saliva, rather than excess production. Patients and their carers, family and professional, may be distressed by this and it can greatly affect communication lead to isolation, due to embarrassment. It is a common symptom – affecting 40% of MND and 65% of PD patients [17, 34].

The action of some anticholinergics drugs (including tricyclics) is on the watery component. For some patients the reduced volume comes at the expense of dry mouth or thick sticky secretions that are difficult to remove. This balance should be considered before starting, with discussion with patients and families, careful titration of the dose, and early review and discontinuation if the medication is not tolerated (Box 5).

Constipation

Constipation is a common problem for people with neurological conditions due to many causes: immobility, poor oral intake, medication such as opioids or anticholinergics, damage to the nerve supply to the bowel and the reduced abdominal muscular power needed to strain. There may also be psychosocial aspects – such as embarrassment in asking for the toilet or immobility making the transfer difficult (Box 6).

Box 5: Management of drooling

Careful attention to posture and explanation to the patient and family is essential and may be sufficient. Medication may be necessary:

- Good mouth care, ensuring the mouth and teeth are kept clean
- Anticholinergic medications reduce saliva production:
  - Glycopyrronium bromide – can be given via a PEG as 200 micrograms TDS or by subcutaneous infusion using a syringe driver, up to 1200 micrograms/24 hours
  - Hyoscine Hydrobromide 300 micrograms sublingually TDS
  - Hyoscine Hydrobromide patches 1mg patch changed every 72 hours
- Tricyclic antidepressants, such as amitriptyline, will have the side effect of causing a dry mouth and can be helpful particularly if there is also a depressive illness.
- Botulinum toxin injections into the salivary glands has been shown to be very effective and may reduce symptoms for several weeks or months.
- Local radiotherapy to the salivary glands can be considered, but this is irreversible and the ensuing dryness can be distressing to some people.
- For some patients the saliva can become very sticky and difficult to clear – pineapple chunks, papaya tablets, Carbocisteine, nebulised saline, or botulinum toxin injections can be helpful.

Box 6: Management of constipation

This should address the particular cause of constipation if possible:

- Increased roughage within the diet, including consideration of supplement feeds
- Ensuring hydration and extra fluids – particularly in patients having enteral feeding by gastrostomy
- Encouraging and assisting mobility, and ensuring privacy
- Reduction of constipating medications if possible
- Oral aperients may be necessary

    A combination of a stimulant laxative and softener/osmotic laxative is helpful, particularly if constipating medications such as opioids cannot be withdrawn

        Macrogols (Polyethyelene glycol) 1–3 sachets daily

        Senna 5–10 ml or 1–2 tablets BD

- Rectal measures may be necessary if sphincter control is difficult

    Regular suppositories or enemas may be helpful for some patients

---

Insomnia

There are many causes of poor sleep – pain/discomfort, anxiety, fear of not being able to attract attention due to immobility, cough, orthopnoea/respiratory failure, cramps, fear of incontinence, restless legs, and confusion.

These will vary with disease processes and in Parkinson's disease sleep disorders are very common, often with hallucinations and confusion and may be related to medication and the development of "off periods" [35, 36].

The management of poor sleep should be directed at the underlying cause and may include simple measures, such as a call button or alternative accessible system to allow the patient to call for attention, or medication changes in PD. Opioids can be helpful for immobile patients who develop pain which affects sleep.

Weakness and Mobility

Patients with progressive neurological disease will face many losses, particularly with mobility. Careful assessment by a physiotherapist and occupational therapist, with specialised knowledge of neurological disease, is essential. The provision of equipment to aid daily living requires sensitive communication and should be a gradual process of discussion, rather than the sudden provision of equipment that the person is not prepared to use and may not accept. Careful explanation is necessary together with forward planning, as equipment needs will change as the disease progresses. Any aids should be adaptable to cope with these anticipated changes and to be able to incorporate the use of other equipment, such as NIV or communication aids [3].

Postural hypotension can be very disabling in MSA, when any movement causes dizziness, syncope, nausea, tremulousness, headache, and "coat hanger pain" (pain across the neck and shoulders). Midodrine may be helpful.

Speech and Communication

Speech may be affected by muscle weakness of the mouth and face, leading to slurring, as well as by respiratory weakness, leading to a very quiet voice. However, communication may also be affected by changes in mood, arm mobility and cognitive change and assessment of the issues may be complex. Careful listening to the person is important and allowing them to complete what they want to say – whether this is by speech or by a communication aid. Assisted communication is sometimes slower than speech, but resist the temptation to talk across the person while they are formulating responses. Treat their non-speech communication as you would treat someone's speech and give it your full focus as it unfolds. Some people find it very tiring to complete every word and sentence and find it helpful if you can anticipate and suggest what they want to say. Others, even if it is tiring, find this off-putting and object as strongly to sentences being completed for them as most speaking people do. Ask people's preferences, and follow them.

The speech and language therapist can assess and provide advice on enhancement of communication. The provision of communication aids can be helpful, from "low tech" paper and pencils to computer systems and iPads, which can include the ability to speak the words the person has typed or entered into the system, to high tech "eye gaze" communication aids, when eye movements may be used to operate a computer screen and allows communication even in the most severely disabled person. The voice generated by the communication aid can be similar to the person's own voice, if they have undertaken voice banking - before speech is lost someone can record phrases and this can be used within a computer system to generate a voice, similar to their own. It is important to assess the cognitive abilities when considering communication aids, as if there is cognitive change it may be very difficult to use any aid effectively.

It is extremely important to enable patients to communicate their wishes and fears while speech is present, although this may require encouragement as these are difficult issues to discuss. This makes it easier to continue these discussions later in the disease progression when communication aids are needed. It is important to ensure that all involved in the person's care understand the importance of communication, as most very disabled patients may remain able to express themselves and communicate with the right support.

Restlessness and Agitation

The causes of restlessness and agitation require careful assessment as it could be due to infection, medication, hypoxia, urinary retention, or constipation, as well as part of the disease progression – for instance in PD [34, 35]. There is often more than one cause. Ensuring the environment is quiet and relaxed is important, as well as exclusion and treatment of reversible causes. In PD, psychotic episodes are common and up to 40% of patients may experience hallucinations [34]. The cause may be related to medication given for PD, and titration of the doses is essential. Clozapine and Quetiapine are widely used in PD for treatment of hallucinations. Risperidone or Olanzapine, often in combination with benzodiazepines, may be helpful. Any of these medications should be used with care in PD and related disease as it can cause increased stiffness and distress.

Cognitive Change

Cognitive change is now recognised in many progressive neurological diseases. Up to 40% of people with MND have evidence of frontal lobe dysfunction and 10–15% have fronto-temporal dementia [36]. In PD about 30-40% of patients develop dementia [35]. Dementia is rarer in MSA but slight to moderate cognitive impairment may be seen in

40% [37]. In PSP over 80% will develop dementia and many will show cognitive change earlier [38]. In MS 40–50% show cognitive change [39]. The changes may be subtle at first and may not be recognised, although changes in personality may have been noticed by the family and close carers.

Careful assessment is essential, as mild changes may not be recognised. However, there may be effects on decision-making and personality, which may affect care and planning ahead. As there is likely to be progression, with the possible reduction in the capacity in decision-making, advance care planning may need to be discussed early in the disease progression, and sometimes soon after diagnosis. It may be very difficult for patients and their families to cope with looking at a difficult future but if they wish to have influence on their care and decisions about their future care they need to be supported in facing these issues (see Chapter 9).

Psychological, Social and Spiritual Distress

People with progressive neurological disease may experience many emotional and psychological issues as they deteriorate (see Box 7).

Box 7: Psychological and spiritual issues

- Fears about the disease – for instance, much is written about the "distressing nature" of MND and other neurological disease. For others social stigma may be an issue. Good information may be helpful, for instance that produced by some voluntary organisations with a disease-specific focus, and patient and carer forums can be invaluable to some.
- Fears about the future and deterioration.
- Coping with the uncertainty and threat to themselves as people – with possible loss of speech and cognition [40]. Careful listening and explanation by the MDT may be able to help patients cope with these issues.
- Inconsistent information – this may come from various teams and many different professionals and it is important to aim to keep clear communication, often through one main MDT which undertakes monitoring and assessment, and through having common approaches to decisions that are shared across networks of services.
- Existential distress due to the loss of function and autonomy and the fears of death. The aim of care should be to enable patients and families to maintain their quality of life. This includes supporting their adjustment to a changing reality, and listening to their fears to help cope with these deeper issues [40]. Both for those with faith and those with none spiritual support can be very helpful in coping with such questions as "why me?"

Depression and Anxiety

Any person with a progressive neurological disease, knowing that the progression will continue and death ensue may have a low mood as part of their adjustment to their situation. Many will develop a depressive illness, estimated as 20-30% in MND and 40% in PD. It may be difficult to make the diagnosis when the patient has severe communication issues and possible cognitive change [35, 36].

Listening to the patient and family and providing counselling support is important. Antidepressant medication may be useful:

- Amitriptyline may be considered, particularly if there is drooling, pain, or poor sleep – at doses of 25—150 mg at night.
- Citalopram 10–20 mg OD has fewer side effects and may be helpful for a patient with emotional lability (in MND) or safer if there is coexistent cardiac disease (for instance in DMD).

As the disease progresses anxiety is common, as fears about extreme debility and dying develop. Listening, information sharing, and correction of misperceptions together with acknowledgement and appropriate reassurances and action plans are vital. Behavioural or cognitive therapies may be helpful and benzodiazepines, such as Temazepam at night or Diazepam, 5–10 mg at night, may be used.

Carer Support

The demands on families and close carers of people with progressive neurological disease can be profound – physically, psychologically, financially, and emotionally. There are often multiple losses faced by both the patient and family with great changes of roles within family units. This is particularly seen when speech and communication are difficult and/or cognitive changes occur, adding increased stresses of all concerned. They will face the similar issues described above – of uncertainty, barriers to communication and personhood, inconsistent information, and existential distress [39]. Families and caregivers may need much support and explanation, in their own rights, as well as enabling them to provide care to the patient.

There may be specific issues for some families, when there is a clear genetic cause, such as in Huntingdon's disease (HD) or in familial motor neurone disease (MND) with a known mutation. It may be possible for family members to have predictive testing which will enable them to know if they are at risk of developing the disease later in life. This predictive testing should only take place with careful genetic counselling, both before and after testing, as there are many implications for someone with a positive test, including coping with uncertainty, consideration of family planning, discussing the test and diagnosis with the wider family who may also be at risk, financial and insurance consequences and planning for future care. These issues may become more prominent as the underlying genetic background of neurological diseases becomes clearer over the coming decades.

Following the death of the person there may be many varying feelings – including ambivalence as there is sadness at the loss, yet relief that the challenges of caring have ended, and the guilt that is often associated with that relief. All involved need time to talk and the primary health care team are well placed to provide the ongoing support and care.

Professional Carers

Many of the challenges and stresses faced by families may be experienced by the professional carers as well. They may feel hopelessness and despondency at seeing the progression of the disease, together with the issues of uncertainty over the timelines of deterioration, loss of personhood of the patient and the existential distress [40]. Involvement in decisions to withdraw life sustaining treatment such as ventilatory support is difficult for many staff, more so because it is sometimes required of teams who rarely experience it. The team approach, including the support and liaison with other teams, is very helpful and discussion and sharing of the feelings experienced in caring for the patient and their family is essential [33]. Regular team meetings when the issues can be shared are helpful and following the death a debriefing meeting allows the ambivalent feelings of team members to be expressed and shared, so that team members are not isolated. Guidance and peer support from teams elsewhere who have experienced similar challenges can help.

End-of-Life Care

People with progressive neurological death will face death, varying from a period of 2–3 years in MND to perhaps many decades in MS, when life may be shortened by only a few years (see Table 1). The joint EAPC / EAN Consensus Statement encourages early discussion about deterioration and dying, particularly if communication or cognition may be compromised later [6]. Moreover, there may be particularly pertinent opportunities to discuss the issues of dying when new interventions are suggested, such as gastrostomy or ventilatory support. At these times it is

necessary to discuss future choices, including end-of-life, to enable informed decisions about the intervention [3].

It is important to recognise that a patient is deteriorating and for this to trigger discussions and preparations for the end-of-life. This need may be identified before patients and families would prefer to discuss it, and clinicians must be skilled in their approach to the issue. Discussion should not be forced on patients and families who do not want it, but it is very important that the opportunity is offered. It should be explained why the discussion is proposed and what the risks might be if it is delayed, such as losing the opportunity to influence their future care. Some people with a preference not to consider the future nonetheless decide to discuss it once they know and understand the benefits of doing so. Others will continue to take an approach to decision-making in the moment or by others.

Recognition of progression may be difficult when there is a slow progression and fluctuating condition, such as in PD. Several ways have been suggested for recognising the later stages of neurological disease (see Box 8).

Key considerations in relation to the end-of-life phase are found in Box 9 (see Chapter 20 for more detail).

Box 8: Recognition of the end-of life phase

- Triggers of consideration of end-of-life:
  - Swallowing problems
  - Recurring infection (particularly aspiration pneumonia)
  - Marked decline in physical status
  - First episode of aspiration pneumonia
  - Cognitive difficulties
  - Weight loss
  - Significant complex symptoms [2]

  These have been shown to increase towards death [41] and the terminal stage could be recognised in 72% of patients [42].

- The "Surprise Question" suggested by the Gold Standards Framework – "Would you be surprised if this patient died in the coming 6 to 12 months?" If the answer to this is "No," this would suggest that the patient could deteriorate and die soon. The Proactive Identification Guidance also provides triggers to consider the end-of-life phase, similar to those outlined earlier (goldstandardsframework.org.uk/pig).

- The Supportive and Palliative Care Indicators Tool (SPICT ™) (see Chapter 1) suggests clinical indicators to help identify people who are deteriorating and for neurological disease these are: progressive deterioration in physical and/or cognitive function, speech and swallowing problems, recurrent aspiration pneumonia, respiratory failure (spict.org.uk/the-spict/).

Hastened Death

People with progressive neurological disease may wish to talk about hastened death – euthanasia and physician assisted dying. These are not legal in the UK and clinicians should be careful to act only in line with relevant law and regulations and do nothing that is intended to hasten death. In some jurisdictions they can be provided legally, within certain criteria, which again should be carefully observed. There are many fears of the mode of dying with neurological disease – including pain, breathlessness, "choking" and distress – and these are widely discussed, particularly when the case for a change in the law allowing assisted dying is presented. Openness and listening to the concerns of the person, and their family, is important so that any issues can be addressed. For instance, discussion of the very small actual risk of choking in MND, ensuring that there are ways to facilitate communication, the provision of a DNACPR form and other measures to protect the person from unwanted interventions or unwanted prolongation of life, the provision of anticipatory medication for any distress and support from the MDT may help to alleviate the fears and reduce the wish for a hastened death (see Chapter 6 – Ethics in Palliative Care).

Conclusion

The care of patients with progressive neurological disease requires:

- Involvement of palliative care services earlier in the disease progression – to allow planning and discussion while the person can communicate and has no cognitive change and can communicate well
- Involvement of many disciplines – working together as a team
- Co-ordinated care
- Careful assessment and management of symptoms
- Support for patients and their families – physical, psycho-social, and spiritual
- Proactive care – and preparation for symptoms or problems that may occur
- Collaboration with voluntary agencies and charities who can provide specialist advice and support
- Good team working and support

Disease Specific Organisations

Motor Neurone Disease Association for England and Wales	mndassociation.org
MND Scotland	mndscotland.org.uk
Multiple Sclerosis Society	mssociety.org.uk
Multiple Systems Atrophy Trust	msatrust.org.uk
Parkinson's UK	parkinsons.org.uk
Progressive Surpranuclear Palsy Association	pspassociation.org.uk
Huntington's Disease Association	hda.org.uk
Muscular Dystrophy UK	musculardystrophyuk.org

References

1. Department of Health. (2005). *National Service Framework for Long-term Conditions*.
2. End of Life Care Programme. (2010). *End of Life Care in Neurological Conditions: A Framework for Implementation*.
3. National Institute for Health and Care Excellence. (2016). NICE guidance on motor neurone disease. NICE. www.nice.org.uk/NG42 (accessed 19 October 2022).
4. National Institute for Health and Care Excellence. (2017). NICE guidance on Parkinson's disease in adults. NICE. www.nice.org.uk/NG71 (accessed 21 October 2022).
5. GBD 2016. (2019). Neurology Collaborators. Global, regional, and national burden of neurological disorders, 1990-2016: a systematic analysis for the Global Burden of Disease Study 2016. *Lancet Neurology* 18: 459-480.
6. Oliver, D.J., Borasio, G.D., Caraceni, A. et al. (2016). A consensus review on the development of palliative care for patients with chronic and progressive neurological disease. *European Journal of Neurology* 23: 30-38.
7. Aridegbe, T., Kandler, R., Walters, S.J. et al. (2013). The natural history of motor neuron disease: assessing the impact of specialist care. *Amyotrophic Lateral Sclerosis* 14: 13-19.
8. Rooney, J., Byrne, S., Heverin, M. et al. (2015). A multidisciplinary clinic approach improves survival in ALS: a comparative study of ALS in Ireland and Northern Ireland. *Journal of Neurology, Neurosurgery, and Psychiatry* 86: 496-503.
9. Creutzfeldt, C.J., Robinson, M.T., and Holloway, R.G. (2016). Neurologists as palliative care providers. Communication and practice approaches. *Neurology* 6: 40-48.
10. Bede, P., Oliver, D., Stodart, J. et al. (2011). Palliative care in amyotrophic lateral sclerosis: a review of current international guidelines and initiatives. *Journal of Neurology, Neurosurgery, and Psychiatry* 82: 413-418.
11. Gao, W., Crosby, V., Wilcock, A. et al. (2016). Psychometric properties of a generic patient-centred palliative care outcome measure of symptom burden for people with progressive long term neurological conditions. *PLOS ONE* 11 (10): e0165379.
12. Higginson, I.J., Hart, S., Burman, R. et al. (2008). Randomised controlled trial of a new palliative care service: compliance, recruitment and completeness of follow-up. *BMC Palliative Care* 7: 7. doi:10.1186/1472-684X-7-7.
13. Higginson, I.J., McCrone, P., Hart, S. et al. (2009). Is short-term palliative care cost-effective in multiple sclerosis? A randomized phase II trial. *Journal of Pain and Symptom Management* 38: 816-826.
14. Solari, A., Giordano, G., Patti, F. et al. (2017). Randomised controlled trial of a home based palliative approach for people with severe muliple sclerosis. *Multiple Sclerosis Journal* 24: 663-674.
15. Veronese, S., Gallo, G., Valle, A. et al. (2017). Specialist palliative care improves the quality of life in advanced neurodegenerative disorders: Ne-PAL, a pilot randomized controlled study. *BMJ Supportive & Palliative Care* 7: 164-172.
16. Gao, W., Wilson, R., Hepgul, N. et al. (2020). Effect of short-term integrated palliative care on patient-reported outcomes among patients severely affected with long-term neurological conditions. A randomized controlled trial. *JAMA open Network* 3 (8): e2015061. doi:10.1001/jmamnetworkopen.2020.15061.
17. Oliver, D. (1996). The quality and care of symptom control – the effects on the terminal phase of ALS/MND. *Journal of the Neurological Sciences* 139 (suppl): 134-136.
18. Lee, M., Walker, R.W., Hildreth, T.J. et al. (2006). A survey of pain in idiopathic Parkinson's disease. *Journal of Pain and Symptom Management* 32: 462-469.
19. Kahraman, T., Ozdogar, A.T., Ertekin, O. et al. (2019). Frequency, type and distribution of pain and related factors in persons with multiple sclerosis. *Multiple Sclerosis and Related Disorders* 28: 221-225.
20. Rana, A.Q., Qureshi, A.R., Siddiqui, O. et al (2019). prevalence of pain in atypical parkinsonism: a systematic review and meta-analysis. *Journal of Neurology* 266: 2093-2102.
21. Sprenger, G.P., van der Zwaan, K.F., Roos, R.A.C. et al. (2019). The prevalence and the burden of pain in patients with Huntington disease: a systematic review and meta-analysis. *Pain* 160: 773-783.
22. Lager, C. and Kroksmark, A.K. (2015). Pain in adolescents with spinal muscular atrophy and Duchenne and Becker muscular dystrophy. *European Journal of Paediatric Neurology* 19: 537-546.
23. Regnard, C., Reynolds, J., Watson, B. et al. (2007). Understanding distress in people with severe communication difficulties: developing and assessing the Disability Distress Assessment Tool (DisDAT). *Journal of Intellectual Disability Research* 51: 277-292.
24. Warden, V., Hurley, A.C., and Volicer, L. (2003). development and psychometric assessment of the Pain Assessment in Advanced Dementia (PAINAD) scale. *Journal of the American Medical Directors Association* 4: 9-15.
25. Oliver, D. (1998). Opioid medication in the palliative care of motor neurone disease. *Palliative Medicine* 12: 113-115.
26. Bourke, S.C., Tomlinson, M., Williams, T.L. et al. (2006). Effects of non-invasive ventilation on survival and quality of life in patients with amyotrophic lateral sclerosis: a randomised controlled trial. *Lancet Neurology* 5: 140-147.
27. Heffernan, C., Jenkinson, C., Holmes, T. et al. (2006). Management of respiration in MND/ALS patients: an evidence based review. *Amyotrophic Lateral Sclerosis and Other Motor Neuron Disorders* 7: 5-15.
28. Oliver, D.J. and Turner, M.R. (2010). Some difficult decisions in ALS/MND. *Amyotrophic Lateral Sclerosis* 11: 339-343.
29. Turner, M.R., Faull, C., McDermott, C.J. et al. (2019). Tracheostomy in motor neurone disease. *Practical Neurology* 19: 467-475.
30. Kaub-Wittemer, D., von Steinbuchel, N., Wasner, M. et al. (2003). Quality of life and psychosocial issues in ventilated

patients with amyotrophic lateral sclerosis and their caregivers. *Journal of Pain and Symptom Management* 24: 890–896.

31. Phelps, K., Regen, E., Oliver, D. et al. (2015). Withdrawal of ventilation at the patient's request in MND: a retrospective exploration of the ethical and legal issues that have arisen for doctors in the UK. *BMJ Supportive & Palliative Care.* doi:10.1136/bmjspcare-2014-000826.

32. Faull, C., Rowe-Haynes, C., and Oliver, D. (2014). Issues for palliative medicine doctors surrounding the withdrawal of non-invasive ventilation at the request of a patient with motor neurone disease: a scoping study. *BMJ Supportive & Palliative Care* 4: 43–49.

33. Association for Palliative Medicine. (2015). Withdrawal of assisted ventilation at the request of a patient with motor neurone disease: guidance for professionals. Association for Palliative Medicine of Great Britain and Ireland.

34. Lee, M.A., Prentice, W.M., Hildreth, A.J. et al. (2007). Measuring Symptom Load in Idiopathic Parkinson's Disease. *Parkinsonism & Related Disorders* 13: 284–289.

35. Poewe, W. (2008). Non-motor symptoms in Parkinson's disease. *European Journal of Neurology* 15 (Suppl 1): 14–20.

36. Goldstein, L. (2006). Control of symptoms – cognitive dysfunction. In: *Palliative Care in Amyotrophic Lateral Sclerosis from Diagnosis to Bereavement*, 2e (ed. D. Oliver, G.D. Borasio, and D. Walsh). Oxford: Oxford University Press.

37. Eschlbock, S., Delazer, M., Krismer, F. et al. (2020). Cognition in multiple systems atrophy: a single center cohort study. *Annals of Clinical and Translational Neurology* 7: 219–228.

38. Golbe, L.I. (2014 April). Progressive supranuclear palsy. *Seminars in Neurology* 34: 151–159. doi:10.1055/s-0034-1381736. Epub 2014 Jun 25.

39. Benedict, R.H.B., Amato, M.P., DeLuca, J. et al. (2020). Cognitive impairment in multiple sclerosis: clinical management, MRI, and therapeutic avenues. *Lancet Neurology* 19: 860–871.

40. Gofton, T.E., Chum, M., Schultz, V. et al. (2018). Challenges facing palliative neurology practice: a qualitative analysis. *Journal of the Neurological Sciences* 385: 225–231.

41. Hussain, J., Adams, D., Allgar, V. et al. (2014). Triggers in advanced neurological conditions: prediction and management of the terminal phase. *BMJ Supportive & Palliative Care* 4: 30–37.

42. Hussain, J., Allgar, V., and Oliver, D. (2018). Palliative care triggers in progressive neurological conditions: an evaluation using a multi-centre retrospective case record review and principal component analysis. *Palliative Medicine* 32: 716–725.

43. Agar, M., Currow, D.C., Shelby-James, T.M. et al. (2008). Preference for place of care and place of death in palliative care: are these different questions? *Palliative Medicine* 22: 787–795.

15 Palliative Care for Infants, Children and Young People

Yifan Liang

Paediatric palliative care (PPC) was recognised as a sub-specialty of paediatrics, in the UK, in 2009. Since this time, there has been an increase in the number of children with life-limiting conditions with an increase in those who are technology dependent [1, 2]. Paediatric palliative care can be daunting for clinicians because of challenging symptoms, potential ethical dilemmas, and the emotional labour of caring for dying children and their families. The majority of children and their families can be cared for in primary and secondary care with support from a paediatric palliative specialist team. An important principle of caring for these most fragile children is to work collaboratively with colleagues and seek advice when the situation is uncertain or challenging. This chapter can only provide a broad overview, but will hopefully encourage, inspire, and stimulate further exploration and learning.

Recipients of Care

The core of PPC is "an active and total approach to care, embracing physical, emotional, social and spiritual elements. It focuses on enhancement of quality of life for the child and support for the family and includes management of symptoms, provision of respite and care through death and bereavement" [3]. It aims for the best quality and enjoyment of life, as well as planning for a good death.

Life-limiting and life-threatening conditions (LLC) affecting children and young people are those from which there is no reasonable hope of cure and from which they will die in childhood or young adulthood. The conditions have been categorised broadly into four groups; Box 1 [4]:

"Life-limitation" is considered for children whom are thought unlikely to reach their 18th birthday, however precise prognostication is not necessary for referral. There are more than 300 diagnoses that these categories encompass

[5]. The largest diagnostic group are children with congenital anomalies, with the greatest need for palliative care support in the first year of life. Prevalence for these conditions is higher in South Asian and black populations (48 and 42 per 10,000) compared with the white population (27 per 10,000) [1]. Families of most deprivation also have higher prevalence. Nearly a third of neonatal deaths are as a result of congenital abnormalities (545 of 1,784 deaths in England and Wales, 2018) [6].

> ## Box 1: Life-limiting and life-threatening conditions (LLC) affecting children and young people.
>
> ### Group 1
> Life-threatening conditions for which curative treatment may be feasible but can fail
> Examples: cancer, organ failures of heart, liver, kidney.
>
> ### Group 2
> Conditions where premature death is inevitable but may include long periods of intensive treatment aimed at prolonging life and allowing participation in normal activities.
> Examples: cystic fibrosis, Duchenne muscular dystrophy.
>
> ### Group 3
> Progressive conditions without curative treatment options Treatment is exclusively palliative and may commonly extend over many years.
> Examples: Batten disease, certain severe metabolic conditions.
>
> ### Group 4
> Irreversible but non-progressive conditions causing severe disability, leading to susceptibility to health complications and an increased likelihood of premature death.
> Examples: severe cerebral palsy, complex disabilities, such as following brain or spinal cord injury.

Handbook of Palliative Care, Fourth Edition. Edited by Richard Kitchen, Christina Faull, Sarah Russell and Jo Wilson.
© 2024 John Wiley & Sons Ltd. Published 2024 by John Wiley & Sons Ltd.

A hurdle to children and families accessing palliative expertise can be clinicians' or families' reluctance to consider it. Children and families can interface and benefit from palliative care at many different points until they die. These points may include support at diagnosis, severe life-threatening deteriorations in condition from which recovery may be possible, episodes of difficult symptomatology and end-of-life care. Hence, PPC may support some children and families over many years, overlapping with disease-oriented treatment and may include transition to adult services. One growing area is perinatal palliative care, with the involvement of PPC clinicians from the antenatal period, supporting families in decision-making, and memory making during a time when many can feel isolated and bewildered [7].

In the UK, the number of children (0–19 years) with life-limiting conditions has been steadily increasing in recent years with a prevalence rise of 25 to 32 per 10,000 (comparing 2000–2001 to 2009–2010) [1]. Over this time there has been an increase in interventions to treat complications, improve and prolong life, with consequent increased survival. This is illustrated by the increasing use of critical care beds by children with LLC, making up the majority of Paediatric Intensive Care Unit (PICU) admissions (57.6%). Each admission being on average significantly longer in duration than children admitted without LLC; accounting for 72.6% of bed days, and 87.5% of those staying more than 28 days. Although mortality rates in PICU continue to fall, children with LLC also contributed to 72.9% of deaths in PICU [8].

Improved critical care expertise to treat and save lives has also changed family expectations and societal attitudes of what is, and can be, possible for all children. An increasing proportion of LLC children are now technology dependent, forming a large proportion of children requiring long-term ventilation (LTV). In England, there are approximately 250–275 tracheostomy-ventilated and 1000–1300 non-invasive ventilated children in the community [2]. These figures illustrate the changed nature of the paediatric population receiving PPC. It also highlights some of the ethical challenges that can arise balancing burdens and benefits of long-term intensive treatments available. There is a small but increasing number of such cases where the courts are asked to make the final judgements on the ongoing clinical management, particularly the continued use of life sustaining treatment.

Delivery of Care

Palliative care best practice is best enabled by a multi-disciplinary team, with the child and family at the centre. At a minimum this should include their general practitioner, hospital or community Consultant paediatrician, a Consultant trained in paediatric palliative medicine and specialist nurses, with ready access to psychology, family support, paediatric pharmacists and allied professionals (such as speech and language therapists, dieticians, physiotherapy, occupational therapy, play or music specialists, counsellor or psychologists, and social workers) [4, 9]. The universal services of primary care, general and community paediatrics are important in the longevity of their relationships with the child and family. The core PPC team should operate as part of a Managed clinical network where linked groups of health professionals across organisations and services work together in a coordinated way with a more formal management structure to support the delivery of care, to have defined objectives, to share expertise and to have a clear governance framework [10].

In the UK, paediatric palliative provision is geographically variable, with different areas having different availability of medical expertise and community nursing teams. Some locations are further from tertiary services and Consultants in paediatric palliative medicine are not evenly distributed. Community nursing provision varies in what levels of support can be offered, and what hours personnel can be available to families. Some larger teams can provide a robust 24/7 service, others are commissioned for this as necessary for specific end-of-life care, while others only offer daytime weekday cover.

In the UK, the first children's hospice was opened in Oxford in 1982 and now there are over fifty [11]. In general, children's hospices were established as third sector organisations independent from the NHS and most receive very little statutory funding, compared to adult hospices [12]. Most hospices offer respite provision to children with LLC and holistic support to families, and the charity Together for Short Lives can help to locate local services [11]. Some are able to provide additional treatment with allied professionals or complementary therapies while others offer outreach and palliative expertise to the community or hospitals. Support by a hospice has the potential benefit of developing long and deep relationships to support honest conversations, end-of-life care and bereavement care in due course. Some families will travel significant distances to be able to access this support and respite care.

There has rightly been a shift in attitudes to consider the priorities, preferences, and wishes of children with LLC and their families with respect to choices, particularly at the end-of-life [13]. The desire to deliver on this and fulfil wishes has galvanised many to work collaboratively across organisational boundaries, be innovative and "think outside the box". This flexibility in working practices for the benefit of families is a strength of multi-professional palliative care teams.

The majority of children with LLC continue to die in hospital and they contribute to over 70% of deaths in PICU [8]. Most neonatal deaths occur in Neonatal intensive care units, including those diagnosed with LLC. This high frequency of in-patient deaths is due to a combination of factors which include; the trajectory of non-malignant LLC being less predictable and a lack of preparation and planning of families by professionals that their child might be deteriorating or nearing the end-of-life. The availability and level of community-based palliative support available to families also influences the choices available for place of end-of-life care; home, hospice, or hospital. Children's hospices will often prioritise an admission for end-of-life care and this setting provides continuous clinical support which some families may prefer. Supporting choices at the end-of-life is important as studies have shown differences in the psychological sequelae of parents and siblings between those whose children have died at home compared to in hospital [14]. Parents of children who died at home reported stronger relationships within the immediate family, better coping, less residual guilt, and fewer indicators of maladjustment [15]. However, families with better interpersonal communications and stronger relationships also tend to be those who favour end-of-life care at home.

An important role of PPC teams is to coordinate delivery of care and to support families to access a variety of services. This may include support for care packages, sourcing equipment needs, assisting education with care plans, liaising with social workers, and applications for statutory benefits. Discharge planning, particularly when rapidly required at the end-of-life is an important coordinating role.

Transition to adult care can be a daunting time as young people and families leave teams that have cared for them often over many years and then have to get to know new health and social care teams. The process should ideally begin early for example, from the age of 14, and any reluctance from clinicians to handover patients overcome. There exist a number of supporting documents to guide clinicians in this process [16]. The increasing cohort of young adults with LLC has resulted in an improving appreciation on both sides of the age divide of the potential benefits that come with transition to adult services. Adult services, including palliative care, serve much larger populations and so can often deliver care more locally to families, have larger teams and some have more robust out of hours' provision. However, managing child and family expectations at this time is also important; often different aspects of care will be attended to by different services and a larger proportion of the coordination will be by the primary care physician and family themselves.

Other considerations include the changing legal status for adolescents with regards to confidentiality and autonomy. It is important to support adolescents in these changes by a gradual adjustment in communication and health decision-making. The method and degree of adjustment is obviously individual, with the principle being to shift decision-making from parents to the individual adolescent. Parents who wish to continue to be their child's primary spokesperson because of mental incapacity, may choose to formalise this through becoming a court-appointed deputy for personal welfare (in England and Wales) [17].

Significant Discussions

Palliative care often requires discussion about significant issues such as explanation of diagnosis, advance care planning, through to end-of-life care and bereavement support. Clinicians often feel anxious about these discussions, with a fear of "getting it wrong", causing upset for families and worries about their own emotional response. Various frameworks exist to support difficult conversations [18]. Pacing any difficult conversation takes skill and being comfortable with periods of silence when families can absorb or contemplate information is important. Primary and secondary care clinicians are often well placed to have these conversations; indeed, families appreciate honest discussions with those who know them and have been key to their journey.

How, how much, and when to share information with the child and siblings can concern parents and the wider family. Often, there may be a wish to shield and protect the child and siblings from distress and upset and a belief that withholding information is the best decision. These concerns are understandable, however, while acknowledging them, children who are appropriately informed have a chance to adjust and prepare for the end of their life. They will have a better understanding of the illness, feel included in decisions about them, and more likely to consent to treatment options. Disclosure of information also results in improved relationships within the family [18]. In surveys of parents whose child had died of malignancy; those who spoke to their children about death did not regret doing so. In contrast, nearly a third of parents regretted not talking to their child about death, with regret more likely in those who sensed their child was aware of imminent death [19].

Children, particularly those who have experiences of healthcare are often more aware of a change in their own condition or clinical deterioration. For example, children who have grown with a condition (such as cystic fibrosis or Duchenne muscular dystrophy) will often be extremely knowledgeable through personal lived experience, peers, social media, and internet searching. Sometimes, children may have an emotional response more in keeping with their chronological age, particularly if they are fearful or in pain. At other times, children choose not to discuss matters in an attempt to protect and not upset other family members, resulting in collusion. Where possible, collusion should be avoided as, inevitably, children are aware of secrecy and upset resulting in fear and isolation. Openness and honesty, although painful, provides the opportunity for families to come together, share and support each other, the chance to make memories and plan goodbyes [19].

It is important to take the child's developmental stage into consideration so that information is tailored to their age, cognitive developmental stage and understanding of the situation, including health experiences to date. It can be useful to establish with parents the tenets of open, honest conversation and the potential boundaries of information likely to be shared at each episode. Information should be delivered at the pace the child requests, once the query and the reason for the question has been clarified. Facts should be explained with consistent, clear and simple language, avoiding euphemisms and abstract concepts. Children and families value the relationship they have with health professionals; unhurried time when they can assimilate information. Allowing opportunity for children to express their feelings and distress gives validity and reassurance [20].

Older children and young people at the developmental junction of gaining independence in thought, identity and sexuality can find dealing with a life-limiting condition especially challenging [16]. At a time when their peers are considering further education options, increasing financial autonomy and exploring relationships, the contrast to their own lives can be very stark. Some may resent complying with treatments, others may become very angry or depressed, while others may have issues with a changed body image as a consequence of illness. Steadfast encouragement and consistency by the PPC team and continued exploration and support of their thoughts through these times is crucial to their development and acceptance of living with LLC, with an emphasis on "the best life possible". Some young people benefit from referral to specialist psychological support.

Advance care planning is an opportunity to explore the current stage in the journey with families, and to document their wishes. It is looking at what is currently appropriate in the event of deterioration and what might be too burdensome. It is also a chance to think ahead and plan for future deterioration and the end-of-life. Ideally, this planning should involve all the professionals involved in the child's care. It is a clear recommendation and quality standard in the NICE guidance on End-of-life care for children [9]. Unlike an adult advance decision (also sometimes called an advance decision to refuse treatment or "living will"), advance care plans (ACP) for children are not legally binding [21].

Discussions often take place over a number of episodes, with explanations of what different support modalities might involve before a consensus is agreed. The ACP is a catalyst for communication and is important to document the discussions and decisions and for parents to know that this should be revisited if the situation changes, annually as a minimum. Recent admission to critical care is often a stimulus to ACP writing, giving both families and clinicians a tangible indication of current fragility. The uncertainty of whether a particular episode of deterioration is the "final" one, is one of the factors resulting in children with LLC making up nearly 73% of deaths in PICU, and the majority continuing to die in hospital. 7% of children with LLC admitted to PICU die in the year following discharge [8].

Living with uncertainty is a tension for both families and clinicians and parallel planning is an important tenet; "hoping for the best whilst planning for the worst" [22]. It is key to differentiate between what might be an acute reversible deterioration and progression of the underlying condition during discussions. It is not unusual for children and families to change their views on requesting aggressive intervention as clinical deterioration progresses and supporting their understanding and emotional response to clinical decline is crucial. Parents may feel that they must advocate for their child's access to critical care support and that "everything must be done". A relationship of trust with caregivers is vital to work together to ensure "everything right for the child" is done. More and more intervention is technically possible, but it is a responsibility to ensure there are opportunities to access what will benefit while not prolonging the dying process.

One of the positives of advance care planning is the opportunity to consider the immensely painful situation of their child dying with someone who knows their child and themselves well. A chance to think about what they would consider the best environment and community for their child's death if it could be planned for, providing the PPC team the insight and the privilege of trying to enable a family's wishes. Many families feel empowered by an ACP, in particular having their wishes respected by professionals of different agencies or settings, and not needing to repeatedly revisit the topic [23].

Another positive in speaking honestly is to discover what a family's priorities are, and if they have specific goals they would like to achieve with their child for example, meeting certain relatives, experiences or trips to undertake. These can be real milestones and important memories to bank, particularly for siblings. Older children may appreciate a sense of control in documenting their thoughts in an ACP or an opportunity to think about their own legacy [16]. Many charities exist to try and support wishes for children with LLC.

Symptom Management

Attention to symptom management is important both to "living well" and "dying well". In surveys of children with progressive malignancies, pain was the most common symptom, present in over 90% of children in the month before death. The most prevalent (more than 50%) other symptoms were weakness, anorexia, weight loss, mobility, nausea, constipation, and vomiting [24]. In non-malignant conditions, with a large range of underlying diagnoses, the symptom profile is more varied, most commonly these are pain, sleep problems, and feeding difficulties. Other common issues are constipation, respiratory problems, seizures, and changes in alertness or interaction. The burden of symptoms can be significant; suffered by a large proportion of children, frequently and sometimes for prolonged periods [25].

Most symptom management only requires the use of a few well-known medications. However, difficult or uncontrolled symptoms affect not only the way a child dies, but

also the bereavement experience of the family so the clinician should consider asking for specialist advice. Medication use in paediatric palliative care is challenged by many medications being unlicensed, with use and doses extrapolated from adult practice [26]. Consequently, medication preparations are often more suited for adults, with tablets or larger dose sizes. Research into medications is ongoing so it is important to seek current references with the most up to date information.

Different formularies exist to assist; the most commonly used in the UK is that of the Association of Paediatric Palliative Medicine formulary [26]. This is regularly updated and peer-reviewed. A guiding principle is "start low, go slow" (with dosages). Many children with LLC are small for age so prescribing by weight is imperative. Polypharmacy is common and drug metabolism (absorption and breakdown) may be compromised, all leading to the need for increased caution. Repeated evaluation is important, and careful titration for the desired effect is always preferable to encountering excessive side effects with generous initial prescribing. It is strongly advised that practitioners do not to prescribe outside their expertise. There is an increasing number of clinicians with specialist expertise in paediatric palliative medicine who can provide specialist paediatric palliative care advice; see Box 2.

Box 2: Principles for effective symptom management [27]

- Listen to the child and their parents
- Communicate closely with professionals across agencies and settings
- Prescribe carefully (by weight), and cautiously (with doses)
- Review effect and re-evaluate frequently
- Pro-actively manage medication side effects
- Know your limits, ask for support and advice early

Routes of Administration

Paediatricians have always been proactive in looking at alternative routes of medication administration. When enteral tolerance is reduced, or speed of onset of action is important, mucosal absorption is a convenient and acceptable route for many children. Buccal midazolam at low doses can ease muscle spasm and at higher doses is a useful anxiolytic in emergency situations such as major terminal haemorrhage or to treat a prolonged seizure. Intranasal or buccal opioids are fast acting for breakthrough pain. For longer duration action, the transdermal route is useful for a number of different medications such as hyoscine, clonidine and opioids. When the enteral route is no longer available continuous subcutaneous syringe drivers can be used to deliver medication effectively [28].

Pain

Pain is the most commonly encountered symptom [29], but is responsive to treatment in the vast majority of cases. As with all symptoms, careful evaluation provides the background for logical prescribing. The likely causes of physical pain will depend on the diagnosis and teasing these out will aid prescribing. Sources of pain in malignancy include neuropathic pain from nerve involvement or compression, ischaemic pain from within the tumour mass, visceral stretch pain, headache from raised intracranial pressure, and tumour ulceration. In severe neuro-disability, pain may be from dystonia, spasticity, gastro-oesophageal reflux, hip subluxation, or scoliosis. It is also important to consider additional acute sources of pain such as urinary tract infections, otitis media, pressure areas, or fractures.

The evaluation should also include identifying contributions of physical, emotional, social, and spiritual components into the whole experience of "total pain" [30]. Prolonged and chronic pain can have wide ranging effects, including affecting sleep, concentration, mental health, and relationships with both friends and family. Often these need to be addressed in tandem by a wider multi-disciplinary team (MDT) such as family support workers, play or music therapists, or psychologists.

Older, verbal children will be able to self-report and there are a number of validated measures [31]. Assessment of pain in non-verbal children can be challenging, and their carers are usually the most familiar with their pain behaviours. Examples of pain behaviours may include characteristic vocalisations or facial expressions, physiological changes as well as less typical pain behaviours specific to the child [32].

There also exist a number of pain assessment tools such as FLACC (Face, Legs, Activity, Cry, Consolability) [33], PPP (Paediatric pain profile) [34] and these should be used in conjunction with the knowledge of carers of individual pain responses. Knowing when the pain occurs can inform prescribing; what the level of background pain is and whether this fluctuates, whether there is incident or procedural pain triggered by predictable stimuli, or breakthrough pain which occurs unexpectedly or before the next routine analgesic dose is due.

The World Health Organisation analgesic ladder was introduced in 1986 to guide the use of analgesics, but this has since been revised since the removal of codeine from paediatric use [35]. Following the first non-opioid step (paracetamol and non-steroidal anti-inflammatory drugs) is now the use of low dose strong opioids (for moderate pain) before the use of strong opioids for severe pain. Clinicians and families are often wary of using opioids, however appropriate use is generally safe. Some worry that death will be hastened but when pain is well managed, patients that are more comfortable may live longer. Respiratory depression is rare if there is careful titration against pain severity. Physiological dependency can occur, requiring increased doses for effectiveness and signs of withdrawal if stopped abruptly. However, when no longer required, opioids can be safely weaned. Such dependency is very different from addiction, which is a complex psychological craving and does not occur with appropriate use. The dose of opioids can increase markedly, especially in the management of end-stage malignancies with sometimes surprising levels of tolerance. Safety advice for children and families are important to emphasise; recreational alcohol will compound respiratory depression, safe storage of medication and careful disposal of used patches are imperative.

The principles of regular analgesia for background pain, rather than waiting for pain to occur before giving analgesia also apply to children. Newer preparations of sustained release enteral morphine and patches with smaller equivalent doses of morphine facilitate conversion from short acting opioids to more convenient administration. Children and families appreciate instructions on what can be given if there is breakthrough pain or before a predictable procedure to minimise distress. Setting realistic targets of what is achievable with medications is important communication with families; the aim for symptom reduction to enable more participation in activities, rather than necessarily total control. It is also important to stress that it may take some time to reach this, as careful titration needs to be slower, particularly in children who may be more sensitive to adverse effects.

Pre-emptive prescribing for opioid side effects and careful explanation prevents issues developing and loss of confidence in new medications. Younger children are generally less nauseated by opioids than older children, and almost all experience some accommodation to this over a few days. Somnolence also gradually improves, and reassurance is important, as this is a common reason for older children discontinuing analgesia. Constipation does not improve with prolonged use and is managed with a stimulant laxative (rather than just a softener). Pruritus is uncommon and occurs particularly with higher dosages; it can be managed with antihistamines [36].

Non-pharmacological management of pain should occur in parallel to medication use. Musculoskeletal pain can be significantly eased by careful positioning (such as with sleep systems), wheelchair adaptations and attention to pressure relief. Additional therapies such as physiotherapy, hydrotherapy, and massage can also significantly reduce musculoskeletal pain. Incident and procedural pain can be minimised with the help of play therapy, guided imagery, and cognitive behavioural therapy [37, 38].

Adjuvant analgesia should be considered alongside opioid use. Management of neuropathic pain includes consideration of a different ladder of medications [32] with gabapentinoids the most commonly used first step. If this is insufficient, further steps include the consideration of tricyclic antidepressants then NMDA antagonists such as ketamine or methadone. Gabapentinoids and NMDA antagonists should only be prescribed by those experienced in their use, accompanied by adequate patient oversight.

For pain secondary to spasticity or dystonia other adjuncts to consider include muscle relaxants, benzodiazepines, and botulinum injections [32]. Pain from malignancy may benefit from targeted radiotherapy or pulsed steroids. Continual high dose steroid use should be avoided whenever possible due to significant side effects. If pain control continues to be difficult, review should include compliance with the suggested regime, pain from potential new sources or increasing side effects. It may be that further dose titration is needed, but there should also be an awareness of possible hyperaesthesia which can occur with increasing opioid doses (when pain worsens with increasing doses). Sometimes psychological aspects causing fear, anxiety, hyperarousal, and an anticipatory state mean pain is not adequately controlled until these are addressed. Chronic pain can result in an up-regulation of receptors and the addition of gabapentinoids or clonidine can be useful as opioid-sparing agents [32, 39].

Gastrointestinal Symptoms

Gastrointestinal symptoms are the next most commonly encountered group of symptoms and include nausea and vomiting, constipation, feed intolerance, and visceral pain [29, 32]. Evaluation of nausea should include trying to work out the most likely cause as this guides treatment

options. Potential sources include gastric stasis and reduced intestinal motility, toxins or chemical disturbances, the vestibular system or psychological aspects such as fear or pain. A receptor model can guide prescribing, as the likely source can be pharmacologically targeted [40].

Drugs, toxins, and chemical disturbances affect the chemoreceptor trigger zone, which is rich in dopamine type 2, and serotonin type 3 receptors. This zone and the other sources of vomiting have neural pathways to the vomiting centre. This centre has histamine, muscarinic acetylcholine, and serotonin receptors. Strong antagonists for receptors are effective antiemetics. Haloperidol works strongly against dopamine receptors and ondansetron against serotonin type 3 receptors and these can be very effective when the chemoreceptor trigger zone is involved. Cyclizine is effective against histamine receptors and hyoscine against acetylcholine receptors. However, the trigger for vomiting is not always clear-cut as there may be a number of contributors. In this situation, a broad based anti-emetic such as Levomepromazine with good action on a variety of receptors is useful; it also has the advantage of good solubility in syringe driver combinations [28].

The symptom burden of nausea and vomiting is often underestimated for children, but can be really miserable for them, causing reduced appetite and affecting nutrition. Effective delivery of an antiemetic is important and a parenteral route may be required until symptoms are under control. Review may indicate a titration dose is needed or the addition of a second antiemetic. Other options in refractory symptoms include the use of steroids or synthetic cannabinoids. Bowel obstruction is rare in the palliative setting for children, but should be managed with a similar drug profile to adult patients with hyoscine, octreotide, and analgesia. Supportive non-medical management of nausea includes avoiding strong food odours and offering small portions of food.

Constipation may be the result of poor motility (most commonly in severe neuro-disability) or secondary to medications (such as anti-chlolinergic medications or opioids). Active prevention with titration of laxatives is important to avoid impaction, which can lead to urinary retention or respiratory embarrassment. Macrogols have become the most commonly used medications in simple childhood constipation. However, many palliative children find the volumes associated with macrogols difficult to tolerate and manage smaller volume stimulants easier. With progressive gut failure, peristalsis can reduce, requiring more active management of constipation.

Gut failure is increasingly encountered in paediatric palliative practice and is particularly seen in older severely neuro-disabled children. This presents with gradual progression of a combination of gastric stasis and worsening intestinal motility, poor feed tolerance, and visceral hyperalgesia. In order to target these factors, prokinetics or jejunal feed administration may be tried. Some success is seen in improving feed tolerance with the utilisation of blended diets and newer prepared feeds are now available. Gabapentinoids have also proved useful in improving feed tolerance [41]. Chronic minor inflammation leads to up-regulation of visceral afferent pathways and visceral hyperalgesia. When this occurs, normal stimuli such as distension or mild gastro-oesophageal reflux can cause significant pain, which can be difficult to manage. Unfortunately, this constellation of symptoms may progress to end stage gut failure where even small volume isotonic fluids are not enterally tolerated and symptom management predominates. The use of parenteral nutrition is another area of ethical debate, which needs consideration on a case-by-case basis. As with all treatment possibilities available, the balance of burdens of intervention versus the potential gains need careful deliberation, particularly as use will not be "a bridge" to a permanent solution.

Seizures

Children may have seizures for a variety of reasons. Many neuro-disabled children have long-standing epilepsy that may be made worse with fever, infection, lack of sleep, or other inter-current stresses. Some children develop seizures as their condition worsens for example, neuro-metabolic conditions. For other patients, notably those with brain tumours, seizures may be a risk with disease progression. It is important to establish why seizures are occurring, as this will influence the appropriate management. Children presenting with a suspected seizure should be assessed by a specialist in the diagnosis and management of epilepsies. The nature of epilepsy means accurate diagnosis can be difficult with estimated error rates up to 30% [42].

For some children with epileptic encephalopathy and frequent seizures, it may not be possible or necessary to totally prevent all seizures, particularly if they are short lived and not distressing. For prolonged generalised seizures fast acting benzodiazepines will be commonly used. It is important to assess, plan, and document a personalised seizure management plan, nuanced for the individual child, communicating doses and medications for carers. For children where seizures are likely to be because of disease progression, treatment may also include management with continuous subcutaneous delivery of midazolam and/or phenobarbitone. Such treatment can be continued for some weeks or months, and can sometimes be withdrawn when enteral medications are instituted or adjusted.

Other Symptoms

Fatigue and dyspnoea are less often reported, but common symptoms. Careful pacing of activities and avoidance of "boom and bust" cycles of activity can ease fatigue. If fatigue is pronounced, honest discussions about priorities to achieve are important. Viewing energy levels as a finite resource for each day can clarify for a child and family what tasks are most important.

Dyspnoea can be a frightening symptom for both the child and family, and calmness and reassurance are integral to management. A hand-held fan near the face, mindfulness techniques and low dose morphine can all improve the sensation of dyspnoea.

Wound management of fungating tumours or pressure areas can be increasingly challenging as a child clinically deteriorates and their nutritional status and mobility decline. Meticulous attention to the risk factors for pressure areas such as shear forces, skin moisture, tissue ischaemia, and nutrition can together make a large difference to the potential for healing. Tissue necrosis can result in exudate, local infection and/or haemorrhage. Odour and body image changes can significantly affect mental well-being. During dressing changes cleaning and removal of adhesive dressings can cause pain and distress needing additional medications.

End-of-Life Care

This area, more than any other, causes worry for clinicians who are acutely aware they have "one chance to get it right". For even the most experienced clinicians, "diagnosing or recognising dying" is not an exact science. Acknowledging uncertainty honestly is important to families. Very often, parents of neuro-disabled children have been told their child is "definitely dying", or "won't recover from this" and yet they have gone on to defy expectations and live, sometimes for many years. It can be hard to trust another pessimistic forecast, and become emotionally "battle-fatigued" from repeated bad news. Clinicians should not feel the need to be certain a patient is dying before considering many of the practical preparations below. The concept of "parallel planning" should be encouraged instead; planning for both the possibility of dying and survival together [3, 22].

Death remains a taboo topic in general conversation, and mostly occurs hidden in healthcare settings with variable portrayals in popular media. Compassionate explanation of what deterioration and dying may look like can be hugely reassuring to a child (if appropriate) and their parents. It is important to explain the physical changes that are expected and the clinical indicators used to diagnose dying. Society generally is now much less familiar with dying; indeed, some clinical staff that have only had paediatric training may not have regular or recent experience of caring for a dying patient. Explanations may include that all the body's processes slow down, requiring less energy and fluids, breathing calms, and there are more periods asleep than awake [43, 44].

Each family will have different priorities and should be encouraged to decide what is right for them, who to have with them, and where they would like to be. This is the chance also to revisit the Advance care plan; to check that their priorities and wishes remain the same. Exploring any faith or spiritual based requirements at the time of death in advance can be helpful. Practical information may also be appreciated such as the steps to take at the time of death; who should be contacted, when, and what the care after death of their child's body should be. This will vary in different geographical locations and families will have different preferences in care after death.

Rationalising treatment plans is also an important aspect; discontinuing unnecessary medications (such as vitamins, or laxatives) if dying is likely. Feeding is very instinctive for parents and careful explanations avert worries that their child may be hungry or starved at a time when feeds are not tolerated. Anticipating symptoms and having written management plans and medications available are important. Some medications and preparations may be harder to obtain in community pharmacies than hospitals. Preparing a family for rare situations is important so they can know what actions can be taken and not be frightened. Sudden situations might include seizures, major haemorrhage, or pneumothorax.

When enteral medications are no longer tolerated and if continuous subcutaneous delivery is needed, explanation of the situation is reassuring to the child and family. Use of a syringe driver is often equated with "the end" for families, but can enable some children to feel better and enjoy life. Some are able to participate in enjoyable activities while attached to a syringe driver, and some improve significantly and can discontinue subcutaneous delivery for a time. There are no differences in syringe driver prescription and preparation for children compared to for adults [41].

When a child dies, there is no immediate rush to verify death. Time and privacy for families at this time enables them to face the moment in the best way for them. After verification, options for place of care include the hospital mortuary, home, a hospice cool room, or a funeral parlour. Some community services have cooling blankets to enable families to keep their child at home for a few days. Sensitive explanation of the changes seen in a body after death helps families to understand the practicalities required to help preserve the body. Families often appreciate guidance on the practicalities following death; obtaining the death certificate, registering the death, and signposting for funeral arrangements.

There is a statutory requirement to report all child deaths in England and Wales to the local Child Death Overview Panel [45]. The process is to understand what happened, why and if there are salient learning points. If the death is not anticipated, the Sudden Unexpected Death in Childhood protocols still apply to children with life-limiting conditions, but investigations may be tailored to account for known diagnoses. In these situations, care should be taken to preserve potential forensic evidence, while compassionately supporting families in their distress. Families can be given the leaflet: *When a Child Dies – a guide for families and carers* [46] to help support them through the Child Death review process.

Bereavement Care

Many families begin to experience the emotions of loss and grief (anticipatory grief) from the time they are given the diagnosis of a life-limiting condition. Loss of dreams they have had for their child and family, loss of current and future well-being. The pain and depression of this experience can be very deep and prolonged. It is also individual, with parents feeling and processing the loss sometimes in very different ways. Families talk of emotional fatigue at being given repeated bad news with each clinical deterioration.

It is important to acknowledge and support families in their anticipatory grief. Emotions may be confused, may surge unpredictably and can be exhausting. Siblings can experience isolation and exclusion as parents come to terms with a diagnosis and deterioration. Supporting siblings in their journey is crucial to their understanding of the situation and mental well-being. Many children's hospices offer sibling support over a prolonged period of time, with the advantage of deeper, longer therapeutic relationships with family support workers.

This emotional support and care for families continues beyond death to support their bereavement. Each grieving family is unique and varies in the level of support they require. Different potential aspects include; deeper spiritual questions (see next section), sibling support, practical needs, and implications for future pregnancies. Some families want to talk and remember with the healthcare team, others see the team as a painful reminder of their loss and prefer minimal involvement. Responding to their wishes, which can fluctuate, is an important role.

With the death of their child, families often talk of the sudden quietness in their lives, and the loss of a community that can include community healthcare teams, special school teams and carers in the home. There can also be an abrupt financial impact with loss of benefits and allowances, which might include recall of accessible vehicles and limited tenancy in adapted housing.

The nature of the life-limiting condition can have implications for both future pregnancies of the parents as well as for siblings. Genetic counselling can be a very significant aspect of ongoing care, particularly if initial diagnostic tests were performed some years earlier. Developments in this field of medicine are rapid, and many new diagnostic tests are emerging.

Children vary widely in their responses to the death of a sibling, depending on their age, the relationship they had, the duration of illness and their personality. During the acute stage of grief, behavioural responses of upset, anger, younger behaviours, or being very mature are all common. Banking and reinforcing memories can be done even after a child has died through activities such as compiling memory books or boxes. This is important to do for siblings of all ages, including those who are very young who will need others to highlight the relationship they had with the deceased as they grow. Bereavement is processing and integrating the life and death of their child into their ongoing story as a family.

A number of charities exist to support children who have been bereaved, with helplines and resources available to purchase. Families value the support of their community as they journey in their bereavement and some choose to access other organisations. Local areas will have different opportunities to support bereavement care and may include children's hospices, adult hospices, bereavement charities, family centres, and counsellors.

Spiritual Care

A child with an LLC often brings into sharp focus bigger questions of meaning, suffering, justice, and hope. These topics in the spiritual dimension can often occur alongside grief, regret, and distress. Healthcare providers may also have similar questions to address themselves (see following section), and feel poorly equipped to speak to concerns. However, a spiritual needs assessment is an important aspect to holistic care [43]. Listening and showing respect for an individual's views form the basis for the assessment; some may have faith-based views, others may be deeply spiritual without acknowledging a formal religion, others may be asking questions for the first time. Some may wish simply to have been heard, others may want more formal support. Support can take many forms and should be tailored; including support from their cultural community, chaplaincy, or religious leader and support to perform or participate in religious rituals. When spiritual concerns are addressed, distress can reduce, coping improves, relationships strengthen, and hope re-emerge.

Staff Support

Working with children with LLC, through death and supporting bereaved families can be emotionally challenging and stressful. It can make us more aware of our mortality and expose weaknesses or our own unresolved hurts and bereavements. It can be stressful clinically managing difficult symptoms and easy to become over-attached. It can also be a hugely rewarding experience, making a real difference to the journey and end-of-life care of children and families.

Integral to maintaining personal resources and resilience is developing self-awareness (particularly through reflective practice and mutual peer support); in which situations we find more emotionally challenging, times and seasons which may remind us of our own losses and bereavements and topics that raise spiritual questions for us. Acknowledging our humanity is not weakness, but rather being sensitive to our own needs. Addressing the needs is important; reflecting on how the experiences with particular families have affected us, helps us to learn from them and strengthens us to care for subsequent families.

When we take the time and energy to do this, we replenish our emotional reserves to not only continue to care for children and their families, but also protect against our own emotional burnout.

Relationships within the palliative care team are crucial to staff support and well-being. Maintaining professional boundaries is often challenging as situations are stressful and highly emotional and altruism is strong amongst staff. Strong, effective and open communication within the team fosters a trusting platform where potential issues can be highlighted and addressed early. Clear working protocols and procedures for a team sets out expectations for families and staff and minimises the risk of overstepping boundaries. Debriefing together as a team provides the opportunity to learn collectively and see how families give back positively, and how these experiences can be used to build on knowledge, resilience, and team capacity. Some teams have also found it beneficial to have regular or *ad hoc* clinical supervision either individually or as a group with chaplaincy or psychology facilitation.

Summary

Children with life-limiting conditions requiring palliative care are a very different population compared to adult recipients of palliative care. Different in terms of their spectrum of diagnoses, setting in families with siblings and different communication needs. However, the tenets of holistic care, compassionate and honest conversations and careful symptom control management apply to patients of all ages. Children and families appreciate care and support given by those with whom they have long-standing relationships. This chapter seeks to support those offering this care and also includes some sources of further information in the references.

References

1. Fraser, L.K., Miller, M., Hain, R. et al. (2012). Rising national prevalence of life-limiting conditions in children in England. *Pediatrics* 129 (4): e923–9.
2. NHS England. Paediatric long term ventilation. https://www.england.nhs.uk/commissioning/wp-content/uploads/sites/12/2015/01/e07-spec-paedi-long-ventilation.pdf (accessed 19 April 2021).
3. Chambers, L. (2018). A guide to children's palliative care. 4th edition. www.togetherforshortlives.org.uk/changing-lives/supporting-care-professionals/resources-and-research (accessed 19 April 2021).
4. Widdas, D., McNamara, K., and Edwards, F. (2013). A core care pathway for children with life-limiting and life-threatening conditions. 3rd Edition. https://www.togetherforshortlives.org.uk/resource/core-care-pathway (accessed 19 April 2021).
5. Hain, R., Devins, M., Hastings, R. et al. (2013). Paediatric palliative care: development and pilot study of a 'Directory' of life-limiting conditions. *BMC Palliative Care* 12 (1): 43.
6. Office for National Statistics (2018). Child and infant mortality in England and Wales. https://www.ons.gov.uk/releases/childandinfantmortalityinenglandandwales2018 (accessed 19 April 2021).
7. Dickson, G. (2019). Perinatal pathway for babies with palliative care needs. 2nd edition. https://www.togetherforshortlives.org.uk/resource/perinatal-pathway-babies-palliative-care-needs (accessed 19 April 2021).
8. Fraser, L.K. and Parslow, R. (2018). Children with life-limiting conditions in paediatric intensive care units: a national cohort, data linkage study. *Archives of Disease in Childhood* 103: 540–547.
9. NICE (2016). End of life care for infants, children and young people with life-limiting conditions: planning and management. https://www.nice.org.uk/guidance/ng61/resources/end-of-life-care-for-infants-children-and-young-people-with-lifelimiting-conditions-planning-and-management-pdf-1837568722885 (accessed 25 April 2021).
10. RCPCH (2012). Bringing networks to life – an RCPCH guide to implementing clinical networks. https://www.rcpch.ac.uk/resources/bringing-networks-life-guide-resources-implement-clinical-networks (accessed 25 April 2021).
11. Together for Short Lives. Children's Hospice Services. https://www.togetherforshortlives.org.uk/wp-content/uploads/2018/01/FamRes-Childrens-Hospice-Services-Factsheet.pdf (accessed 25 April 2021).
12. Together for Short Lives. A more equitable and sustainable approach to statutory funding in England. https://www.togetherforshortlives.org.uk/changing-lives/speaking-up-for-children/policy-advocacy/statutory-funding-in-england (accessed 25 April 2021).
13. National Palliative and End of Life Care Partnership. Ambitions for palliative and end of life care. A national framework for local action 2015–2020. www.endoflifecareambitions.org.uk (accessed 25 April 2021).
14. Mulhern, R.K., Lauer, M.E., and Hoffmann, R.G. (1983). Death of a child at home or in the hospital: subsequent psychological adjustment of the family. *Pediatrics* 71 (5): 743–747.
15. Lauer, M.E., Mulhern, R.K., Schell, M.J. et al. (1989). Long-term follow-up of parental adjustment following a child's death at home or hospital. *Cancer* 63 (5): 988–994.
16. Chambers, L. (2015). Stepping up: a guide to developing a good transition to adulthood for young people with life-limiting and life-threatening conditions. https://www.togetherforshortlives.org.uk/resource/transition-adult-services-pathway (accessed 25 April 2021).
17. Office of the Public Guardian. SD4 how to be a health and welfare deputy (web version).www.gov.uk/government/publications/deputy-guidance-how-to-carry-out-your-

duties/sd4-how-to-be-a-health-and-welfare-deputy-web-version (accessed 25 April 2021).

18. Stein, A., Dalton, L., Rapa, E. et al. (2019). Communication with children and adolescents about the diagnosis of their own life-threatening condition. *Lancet* 393: 1150–1163.

19. Kreicbergs, U., Valdimarsdóttir, U., Onelöv, E. et al. (2004). Talking about death with children who have severe malignant disease. *The New England Journal of Medicine* 351: 1175–1186.

20. Beale, E.A. (2005). Silence is not golden: communicating with children dying from cancer. *Journal of Clinical Oncology* 23: 3629–3631.

21. NHS. Advance decision (living will). https://www.nhs.uk/conditions/end-of-life-care/advance-decision-to-refuse-treatment (accessed 25 April 2021).

22. Thompson, A. (2015). Paediatric palliative care. *Paediatrics & Child Health* 25: 458–464.

23. Harrop, E.J., Boyce, K., Beale, T. et al. (2018). Fifteen-minute consultation: developing an advance care plan in partnership with the child and family. *Archives of Disease in Childhood. Education and Practice Edition* 103: 282–287.

24. Goldman, A. (2006). Symptoms in children/young people with progressive malignant disease: united kingdom children's cancer study group/paediatric oncology nurses forum survey. *Pediatrics* 117: e1179–e1186.

25. Steele, R., Siden, H., Cadell, S. et al. (2014). Charting the territory: symptoms and functional assessment in children with progressive, non-curable conditions. *Archives of Disease in Childhood* 99: 754–762.

26. Association for Paediatric Palliative Medicine (2020). Association for paediatric palliative medicine master formulary 2020. 5th edition. https://www.appm.org.uk/guidelines-resources/appm-master-formulary (accessed 25 April 2021).

27. McCluggage, H. and Jassal, S.S. (2009). Chapter 8 Symptom management. In: *Palliative Care for Children and Families* (ed. J. Price and P. McNeilly). Basingstoke, UK: Palgrave Macmillan.

28. Dickman, A. and Schneider, J. (2016). *The Syringe Driver: Continuous Subcutaneous Infusions in Palliative Care*, 4th edition. Oxford University Press.

29. Wolfe, J., Grier, H.E., Klar, N. et al. (2000). Symptoms and suffering at the end of life in children with cancer. *The New England Journal of Medicine* 342: 326–333.

30. Richmond, C. (2005). Dame Cicely Saunders. *British Medical Journal* 33: 238.

31. Birnie, K.A., Hundert, A.S., Lalloo, C. et al. (2019). Recommendations for selection of self-report pain intensity measures in children and adolescents: a systematic review and quality assessment of measurement properties. *Pain* 160: 5–18.

32. Hauer, J. and Houtrow, A.J. (2017). AAP section on hospice and palliative medicine, council on children with disabilities, pain assessment and treatment in children with significant impairment of the central nervous system. *Pediatrics* 139 (6): e20171002.

33. Crellin, D.J., Harrison, D., Santamaria, N. et al. (2015). Systematic review of the face, legs, activity, cry and consolability scale for assessing pain in infants and children is it reliable, valid, and feasible for use? *Pain* 156 (11): 2132–2151.

34. Hunt, A., Goldman, A., Seers, K. et al. (2004). Clinical validation of the paediatric pain profile. *Developmental Medicine and Child Neurology* 46 (1): 9–18.

35. Tobias, J.D., Green, T.P., Cote, C.J. et al. (2016). Codeine: time to say "No". *Pediatrics* 138 (4): e20151648.

36. Reich, A. and Szepietowski, J.C. (2010). Opioid-induced pruritus: an update. *Clinical and Experimental Dermatology* 35 (1): 2–6.

37. Wren, A.A., Ross, A.C., De Souza, G. et al. (2019). multidisciplinary pain management for paediatric patients with acute and chronic pain: a foundational treatment approach when prescribing opioids. *Children* 6 (2): 33.

38. Jassal, S.S. (2016). Basic symptom control in paediatric palliative care. The Rainbows Hospice for Children and Young Adults guidelines. 9th edition. https://www.togetherforshortlives.org.uk/resource/basic-symptom-control-paediatric-palliative-care (accessed 25 April 2021).

39. Friedrichsdorf, S.J. and Goubert, L. (2019). Paediatric pain treatment and prevention for hospitalized children. *Pain Reports* 5 (1): e804.

40. Mannix, K. (2006). Palliation of nausea and vomiting in malignancy. *Clinical Medicine (London)* 6 (2): 144–147.

41. Hauer, J. (2018). Feeding intolerance in children with severe impairment of the central nervous system: strategies for treatment and prevention. *Children* 5: 1.

42. NICE (2013). Epilepsy in children and young people. NICE Quality standard QS27. www.nice.org.uk/guidance/qs27 (accessed 25 April 2021).

43. Chambers, L. (2019). Caring for a child at end of life: a guide for professionals on the care of children and young people before death, at the time of death and after death. https://www.togetherforshortlives.org.uk/wp-content/uploads/2019/11/TfSL-Caring-for-a-child-at-end-of-life-Professionals.pdf (accessed 25 April 2021).

44. Chambers, L. (2019). Caring for your child at end of life: a guide for parents and carers. www.togetherforshortlives.org.uk/wp-content/uploads/2019/11/TfSL-Caring-for-a-child-at-end-of-life-Parents.pdf (accessed 25 April 2021).

45. HM Government (2018). Working together to safeguard children. https://assets.publishing.service.gov.uk/government/uploads/system/uploads/attachment_data/file/942454/Working_together_to_safeguard_children_inter_agency_guidance.pdf (accessed 25 April 2021).

46. The Lullaby Trust. When a child dies – a guide for families and carers. https://www.lullabytrust.org.uk/wp-content/uploads/lullaby-cdr-booklet.pdf (accessed 25 April 2021).

16 Frailty, Dementia and Multi-Morbidity

Sarah Russell

Introduction

The palliative and end-of-life care needs of people living and dying with frailty, dementia, and multi-morbidity is a global issue, because of the rising incidence, prevalence, and mortality of chronic illness, an ageing population and increased multi-morbidity [1]. By 2040, healthcare systems will need to adapt and adjust to the higher need for palliative care because of age-related growth in deaths from chronic illness [1]. This is pertinent as despite evidence of the benefits of early palliative care; referral and access to services remains limited, for the non-cancer population [2].

In this chapter, some of the palliative and end-of-life care needs of people living with frailty, dementia, and/or multi-morbidity is described. There are two underpinning principles. First, attention should be paid to the specific needs of people living and dying with these conditions. Second, provision should be made for early, focussed, tailored integrated approaches to the assessment and support of the needs of people living and dying with frailty, dementia, and/or multi-morbidity.

Frailty

Frailty is a health state in which people experience an accelerated decline in physiological reserve leaving them less resilient to relatively minor stressor events [3]. While all adults are at risk of developing frailty:

> risk levels are substantially higher among those with comorbidities, low socioeconomic position, poor diet, and sedentary lifestyles. [4 p.1365]

While the onset of frailty can be before the age of 65 years, not all adults develop frailty, even at advanced ages [3]. In high income countries, the overall prevalence of frailty for people 65 years and older is approximately 10%, with 25%–50% prevalence for those over 85 years [5, 6]. Frailty is progressive and typically erodes functional, cognitive, and/or emotional reserves [7]. While severe frailty is easier to diagnose, lesser degrees of frailty may be difficult to differentiate from normal ageing [7]. Furthermore, individuals can fluctuate between states of severity of frailty [8]. As frailty progresses, there is an increased symptom burden and reduced quality of life [9]. This includes higher risk of falls, delirium, disability, mortality, and use of hospital services [10, 11]. Frailty is multi-dimensional [4], with a variety of measurement tools [5, 12]. Most tools were developed in western countries, highlighting the need to consider diversity and cross-cultural studies in models and tool development [12]. Two widely used frailty dimensions are the phenotype and the cumulative deficit model [4].

Phenotype: conceptualises frailty as a biological syndrome [10], suggesting that a person is frail if they present with three or more of five criteria such as exhaustion, weight loss, weakness/loss of muscular strength, reduced gait speed, and reduced energy/physical activity [10]. Scores range from robust, pre-frail or frail [10].

Cumulative Deficit Frailty: is concerned with health deficits accumulation assessed through, for example, The Frailty Index (FI) contains 36 or more deficits, to give a score between no frailty and extreme frailty [11]. As deficits accumulate, people become increasingly vulnerable to adverse

Handbook of Palliative Care, Fourth Edition. Edited by Richard Kitchen, Christina Faull, Sarah Russell and Jo Wilson.
© 2024 John Wiley & Sons Ltd. Published 2024 by John Wiley & Sons Ltd.

outcomes [12, 13]. An electronic version of this (the eFI) is used in the UK in primary care for patients aged 65 years and over in order to identify patients at risk of severe frailty and therefore requiring for example, an annual medicines review and falls assessment see: https://www.england.nhs.uk/ourwork/clinical-policy/older-people/fraility/efi

A measure recommended by the British Geriatrics Society is the Comprehensive Geriatric Assessment (CGA):

a multi-dimensional diagnostic and therapeutic process that is focused on determining a frail older person's medical, functional, mental, and social capabilities and limitations with the goal of ensuring that problems are identified, quantified, and managed appropriately. [14 p. 6]

Widely used to summarise a CGA, the Rockwood clinical frailty scale is also often utilised and includes seven levels from "very fit to severely frail" with additional two additional levels of eight "very severely frail" and nine "terminally ill" [15].

Frailty, Palliative and End-of-Life Care

There are few targeted frailty and end-of-life care specialist services, despite people with people with frailty requiring levels of palliative care similar to those living with cancer [5] (Table 1).

Advance care planning rates for frail, older people are low. A recent systematic review reported:

although 74%–84% of capacitous older inpatients are receptive to ACP, rates of ACP are 0%–5% [16 p. 164].

Furthermore, since fluctuating function and frequent acute illness episodes affects the stability of choice-making, it important to understand the individual context of wishes and decisions such as family support, long term goals, recovery from illness, and changes in health awareness [1, 17, 18]. Other commentators point out the importance of re-conceptualising advance care planning to include current and future care, with emphasis on the significance of relational decision-making, family relationships, and engagement [19, 20]. Moreover, there can be differences in attitudes towards dying and talking about death between frail patients and those with cancer or organ failure, in part related to the unpredictability of death and dying in frailty [21].

Frailty is characterised by a slow and gradual decline interspersed with crises or episodes of rapid deterioration [22] which makes it difficult to identify when someone is entering the final twelve months of their life [23]. Furthermore, the dying trajectory is characterised by high levels of disability in the last year of life [24]. This uncertain prognostication landscape emphasises the need for specific assessments and services tailored to patient and family needs and end-of-life preferences [5]. Frailty approaches can be helpful to focus care, as "framing

Table 1 Palliative care needs and outcomes in frailty.

Physical	Pain, shortness of breath, drowsiness, weakness, fatigue, loss of appetite, pressure ulcers, insomnia.
Psychosocial	Emotional distress (sustained, intense, progressive, and not related to acute concurrent conditions), psychological burden (anxiety, low mood confusion, and loneliness), low perceived social support, low levels of hope, desire for death, losses of dignity, suffering, hopelessness and dissatisfaction, anxiety, depression, and loss of wellbeing towards the end-of-life, recognising nearing the end-of-life, without a specific life-threatening diagnosis.
Function	Decreased function, dependence for assistance with bathing, eating, mobility, and continence especially when cognitively impaired and at the end-of-life.
Place of Death and Preferences for Care	Variation depending upon internationally different healthcare systems, with increased hospitalisation in some systems and in others more likely to die in nursing home or own home. Preferences for treatment or treatment intensity also mixed, more likely to express a preference for reduced treatment or interventions at the end-of-life, however these preferences are not always observed at critical phases of care.
Satisfaction and Access to Care	Lower satisfaction with care and less likely to access palliative care.

Drawn from [5]

discussions in the context of degree of frailty provides a unifying concept" [13 p. 171], rather than concentrating on diagnosing dying or biological age alone. Rajabali et al. [25] argue that recognition of an individual's frailty status informs treatment decisions, goals of care, and recovery expectations.

Considering the relationship between frailty, chronic disease, and palliative care needs is useful. For example, clinical frailty scales (rather than diagnosing dying) have been used to trigger palliative care referral in intensive care units, chronic respiratory disease, and end-stage renal disease [26–28]. Amblàs-Novellas [29] also advocates a needs-based care provision (rather than diagnosis or prognosis) commentating:

a progressive approach, then, in which palliative care is provided as long as patients' needs evolve. [29 p.190]

Dementia

The palliative and end-of-life care needs of people living and dying with dementia is significant. Globally, dementia affects 50 million people worldwide with an estimated increase to 152 million by 2050 [30]. In England and Wales, by 2040, deaths from dementia are projected to rise from 59,199 to 219,409 per year [1]. Dementia is often associated with older people, but it is not a normal part of ageing [31]. It is the fourth cause of major disability among people aged 75 and older [32], and its relationship with multi-morbidity (including frailty) in older people should not be discounted [31]. One of the significant challenges is that dementia is not always considered to be life limiting in practice, leading to lack of (and referral to) specialised palliative and end-of-life care services [31].

Dementia encompasses a range of disorders for example, Alzheimer's, vascular dementia, and dementia with Lewy bodies which affect the cognitive (and other) functions of the brain and is a complex biopsychosocial constellation of progressive, neurodegenerative symptoms [33]. Dementia is ultimately fatal and is characterised by profound cognitive impairment, inability to communicate verbally, and complete functional dependence [34]. While dementia is an organic, progressive neurodegenerative disorder, Kitwood [35] points out that people exist in a social, relational context, and that positive and enriching interpersonal relationships can prevent the disabling effects of dementia and promote a sense of well-being.

Dementia, Palliative and End-of-Life Care

Optimal palliative care should be provided across all stages of dementia, however the end-of-life care period for those living with dementia can be difficult to define [36]. People with dementia may live with the progressive, life-limiting disease for years, with their last year, months, or weeks of life difficult to predict. There is a lack of studies regarding the needs and care of those with early-stage or moderate dementia who may be dying from other life-limiting diseases or co-morbidities [37]. In addition, different profiles of symptoms and carer experiences, of those dying from advanced dementia, or in people with young onset and rapidly progressive dementias, highlight the need not to treat all dementias the same [37].

There is an inconsistency in the use of dementia and end-of-life assessment tools, with a predominance of single measure tools which focus on cognition or function which fail to recognise the complexities and individual unmet needs relevant to dementia and end-of-life [33]. Many of the assessment tools are designed to measure dementia severity rather than palliative and end-of-life needs, raising questions about their use in the end-of-life context [33]. More dementia specific assessment tools such as the Integrated Palliative Care Outcome Scale for Dementia (IPOS-Dem) are helpful. IPOS-Dem is a proxy-reported outcome measure allowing comprehensive and specific assessment of symptoms and concerns experienced by people with dementia [14]. There is evidence that IPOS-Dem improves aspects of caring quality for people with dementia as it takes a person-centred approach asking about the person's most important concerns, and then assessing symptoms and unmet needs, to enable carers and nonclinical staff to identify needs, plan, and improve care [14, 37].

While end-of-life care in dementia can be complicated by its potentially long and unpredictable trajectory [33], people with dementia may never reach its advanced stages and can die from other causes earlier in the trajectory [38]. This is relevant as the dementia trajectory is variable with progressive decline, punctuated by acute events such as an infection, falls, and hospital admissions, where the person may recover or experience an increased rate of decline in health until the end-of-life [39]. A 2021 study reported that only one third of people with dementia were recognised as having palliative care needs in the last year of life [40]. Furthermore, identification of palliative care needs before the last 90 days was associated with a lower risk of having multiple non-elective admissions to hospital [40].

Advance Care Planning and Dementia

Advance care planning is often instigated late in the dementia disease trajectory [41], despite evidence that it reduces aggressive or burdensome disease orientated treatments [36, 37]. Challenges include the fluctuating capacity of the person with dementia their ability to retain information, weigh up concerns, make judgements as well as difficulty in imagining and articulating their future wishes and decisions [41]. Family carers may not always be able to accurately predict preferences and choices [41] and practitioners may lack confidence in starting conversations due to lack of knowledge of disease progression and the communication needs of a person with dementia [42]. Chapter 7 (Conversations and Communication) suggests some communication recommendations and early advance care planning conversations are advised.

In 2014, Van der Steen and colleagues [36] published a white paper defining optimal palliative care in older people with dementia. Eleven key principles underpin the document illustrating that patients and families may need palliative care specific to dementia (Box 1) and services should be designed around these principles.

Box 1: Principles of Optimal palliative care in dementia [36].

1) Applicability of palliative care
2) Person-centred care, communication, and shared decision-making
3) Setting care goals and advance planning
4) Continuity of care
5) Prognostication and timely recognition of dying
6) Avoiding overly aggressive, burdensome, or futile treatment
7) Optimal treatment of symptoms and providing comfort
8) Psychosocial and spiritual support
9) Family care and involvement
10) Education of the healthcare team
11) Societal and ethical issues

There are specific palliative and end-of-life care needs for people (and their families) living and dying with dementia (Table 2), which is helpful for services and practitioners to consider.

Table 2 Symptom control considerations.

Pain		
Underdiagnosed and assessed by professionals [43]	Consider observational pain assessment tools e.g. Abbey, ADD, CNPI, DS-DAT, DOLO-Plus 2, EPCA, MOBID2, NOPPAIN, PACSLAC, PAINAD, PADE, and PAINE [44]	Consider polypharmacy, drug interactions, renal, and hepatic insufficiency [45]
High prevalence with multiple causes such as musculoskeletal, gastrointestinal, cardiac conditions, genitourinary infections, wounds, oral facial, and pressure ulcers [46]	Abbey Pain Scale and DOLO-Plus2 valuable to assist in the assessment of pain for people who are unable to clearly articulate their needs. Other tools for the assessment of distress (where distress may be a manifestation of pain) include "DS-DAT", however individual judgement and assessment is important [47]	Consider non-pharmacological interventions e.g. music therapy, reflexology, tailored pain intervention, painting, and singing, personal assistive robot, cognitive-behavioural therapy, play activity, and person-centred environment programme [48]
The location of the neuropathology may affect the sensation and experience of pain [46]	May be difficult to convey or assess due to communication problems due to cognitive decline [46]	Consider consent issues for assessment, management, and prescribing.
Breathlessness		**Agitation**
Often associated with co-morbidity [49] Use usual assessment tools and management		Restlessness, pacing, shouting, and verbal or physical aggression; it is complex and multifactorial with a range of biological, psychological, and social causes. It may be a direct result of neurodegeneration, affecting brain circuits that control behaviour, and also an expression of unmet needs (e.g., pain or thirst, lack of communication or comfort) [37, 43, 49]

(Continued)

Table 2 *(Continued)*

Changing Behaviours		
Waking during the night, or sleeping excessively during the day [43]		Identify usual behaviours, changes, possible causes of changed behaviour.
Infection and Delirium		
Consider urinary tract infections and pneumonia [43]	Do not confuse with dementia, however acute delirium may develop in an individual with pre-existing cognitive impairment [45]	Consider PINCHME Mnemonic (Pain, Infection, Constipation, Hydration, Medication, Environment) and that hypoactive (drowsy) delirium maybe conflated with signs of dying.
Often complicated by other behavioural manifestations [50]	Consider Confusion Assessment Method (CAM) e.g., three of the following four possible features: (1) acute onset and fluctuating (2) inattention plus either (3) disorganised thinking or (4) altered level of consciousness [45]	Assess for hypo and hyper delirium. Avoid use of Haloperidol, Olanzapine, Risperidone, Quetiapine in Parkinson's Disease and in Lewy Body Dementia [45]
Nutrition and Hydration		
In early stages an individual may forget to eat and drink and experience changes in perceptions of food, including altered taste and smell. As dementia develops, apraxia, dysphagia, or a lack of attention might make it difficult for the person to feed themselves. May find it difficult to recognize food, or does not feel hungry. Associated problems include aspiration, pneumonia, weight loss, malnutrition, and dehydration [51]		Presence of dysphagia and associated risk of aspiration are indicators that prognosis is limited and should trigger a discussion of treatment goals in this context [51, 52]
Consider the goal of care, the communication difficulties of the person with dementia, communication with family members, early advance care planning, strain on carers and practitioners in helping someone to eat while they may choke, other ways to provide texture and taste to a dying person [51]		The use of artificial nutrition and hydration should be carefully considered [52]
Skin Care		
Increased risk of pressure ulcers and damage [43]		
Continence		
Higher prevalence of bowel and bladder incontinence [53]		Consider medications, dietary tolerance, comfort, dignity, and exercise
Depression		
Increased risk of and should be carefully assessed [43]		
Carer Burden		**Dementia Grief**
Concerns over being a "burden" to relatives and high levels of carer burden [54]		Specific type of anticipatory grief in response to compounded serial losses of varying magnitude and marked by the ambiguity that characterize the experiences of loss in dementia [55]
Increased emergency department visits		
Common clinical reasons include infection, injury, and respiratory problems. High-strength evidence that ethnic minority groups, greater number of comorbidities, neuropsychiatric symptoms, living in more rural areas, and previous hospital transfers are associated with increased attendance [56]		Patients admitted with a Clinical Frailty Score of 7–9 have an inpatient mortality rate of 11–31%, readmission rates of 10–14% and a one-year mortality rate of 50% [57]

Family Carers

The needs of family or informal carers of those living and dying with dementia should not be underestimated, including the transition stages when the person with dementia moves from one stable period/state to another [58]. Recent studies report that informal carers experience physical, emotional, and economic stressors, and are likely to experience mental and physical disability themselves and have higher risk of mortality compared to carers of patients with other types of chronic illness [59]. Furthermore, support for informal carers as "co-workers" in supporting patients (to ensure they have the information, skills, and equipment for this role) as well as "clients" in their own right (to preserve their own wellbeing and health) is essential [60]. Research using the Carer Support Needs Assessment Tool (CSNAT) for family carers in dementia looks promising enabling family carer and the service provider to discuss support needs and strategies to address them [61]. Table 3 provides some useful palliative and end-of-life resources.

Table 3 Useful palliative and end-of-life care resources in dementia.

North West Coast Strategic Clinical Network, Palliative Care Guidelines in Dementia 2nd Edition Version 3.9 – March 2018 (accessed 18/09/2021)
https://www.england.nhs.uk/north/wpcontent/uploads/sites/5/2018/06/palliative-care-guidelines-in-dementia.pdf

NHS Scotland, Healthcare Improvement Scotland: Scottish Palliative Care Guidelines https://www.palliativecareguidelines.scot.nhs.uk/guidelines/pain/pain-assessment-cognitive-impairment.aspx
(accessed 18/09/2021)

Irish Hospice Foundation: Guidance Documents to Improve Palliative Care for People with Dementia
https://hospicefoundation.ie/other/ihf-launch-seven-guidance-documents-improve-palliative-care-people-dementia (accessed 18/09/2021)

Alzheimer's Society, End-of-Life Care for a person with dementia
https://www.alzheimers.org.uk/get-support/help-dementia-care/end-life-care-dementia (accessed 18/09/2021)

Dementia UK Advice Leaflets
https://www.dementiauk.org/our-advice-leaflets (accessed 18/09/2021)

British Geriatrics Society End-of-Life Care in Dementia in Frailty and End-of-Life Resource Series https://www.bgs.org.uk/resources/resource-series/end-of-life-care-in-frailty (accessed 18/09/2021).

NHS England: My Future Wishes, Advance Care Planning for people with demean in all care settings https://www.england.nhs.uk/publication/my-future-wishes-advance-care-planning-acp-for-people-with-dementia-in-all-care-settings (accessed 18/09/2021)

NICE Decision Aid: Enteral (tube) feeding for people living with severe dementia
https://www.nice.org.uk/guidance/ng97/resources/enteral-tube-feeding-for-people-living-with-severe-dementia-patient-decision-aid-pdf-4852697007 (accessed 18/09/2021)

UCL and Marie Curie Palliative Care Research Department: Supporting family carers of people living with dementia to make difficult decisions during COVID-19
https://www.ucl.ac.uk/psychiatry/sites/psychiatry/files/endemic_decision_aid_26_08_20_v.2.pdf (accessed 18/09/2021)

UCL and Marie Curie Palliative Care Research Department: Rules of Thumb for End-of-Life Care for People with Dementia.
https://www.ucl.ac.uk/psychiatry/sites/psychiatry/files/rules_of_thumb_davies_iliffec.pdf (accessed 15/10/2021)

UCL and Marie Curie Palliative Care Research Department: The Compassion Intervention Manual: A model of enhanced integrated care for people with advanced dementia. https://www.ucl.ac.uk/psychiatry/sites/psychiatry/files/the-compassion-intervention-manual.pdf (accessed 18/09/2021)

UCL and Marie Curie Palliative Care Research Department: Caring for family or friends with dementia: Could these feelings be grief? https://www.ucl.ac.uk/psychiatry/research/marie-curie-palliative-care-research-department/research/centre-dementia-palliative-care-23 (accessed 18/09/2021)

Multi-morbidity, Palliative and End-of-Life Care

Multi-morbidity is defined as where two or more chronic conditions co-exist [62]. A study in Scotland reported that by 2040 people dying from multiple chronic progressive diseases across different disease groups will rise by 60%, accounting for nearly half of all palliative care deaths [63]. Earlier in this chapter some of the palliative and end-of-life care needs for people living with frailty and dementia have been described. Some of that population live with multi-morbidity indicating the importance of assessing each morbidity separately as well as together. This is relevant as recent studies report that a significant amount of people with frailty also present with multi-morbidity [4].

Melis and colleagues [64] report that baseline chronic multi-morbidity is significantly associated to accelerated decline in daily functioning but not in cognition in dementia patients. Oosterveld et al. [65] argue that physical health and Alzheimer's Disease manifestation are associated, emphasising the importance of adequate assessment of co-morbid medical conditions and frailty in patients with Alzheimer's Disease. Other indications of the relationship of multi-morbidity on dementia include the acceleration of cognitive decline and type 2 diabetes [66], the significant association of cerebrovascular disease, chronic kidney disease, and diabetes with dementia [67]. There are also strong correlations between multi-morbidity and dementia with adverse health outcomes as well as a proxy for loss of independent living [68].

One of the challenges is that the population of older people with multi-morbidity has not been routinely recognised as having specialist (and considerable) palliative care needs [69]. This population can have poorly controlled symptoms, functional dependence, poor quality of life and distressed caregivers, but a prolonged life expectancy [70]. Nicholson et al. [69] argue that older people with progressive long-term conditions may have different palliative care needs compared to young people with malignancy and suggest that more work is needed to understand whether there are specific palliative care symptom clusters, which are commonly associated with older people with multi-morbidity, in order to determine the response to need.

Prescribing and Deprescribing in Frailty, Dementia and Multi-Morbidity

Safe, effective prescribing at the end-of-life for people with frailty, dementia, and multi-morbidity means paying close attention to polypharmacy, co-morbidities, and the goal of prescribing. The risk, benefits and possible harm or burden of prescribed medications must be assessed as should the medications used beyond licence, by routes that are effective but unlicensed. Practitioners should consider renal and liver function, route of administration and interaction with specific conditions and other drugs. National, regional, local, and organisational policies will provide specific advice.

People living with frailty, dementia and multi-morbidity are often subject to poly pharmacy with subsequent potential harm, with serious adverse events including, falls, cognitive impairment, functional decline, hospitalisation, length of stay, and death [71]. There is further evidence that older people approaching end-of-life are among the greatest consumers of prescription medications [72]. Deprescribing involves a stepwise, patient-centred process that reduces the risks and burden of taking multiple medications [73]. It reduces adverse events, reduced tablet burden, prioritisation of the most essential medications, reduced costs and, most importantly, enhanced quality of life [73]. Curtin et al. [72] advocate the use of the STOPPFrail list of potentially inappropriate prescribing indicators, advocating that symptom control is the priority rather than prevention of illness progression. All deprescribing (reducing or stopping) needs to be individualised to each patient.

Case Study: Thinking ahead to End-of-Life

Mabel (pseudonym) is a 97-year-old grandmother, living with her husband (Ed) in their own home. She has been living with dementia and renal failure for 9 years and type 2 diabetes for over 40 years. Recently she has had several falls at home resulting in a hospital admission and surgery for a fracture of her right neck of femur. In the immediate post-operative period she was confused, distressed, and agitated. Her Estimated Glomerular Filtration Rate (eGFR) is below 50, her C-reactive protein (CRP) is very high, her diabetic control is poor and she has signs of a hospital acquired pneumonia. An assessment of Mabel with her, and her husband using IPOS-Dem reveals that Mabel no longer goes out of the house, sleeps most of the time in the day, is restless and walks around the house at night, she eats and drinks very little, falls or stumbles every day, and they do not monitor her diabetes. Her husband also reports that she is having more difficulty finding the right words and he often finds her sitting in the bathroom trying to put on her clothes. He is mentally and physically exhausted but wants for her to return home for "whatever time we have together".

What are the considerations? For example:

1. Full assessment of their psychological, emotional, physical, social, and spiritual needs.

2. Invite a conversation about future end-of-life preferences (advance care planning) and what is most important to them now and in the future.

3. Check if any advance care planning has already taken place for example, Lasting Power of Attorney, Advance Decision to Refuse Treatment, decision about cardiopulmonary resuscitation.

4. Review medications and consider renal function – deprescribe if necessary.

5. Discuss and review with Mabel and Ed what their expectations and assumptions are about what support and help they need at home.

6. Coordinate with multi-professional colleagues both within and outside of the hospital setting to maximise Mabel's physical function and her independence and emotional wellbeing for example, equipment, package of care, community nurses, and/or specialist palliative/hospice care referral.

7. Discuss the "what if's" and "what next" of when Mabel deteriorates at home – would she come back into hospital, what would a Community and Hospital Treatment Escalation Plan (a document for healthcare practitioners to communicate urgent treatment decisions) contain?

8. Consider if anticipatory "Just in Case" medications (drugs for symptom control to be administered in the community) are necessary on discharge home.

9. Ensure all of the above is communicate to community colleagues using the local policy and procedures.

Practice and Service Models for People Living and Dying with Frailty, Dementia and Multi-Morbidities

Service models will need to adapt to the needs of people living and dying with frailty, dementia, and multi-morbidity, bringing together the knowledge, skills, and tools from a variety of multidisciplinary teams and settings. For example, if living and dying well is a priority for our population, then palliative care and geriatric practice have much to offer each other [74]. Both include person-centred care, education, and a multi-professional workforce. While it is pertinent to be alert to subtle differences so that we do not impose a model of palliative care developed for cancer onto the care of frail older people [75], a 2019 review concluded that both Integrated Geriatric Care or Palliative Care were effective in improving end-of-life for older people [9]. Different specialities need to adjust to different ways of working together (integration) based upon the complex needs of patients across a longer (and maybe uncertain) time continuum.

Short-term Integrated Palliative and Supportive Care (SIPS) [76] point out the value of episodic involvement of specialist palliative care for patients with non-malignant conditions. Involvement may be for complex symptoms (including emotional distress), discussing the future, increased healthcare utilisation and unmet carer needs [76]. Furthermore, person-centred care should drive access to services with service use triggered by individual need rather than prognostication [9].

Comprehensive Geriatric assessment (CGA) is a multidisciplinary diagnostic process intended to determine a frail elderly person's medical, psychosocial, and functional capabilities and limitations to develop an overall plan for treatment and long-term follow-up [77]. Recent studies report that adding in specific advance care planning components to CGA has utility for frail hospitalised geriatric patients [78]. Additionally, including routine CGA for older cancer patients undergoing systemic medical cancer treatment aids identification of frail patients needing early supportive and palliative care [79].

"Age Attuned Hospice Care" is an approach proposed by Nicholson and Richardson [19] that balances continuity with ongoing adaptation to loss. They argue that the model (Box 2) is particularly relevant as specialist palliative care often focuses its attention on people either with dominating single diseases, like cancer, or giving care at the very end-of-life [80]. The proposal is that the focus should be on

> helping people to live well even when their condition(s) is advancing and cannot be cured. [19 p. 8]

The Bromley Care Co-ordination Centre (Box 3) in Kent, London is a nurse-led service primarily for older people with palliative care needs who do not meet the criteria for referral to specialist palliative care services providing timely and coordinated end-of-life care to patients with progressive illness and/or frailty, thought to be in the last year of their life [69]. It offers 24/7 telephone support and home visits to patients providing symptom control pain control and psychological support. It has led to working with a different skill mix developing a "stratification" tool introducing the role of care navigators and volunteers [81].

> ## Box 2: Summary of age attuned hospice care [19].
>
> **Level 1: Clinical interactions and support for people, their families and carers**
>
> Use specific assessment tools, prioritise use of advance care plans capturing current goals and future wishes, regular review, and reflect small incremental changes, recognise family carers as experts in care as well as recipients of care, provide targeted education programmes for the workforce.
>
> **Level 2: Partnership across the system**
>
> Understand the population and those likely to die in next few years, proactively develop new relationships with other care providers, jointly develop referral triggers and pathways, think where you can most make a difference, work together across professional and service boundaries to engage with older people to explore their needs and requirements for care.
>
> **Level 3: Supporting societal change**
>
> Confirm the value of older people within the service you provide. Use images, stories, and quotations that reinforce their central place in current and future care, encourage people to tell stories about their life and their legacy; encourage others simultaneously to listen and reflect on what they hear with the intention of amending and expanding their life view, find opportunities for intergenerational activity and care, focus strong reciprocal learning or attachment, encourage community participation in care, provide training and support to ensure people feel confident in their roles, and know where to go if they face something they feel unprepared for, create learning networks.

> ## Box 3: Bromley care co-ordination centre [81].
>
> - 2200 referrals (55% from GP 26% from Hospital 19% other)
> - Of those who have died 70% have died in their own home/care home
> - Average age of patients referred 86 years
> - Non-cancer to cancer diagnoses ratio = 85%: 15%
> - 86% of patients have no other current healthcare intervention apart from the GP and occasionally a social care agency/provider
> - 39% of patients live alone

Admiral Nurses are specialist dementia nurses who use a case management approach to support people facing dementia using range of psychosocial, educational, and practical approaches to support families living with dementia [82]. It is the only defined model of case management that integrates health and social care for all members of the family unit affected by dementia in the UK [83]. Emerging evidence reports that the person-centred approach benefits those living and dying with dementia through specialist knowledge and information, holistic assessment, focussing on the experience of carers, supporting them with decision making, and helping to anticipate prevent and avert crisis [9].

Hospice Enabled Dementia Care guidance from the national charity Hospice UK stresses the important requirement for

palliation of symptoms and provision of comfort for anyone with dementia regardless of anticipated prognosis. [84 p. 3]

The call for action for hospices included a corporate commitment to engage with the agenda of dementia care, efforts to establish new partnerships, creativity in the provision of care, and services to meet the specific needs of people with dementia, an evidence-based approach to care and the care environment, investment in training of staff and volunteers [84]. Since its publication there has been an increase in hospices in the UK providing services to enable people with dementia to live and die well as well as establishment of integrated communities of practice (knowledge networks).

Conclusion

This chapter has explored the evidence for the palliative and end-of-life care needs of people living with frailty, dementia, and multi-morbidity. Examples of practice have been suggested which focus on the specific needs of people living and dying with these conditions as well as illustrating the need for early, focussed, tailored integrated approaches to the assessment and support of the palliative and end-of-life care needs of people living with frailty, dementia, and multi-morbidity.

References

1. Etkind, S.N., Bone, A.E., Gomes, B. et al. (2017). How many people will need palliative care in 2040? past trends, future projections and implications for services. *BMC Medicine* 15 (1): 102.

2. Allsop, M.J., Ziegler, L.E., Mulvey, M.R. et al. (2018). Duration and determinants of hospice-based specialist palliative care: a national retrospective cohort study. *Palliative Medicine* 32 (8): 1322–1333.

3. Clegg, A., Young, J., Iliffe, S. et al. (2013). Frailty in elderly people. *The Lancet* 381 (9868): 752–762.

4. Hoogendijk, E.O., Afilalo, J., Ensrud, K.E. et al. (2019). Frailty: implications for clinical practice and public health. *The Lancet* 394 (10206): 1365–1375.

5. Stow, D., Spiers, G., Matthews, F.E., and Hanratty, B. (2019). What is the evidence that people with frailty have needs for palliative care at the end of life? a systematic review and narrative synthesis. *Palliative Medicine* 33 (4): 399–414.

6. Wilhelmson, K., Andersson Hammar, I. et al. (2020). Comprehensive geriatric assessment for frail older people in Swedish acute care settings (CGA-Swed): a randomised controlled study. *Geriatrics* 5 (1): 5.

7. Moody, D., Lydon, H., and Stevens, G. (2017). Toolkit for general practice in supporting older people living with frailty. NHS England/Long term conditions team. Quarry Hill, Leeds.

8. Markle-Reid, M. and Browne, G. (2003). Conceptualizations of frailty in relation to older adults. *Journal of Advanced Nursing* 44 (1): 58–68.

9. Evans, C.J., Ison, L., Ellis-Smith, C.L. et al. (2019). Service delivery models to maximize quality of life for older people at the end of life: a rapid review. *The Milbank Quarterly* 97 (1): 113–175.

10. Fried, L.P., Tangen, C.M., Walston, J. et al. (2001). Frailty in older adults: evidence for a phenotype. *The Journals of Gerontology. Series A, Biological Sciences and Medical Sciences* 56: M146–M156.

11. Rockwood, K. and Mitnitski, A. (2007). Frailty in relation to the accumulation of deficits. *The Journals of Gerontology. Series A, Biological Sciences and Medical Sciences* 62: 722–727.

12. Huang, E.Y. and Lam, S.C. (2021). Review of frailty measurement of older people: evaluation of the conceptualization, included domains, psychometric properties, and applicability. *Aging Medicine* 4 (4): 272–291.

13. Koller, K. and Rockwood, K. (2013). Frailty in older adults: implications for end-of-life care. *Cleveland Clinic Journal of Medicine* 80 (3): 168–174.

14. Ellis, G., Gardner, M., and Tsiachristas, A. (2017). Comprehensive geriatric assessment for older adults admitted to hospital. *Cochrane Database of Systematic Reviews* 9 (9): CD006211.

15. Theou, O., Pérez-Zepeda, M.U., van der Valk, A.M. et al. (2021). A classification tree to assist with routine scoring of the clinical frailty scale. *Age and Ageing* 50 (4): 1406–1411.

16. Hopkins, S., Bentley, A., Phillips, V., and Barclay, S. (2020). Advance care planning with frail older patients in the acute hospital setting: a systematic review. *BMJ Supportive & Palliative Care* 10: 164–174.

17. Etkind, S.N., Bone, A.E., Lovell, N. et al. (2018). Influences on care preferences of older people with advanced illness: a systematic review and thematic synthesis. *JAGS* 66 (5): 1031–1039.

18. Etkind, S.N., Lovell, N., Bone, A.E. et al. (2020). The stability of care preferences following acute illness: a mixed methods prospective cohort study of frail older people. *BMC Geriatrics* 20 (1): 1–3.

19. Nicholson, C. and Richardson, H. (2019). Age attuned palliative care: an opportunity to better end of life care for older people. St Christophers Hospice London, Kings College London.

20. Combes, S., Gillett, K., Norton, C., and Nicholson, C.J. (2021). The importance of living well now and relationships: a qualitative study of the barriers and enablers to engaging frail elders with advance care planning. *Palliative Medicine* 35 (6): 1137–1147.

21. Kendall, M., Carduff, E., Lloyd, A. et al. (2015). Different experiences and goals in different advanced diseases: comparing serial interviews with patients with cancer, organ failure, or frailty and their family and professional carers. *Journal of Pain and Symptom Management* 50: 216–224.

22. Harwood, R.H. and Enguell, H. (2022). End-of-life care for frail older people. *BMJ Supportive & Palliative Care* 12 (e3): e293–e298.

23. Hall, A., Boulton, E., Kunonga, P. et al. (2021). Identifying older adults with frailty approaching end-of-life: a systematic review. *Palliative Medicine* 35 (10): 1832–1843.

24. Lunney, J.R., Lynn, J., Foley, D.J. et al. (2003). Patterns of functional decline at the end of life. *JAMA* 289: 2387–2392.

25. Rajabali, N., Rolfson, D., and Bagshaw, S.M. (2016). Assessment and utility of frailty measures in critical illness, cardiology, and cardiac surgery. *The Canadian Journal of Cardiology* 32: 1157–1165.

26. Hope, A.A., Enilari, O.M., and Chuang, E. (2021). Prehospital frailty and screening criteria for palliative care services in critically ill older adults: an observational cohort study. *Journal of Palliative Medicine* 24 (2): 252–256.

27. Brighton, L.J., Bone, A.E., and Maddocks, M. (2020). Supportive and palliative care for people with chronic respiratory disease and frailty. *Current Opinion in Supportive and Palliative Care* 14 (3): 206–212.

28. Chao, C.T., Wang, J., Huang, J.W. et al. (2019). Frailty predicts an increased risk of end-stage renal disease with risk competition by mortality among 165,461 diabetic kidney disease patients. *Aging and Disease* 10 (6): 1270.

29. Amblàs-Novellas, J., Espaulella, J., Rexach, L. et al. (2015). Frailty, severity, progression and shared decision-making: a pragmatic framework for the challenge of clinical complexity at the end of life. *European Geriatric Medicine* 6 (2): 189–194.

30. Barbarino, P., Lynch, C., and Bliss, A. (2020). *From Plan to Impact III: Maintaining Dementia as a Priority in Unprecedented Times*. London: Alzheimer's Disease International.

31. Stein, K.V., Barbazza, E.S., Tello, J., and Kluge, H. (2013). Towards people-centred health services delivery: a framework for action for the World Health Organisation (WHO) European Region. *International Journal of Integrated Care* 13: e058.

32. Vos, T., Lim, S.S., and Abbafati, C. (2020). Global burden of 369 diseases and injuries in 204 countries and territories, 1990–2019: a systematic analysis for the global burden of disease study 2019. *The Lancet* 396 (10258): 1204–1222.

33. Browne, B., Kupeli, N., and Moore, K.J. (2021). Defining end of life in dementia: a systematic review. *Palliative Medicine* 35 (10): 1733–1746.

34. Murphy, E., Froggatt, K., and Connolly, S. (2016). Palliative care interventions in advanced dementia. *Cochrane Database of Systematic Reviews* 12 (12): CD011513.

35. Kitwood, T.M. (2007). *Dementia Reconsidered: The Person Comes First*. Buckingham: Open University Press.

36. Van der Steen, J.T., Radbruch, L., and Hertogh, C.M. (2014). White paper defining optimal palliative care in older people with dementia: a delphi study and recommendations from the European Association for palliative care. *Palliative Medicine* 28 (3): 197–209.

37. Sampson, E.L., Anderson, J.E., and Candy, B. (2020). Empowering better end-of-life dementia care (EMBED-care): a mixed methods protocol to achieve integrated person-centred care across settings. *International Journal of Geriatric Psychiatry* 35 (8): 820–832.

38. Brunnström, H. and Englund, E. (2009). Cause of death in patients with dementia disorders. *European Journal of Neurology* 16 (4): 488–492.

39. Murray, S.A., Kendall, M., Boyd, K. et al. (2005). Illness trajectories and palliative care. *BMJ* 330 (7498): 1007–1011.

40. Leniz, J., Higginson, I.J., Yi, D., Ul-Haq, Z. et al. (2021). Identification of palliative care needs among people with dementia and its association with acute hospital care and community service use at the end-of-life: a retrospective cohort study using linked primary, community and secondary care data. *Palliative Medicine* 31: 02692163211019897.

41. Harrison Dening, K., King, M., Jones, L. et al. (2016). Advance care planning in dementia: do family carers know the treatment preferences of people with early dementia? *PLoS One* 11 (7): e0159056.

42. Harrison Dening, K. (2018). Advance care planning and people with dementia. In: *Advance Care Planning in End of Life Care* (ed. K. Thomas, B. Lobo, and K. Detering). Oxford University Press.

43. Sampson, E.L., Candy, B., Davis, S. et al. (2018). Living and dying with advanced dementia: a prospective cohort study of symptoms, service use and care at the end of life. *Palliative Medicine* 32 (3): 668–681.

44. Kunz, M., de Waal, M.W., and Achterberg, W.P. (2020). The pain assessment in impaired cognition scale (PAIC15): a multidisciplinary and international approach to develop and test a meta-tool for pain assessment in impaired cognition, especially dementia. *European Journal of Pain* 24 (1): 192–208.

45. Wessex Palliative Care Physicians (2019). The palliative care handbook: a good practice guide. https://www.futureplanning.org.uk/uploads/8/0/4/0/80407130/gb_9th_edition_2019_copy_amended_aug_2020.pdf (accessed 18 September 2021).

46. Achterberg, W., Lautenbacher, S., Husebo, B. et al. (2020). Pain in dementia. *Pain Reports* 5 (1): e803.

47. North West Coast Strategic Clinical Network. Palliative care guidelines in dementia 2nd edition version 3.9 – March 2018. https://www.england.nhs.uk/north/wpcontent/uploads/sites/5/2018/06/palliative-care-guidelines-in-dementia.pdf (accessed 18 September 2021).

48. Liao, Y.J., Parajuli, J., Jao, Y.L. et al. (2021). Non-pharmacological interventions for pain in people with dementia: a systematic review. *International Journal of Nursing Studies* 124: 104082.

49. Sampson, E.L., Stringer, A., La Frenais, F. et al. (2019). Agitation near the end of life with dementia: an ethnographic study of care. *PloS one* 14 (10): e0224043.

50. Livingston, G., Sommerlad, A., Orgeta, V. et al. (2017). Dementia prevention, intervention, and care. *Lancet* 390 (10113): 2673–2734.

51. Barrado-Martín, Y., Hatter, L., Moore, K.J. et al. (2021). Nutrition and hydration for people living with dementia near the end of life: a qualitative systematic review. *Journal of Advanced Nursing* 77 (2): 664–680.

52. British Medical Association, Royal College of Physicians. (2021). Clinically assisted nutrition and hydration (CANH) and adults who lack the capacity to consent guidance for decision-making in England and Wales. BMA. London.

53. Miu, D.K., Lau, S., and Szeto, S.S. (2010). Etiology and predictors of urinary incontinence and its effect on quality of life. *Geriatrics & Gerontology International* 10 (2): 177–182.

54. Van der Lee, J., Bakker, T.J., Duivenvoorden, H.J., and Dröes, R.M. (2014). Multivariate models of subjective caregiver burden in dementia: a systematic review. *Ageing Research Reviews* 15: 76–93.

55. Blandin, K. and Pepin, R. (2017). Dementia grief: a theoretical model of a unique grief experience. *Dementia* 16 (1): 67–78.

56. Williamson, L.E., Evans, C.J., Cripps, R.L. et al. (2021). Factors associated with emergency department visits by people with dementia near the end of life: a systematic review. *Journal of the American Medical Directors Association* 22 (10): 2046–2055.

57. British Geriatrics Society (2020). End of life care and frailty. Clinical Guidelines. https://www.bgs.org.uk/resources/end-of-life-care-in-frailty-dementia (accessed 18 September 2021).

58. Davies, N., Maio, L., Rait, G., and Iliffe, S. (2014). Quality end-of-life care for dementia: what have family carers told us so far? a narrative synthesis. *Palliative Medicine* 28 (7): 919–930.

59. Schulz, R. and Sherwood, P.R. (2008). Physical and mental health effects of family caregiving. *The American Journal of Nursing* 108 (9 Suppl): 23–27.

60. Ewing, G. and Grande, G., National Association for Hospice at Home. (2013). Development of a Carer Support Needs Assessment Tool (CSNAT) for end-of-life care practice at home: a qualitative study. *Palliative Medicine* 27 (3): 244–256.

61. Aoun, S.M., Toye, C., Slatyer, S. et al. (2018). A person-centred approach to family carer needs assessment and support in dementia community care in Western Australia. *Health & Social Care in the Community* 26 (4): e578–86.

62. NICE (2016). Multimorbidity: clinical assessment and management NG56 overview | Multimorbidity: clinical assessment and management | Guidance | NICE. https://www.nice.org.uk/guidance/ng56 (accessed 28 September 2021).

63. Finucane, A.M., Bone, A.E., Etkind, S. et al. (2021). How many people will need palliative care in Scotland by 2040? a mixed-method study of projected palliative care need and recommendations for service delivery. *BMJ open* 11 (2): e041317.

64. Melis, R.J., Marengoni, A., Rizzuto, D. et al. (2013). The influence of multimorbidity on clinical progression of dementia in a population-based cohort. *PloS one* 8 (12): e84014.

65. Oosterveld, S.M., Kessels, R.P., Hamel, R. et al. (2014). The influence of co-morbidity and frailty on the clinical manifestation of patients with Alzheimer's disease. *Journal of Alzheimer's Disease* 42 (2): 501–509.

66. Biessels, G.J., Staekenborg, S., Brunner, E. et al. (2006). Risk of dementia in diabetes mellitus: a systematic review. *Lancet Neurology* 5: 64–74.

67. Russell, S.G., Quigley, R., and Thompson, F. (2022). Factors associated with the increased risk of dementia found in the Torres Strait. *Australasian Journal on Ageing* 41 (1): 88–96.

68. Tonelli, M., Wiebe, N., Straus, S. et al. (2017). Multimorbidity, dementia, and healthcare in older people: a population-based cohort study. *Canadian Medical Association Open Access Journal* 5 (3): E623–31.

69. Nicholson, C., Davies, J.M., and George, R. (2018). What are the main palliative care symptoms and concerns of older people with multimorbidity? a comparative cross-sectional study using routinely collected phase of illness, Australia-modified Karnofsky performance status and integrated palliative care outcome scale data. *Annals of Palliative Medicine* 7 (Suppl 3): S164–75.

70. Powell, V.D. and Silveira, M.J. (2021). Palliative Care for Older Adults with multimorbidity in the time of COVID-19. *Journal of Aging & Social Policy* 33 (4–5): 500–508.

71. Christensen, M. and Lundh, A. (2016). Medication review in hospitalised patients to reduce morbidity and mortality. *Cochrane Database of Systematic Reviews* 2 (2): CD008986.

72. Curtin, D., O'Mahony, D., and Gallagher, P. (2018). Drug consumption and futile medication prescribing in the last year of life: an observational study. *Age and Ageing* 47 (5): 749–753.

73. Thompson, J. (2019). Deprescribing in palliative care. *Clinical Medicine* 19 (4): 311.

74. Russell, S., Coxon, G., and Taylor, R. (2019). Are care homes the hospices of the future? British Geriatrics Society. https://www.bgs.org.uk/comment/2378 (accessed 10 October 2021).

75. Payne, S., Seymour, J. and Ingleton, C. (2008). *Palliative Care Nursing: Principles and Evidence for Practice*. McGraw-Hill Education (UK).

76. Bone, A.E., Morgan, M., Maddocks, M. et al. (2016). Developing a model of short-term integrated palliative and supportive care for frail older people in community settings: perspectives of older people, carers and other key stakeholders. *Age and Ageing* 45 (6): 863–873.

77. Conroy, S., Carpenter, C., and Banerjee, J. (2021). The silver book II. Quality urgent care for older people. British Geriatrics Society, London. https://www.bgs.org.uk/resources/resource-series/silver-book-ii (accessed 10 October 2021).

78. Yip, K.F., Wong, T.H., and Alhamid, S.M. (2020). Integrating advance care planning as part of comprehensive geriatric assessment for hospitalised frail elderly patients: findings of a cross-sectional study. *Singapore Medical Journal* 61 (5): 254.

79. Kirkhus, L., Šaltytė Benth, J., Grønberg, B.H. et al. (2019). Frailty identified by geriatric assessment is associated with poor functioning, high symptom burden and increased risk of physical decline in older cancer patients: prospective observational study. *Palliative Medicine* 33 (3): 312–322.

80. Bennett, M.I., Ziegler, L., and Allsop, M. (2016). What determines duration of palliative care before death for patients with advanced disease? a retrospective cohort study of community and hospital palliative care provision in a large UK city. *BMJ open* 6 (12): e012576.

81. Noble, J., Nicholson, C., Harris, L. et al. (2018). Learning from a new model of end of life care for older people with frailty/multi-morbidities – The challenges and opportunities for specialist palliative care services. *BMJ Supportive & Palliative Care* 8: 360.

82. Bunn, F., Pinkney, E., Drennan, V., and Goodman, C. (2013). An evaluation of the role of the admiral nurse: a systematic evidence synthesis to inform service delivery and research. University of Hertfordshire, Report for Dementia UK.

83. Dening, K.H. and Aldridge, Z. (2019). Admiral nurse case management: a model of caregiver support for families affected by dementia. *OBM Geriatrics* 3 (2): 1–13.

84. Hospice UK (2015). Hospice enabled dementia care the first steps. A guide to help hospices establish care for people with dementia, their families and carers. Hospice UK, London. https://professionals.hospiceuk.org/what-we-offer/clinical-and-care-support/hospice-enabled-dementia-care?page=2 (accessed 17 August 2021).

17 Palliative Care in Advanced Heart Failure

Amy Gadoud

Introduction

Heart failure (HF) is a global problem with a prevalence of 38 million worldwide, a number that is increasing with the ageing population despite advances in cardiovascular medicine and surgery [1]. It is the most common diagnosis of patients admitted to hospital over 65 years in high-income countries [1]. In the UK there are as many people with advanced HF as there are with the four most common cancers combined [2]. As risk factors for cardiovascular disease in low- and medium-income counties increase, the prevalence of HF is also increasing in these settings [1].

The prognosis following a diagnosis of HF remains poor and lags behind other serious conditions such as cancer [3]. These patients have a significant symptom burden, poor quality of life, and other palliative care needs, often over a longer period than for patients with cancer [4, 5]. The economic cost of HF, largely driven by unscheduled hospital admissions, is considerable [6–8].

National and international guidance calls for the integration of palliative care alongside other health services for patients with HF [9–12]. But despite these recommendations, the palliative care needs of many patients with HF are not recognised or well managed [13].

This chapter will address both the common physical symptoms and psychosocial distress that patients with advanced HF face and will examine the barriers that often limit access to quality symptom management and palliative care for these patients living with advanced HF. A case study is used to integrate this approach into a patient's journey.

Definition and Characteristics

The European Society of cardiology defines HF as a clinical syndrome consisting of cardinal symptoms of breathlessness, ankle swelling, and fatigue that may be accompanied by physical signs (e.g. elevated jugular venous pressure, pulmonary crackles, and peripheral oedema). It is due to a structural and/or functional abnormality of the heart that results in elevated intracardiac pressures and/or inadequate cardiac output at rest and/or during exercise [14].

The aetiology of HF varies according to geography. In Western-type and developed countries, coronary artery disease (CAD) and hypertension are predominant factors [14]. Rheumatic heart disease remains a major cause of HF in developing countries; as countries undergo socio-economic development, the epidemiology of HF becomes increasingly similar to that of Western Europe and North America [15].

The severity of HF is useful to classify, such as described by the New York Heart Association (NYHA) [16], and HF has been divided into distinct phenotypes based on the measurement of left ventricular ejection fraction (LVEF). The rationale behind this relates to the original treatment trials in HF that demonstrated substantially improved outcomes in patients with reduced LVEF. However, HF spans the entire range of LVEF (a normally distributed variable), and additionally measurement by echocardiography is subject to substantial variability. The European Association of Cardiology use the following classification of HF (Box 1).

Handbook of Palliative Care, Fourth Edition. Edited by Richard Kitchen, Christina Faull, Sarah Russell and Jo Wilson.
© 2024 John Wiley & Sons Ltd. Published 2024 by John Wiley & Sons Ltd.

The Growing Need

In developed countries, the age-adjusted incidence of HF may be falling, presumably reflecting better management of cardiovascular disease, but due to ageing, the overall incidence is increasing [14]. HF is a common condition with a prevalence of 1 to 2% in the developed world and increasing to greater than 10% in elderly cohorts [17, 18]. As studies only usually include recognised/diagnosed HF cases, the true prevalence is likely to be higher [14].

Studies from several European countries and the United States (US) have shown that HF hospitalisation rates peaked in the 1990s, and then declined [14]. However, in a recent study of incident HF conducted between 1998 and 2017 in the United Kingdom (UK), first hospitalisations increased by 28% for both all-cause and HF admissions [19] during the study period. These increases were higher in women, perhaps related to higher comorbidity rates.

During 2000–1, there were 84,151 admissions for people with HF in the UK [20]. This had risen to 141,566 UK admissions in 2009 [21]. This is estimated to represent 2% of all NHS inpatient bed-days and 5% of all emergency medical admissions to hospital. Due to population growth, ageing, and the increasing prevalence of comorbidities, the absolute number of hospital admissions for HF across Europe is expected to increase considerably in the future, perhaps by as much as 50% in the next 25 years [14].

It is estimated that the total annual cost of HF to the NHS is around 2% of the total NHS budget: approximately 70% of this total is due to the costs of hospitalisation [22]. The average number of admissions in the last six months of life for patients with HF is two, but there is wide variation [23].

Prognosis due to HF is poor. The five-year prognosis is worse than that for many cancers [24]. There have been improvements in mortality due to improved medical management. Implantable cardioverter-defibrillator (ICD) placement reduces the risk of sudden death and as its use becomes more common, more patients will develop progressive advanced HF [25]. Prognosis remains poor and data from a Canadian study assessing prognosis of patients newly admitted with HF still showed a 5-year mortality of 68.7% (median survival 2.4 years) and in those with an ejection fraction of less than 30% there was a median survival of only 3 months [26].

Barriers and Challenges in Integrating Palliative Care for Patients with HF

Disease Trajectory "Prognostic Paralysis"

Different disease trajectories have been described for cancer, single organ failure, and general frailty [27]. These are important on a population level and for understanding the natural history of these diseases. There is much uncertainty when dealing with prognostication at the end-of-life which has resulted in some clinicians feeling powerless and unable to act, described as prognostic paralysis [28]. Population level studies have described the HF trajectory as gradual decline, punctuated by episodes of acute deterioration, any of which may result in death or recovery. Death is described as seemingly sudden compared with the more predictable terminal phase seen with some cancers [27]. However, there is much inter-patient variability and so this "typical" disease trajectory may be less helpful with the specific individual patient seen on the ward or in the clinic [29].

In contrast to cancer where palliative care may be welcomed alongside treatments that may alter the natural history of the illness to a similar trajectory to a chronic illness interspersed by acute deteriorations, there appear to be more barriers to integrating palliative care in HF according to patient need.

Recognition of Advanced Disease

The disease course of HF is often one of a gradual deterioration interrupted by exacerbations that towards end-stage may have no precipitant. As the disease worsens, exacerbations may become more frequent and less responsive to treatment, resulting in "revolving door" admissions [30, 31]. In addition, the patient may become less tolerant to maintenance treatment due to renal failure or hypotension [32, 33]. A retrospective review has demonstrated that patients with HF have symptom burden, measured by functional status for a longer period of time than cancer patients [4].

Communication with Patients

Recognition of advanced disease is only the first step in improving patient care. The second step is to sensitively and appropriately communicate this to patients and their families. In the SUPPORT study however, even when clinicians were given detailed accurate information about the patient's likely prognosis, many failed to recognise and act on that information, and only 15% discussed it with the patients and/or their families [34, 35]. A systematic review of literature by Barclay and colleagues concerning conversations about end-of-life care between patients with HF and health-care professionals suggests that clinicians wait for cues from patients before raising end-of-life issues, while patients commonly wait for clinicians to raise these issues: as a result, the conversations rarely take place [36]. Interviews with 106 hospitalised patients with HF across five tertiary centres in Canada confirmed that patients valued honest communication by the doctor as among the most important issues in relation to end-of-life care [37]. These views are reflected in a large study of 2331 cancer patients, 1046 of whom were being treated palliatively, 87% wanted all possible information, good or bad, including a similar proportion in the palliative group [38]. In cancer palliative care, significant strides have been made with training in communication skills [39]. Truth telling tailored to an individual's requirements, while maintaining realistic hope is a skill, and although it is difficult, it is usually the best way to work together to plan future appropriate management, and does not destroy hope, a fear expressed by clinicians [40]. Cardiologists in a focus group study confirmed that they rarely raised end-of-life issues with patients, citing lack of confidence and training in discussing end-of-life issues as a significant barrier. It also takes time, and may require restructuring of services, for example out-patient cardiology clinics [41]. Disease specific communication guidelines for cardiology have very recently been produced and will enable patients, if they wish, to discuss their poor prognosis and be involved in decisions about their future care despite uncertain disease trajectories by [42] "hoping for the best, and preparing for the worst" [43].

Societal and Professional Lack of Understanding of Diagnosis and Needs

There is a risk that clinicians as well as patients feel the symptoms in HF are inevitable [44] and untreatable making a full assessment of palliative care needs less likely. It is known that patients and carers have a poor understanding of HF [45], the stage of their illness, its treatments and aims of treatments, and the poor prognosis [46–50]. Patients report being given little information, or what is given is discussed in complex language that is difficult to understand, and the term "HF" itself is perceived as a barrier by some clinicians [46]. In addition, if palliative care is perceived as something that is required only for the imminently dying or for cancer patients this can be a significant barrier. Clinicians find it difficult for many reasons to recognise that a patient is approaching the end of their life. There are societal norms with the avoidance of death and professional codes such as the duty of the doctor to preserve life and may result in clinicians seeing death as a failure. Increased therapeutic options may make it tempting for clinicians to strive for any prolongation of life, even if this is futile, or merely prolongs the dying itself.

Fragmentation of Care

Many different disciplines are involved in patients with advanced HF: cardiology, general medicine, care of the elderly, emergency medicine, primary care, and palliative care across community, hospital, and hospice settings. A qualitative study by Hanratty and colleagues in 2002 demonstrated poor coordination of services between hospital and community, lack of clarity regarding different speciality clinicians' roles, and the need for improved communication between all the professionals involved in patients with HF and palliative care needs [41].

Many patients would prefer to remain at home, especially at the end-of-life, and see their GPs as the most important person coordinating their care [41]. This is a role that GPs are able and willing to undertake, but for HF it has been suggested they would like education regarding HF management and communication issues [51]. Cardiologists lack experience in palliative care [41, 52]. Palliative care specialists also require education, for example, regarding medications and cardiac devices. This is important as there is a need to continue some disease modifying medications for patients with HF to control symptoms [53]. Some palliative care specialists have also expressed concern that scarce resources will be overwhelmed [54] although established integrated services have not reported this to be the case [55, 56]. Cancer palliative care services tend to be better developed. As a large number of professionals are involved in HF care it can make it difficult to understand who is responsible for initiating discussions about end-of-life care. Due to the barriers to communication that have already been discussed, it could mean that each professional leaves it to someone else meaning it never happens.

An important area with regard to fragmentation of care is out-of-hours care. In cancer palliative care, there are already concerns about poor coordination in out-of-hours care [57–59]. In the UK out-of-hours GPs are a separate service and in order to facilitate good out-of-hours palliative care, generally a specific communication or handover is required. Advanced HF because of difficulty of recognising advanced disease may mean this handover is less likely to happen creating another barrier to effective palliative care for HF patients.

Case Study Part 1

BB is a 94-year-old female who lives alone in a two-story house with three supportive adult children nearby. She has New York Heart Association (NYHA) class 4 HF, hypertension, coronary artery disease with previous coronary artery bypass graft, and implantable cardioverter-defibrillator (ICD) with biventricular pacemaker inserted three years ago, osteoporosis with recent T12 compression fracture, chronic kidney disease with baseline glomerular filtration rate of 40 ml/min, and recurrent urinary tract infections.

Two years ago, she had significant decompensation of HF and was hospitalised for two months. Both BB and her family were told repeatedly during that admission to "prepare for the worst". The echocardiogram at discharge showed very poor LV function. She was discharged home with significantly reduced functional status but it improved gradually over the next few months. She remained confined to her house, however, only leaving it to go for primary care/hospital appointments. In the last six months, her condition has deteriorated again with three hospital admissions.

Needs Assessment Not Prognostication as the Route to Improving Outcomes

The trajectory of HF can be quite variable but typically includes a slow progressive overall decline accompanied by a gradual worsening of breathlessness, fatigue, and function with a decreased quality of life. With time, patients will experience exacerbations of acute HF and the frequency of cardiac decompensation increases with a need for more hospitalisations and further decline in quality of life. Families and patients grow accustomed to this course of illness and often do not foresee dying, thus, patients frequently die in an acute facility [60].

Further, sudden cardiac death occurs in approximately half of all deaths in patients with HF [61]. The variable trajectory coupled with high rates of sudden unpredictable cardiac death makes prognostication very difficult [62].

Accurate prognostication can aid clinical decision making and help patients and families with expectations and advance care planning (ACP) [63]. As with other disease states, patients and families tend to overestimate likelihood of survival. Although informing patients of their likely prognosis is important, such predictions are not exact at the individual level, and the notion of uncertainty must enter into the discussion [12].

Indeed, given the unpredictable trajectory of HF, prognostic tools are of limited value for identifying patients with a high risk of mortality who can benefit from palliative care [64]. The National Institute for Health and Care Excellence (NICE) guidelines do not recommend prognostic risk tools to determine if patients with HF need palliative care referral [22]. These guidelines recommend if the symptoms of a person with HF are worsening despite optimal specialist treatment, discuss their palliative care needs with the specialist HF multidisciplinary team and consider a needs assessment for palliative care [22].

A recent systematic review identified six palliative care needs assessment and measurement tools for patients with HF [65]. The review concluded that despite limited evidence, the Needs Assessment Tool: Progressive Disease—Heart Failure (NAT: PD-HF) is the most appropriate palliative care needs-assessment tool for use in HF populations [66–68]. It covers most of the patient needs and has the best psychometric properties and evidence of

---

Case Study Part 2

In the past six months, she had three hospital admissions and her primary care family physician reviews her at home. Previously they had a good professional relationship but he has not seen her recently. He also notes multiple call outs to out of hours GP or paramedic services. The most recent discharge from hospital was two weeks ago. Discharge letter reads: "decompensated HF. IV Furosemide for 2 days and discharged home on usual cardiac meds." He notes she was under a different team each admission who stabilised her HF and then quickly discharged her from hospital. The letter ends with "BB not keen on hospital and family happy to support her at home." The primary care physician reviews that her creatinine is currently 300 and has been rising for last year. She has a chronic low Na and is no longer able to tolerate her angiotensin-converting-enzyme inhibitor (ACEI) due to hypotension. She is on a large dose of diuretics. She has had a comprehensive cardiology review and primary care physician is happy that her medical and device therapy are optimised. The primary care physician gained her agreement for referral to the community palliative care team.

identification ability and appropriateness. Psychometric testing of the tools in patients with HF and evaluating the tools to identify those with palliative care needs require more investigation [65]. NAT:PD-HF is completed by health-care professionals, has been adapted for use in HF populations and identifies palliative care needs which the health-care professionals can meet themselves or refer to palliative care or other services to receive assistance with a particular concern [65, 66].

Palliative Care Delivery in HF

Five systematic reviews that show palliative care interventions are effective for patients with HF [69–73]. Two of the reviews included a variety of study designs as well as RCTs and improved patient centred outcomes and support the use of multidisciplinary palliative care teams for patients with HF [69, 70]. The three reviews that only included RCTS showed a reduction in depression [72,73], hospitalisations [73], and readmissions [71].

Case Study Part 3

BB and her family explain to the community palliative care team that they are keen for her to spend as much time at home rather than in hospital. The team discussed resuscitation including deactivating her ICD. One of her daughters finds these conversations difficult. As she explained: "Doctors don't know anything. They thought she was dying two years ago and she got better."

Over a couple of conversations with the palliative care team, BB, her family and the team decided it is appropriate for BB not to be resuscitated and for her ICD to be switched off but keep the biventricular function. This is organised via local protocols. BB attended day hospice once a week for an eight-week block. She found the peer support and her discussions with the spiritual care coordinator particularly beneficial. The physiotherapist reviewed her breathing exercises, and BB was confident to do them at home along with using her hand-held fan. Breathlessness was further palliated by low-dose opioid, which also controlled her back pain from the T12 compression fracture secondary to her osteoporosis. BB and her family appreciated being able to call the out-of-hours hospice/community palliative care telephone line when she was breathless at night and had not felt the need to phone emergency services. Appropriate advance care planning documents including treatment escalation orders, detailing the plan to manage BB symptoms at home were completed. Admission to hospital would be avoided unless comfort measures failed. BB indicated that her preference would be to die at home.

An integrated approach is recommended in European and United States (US) guidelines [9–12]. This is provision of palliative and supportive care along with disease modifying interventions as part of comprehensive HF care. Goodlin describes five stages of HF care from initial symptoms to end-of-life. She describes how at each stage there are HF interventions, decision making/advance care planning, and supportive care (communication, education, psychosocial and spiritual issues, and symptom management). Despite having five stages, the stages are not consecutive: sudden death can occur at any point along the disease trajectory and transplant and other acute interventions can put a patient back to an earlier stage[53].

Interventional Aspects of Care

Implantable cardiac defibrillators (ICD) and cardiac resynchronisation therapy defibrillators (CRTD) are currently the gold standard in treatment of HF [74]. Both devices reduce mortality in HF by preventing sudden cardiac death due to ventricular arrhythmia [14]. In end-stage HF, consideration of deactivation of ICD or CRTD devices is of paramount importance. HF patients approaching death may have unstable ventricular rhythms causing recurrent shocks with pain and distress. It is therefore recommended that the defibrillator function of these devices is disabled [10]. The exact timing of this will vary depending on the individual patient, their arrhythmia burden, and previous device therapies but generally when considering do not attempt cardiopulmonary resuscitation decisions as part of wider goals of care decisions [42, 75]. Indeed, it is recommended that discussions about future deactivating ICDs take place prior to their insertion [75]. The concept of device deactivation must be conveyed sensitively to the patient and their carers. Patients may have misconceptions about how their device works and may even anticipate instantaneous death on deactivation of the defibrillator [76]. Importantly, disabling the defibrillator function of an ICD or CRTD does not affect the pacing function of the device. A cardiac resynchronisation therapy (CRT) pacemaker, as well as improving survival, improves symptoms and quality of life while reducing hospital admission and so should usually be continued [14]. If reprogramming of an ICD is not possible and patient is close to death and receives shocks, a magnet over the ICD will temporarily suspend antitachycardia therapies while not disabling antibradycardia pacing [77].

Cardiac transplantation is an established therapy associated with good long-term survival and marked improvement in functional capacity in appropriate patients. It is only available to limited patients with about 5,000 patients worldwide receive heart transplants each year. Best utilisation of available donor organs dictates that patients selected for transplant should be both ill enough to require transplantation but well enough to have good long-term outcome after transplantation. Most transplant centres exclude patients >70–75 years of age and those with advanced comorbidities [9].

A left ventricular assist device is a battery-operated blood pump that is implanted into either ventricle to decrease the workload of the struggling ventricle. They provide mechanical circulatory support and can serve as a bridge to transplant or used on a long-term basis but are costly and available to very few at present. It is now recommended, apart from in emergency situations, that a palliative medicine consultation is conducted prior to insertion and palliative care specialists are part of the mechanical circulatory support team [9, 12].

Symptom Management

Patients with HF have a symptom burden similar to those with malignant disease. To ensure good palliation of symptoms and best patient care, a systematic symptom assessment should be performed. Special attention should be given to patient preferences and goals of care.

Optimal HF management combines both symptom- and disease-modifying therapies and as patient goals of care change, the benefits of some medications will need to be revisited. Many patients with HF have refractory symptoms such as pain, breathlessness, fatigue, cough, nausea, limited mobility, falls, depression, anxiety, insomnia, constipation, and loss of appetite [5, 33, 78]. In the community, these persons experience a loss of independence with increased dependence on others [5]. The management of symptoms should consider patient goals and preferences, subjective experience, and disease-specific factors such as available and appropriate therapies, performance status, and prognosis.

HF patients require the same approach to symptom assessment and management as all palliative care patients, and the concepts of "total pain" or "total breathlessness" [79] remind us of the need to holistically assess all domains including psychosocial, spiritual, carer concerns and information and communication needs as well as physical [76].

Good symptom control requires both recognising and treating any co-morbidities while optimising HF medical and device therapy management as appropriate depending on the stage of disease and the wishes of the patient [76].

The HF population is not well represented in studies investigating the palliation of pain and other symptoms. It is, however, reasonable to extrapolate from evidence and guidance from other palliative care populations, unless there is evidence of contraindication. It is also important to consider multi-morbidity such as renal failure which is common in patients with HF patients [76].

Breathlessness

Breathlessness is the most common reason for patients with HF to seek medical attention and hospital admission [80]. Compared with primary or metastatic lung cancer, persons with HF and other non-cancer causes of breathlessness have significantly higher levels of breathlessness in the last three months of life, which remains relatively constant until death [81]. Non-pharmacological management is important. This includes providing a fan to the facial area, breathing training and exercise programmes, and anxiety management [82].

Exercise has been clearly shown to improve quality of life in HF [83, 84]. However, studies of patients with the most severe symptoms are lacking [83]. Evidence for other non-pharmacological interventions for breathlessness in HF is mostly extrapolated from trials in patients with chronic obstructive pulmonary disease (COPD) [85]. Psychological interventions, specifically in HF patients, have shown some benefit [85–87].

An adequately powered RCT of morphine compared with placebo demonstrated an improvement in refractory breathlessness in those taking morphine in a palliative care population [88]. There are fewer studies specifically in HF populations. Therefore, extrapolating from evidence in other populations, low dose opioids are both efficacious and safe [89]. Relatively low doses are often sufficient [9].

Benzodiazepines are commonly used to palliate refractory breathlessness, but a Cochrane review demonstrated insufficient evidence and concluded that until more adequately powered studies were conducted, benzodiazepines should be considered second- or third-line treatment only [90]. They should be used cautiously because of risk of side effects in advanced HF especially considering comorbidities such as renal failure.

Despite being commonly prescribed, there is no evidence for supplementary oxygen in the palliation of refractory breathlessness in the absence of significant hypoxaemia [91, 92]. However, very few patients with HF were included in these studies. European guidance specifically for heart failure patients state there is little benefit of supplementary oxygen in pts with HF alone [10].

For further information on breathlessness see Chapter 12: The Management of Respiratory Symptoms and Advanced Chronic Obstructive Pulmonary Disease.

Pain

Patients with advanced HF commonly experience pain, present in up to 90 % of patients with NYHA class IV [10]. As with all pain the underlying cause should be determined and treated as appropriate, for example, anti-anginal medication as tolerated for ischaemic chest pain. For other pains opioids are generally used, avoiding renally excreted opioids in renal failure [9]. NSAIDs are generally contraindicated due to adverse effects on renal function, sodium and fluid retention, and gastrointestinal side effects [9]. Tricyclic antidepressants (TCAs) and gabapentinoids may be useful for peripheral neuropathy for example due to diabetes related neuropathy although TCAs should be used with caution as they may prolong the QT interval leading to tachyarrhythmias.

Fatigue

The management of fatigue should include an attempt to identify reversible causes such as anaemia, infection, obstructive sleep apnoea, electrolyte abnormalities, and renal failure. One should exclude depression, thyroid abnormalities, and psychosocial contributors, and ensure the optimal treatment of HF.

Exercise may be helpful for fatigue but should be tailored to an individual's performance status and stage of heart failure [10]. Educating patients on how to time their activities to periods of peak energy may be useful. There is no evidence for the use of stimulants such as methylphenidate for heart failure related fatigue evidence. It may be reasonable to consider these therapies but important to be mindful of potential adverse effects such as an increased heart rate and blood pressure [9].

Anaemia

Iron deficiency and anaemia are common in patients with HF, being independently associated with reduced exercise capacity, recurrent HF hospitalisations, and high cardiovascular and all-cause mortality. Treatment is complex and generally consists of IV iron therapy. Erythropoietin stimulating agents are not indicated for the treatment of anaemia in HF. For further details the reader is directed to

recent European guidance [14]. As with all palliative therapeutic strategies, one must consider patient goals and potential benefits and risks of therapy.

Oedema/Ascites

The management of oedema requires excellent skin care to prevent pressure and other skin ulcers and cellulitis. Compression stockings may be useful but many patients find them uncomfortable to use [9] and raising legs when not mobilising will give symptomatic relief.

Optimal management of HF is necessary and discontinuing medications associated with fluid retention such as dihydropyridine calcium channel blockers, thiozolidinediones, NSAIDs, corticosteroids, and others may help. Optimal dosing of diuretics considering electrolyte balance depending on goals and prognosis is the mainstay of medication management. Similarly, ascites secondary to right-sided HF is best managed with diuretics; paracentesis including indwelling catheters could be considered rarely if refractory [10].

Psychological /Psychosocial

Depression and anxiety is very common in heart failure and present is more than 50% of patients and more common in patients with severe disease, for example present in 40 to 70% of hospitalised patients with NYHA class III or IV symptoms [10].

The presence of depression is associated with higher symptom burden and increased risk of adverse outcome such as hospitalisations and mortality [9].

Treatment of depression must be holistic, addressing physical, psychological, spiritual, and social needs. People with HF at the end-of-life face social isolation, hopelessness, significant frustration, challenges of working with the formal health-care system, life disruption, high symptom burden, and uncertainty about prognosis and symptoms [5, 93].

Non-pharmacological management includes open communication, cardiac rehabilitation, exercise, and psychological therapies including cognitive behavioural therapy. Selective serotonin reuptake inhibitors (SSRIs) are recommended first line as pharmacological agents for depression and are safe and relatively well tolerated [10].

Further, it is important not to forget the challenges that caregivers experience. Many caregivers of elderly patients with HF are themselves elderly and often experience poor health. These caregivers have high rates of depression.

Case Study Part 4

Following her eight weeks at the day hospice she was discharged from palliative care services with excellent symptom control at rest. She remained fatigued but focused what energy she had on her most important tasks. She was screened for depression but her mood remained stable in spite of recognising her uncertain prognosis. She continued with a Palliative Performance Scale (PPS) of 40% and was unable to descend her stairs. Occupational Therapy Services reviewed her home and provided appropriate equipment and a hospital bed downstairs. Home care was organised to support BB and her family with her care needs.

Her home care nurse and primary care physician monitored her closely at home. She had no further admissions to hospital.

Case Study Conclusion

The palliative care team did not hear from BB for two months. They telephoned to find she was as stable as at her discharge, with good symptom control and acceptable quality of life and was planning for Christmas. Her primary care physician and home care nurse had been seeing to her needs. She remained stable for a number of additional months with daily visits from her daughters and received twice daily home support help. She slowly deteriorated with a PPS of 30%, and then a more rapid deterioration with changes week by week. She recognised she was dying.

She was well supported by her family, primary care physician, and home care nurse and utilised the support of the palliative response team who assisted with a change of medication administration to SC route, titration of doses to comfort, and provided glycopyrrolate subcutaneously at a PPS of 10% for the treatment and relief of upper respiratory secretions. The three daughters had gathered around their mother for her last weeks and received grief and bereavement counselling.

Discontinuing Medical Therapies

Large randomised double-blind placebo-controlled trials have irrefutably demonstrated the prognostic benefit of HF medical therapy, such as angiotensin converting enzyme (ACE) inhibitors, beta blockers and mineralocorticoid receptor antagonists. These drugs have also been unequivocally shown to alleviate symptoms, reduce hospital admissions, and improve quality of life [14].

It follows that in HF patients with escalating palliative care needs, conventional HF medical therapy should be continued wherever possible. Medication should be reviewed regularly, and the relative benefits with respect to survival and symptom management considered. Advanced HF patients are prone to hypotension and hypovolaemia. As a transition to a more palliative approach is taken, one must weigh the risks and benefits of what medications are continued and for what benefit. Diuretics remain important throughout the disease trajectory with respect to alleviating peripheral oedema and preventing pulmonary oedema [94]. Intermittent intravenous diuretic therapy is often considered appropriate in advanced HF, but aggressive diuretic management in hospital is not recommended in the terminal stages. Subcutaneous infusion of diuretics may be of benefit [95, 96]. Continuing digoxin in end-stage HF may have symptomatic benefit by reducing heart rate and breathlessness without adversely affecting blood pressure [97].

Advance Care Planning and End-of-Life Care

Advance care planning should be part of routine care for all patients with HF. It should be wide ranging, including all aspects important to each patient and those close to them. It should also include medical anticipatory care planning, where likely deteriorations are discussed and patient centred plans made and documented. It is often helpful to frame as "hope for the best and plan for the worst"[42].

When death is imminent and comfort is the primary goal, a reassessment of symptom burden, psychosocial, informational, and other needs must be done. Opioids with or without benzodiazepines via subcutaneous (SC) route of administration for breathlessness are used. Medications must be re-evaluated. Grief and bereavement support for families should be available.

Conclusion

The prevalence of HF patients is increasing and so are their symptom, caregiver, informational, social, psychological, and spiritual needs. Earlier identification of these palliative care needs will help bring improved quality of life to this growing population. Recognition of end-stage disease is crucial to meet patient goals and optimise care, but palliative care is not simply "terminal care" in this population and should be introduced earlier along with active care depending on identified needs. Discussions with patients and families about the anticipated course of the disease, prognostic uncertainty, goals of care, and advance directives (advance decisions) including preference for resuscitation orders, deactivation of defibrillation devices, and place of death need to be revisited along the trajectory. A patient and family-centred multidisciplinary approach with improved integration and communication between primary, palliative, and cardiology care will likely serve patients best.

References

1. Braunwald, E. (2015). The war against heart failure: the Lancet lecture. *The Lancet* 385 (9970): 812–824.
2. Conrad, N. et al. (2017). Temporal trends and patterns in heart failure incidence: a population-based study of 4 million individuals. *The Lancet* 391 (10120): 572–580.
3. Taylor, C.J. et al. (2019). Trends in survival after a diagnosis of heart failure in the United Kingdom 2000–2017: population based cohort study. *BMJ* 364: l223.
4. Teno, J.M. et al. (2001). Dying trajectory in the last year of life: does cancer trajectory fit other diseases? *Journal of Palliative Medicine* 4 (4): 457–464.
5. O'Leary, N. (2009). The comparative palliative care needs of those with heart failure and cancer patients. *Current Opinion in Supportive and Palliative Care* 3 (4): 241–246.
6. Unroe, K.T. et al. (2010). Resource use in the last 6 months of life among medicare beneficiaries with heart failure, 2000–2007. *Archives of Internal Medicine* 171 (3): 196–203.
7. Kaul, P. et al. (2010). Resource use in the last 6 months of life among patients with heart failure in Canada. *Archives of Internal Medicine* 171 (3): 211–217.
8. Gibson, R. (2011). Resource use in the last 6 months of life: what does it mean for patients? *Archives of Internal Medicine* 171 (3): 194–195.
9. Whellan, D.J. et al. (2014). End-of-life care in patients with heart failure. *Journal of Cardiac Failure* 20 (2): 121–134.
10. Hill, L. et al. (2020). Integration of a palliative approach into heart failure care: a European Society of Cardiology Heart Failure Association position paper. *European Journal of Heart Failure* 22 (12): 2327–2339.
11. National Heart Foundation of Australia and Cardiac Society of Australia and New Zealand Heart Failure Guidelines Working Group. et al. (2018). National Heart Foundation of Australia and Cardiac Society of Australia and New Zealand: guidelines for the prevention, detection, and management of heart failure in Australia 2018. *Heart, Lung & Circulation* 27 (10): 1123–1208.
12. Braun, L.T. et al. (2016). Palliative care and cardiovascular disease and stroke: a policy statement from the American Heart Association/American Stroke Association. *Circulation* 134 (11): e198–225.
13. Gadoud, A. et al. (2014). Palliative care among heart failure patients in primary care: a comparison to cancer patients using English family practice data. *PLoS One* 9 (11): e113188.
14. McDonagh, T.A. et al. (2021). 2021 ESC Guidelines for the diagnosis and treatment of acute and chronic heart failure. *European Heart Journal* 42 (36): 3599–3726.
15. Mendez, G.F. and Cowie, M.R. (2001). The epidemiological features of heart failure in developing countries: a review of the literature. *International Journal of Cardiology* 80 (2): 213–219.
16. Dolgin, M. (1994). *Nomenclature and Criteria for Diagnosis of Diseases of the Heart and Great Vessels*. Boston, MA. [u.a.]: Little, Brown and Co.
17. Davis, R.C., Davies, M.K., and Yip, G.Y.H. (2006). History and epidemiology. In: *ABC of Heart Failure* (ed. R.C. Davis, M.K. Davies, and G.Y.H. Yip), 1–4. Oxford: Blackwell Publishing Ltd.
18. Mosterd, A. and Hoes, A.W. (2007). Clinical epidemiology of heart failure. *Heart* 93 (9): 1137–1146.
19. Lawson, C.A. et al. (2019). 20-year trends in cause-specific heart failure outcomes by sex, socioeconomic status, and place of diagnosis: a population-based study. *The Lancet Public Health* 4 (8): e406–e420.
20. BHF. (2000). Cost of heart failure to the NHS. (cited 9 November 2010) https://www.bhf.org.uk/-/media/files/research/heart-statistics/bhf-cvd-statistics-englandfactsheet.pdf?rev=37d0929ec6904079909248f02bf8e0ce&hash=E406B45B46FAB27AE2C0031943184E09.
21. Townsend, N. et al. (2012). Coronary heart disease statistics 2012 Edition. London: British Heart Foundation.
22. National Clinical Guideline Centre for Acute and Chronic Conditions. (2010). NICE Clinical Guideline 108: chronic heart failure – management of chronic heart failure in adults in primary and secondary care. London: National Institute for Health and Clinical Excellence.
23. National End of Life Care Intelligence Network. (2013). Deaths from cardiovascular diseases implications for end of life care in England. (cited 24 February 2013) http://www.endoflifecare-intelligence.org.uk/resources/publications/deaths_from_cardiovascular_diseases.aspx.
24. Stewart, S. et al. (2001). More "malignant" than cancer? Five-year survival following a first admission for heart failure. *European Journal of Heart Failure* 3 (3): 315–322.
25. Caverly, T.J. et al. (2012). Patient preference in the decision to place implantable cardioverter-defibrillators. *Archives of Internal Medicine* 172 (14): 1104–1107.
26. Ko, D.T. et al. (2008). Life expectancy after an index hospitalization for patients with heart failure: a population-based study. *American Heart Journal* 155 (2): 324–331.
27. Murray, S.A. et al. (2005). Illness trajectories and palliative care. *BMJ* 330 (7498): 1007–1011.
28. Stewart, S. and McMurray, J.J. (2002). Palliative care for heart failure. *BMJ* 325 (7370): 915–916.

29. Gott, M. et al. (2007). Dying trajectories in heart failure. *Palliative Medicine* 21 (2): 95–99.

30. Boyd, K. and Murray, S.A. (2010). Recognising and managing key transitions in end of life care. *BMJ* 341: c4863.

31. Brown, R. and Clark, A.L. (2013). Reducing the cost of heart failure while improving quality of life. *British Journal of Cardiology* 20: 45–46.

32. Goodlin, S.J. et al. (2004). Consensus statement: palliative and supportive care in advanced heart failure. *Journal of Cardiac Failure* 10 (3): 200–209.

33. Jaarsma, T. et al. (2009). Palliative care in heart failure: a position statement from the palliative care workshop of the Heart Failure Association of the European Society of Cardiology. *European Journal of Heart Failure* 11 (5): 433–443.

34. Christakis, N. (1999). *Death Foretold: Prophecy and Prognosis in Medical Care*. Chicago and London: University of Chicago Press.

35. Connors, A.F. et al. (1995). A controlled trial to improve care for seriously Ill hospitalized patients. *JAMA: The Journal of the American Medical Association* 274 (20): 1591–1598.

36. Barclay, S. et al. (2011). End-of-life care conversations with heart failure patients: a systematic literature review and narrative synthesis. *British Journal of General Practice* 61: 49–62. doi: 10.3399/bjgp11X549018.

37. Strachan, P.H. et al. (2009). Mind the gap: opportunities for improving end-of-life care for patients with advanced heart failure. *Canadian Journal of Cardiology* 25 (11): 635–640.

38. Jenkins, V., Fallowfield, L., and Saul, J. (2001). Information needs of patients with cancer: results from a large study in UK cancer centres. *British Journal of Cancer* 84 (1): 48–51.

39. Maguire, P. et al. (1996). Helping health professionals involved in cancer care acquire key interviewing skills—the impact of workshops. *European Journal of Cancer* 32 (9): 1486–1489.

40. Fallowfield, L.J., Jenkins, V.A., and Beveridge, H.A. (2002). Truth may hurt but deceit hurts more: communication in palliative care. *Palliative Medicine* 16 (4): 297–303.

41. Hanratty, B. et al. (2002). Doctors' perceptions of palliative care for heart failure: focus group study. *BMJ* 325 (7364): 581–585.

42. Allen, L.A. et al. (2012). Decision making in advanced heart failure. *Circulation* 125 (15): 1928–1952.

43. Back, A.L., Arnold, R.M., and Quill, T.E. (2003). Hope for the best, and prepare for the worst. *Annals of Internal Medicine* 138 (5): 439–443.

44. Rogers, A. et al. (2002). A qualitative study of chronic heart failure patients' understanding of their symptoms and drug therapy. *European Journal of Heart Failure* 4 (3): 283–287.

45. Banerjee, P. et al. (2010). Do heart failure patients understand their diagnosis or want to know their prognosis? Heart failure from a patient's perspective. *Clinical Medicine, Journal of the Royal College of Physicians* 10: 339–343.

46. Barnes, S. et al. (2006). Communication in heart failure: perspectives from older people and primary care professionals. *Health & Social Care in the Community* 14 (6): 482–490.

47. Murray, S.A. et al. (2002). Dying of lung cancer or cardiac failure: prospective qualitative interview study of patients and their carers in the community. *BMJ* 325 (7370): 929.

48. Murray, S.A. et al. (2004). Exploring the spiritual needs of people dying of lung cancer or heart failure: a prospective qualitative interview study of patients and their carers. *Palliative Medicine* 18 (1): 39–45.

49. Rogers, A.E. et al. (2000). Knowledge and communication difficulties for patients with chronic heart failure: qualitative study. *BMJ* 321 (7261): 605–607.

50. Harding, R. et al. (2008). Meeting the communication and information needs of chronic heart failure patients. *Journal of Pain and Symptom Management* 36 (2): 149–156.

51. Barnes, S. et al. (2006). Characteristics and views of family carers of older people with heart failure. *International Journal of Palliative Nursing* 12 (8): 380–389.

52. Selman, L. et al. (2007). Improving end-of-life care for patients with chronic heart failure: "let's hope it'll get better, when I know in my heart of hearts it won't". *Heart* 93 (8): 963–967.

53. Goodlin, S.J. (2009). End-of-life care in heart failure. *Current Cardiology Reports* 11 (3): 184–191.

54. Gibbs, L.M., Khatri, A.K., and Gibbs, J.S.R. (2006). Survey of specialist palliative care and heart failure: September 2004. *Palliative Medicine* 20 (6): 603–609.

55. Daley, A., Matthews, C., and Williams, A. (2006). Heart failure and palliative care services working in partnership: report of a new model of care. *Palliative Medicine* 20 (6): 593–601.

56. Johnson, M. and Houghton, T. (2006). Palliative care for patients with heart failure: description of a service. *Palliative Medicine* 20 (3): 211–214.

57. Shipman, C. et al. (2000). Providing palliative care in primary care: how satisfied are GPs and district nurses with current out-of-hours arrangements? *British Journal of General Practice* 50 (455): 477–478.

58. Munday, D., Dale, J., and Barnett, M. (2002). Out-of-hours palliative care in the UK: perspectives from general practice and specialist services. *Journal of the Royal Society of Medicine* 95 (1): 28–30.

59. Worth, A. et al. (2006). Out-of-hours palliative care: a qualitative study of cancer patients, carers and professionals. *British Journal of General Practice* 56 (522): 6–13.

60. Johnson, D.M.J. (2010). Extending palliative care to patients with heart failure. *British Journal of Hospital Medicine* 71 (1): 12–15.

61. Dickstein, K. et al. (2008). ESC Guidelines for the diagnosis and treatment of acute and chronic heart failure 2008‡. *European Journal of Heart Failure* 10 (10): 933–989.

62. Lloyd-Jones, D. et al. (2010). Executive summary: heart disease and stroke statistics—2010 update. *Circulation* 121 (7): 948–954.

63. Boyd, K.J. et al. (2009). Making sure services deliver for people with advanced heart failure: a longitudinal qualitative study of patients, family carers, and health professionals. *Palliative Medicine* 23 (8): 767–776.

64. Haga, K. et al. (2012). Identifying community based chronic heart failure patients in the last year of life: a comparison of the Gold Standards Framework Prognostic Indicator Guide and the Seattle Heart Failure Model. *Heart* 98 (7): 579–583.

65. Remawi, B.N. et al. (2021). Palliative care needs-assessment and measurement tools used in patients with heart failure: a systematic mixed-studies review with narrative synthesis. *Heart Failure Reviews* 26 (1): 137–155.

66. Waller, A. et al. (2013). Facilitating needs-based support and palliative care for people with chronic heart failure: preliminary evidence for the acceptability, inter-rater reliability, and validity of a needs assessment tool. *Journal of Pain and Symptom Management* 45 (5): 912–925.

67. Janssen, D.J. et al. (2019). Timely recognition of palliative care needs of patients with advanced chronic heart failure: a pilot study of a Dutch translation of the needs assessment tool: progressive disease – heart failure (NAT:PD-HF). *European Journal of Cardiovascular Nursing* 18 (5): 375–388.

68. Campbell, R.T. et al. (2018). Which patients with heart failure should receive specialist palliative care? *European Journal of Heart Failure* 20 (9): 1338–1347.

69. Diop, M.S. et al. (2017). Palliative care interventions for patients with heart failure: a systematic review and meta-analysis. *Journal of Palliative Medicine* 20 (1): 84–92.

70. Datla, S. et al. (2019). Multi-disciplinary palliative care is effective in people with symptomatic heart failure: a systematic review and narrative synthesis. *Palliative Medicine* 33 (8):1003–1016. 269216319859148.

71. Xu, Z. et al. (2018). Effect of palliative care for patients with heart failure. *International Heart Journal* 59 (3): 503–509.

72. Zhou, K. and Mao, Y. (2019). Palliative care in heart failure: a meta-analysis of randomized controlled trials. *Herz* 44 (5): 440–444.

73. Sahlollbey, N. et al. (2020). The impact of palliative care on clinical and patient-centred outcomes in patients with advanced heart failure: a systematic review of randomized controlled trials. *European Journal of Heart Failure* 22 (12): 2340–2346.

74. Spartalis, M. et al. (2021). Contemporary ICD use in patients with heart failure. *Cardiology and Therapy* 10 (2): 313–324.

75. Pettit, S.J. et al. (2012). ICDs in end-stage heart failure. *BMJ Supportive & Palliative Care* 2 (2): 94–97.

76. Gadoud, A., Jenkins, S.M., and Hogg, K.J. (2013). Palliative care for people with heart failure: summary of current evidence and future direction. *Palliative Medicine* 27 (9): 822–828.

77. Padeletti, L. et al. (2010). EHRA Expert Consensus Statement on the management of cardiovascular implantable electronic devices in patients nearing end of life or requesting withdrawal of therapy. *Europace* 12 (10): 1480–1489.

78. Howlett, J. et al. (2010). End-of-life planning in heart failure: it should be the end of the beginning. *Canadian Journal of Cardiology* 26 (3): 135–141.

79. Abernethy, A.P. and Wheeler, J.L. (2008). Total dyspnoea. *Current Opinion in Supportive and Palliative Care* 2 (2): 110–113.

80. Opasich, C. and Gualco, A. (2007). The complex symptom burden of the aged heart failure population. *Current Opinion in Supportive and Palliative Care* 1 (4): 255–259.

81. Currow, D.C. et al. (2010). Do the trajectories of dyspnea differ in prevalence and intensity by diagnosis at the end of life? A consecutive cohort study. *Journal of Pain and Symptom Management* 39 (4): 680–690.

82. Goldfinger, J.Z. and Adler, E.D. (2010). End-of-life options for patients with advanced heart failure. *Current Heart Failure Reports* 7 (3): 140–147.

83. Davies, E.J. et al. (2010). Exercise training for systolic heart failure: Cochrane systematic review and meta-analysis. *European Journal of Heart Failure* 12 (7): 706–715.

84. O'Connor, C.M. et al. (2009). Efficacy and safety of exercise training in patients with chronic heart failure: Hf-action randomized controlled trial. *JAMA: The Journal of the American Medical Association* 301 (14): 1439–1450.

85. Bausewein, C. et al. (2008). Non-pharmacological interventions for breathlessness in advanced stages of malignant and non-malignant diseases. *Cochrane Database of Systematic Reviews* (2): CD005623.

86. Galbraith, S. et al. (2010). Does the use of a handheld fan improve chronic dyspnea? A randomized, controlled, crossover trial. *Journal of Pain and Symptom Management* 39 (5): 831–838.

87. Sullivan, M.J. et al. (2009). The Support, Education, and Research in Chronic Heart Failure Study (SEARCH): a mindfulness-based psychoeducational intervention improves depression and clinical symptoms in patients with chronic heart failure. *American Heart Journal* 157 (1): 84–90.

88. Abernethy, A.P. et al. (2003). Randomised, double blind, placebo controlled crossover trial of sustained release morphine for the management of refractory dyspnoea. *BMJ* 327 (7414): 523–528.

89. Currow, D.C. et al. (2011). Once-daily opioids for chronic dyspnea: a dose increment and pharmacovigilance study. *Journal of Pain and Symptom Management* 42 (3): 388–399.

90. Simon, S.T. et al. (2010). Benzodiazepines for the relief of breathlessness in advanced malignant and non-malignant diseases in adults. *Cochrane Database of Systematic Reviews* 1.

91. Cranston Josephine, M. et al. (2013). Oxygen therapy for dyspnoea in adults. *Cochrane Database of Systematic Reviews* (1): CD007354.

92. Abernethy, A.P. et al. (2010). Effect of palliative oxygen versus room air in relief of breathlessness in patients with refractory dyspnoea: a double-blind, randomised controlled trial. *Lancet* 376 (9743): 784–793.

93. Hopp, F., Thornton, N., and Martin, L. (2010). The lived experience of heart failure at the end of life: a systematic literature review. *Health and Social Work* 35: 109–117.

94. Faris Rajaa, F. et al. (2012). Diuretics for heart failure. *Cochrane Database of Systematic Reviews* (2):CD003838.

95. Zacharias, H. et al. (2011). Is there a role for subcutaneous furosemide in the community and hospice management of end-stage heart failure? *Palliative Medicine* 25 (6): 658–663.

96. Beattie, J.M. and Johnson, M.J. (2012). Subcutaneous furosemide in advanced heart failure: has clinical practice run ahead of the evidence base? *BMJ Supportive & Palliative Care* 2 (1): 5–6.

97. Ward, C. et al. (2009). Palliative and supportive care for patients with advanced and terminal heart failure. In: *A Practical Guide to Heart Failure in Older People* (ed. C. Ward and M. Witham), 241–270. Chichester, UK: Wiley-Blackwell.

18 Palliative Care in Advanced Renal Disease

Jo Wilson and Jenny Cross

Introduction

The requirement for palliative care in non-malignant conditions including advanced renal disease is established [1, 2]. People living with advanced renal disease (ARD) are often more symptomatic than those living with malignant conditions [3], and they report a reduction in quality of life and in psychological distress akin to cancer patients [4]. This chapter provides advice for practitioners on the management of symptoms in patients with ARD.

There are increasing numbers of patients with renal disease [5], and our ageing population has an emergent problem of complex interacting comorbidity involving obesity, diabetes, and heart disease for which renal failure is a common result. In this we recognise the detrimental impact of poverty [6] with chronic disease and patients who may suffer repeated admissions to hospital to manage their illnesses [7]. This brings us to the concepts of "supportive care," "advance care planning" (ACP) and "frailty." Supportive care is defined as "helping the patient and their family to cope with the illness journey – from pre-diagnosis, through the process of diagnosis and treatment, to cure, to continuing illness or death and bereavement" [8]. Advance care planning (Chapter 9: Recognising Deterioration, Preparing and Planning for Dying) allows the dual consideration of the future, while actively engaging in how to enjoy life currently and making realistic plans for the future bereavement experience of the family. The assessment of frailty (Chapter 16: Frailty, Dementia and Multi-Morbidity) and a comprehensive geriatric assessment permits a focus on rehabilitation to optimise life experience in this period. We consider these topics in this chapter, in the context of the assessment of mental capacity in decision-making and the vital role

family/informal carers play in the care of people with ARD. We consider the relationship of the patient and family to health-care professionals and the requirement for teams working across the health and social care system to meet the needs of the individual, before giving recommendations for clinical practice. The chapter concludes by considering death (whether sudden or planned) and anticipated death following the withdrawal of dialysis and the care required for the deceased and to the bereaved family.

Context

Chronic kidney disease (CKD) is common. It is classified into five stages (Table 1) based on the estimated glomerular filtration rate (eGFR) and the presence of protein in the urine.

CKD in its early stages [1, 2, 5] is generally totally asymptomatic and largely irreversible, and care is focused upon establishing a diagnosis of the underlying cause, reducing the associated cardiovascular risk and retarding progression. Symptoms are more likely as disease progresses towards stage 5 which may require renal replacement therapy (RRT). RRT is therapy which replaces the normal blood filtering function of the kidneys. Renal disease is common. 11–15% of adults over the age of 35 have some level of CKD, while 7% have the most severe stages [5]. Advanced renal failure refers to those with stage 4–5 CKD with or without proteinuria.

Advanced Renal Disease or End Stage Renal disease (ESRD) or End Stage Kidney Disease (ESKD) all refer to a condition in which renal function has deteriorated such that it is insufficient to allow a person to remain well and is persistent over a 90-day period [1]. The modern unifying

Handbook of Palliative Care, Fourth Edition. Edited by Richard Kitchen, Christina Faull, Sarah Russell and Jo Wilson.
© 2024 John Wiley & Sons Ltd. Published 2024 by John Wiley & Sons Ltd.

Table 1 Stages of CKD (Based on [1] and [5]).

Chronic Kidney Disease Stage	eGFR	Presence of Albumin in the Urine	Description of renal function
1	>90	Yes	Normal
2	89–60	Yes	Mildly reduced
3a	59–45	Regardless of albuminuria	Moderately reduced
3b	44–30	Regardless of albuminuria	Moderately reduced
4	29–15	Regardless of albuminuria	Severely reduced
5	<15	Regardless of albuminuria	Severely reduced

term is Advanced Renal Disease (ARD). Symptoms are non-specific and their onset is pernicious, often passing unnoticed. Where reported, symptoms of illness such as nausea, itch, and fatigue demonstrate a considerable increase often only in the month before death [3].

Renal Replacement Therapy (RRT)

The decision to choose renal replacement therapy is ideally made well in advance (minimum of six months) when the GFR is <20mls/min to allow preparation of vascular access and shared decision making about modality [1]. Medical therapies begin in parallel, and RRT starts when potassium, phosphate, or fluid cannot be controlled by diet, fluid restriction, and pharmacological interventions. The mean GFR at the time of dialysis is 8 mls/min in the UK [9]. There are now four forms of therapy to consider: conservative or maximum conservative management (MCM), haemodialysis, peritoneal dialysis, and transplantation. It is important to note that these are not necessarily "either/or" treatments, and several may be utilised over the lifetime of a patient with renal disease. They can though appear as "either/or" due to the progressive nature of ageing and accumulating co-morbidities making one modality, most commonly transplantation, unlikely to be beneficial.

Haemodialysis (HD)

HD is the most familiar of the renal replacement therapies. In this therapy the patient's blood is filtered via a porous membrane to clear it of by-products of metabolism. Most UK patients (95%) receive this therapy in a hospital facility three times a week. Each HD sessions lasts approximately

four hours. When a patient first starts HD, they often still pass residual urine, and this allows some flexibility in the hours and frequency of treatment in the first 6–9 months or so. The dose time and frequency of HD is re-assessed and planned accounting for gradually waning residual renal function. Patients who have residual function, have considerable flexibility in what they can eat and drink, and will survive even if they miss treatment sessions sometimes for weeks or even months. Once urine output is lost, so is this flexibility, and missing dialysis sessions or dialysis withdrawal will rapidly result in death in days or a small number of days or weeks. HD is not easy to tolerate, nor without physiological consequences. It requires an operative procedure to place a fistula connecting an artery to a vein in the forearm and these commonly fail or require further intervention and further anaesthetics and hospital stays [10]. HD itself can contribute to the accelerated loss of renal function. This is thought to relate to hypotensive episodes on dialysis, but even in their absence there is evidence of critical organ hypoperfusion during dialysis [11]. The reality of a day on HD is a long and tiring one. Treatment shifts start at 07.00 am and the last shift ends at midnight. The demand for HD machines is such that patient choice of time is not always possible. NHS-provided transport to and from treatment is one of the biggest challenges, particularly in city centres, and is the single commonest cause of patient complaint. Most frail elderly patients report that a dialysis day is a null day, where they do little other than attend treatment, and sleep on return home. A minority of patients can conduct their own dialysis at home often with a family member or partner to assist.

Peritoneal Dialysis (PD)

PD offers a gentler option. It requires daily treatment at home but has the advantage that it uses the abdominal cavity, rather than the circulatory system to achieve dialysis, using ultra-pure dialysate fluid installation through a semi-permanent indwelling dialysis catheter. The dialysate fluid is delivered monthly to a patient's home and is a more flexible option if travel or family are a priority. It is associated with better preservation of residual kidney function and avoids the need to attend hospital three times weekly with the attendant frustrations of transport and risks of nosocomial infection. The treatment is performed daily and is effective in smoothing fluid removal, it is the preferred treatment modality for those with a history of ischaemic heart disease, left ventricular dysfunction, or heart failure. It also allows considerable flexibility in dietary restriction, as it is more effective in clearance as it is performed daily.

Transplantation

Renal transplantation is the preferred option for many patients, as this negates the limitations of renal replacement therapy in terms of dialysis dietary and fluid restrictions; however it does require the patient to be compliant with immunosuppressive therapy for the lifetime of the graft. It also requires patients to be fit for transplantation surgery. Patients require substantial physiological reserve such as normal heart function, the ability to ascend two flights of stairs or to achieve a six-minute rapid walk test to even be considered for assessment. Mortality at five years is more than doubled for those patients with a poor functional status at the time of transplant compared with those without [12]. Only 25% of patients on HD are sufficiently robust to be considered for activation on the transplant waiting list and the majority of these are under 70 years. Although there is no age cut off, comorbidity precludes them from this operation, therefore transplant in the over 80 years, is a rare event. Surprisingly, transplantation in the older age group above 50 does not offer a survival advantage over dialysis but certainly has a substantial benefit in terms of quality of life. If a patient is transplanted, the graft might be expected to last 12–17 years. Again because of the requirement for immunosuppression and the persistence of the underlying primary disorder, transplant is also associated with progression of cardiovascular disease which can be accelerated by the presence of immunosuppression particularly steroids. It should be noted that some grafts can last 30 years, and patients may be become frail and comorbid while the graft fails in parallel. It can be a critical time for decision making when the graft fails, and not all patients wish to be dialysed.

Maximal Conservative Management (MCM)

Maximal conservative management is the support of patients with ARD without resorting to RRT and describes conservative renal care that is now routinely provided in UK renal units. It involves the management of patient's renal failure with diet, fluid, and pharmacological and lifestyle interventions. Medical therapy includes the treatment of underlying renal pathology and other manoeuvres to prolong residual renal function, such as anti-hypertensive medication. As renal function declines, the treatment of renal anaemia with erythropoietin and optimization of fluid balance with diuretics can become more important. Symptom management is the focus [13].

While understanding that renal units have historically had differing approaches to offering MCM as a valid option [14], most units have offered this treatment option, since 2009, to patients who have restricted activities of daily living and diabetes [15] and other co-morbidities [16]. These patients have tended to be older. For many years now some renal clinicians have been interested in understanding the survival versus quality-of-life risk/benefit ratio of patients being offered MCM. Dialysis prolongs survival of elderly patients who have ARD with significant comorbidity by approximately two years. However, those patients who choose conservative management commonly survive beyond a year and surprisingly achieving similar numbers of hospital-free days compared to patients who chose haemodialysis [17]. These patients also have more access to palliative care and are more likely to die outside of a hospital setting [18]. Currently there is a large NIHR funded multi-centre "Prepare for Kidney Care" Study underway [19, 20]. This study recognises that previous evidence was from small observational studies, where like was not being compared with like. This study is designed to assist clinicians and patients with data on survival and health related quality of life benefits associated with different approaches to managing end stage chronic kidney disease in patients aged 80 years and over and those aged 65 years and multiple co-morbidities.

Frailty

The relationship between frailty and ARD is important. Frailty is a state of health where even minor insults can result in decline in physical or mental well-being. People who are frail are at highest risk of adverse outcomes such as falls, disability, admission to hospital or the need for long-term care [21]. Frailty can be assessed using a clinical frailty scale (CFS) which is based on a person's functional status two weeks prior to the assessment [22]. The CFS is only validated in those over the age of 65 and has not been validated for those with Learning Disabilities. However, as the glomerular filtration rate (GFR) decreases the prevalence of frailty with ARD is high irrespective of age [23].

While there is interest in whether frailty predicts mortality [24], the intention of the assessment of the frailty score is to open opportunities for a comprehensive geriatric assessment (CGA) [25] and opportunities for the patient to rehabilitate, increasing the likely hood of independence and improving quality of life. A CGA has been demonstrated to reduce hospital admission rates [26] and increase the likelihood of the person remaining in their own home [27].

Physical frailty is often associated with sarcopenia – the loss of muscle mass [28] and is common in those with CKD. The combination of sarcopenia and frailty are both negative prognosticators for quality of life, morbidity and mortality [29]. Like frailty however, the assessment of sarcopenia, allowing interventions such as introduction of movement, nutrition, may allow for recovery or prevention of decline [29].

Decision-making in elderly patients considering dialysis is complex. A recent Dutch study of 196 participants greater than 65 years of age starting dialysis (GoLD study) found that 94% had geriatric impairments (cognition, mood, mobility, functional performance, comorbidity burden, and nutritional status) [30]. Of those, 77% starting dialysis, and 88% of those in the MCM group had two or more impairments. The most frequent were in functional performance, cognition and severe co-morbidity. In the 89 patients who chose conservative management the prevalence of geriatric impairments was even higher (88%). In the "Frail Elderly person on Dialysis" study 33% had fallen in the previous three months, 14% sustained a fracture [31] and it is well known that fractures in the elderly carries its own mortality [32]. The Cognitive-HD study found that patients with cognitive impairments on haemodialysis had premature mortality compared with those who did not [33]. Renal clinicians in the UK are evaluating ways to make the CGA a standard part of renal care [34] and are evaluating the impact this approach may have on outcomes [35]. Just because we technically can dialyse elderly frail patients does not mean that it is in their interests that it is started if the above information is shared.

Advance Care Planning

While the concept of advance care planning is supported [36], renal clinicians can find the concept of uncertainty and advance care planning challenging and have linked this to lack of communication training, and lack of experience in conservative management of patients with ARD [37]. Others have linked this to systemic challenges such as finding time when patients are/are not on dialysis to have difficult conversations with carers and family present [38], or to having documentation and processes that are simple, individually tailored, culturally appropriate, and involves key contacts/family [39].

People with ARD though have what is described as "high burden, time consuming, invasive and exhaustive tasks, impacting on all aspects of patient's and care givers

lives" [40]. The act of remaining well, while on dialysis is hard work from getting to dialysis, understanding and making decisions about disease management, compliance with diet and fluid, and all of this is affected by socioeconomic factors, such as poverty and housing. Loss of independence is a common sequelae with frequent social support to assist during episodes of poor health. It's not all bad. Dialysis keeps you alive at the very least and at its best can provide good physical health allowing you to maintain a full life. Some patients report, dialysis has a social quality, making friends at dialysis, and providing a structured routine which can make patients feel cared for [40].

While waiting for the "right time" to begin advance care planning conversations, we often witness the inexorable progression of the underlying conditions where, despite ongoing technically impeccable dialysis treatment, patients fail to thrive and symptomatically deteriorate, developing end-of-life symptoms like breathlessness, weight loss, hypotension, and progressive cognitive decline despite treatment. Patients on dialysis experience intermittent confusion, and microstrokes or frank stroke events, the latter is one of the most feared outcomes for patients and is a common event in a dialysis population. There is fatigue and discomfort associated with transport to/from/dialysis that occur in parallel with increasing requirements for social and financial support. Cardiac arrest on dialysis is an infrequent event [41], and if a death is anticipated, then effective processes for decision-making need to be in place to avoid death occurring on dialysis if this can reasonably be avoided. While some haemodialysis centres have developed procedures for the verification of death, and transfer of the deceased to a public mortuary, a dialysis centre is rarely the place for relatives to spend time with the deceased. This situation may also distress other patients who are dialysing in the vicinity.

Part of the challenge with advance care planning in any disease is to see ACP, not as an additional "to do," but as the building and maintenance of a relationship where the evolving goals of the patient are clearly understood and documented for all to see. This means all (renal physician/urse/GP or palliative care/allied healthcare professionals) have the capacity to advance care plan, but it is likely that one will need to lead and the other to support. It should also be noted that people on dialysis have an additional option, denied to the rest of us, of HD withdrawal: this effectively allows them to die at a time of their choosing [42]. It is rare that patients or families spontaneously raise this.

Relationship of Patients to Renal Physicians and General Practitioner (GP)

For renal patients, and especially those who are receiving RRT through dialysis or transplant, their primary relationship may be with their renal team, rather than their GP. Since this relationship is often over a lifetime, the complexity of active renal care means that GPs are often fearful of interfering or prescribing. There is also inconsistency for GPs about when to refer patients with CKD 5 to renal services [14]. However, the reverse is also true, that while renal physicians are experts in optimising the technical aspects of renal care patients, they are not expert in general practice. If a renal physician is regarded as leading care, then patients may inadvertently be denied access to holistic GP review including frailty assessment and interventions, and a provision of a package of care. Integrating individualised care across renal, general practice, and palliative care teams is important for holistic care.

Families/Informal Support

The care of the family is a critical part of management of ARD. Most patients with ARD highlight the support provided by family, friends, staff, other patients, and church communities [40]. ARD does affect family life, and carer mental health, which is affected by the quality of the relationship, whether there is conflict, the degree to which dialysis negatively impacts on daily life, and the number of caring responsibilities [43]. Carers can prefer to avoid death talk and concentrate on hopefulness of living [44].

RRT is a lifelong series of therapy in one form or another, and patients and their support networks often accommodate to live with renal disease. Relatives adjust their jobs and lifestyle to accommodate caring duties and can become more reliant upon state financial support. They accept the financial and social impact, often over decades, which may include them being dependent for housing and carers income on the individual for whom they care. So, accepting that a loved one with ARD may be approaching the end of their life can be distressing for relatives, because of the potential bereavement, and how that bereavement impacts the lives of those left living in relation to finance and living accommodation. In a study only USA clinicians mentioned this financial aspect [45], but we have found it to occur in the UK. The same study described nephrologist's experience of conversations with families about withdrawing dialysis has shown that these conversations are not necessarily easy and can be highly charged. The factors that either block or facilitate are the emotional attachment of the family to the patient, awareness of the needs of the person receiving dialysis, trust in the physician and health-care system, acceptance of the patient's previously declared wishes, and financial dependency on the patient [45].

There is limited literature, on the experience of families when dialysis is withdrawn. What literature there is suggests that families positively adapt to this—way of dying—in bereavement [46].

While the withdrawal of dialysis can be a critical decision-making time, those who have chosen conservative management and actively decided not to dialyse may still face a time of crisis, when acute symptoms develop in the period leading to death. It is vital that prior to this time, the GP and palliative care team adopt an anticipatory approach prescribing medicines for comfort at the end-of-life to support the dying person and their family in their home setting to avoid Emergency Department (ED) attendance, often out of hours, without family present. This is now especially important now in the context of COVID-19. The clinical team may be less familiar with the wishes of the patient, and when faced with fluid overload and breathlessness they may start dialysis in an unplanned manner compounding the challenges of the dying person and family. Ten percent of MCM patients convert at the last minute to an RRT unplanned start very often at the time of a crisis admission [47].

This brings us to advance care planning, which is employed to record the preferences and decisions of the person during the period when they are well and have capacity to express those preferences and decisions in an informed way to family and health workers. Recording an "advance statement of wishes," or an "advance decision to refuse treatment," appears to be associated with a greater chance that the patient's wishes are enacted at the end-of-life [48]. Informal recording of a patients advanced wishes without family involvement can result in the patient reversing previous decisions to plan their end-of-life care or having decisions reversed in order to help their family who may prefer life prolongation [49]. In a best-interest scenario however, the family and key contacts are critical to understanding the patient's known wishes. The clinical and relationship work that needs to be taken to make a best interest's decision is very well described [50], and the fewer times this process needs to occur in a time pressured, acute trust setting the better.

How Do We Spot These Patients?

Tools have been developed to help consider who may be approaching the last years of their lives. These tools are the

Clinical Frailty Score [22], and the Supportive and Palliative Care Indicator Tool (SPICT) [51]. Tools have also been developed to help decision make about who would benefit from dialysis [52, 53]. When used consistently, with patients and families, they can help bring patients to a place where conversations can begin advance care planning. Most clinicians have a "gut instinct" that patients are deteriorating. This can be systematically evidenced by assessing factors such as hospital admissions, mobility, frailty, dependence, cognitive decline over time to establish where a patient is in the disease trajectory, which will inform an MDT discussion prior to discussion with the patient and family [54].

We recognise that it is not as simple as "identifying the person" for discussion. The person may be recognisable to the clinician e.g., those ageing individuals on dialysis who despite optimised therapy are not thriving. They are recognised over weeks or months repeatedly suffering hypotensive episodes on dialysis, poor appetite, weight loss with a characteristic low phosphate and potassium, all features of poor nutrition despite therapy. They lose lean body mass resulting in progressive reduction in dry weight, and often report a progressive deterioration in mobility and independence or cognitive decline. These are manifestations of both the progression of the underlying multi system disorder that contributed to renal failure and the impact of renal failure on the body usually as a result of accelerated atherogenesis and small vessel disease related to uraemia. This is one of the most challenging situations to manage as the global deterioration observed by the patient and family is often mistakenly interpreted as something wrong or lacking in the technicalities of treatment and the discussion begins as a problem to be solved by changing the dialysis. In fact, it's more akin to those with advanced cancer deteriorating despite chemotherapy, that is we have reached a point where the treatment is not working as it did before and within limits the patients experience of symptoms may not improve despite our efforts.

Advance Care Planning Recommendations

Advance care planning has not yet been an integral part of the routine care of older patients with end stage renal disease [37]. Renal teams are working towards practices that include the setting of common clinical treatment goals, and ceilings of treatment, for patients requiring renal replacement therapy [55]. There is also work to sustain the multi-disciplinary working to achieve this [56] and renal units are increasingly moving to include frailty and

geriatric assessment into routine dialysis care [34]. This means that the earlier recognition of increasing frailty by renal teams means GPs, community teams and palliative care can be involved and work together to address the rehabilitative and supportive care needs of people with ARD and help them die in their preferred place of care [18].

We recommend that early in the patient's renal disease, clinicians focus on "what matters to the patient?" [57], and "who matters to the patient," to direct care planning and who to involve to prepare for the possibility of loss of capacity. We recommend patients consider Lasting Powers of Attorneys for health [58] and to consider "how to both live and die well" [59]. In these on-going documented conversations, different clinicians can progress them and ensure that treatments offered address the patient's priorities as best they can. Culture, language, faith and previous experiences of health-care decision-making can impact on advance care planning [60], and patients should be offered translators, or spiritual care support that are acceptable to them.

We recommend that clinician's work to build trusting relationships with patients and their families and begin conversations about planning for the future if treatments, including RRT, become ineffective or impossible to administer safely. Having these conversations appear to be both acceptable to patients and well tolerated when conducted in the presence of family at a time when patients are relatively well, allowing families to be aware of a patient's wishes and preferences even if they do not agree with them [39]. Dialysis is a treatment like any other. It is helpful to frame this for patients and families at the outset, and to be clear that the if the treatment is no longer working or is not benefitting the patient, then a conversation will occur about stopping the treatment.

When the process of advance care planning for the person occurs, we need to ask what future bereavement may look like for the carers and support them to independently prepare. We would recommend that we focus on the concept of "uncertainty" [61], "living well and making preparation for the future" [59] and specifically the concept of parallel planning. This is well defined in paediatric palliative care [62] as "planning for end-of-life care while taking account of the often-unpredictable course of life limiting conditions; it involves making multiple plans of care and using the one that best fits the [person's] circumstances at the time." While clinicians are constantly asked to hone their communication skills [45], we would argue that a key skill is MDT working of renal, palliative care, and general practice. We all need to build relationships with the patient and family until the point of needing to either withdraw dialysis, or manage the end-of-life subsequent to MCM, and then flex our skills to best support the patient and family.

Symptom Management

Symptom Management in ARD

Patients with ARD, who are not on dialysis, can suffer from up to 20 symptoms in their last month of life. The most common are pain, fatigue, pruritus, breathlessness, dry mouth, muscle cramps, restless legs, lack of appetite, poor concentration, dry skin, sleep disturbances, and constipation [3]. Patients on dialysis can also suffer from calciphylaxis. Calciphylaxis is the term used for a condition called calcific uraemic arteriolopathy. It is a chronic (long term) condition that occurs as a result of a build-up of calcium and phosphate within the small arteries (blood vessels) of the body. This build-up of calcium and phosphate causes a brittle, chalky material to form that can often look like bone. The condition is rare, and treatment is difficult, often only partially effective and the condition is associated with a 50% mortality. Calciphylaxis can affect the heart, blood vessels, and other tissues in the body. It can lead to infarction of large areas of the skin which painfully break down and often do not heal. Specialist renal advice for management and specialist palliative care advice for symptom management is helpful.

Many drugs used routinely in palliation are renally cleared and tend to accumulate in the presence of renal failure and it is therefore important to understand the degree of renal failure and to be clear whether these agents are being used to manage chronic symptoms in ARD where death is not imminent (weeks to months of life) and when the person is dying (last hours and days of life) as it affects the choice of drugs.

Prescribing chronically in renal failure requires careful consideration of the eGFR. Even when drugs are "renally safe," it is recommended that slower titration than usual is advisable, particularly in the elderly and/or frail patient, and particularly for those with Central Nervous System (CNS) effects. For patients on dialysis, it is recommended that there is a discussion with the dialysis team. It is also important to consider such things as concurrent symptoms, co-morbidities, other drugs, and patient preference [63].

Polypharmacy is common in patients with ARD [64] and there is opportunity to withdraw drugs by considering the time frame over which a drug might be expected to deliver benefit against the patients stated priorities. This review should include long-term renal medicines that protect bone health (calcium and vitamin D preparations), drugs to maintain haemoglobin (erythropoietin and IV Iron), fluid control (diuretics), blood sugar control (hyopglycaemics), to manage cardiovascular disease (aspirin and anti-hypertensives) and to maintain dialysis access (warfarin) [63].

It is also important to consider the lived experience of the patient with any medication regime. People find it hard to take large numbers of medication and live with potential side effects without understanding the reason for the medications, family support, and sometimes prompts to help them remember to take essential medications [65].

There is expert prescribing advice in the Palliative Care Formulary available on Medicines Complete https://about.medicinescomplete.com/ and the Renal Drug Handbook [66]. It is vital that clinicians are aware of opioid equivalence guidelines and if unsure seek pharmacy and palliative care advice https://bnf.nice.org.uk/guidance/prescribing-in-palliative-care.html. Please note there is also helpful patient advice available for symptoms such as "restless legs" to download from https://www.kidneycareuk.org/about-kidney-health/order-or-download-booklets/

Depression

Depression is well known to affect adults with ARD [67] due to biological and psychosocial changes associated with ARD. Antidepressant doses should start with low starting doses and cautious titration, as side effects can take weeks to occur. From a renal point of view the first-line antidepressant of choice is Sertraline. Citalopram can be used but has an increased risk of ventricular arrhythmia. Some renal units prefer to use Mirtazepine despite its potential for accumulation [63].

Pain

The management of pain is in line with other pain management guidelines (WHO), but the plan needs to be individual for each patient.

Non-opioid Analgesics

Non-opioid analgesics are appropriate for mild to moderate pain, especially in patients experiencing musculoskeletal discomfort. Paracetamol (acetaminophen) is a good first choice. For patients with an eGFR >20, Paracetamol should be taken in divided doses of 1 gram, 6 to 8 hourly to a max of 4g/day. If the eGFR is <10 or the patient is undergoing renal replacement therapies, then the dosing is 500mg-1g every 6 to 8 hours (usually to a max of 3g/day). In all cases if a person weighs less than 50kg then the dose should be reduced to 500mg per dose and a ceiling of 3g/day [66].

Non-steroidal anti-inflammatory medications (NSAIDs) can be highly effective analgesics but should be avoided in renal patients, unless they are anuric and on dialysis in which case they can be used at normal doses [63] with a proton pump inhibitor prescription to mitigate the risk of gastric bleeding. If generalists wish to consider NSAIDs they are advised to discuss with the renal team first.

Opioid Analgesics

In renal impairment, opioids vary in their potential for toxicity and while the evidence base is limited, there is "expert opinion" [63]. Opioids, if required, should be started at low dose and given less frequently, titrating to response. All opioids result in a degree of CNS depression, but this takes time and may not be immediately obvious. Additionally, drugs can potentiate effects e.g., opioids and benzodiazepines. The Palliative Care Formulary gives wise advice "because of the risks associated with using an unfamiliar opioid, a pragmatic approach is important. Thus, the cautious use of a familiar opioid (including morphine) may be preferable to an unfamiliar (albeit a 'renally safer') one. The ease of obtaining, administering, and titrating the opioid are also important considerations, particularly in a community setting" [63], P727.

Opioid accumulation in renal impairment often presents with an encephalopathy, myoclonic jerks, and confusion in addition to the more common observation of sedation. Ironically this can be in the context of ongoing uncontrolled pain. In palliative care it is preferable not to administer Naloxone if opioid toxicity is not life-threatening, but to pause the opioid then reintroduce at a lower dose less frequently, allowing time for the medication to "wash out." However, if monitoring is required to ensure the respiratory rate does not drop below 8 breathes/minutes, or if patients drop their breathing rate below this, they will require hospitalisation and the administration of Naloxone [63].

What opioids are recommended for people with renal failure in the palliative phase of their illness, depends on holistic individual assessment, whether the pain is chronic or acute in nature and how well they are able to manage the route of administration of opioid. It is recommended to discuss any plan with the renal and palliative care teams.

In mild renal impairment (eGFR >60), weak and strong opioids with active metabolites—codeine, hydromorphone, morphine, oxycodone, and tramadol—can be used

with caution reducing dose and frequency and deciding to monitor effect and giving advance warning to the patient and carers of effects to look out for.

In severe renal impairment (eGFR<30), it is generally preferable to use an opioid with no active metabolites such as alfentanil, buprenorphine, or fentanyl. There are practical considerations to their use including the fact that these are "strong opioids", and they have very limited availability of oral routes. Often it is preferable to use Oxycodone at a low dose as required (1-2mg PO every 6-8 hours). If swallowing medicines becomes challenging and the patient is in a stable state pain wise, and is already on opioids, then a Fentanyl TD patch is a good choice in severe renal impairment as it has a low side effect profile in terms of nausea, sedation, and pruritus (non-histamine releasing). The patch is popular with patients due to its transdermal route and long 72-h duration of action. Disadvantages include fixed dose limitations and the previous requirement to have been on opioids as the 12mcg/h patch is equivalent to 30mg oral morphine/24 hours [63]. Therefore, conversion to a Fentanyl patch always occurs following titration with an alternative, short-acting opioid, or other agents such as a Buprenorphine transdermal patch. Patients who are showing signs of opioid toxicity on a fentanyl patch, should have their patch removed. They will have opioid in their systems for 48–72 hours [63] following patch removal and will require prolonged monitoring.

In moderate renal failure (eGFR less than 60 and greater than 30), it is preferable to use immediate release Oxycodone Hydrochloride in small doses (1-2mg PO every 6-8 hours) and then continue if tolerated. As an alternative, Buprenorphine transdermal patch has become popular for use in the UK for the management of pain in frail patients. This is a partial opioid agonist and is available in in lower equivalent doses than a Fentanyl patch. In the United Kingdom, the buprenorphine transdermal patch is available in 5, 10, and 20 mcg/h strengths and comes in a 7-day patch formulation (as well as higher doses that are given twice weekly). Buprenorphine transdermal 5 mcg/h patches can be initiated in an opioid naïve patient (this is equivalent to 12mg oral morphine/24 hours) [68].

Adjuvants

Adjuvant medications are typically combined with analgesics for improved control of complex pain and may be derived from a range of separate drug categories. Adjuvants used for neuropathic pain management typically affect the CNS and may require dose reduction.

Gabapentin is used for pruritus and restless legs associated with ARD, and this may make its use for neuropathic pain a sensible multi-purpose option. Gabapentin accumulates in ARD, resulting in profound sedation, encephalopathy, and myoclonic jerks. For non-dialysis or PD patients, start with 100mg at night and titrate slowly. For HD patients with a urine output 100mL/24h, start with 100mg at night: consider either a supplementary dose after each HD session or timing the daily dose after HD. For anuric HD patients, start with 100mg stat and 100mg after every HD session; a regular maintenance dose is not generally required for anuric HD patients [63].

Tricyclic medications are useful but require careful monitoring, especially in patient with cardiac disease. Amitriptyline is a common choice and should be started at 10 mg at bedtime and titrated upward for effect. Amitriptyline is not used first line as an antidepressant, and this must be considered. It also has a long half-life and time taken to reach a steady state and therefore undesirable side effects may only become apparent weeks after regular use [63].

Carbamazepine is licensed for temporal mandibular joint pain and peripheral neuropathy and requires little dose adjustment. The usual starting dose of 200 mg twice daily is generally well tolerated in renal populations and can be further titrated as required. There needs to be consideration of other drug-drug interactions prior to starting the prescription [63].

Gastro-intestinal Symptom Management

ARD patients experience a variety of gastro-intestinal complaints. Chronic anorexia, nausea and vomiting, diarrhoea, or constipation often go under-recognised and undertreated in renal patients but are a frequent source of distress in advancing disease.

Diarrhoea on dialysis is common. Infective causes should still be excluded. The commonest cause is GI diabetic neuropathy. However, it can relate to the dialysis process itself or medications, commonly proton pump inhibitors or phosphate binders although constipation is much more common with the latter. Persistent diarrhoea should initially be investigated for a coincidental cause unrelated to the chronic renal disease and if no other correctable cause is found it should be treated symptomatically with Loperamide or the lowest tolerated dose of an appropriate opioid. Bear in mind that Fentanyl, which is favoured in renal patients, causes less constipation than other opioids and so may not prove useful in reducing the tendency to diarrhoea.

Conversely, constipation is also common in ARD. Aetiologies include fluid restriction, avoidance of high potassium foods which are also often high fibre foods, decreased mobility, and constipating medications such as phosphate binders. Patients should maximise fibre in their diet as far as this can be tolerated and require laxatives to be prescribed and titrated to effect alongside opioid medication. Bisacodyl, Sodium Docusate, Lactulose, Macrogols (polyethylene glycols), and Senna are safe in end stage renal failure with doses unchanged. Macrogols should be used with caution due to the volume of water required, and bulking agents e.g. Ispaghula husk is avoided completely.

Nausea and Vomiting

Nausea and vomiting are common symptoms in uraemia and occur in 5–15% of patients during haemodialysis. It is important to consider reversible causes which may relate to comorbidities such a dysmotility associated with diabetes, peptic ulcer disease, and the frequent use of aspirin as cardiovascular protection, severe constipation in the presence of opiates and poly pharmacy as this will guide the appropriate anti-emetic with a motility action or a central effect. Cyclizine and Ondansetron are generally safe and prescribed without dose adjustment [63]. Domperidone, Metoclopramide, Haloperidol, and Levomepromazine should be used cautiously, and dose reduced [63] due to their accumulation and extra-pyramidal effects. These can occur weeks after starting the medicines. Once again, the principal of choosing a drug with which you have experience is probably more important than choosing a drug that is thought to be renally safer as this is seldom absolute.

Dyspnoea (Air Hunger)

The incidence of dyspnoea is low in dialysed patients because volume overload and acidosis can largely be controlled, but it is more common in conservative care. ARD combines with comorbid disease such as heart failure or chronic obstructive pulmonary disease to create a vicious cycle of breathlessness and immobility, leading to muscle weakness and excess lactate, leading to further breathlessness [69]. We are cautioned against the "lazy use of prescribing" to alleviate the symptoms of breathlessness because non-drug interventions which include relationship development, exercise, crisis management, and assisting with the emotional components of breathlessness all of which are appropriate for every patient, but "seem hard" [69].

Dyspnoea, requires assessment of the cause, including looking at comorbid disease, anaemia management, the identification of chronic hypoxia considering home oxygen, diuretics, and isolated ultrafiltration (hemodialysis for fluid removal only). Equally important are general comfort measures such as lowered room temperature, brisk airflow via a fan or opened window (only in a single living environment in COVID-19 infections), loose clothing, and elevated head of bed [70].

Patients report a reduction in the perception of breathlessness with regularly administered low dose opioids that lead to steady state blood levels. There is little evidence to support the early reports that Oxycodone as more effective than other opiates but there is good evidence for low dose Morphine Sulfate [71], which should be dose and frequency reduced for patients with ARD.

Delirium

The incidence of delirium is high in all palliative populations, but renal patients face additional risk as GFR falls. Patients with pre-existing cerebral vascular disease or dementia are especially vulnerable to the CNS consequences of metabolic aberration, altered drug metabolism, or haemodialysis. All delirium should be precipitate a review of reversible causes which include sepsis, hypoxia, and medication effects, and a specialist geriatrician advice considered. Pharmaceuticals with CNS effects such as opioids, benzodiazepines, steroids, or Gabapentin should be reviewed and dose adjusted or removed, where possible.

Low doses of antipsychotic medication should be used and titrated slowly due to the risk of an enhanced CNS effect. Side effects can take weeks to present, and the drugs can be potentiated by using opioids. There is also the risk of ventricular arrhythmias. From a renal perspective, Olanzapine is the first-line choice in ARD and Haloperidol can be used, if the dose is halved if used chronically. For patients on dialysis, Haloperidol, Olanzapine, and Quetiapine do not require any additional dose reduction but risperidone is unpredictably cleared and should be avoided [63].

However, neuroleptics should be considered in any patient with severe agitation or terminal delirium. Haloperidol 500micrograms nocte and as required may settle early delirium [63] but when anti-psychotics are inefficient at managing agitation then benzodiazepines can be useful especially in the last days of life [63]. Lorazepam is a good first-line choice if the patient can manage a sublingual preparation. Clonazepam (cautious use) can be used if restless legs are a feature. Diazepam should be avoided due to the risk of accumulation, but the shorter acting Midazolam 2.5mg SC as required or via syringe pump (CSCI) may be needed.

Seizures and Myoclonic Jerking

Although seizure activity in terminal uraemia does occur, it is less frequent than commonly assumed. Grand mal seizures occur in approximately 10% of ARD patients and some require antiseizure prophylaxis post first seizure [63]. Phenytoin is commonly prescribed, but dose reduction and careful blood level monitoring is required. Myoclonic jerks are very common in advanced uraemia and are attributed to uraemic toxic encephalopathy and is more common in the presence of pharmaceutical by-products including cephalosporins, Gabapentin, and opioids. Twitching tends to become more pronounced in the imminently dying patient, and can cause distress to the patient, family, and medical team. This symptom is well controlled with benzodiazepines such as Midazolam 2.5mg SC as required or via CSCI.

Skin

Skin problems are common in CKD with most patients experiencing one or more dermatological disorders. Manifestations range from mild to severe and include changes such as easy bruising, Raynaud's phenomenon, peripheral vascular breakdown, and metastatic calcification. However, the most common complaints are pruritus and xerosis.

Pruritus

Pruritus occurs in up to 50% of renal patients during their illness. Pruritus related to ARD increases with the severity and duration of renal failure but tends to resolve with RRT. However, it may additionally occur during dialysis if the patient develops allergies to one or more dialysis compounds. Pruritus can be local but is more often generalised. Mild to moderate itching is usually managed through a combination of topical emollients, and moisturisers, and non-drug treatment such as avoiding soap, and scratching and drying the skin by patting gently [63]. If localised, topical agents such as capsaicin may also help. Progressive pruritus requires the addition of Gabapentin. The dose requires tailoring. For non-dialysis or PD patients PO; start with 100mg on alternate nights and titrate slowly. For anuric HD patients start with 100mg stat and 100mg after each HD session [63].

Xerosis

Xerosis, or dry roughened skin, also contributes to pruritus in renal disease. Of dialysis patients, 50–75% complain of xerosis, which typically occurs along the extensor surfaces of arms and legs. It is thought to relate to dysfunction of the dermal barrier, which predisposes patients to painful fissures, ulcers, and infections. Most dialysis patients improve with routine moisturisers and keratolytics e.g., Aqueous cream.

Dying

The care of the dying patient is covered in Chapter 20: Care in the last days of life and after death. With respect to the person dying with advanced renal failure most clinicians consider that there are two groups:
• Those already of dialysis in whom a decision to stop dialysis has been made.
• Those with ARD being treated with MCM and who are rapidly approaching death.
However, we recognise a third group, where the withdrawal of dialysis has been discussed with the person and their family and for whom withdrawal of dialysis is unacceptable. The numbers of these patients are very small, but their care needs are very intensive. These patients need daily review pre the dialysis session, and ultimately there comes a time when they just cannot be dialysed as their blood pressure is too low, despite blood pressure support such as Midodrine. At this point there is a very rapid turn to helping the patient and family be cared for in the person's home or where the care needs of the patient and the pre-bereavement needs of the family can best be met—this may be hospital, hospice, or care home.

When a person stops dialysis, the mean survival is 8–10 days but can be weeks to months, dependent on the amount of residual urine function [72]. The patient and family need to be prepared for this. For patients being managed conservatively the time to death from recognising imminent dying can be more variable. Indicators that death is approaching are increasing symptoms that are not amenable to intervention (the person is deteriorating despite best treatment), increasing numbers of symptoms, a steep physical and sometimes cognitive decline [73], and increasing care needs.

Patients with ARD can be very symptomatic [3]. Common symptoms in the last month of life are:

1. breathlessness (may relate to fluid overload and acidosis)
2. myoclonic jerks and seizures (relate to both increased drug toxicity and uraemia)
3. delirium (also relates to both increased drug toxicity and uraemia).
Other symptoms particularly associated with ARD may continue to be a major problem, e.g. pruritus and restless legs. Clonazepam in low doses is often helpful in relieving restless legs, myoclonus, and neuropathic pain.

Occasionally, with severe fluid overload, if the patient still has a dialysis line in place, it may be appropriate to have a few hours of ultra-filtration to correct the overload. Regarding prescribing at end-of-life please see Table 2 and Chapter 20: Care in the Last Days of Life and after Death. In ARD there are a few specific considerations. Starting doses must consider the risk of accumulation and thus maybe lower than in other circumstance. Where a CSCI is prescribed all as required doses should be prescribed q1h [63]. Referral to Palliative Care is recommended if assessment is complicated and advice required.

Care after Death

It is vital that there is the physical care of the deceased in line with guidance [75], and the immediate support of the bereaved. This would include how to register the death, and guidance to processes after the death. In the UK these are available https://www.gov.uk/when-someone-dies. We have already discussed how the care of the person with ARD is very much a family and community concern, and in bereavement the caregivers are likely to need support. If the person has been home dialysing there is likely to be nutritional supplements, filtration fluid to remove from the home, and the need to return controlled drugs to the pharmacy for safe disposal. There may be equipment that needs collection from the home. If the person has been dialysing in a hospital, then other patients and staff may well experience bereavement too and may wish to have an opportunity to remember the patient and discuss them.

Summary

This chapter has considered the context of ARD and the factors that can impact on the rising incidence of this. It has considered the varying forms of RRT and the impact of this

Table 2 Drug suggestions for symptom management at end-of-life in renal failure (based on [63,74]).

Symptom	Drug	Supplementary advice
Pain	Alfentanil 50–100microgram SC PRN Morphine 1.25–2.5mg SC PRN Oxycodone 1–2mg SC PRN	Some centres prescribe Alfentanil SC instead of Morphine or Oxycodone. If staff are not familiar with Alfentanil it is safer to use the commonly prescribed and familiar Morphine / Oxycodone. In a community setting these familiar opioids are much easier to access in a prompt manner.
Breathlessness	Alfentanil 50–100microgram SC PRN Morphine 1.25–2.5mg SC PRN Oxycodone 1–2mg SC PRN **Additionally:** Midazolam 1.25–2.5mg SC PRN	The prescribed strong opioid can be used for breathlessness and pain. Where there is anxiety add in a benzodiazepine.
Nausea and vomiting	Haloperidol 0.5–1mg SC PRN **Alternatively:** Levomepromazine 2.5–5mg SC PRN	
Agitation, restlessness	Midazolam 1.25–2.5mg SC PRN	
Delirium	Haloperidol or levomepromazine ± midazolam, starting with similar doses to above.	
Excessive respiratory secretions	Hyoscine butylbromide 20mg SC PRN Glycopyrronium 200mcg SC PRN	

Usually PRN doses are prescribed hourly. However, this may need to be less frequent dependent on degree of renal failure and symptoms. Of note, if three or more PRN doses are required over 24 hours, consider giving medication in a CSCI.

for patients and their carers. It has identified the need for frailty assessment and the consideration of the ability of the patient to have episodes of improvement or non-deterioration in the last year of life. It has strongly argued for an MDT approach to the care of the patient living with ARD and in the advance care planning. This MDT needs to include the renal team, general practice, palliative care as well as the wider MDT including social care support as well as the patient and those important to them. The care needs to helping the patient think about the context of their actual dying, and to extend to helping carers prepare for how they might sustain themselves—physically, emotionally, financially, and socially in bereavement. The chapter has concluded with a review of pharmacological symptom management approaches.

References

1. Brown, E., Murtagh, F., and Murphy, E. *Kidney Disease: From Advanced Disease to Bereavement*, 2e (ed. M. Watson). OUP. 2012

2. Murtagh, F.E.M. Palliative care in kidney disease. In: *Textbook of Palliative Care* (ed. R.D. MacLeod and L. Van den Block). Cham: Springer International Publishing. 2019. P1153-1166

3. Murtagh, F.E.M., Addington-Hall, J.M., Edmonds, P.M., Donohoe, P., Carey, I., Jenkins, K., and Higginson, I. Symptoms in the month before death for stage 5 chronic kidney disease patients managed without dialysis. *Journal of Pain and Symptom Management* 2010; 40(3): 342–352.

4. Saini, T., Murtagh, F.E., Dupont, P.J., McKinnon, P.M., Hatfield, P., and Saunders, Y. Comparative pilot study of symptoms and quality of life in cancer patients and patients with end stage renal disease. *Palliative Medicine* 2016; 20(6): 631–636.

5. Ng Fat, L., Mindell, J., and Roderick, P. Health survey for England 2016. Kidney and liver disease. https://files.digital.nhs.uk/publication/m/e/hse2016-adult-kid-liv.pdf [Accessed 4 Sept 2022]

6. Barnett, K., Mercer, S.W., Norbury, M., Watt, G., Wyke, S., and Guthrie, B. Epidemiology of multimorbidity and implications for health care, research, and medical education: a cross-sectional study. *The Lancet* 2012; 380(9836): 37–43.

7. Mumford, E., Wilson, J., and Burns, A. Priorities MDT: a single centre experience of complex decision making in renal patients approaching the end of life in British Renal Society Conference. 2017.

8. NICE. Improving supportive & palliative care for adults with cancer. https://www.nice.org.uk/guidance/csg4/resources/improving-supportive-and-palliative-care-for-adults-with-cancer-pdf-773375005 [accessed 4 Sept 2022]

9. Stel, V.S., Tomson, C., Ansell, D., Casino, F.G., Collart, F., Finne, P. et al. Level of renal function in patients starting dialysis: an ERA-EDTA Registry study. *Nephrology Dialysis Transplantation* 2010; 25(10): 3315–3325.

10. Al-Jaishi, A.A., Oliver, M.J., Thomas, S.M., Lok, C.E., Zhang, J.C., Garg, A.X. et al. Patency rates of the arteriovenous fistula for hemodialysis: a systematic review and meta-analysis. *American Journal of Kidney Diseases* 2014; 63(3): 464–478.

11. Van Buren, P.N. Redefining the burden of intradialytic hypotension in the modern era of hemodialysis. *American Journal of Nephrology* 2019; 9(49): 494–496.

12. Nastasi, A.J., McAdams-DeMarco, M.A., Schrack, J., Ying, H., Olorundare, I., Warsame, F. et al. Pre-kidney transplant lower extremity impairment and post-kidney transplant mortality. *American Journal of Transplantation: Official Journal of the American Society of Transplantation and the American Society of Transplant Surgeons* 2018; 18(1): 189–196.

13. Brown, E.A. Maximal conservative management. *Medicine* Elsevier Ltd; 2015; 43 (8): 493–495.

14. Roderick, P., Rayner, H., Tonkin-Crine, S., Okamoto, I., Eyles, C., Leydon, G. et al. A national study of practice patterns in UK renal units in the use of dialysis and conservative kidney management to treat people aged 75 years and over with chronic kidney failure. *Health Services and Delivery Research* 2nd ed. 2015; 3(12): 1–186.

15. Smith, C., Da Silva-Gane, M., Chanda, S., Warwicker, P., Greenwood, R., and Farrington, K. Choosing not to dialyse: evaluation of planned non-dialytic management in a cohort of patients with end-stage renal failure. *Nephron Clinical Practice* 2003; 95:c40-c46 DOI:10.1159/000073708

16. Wong, C.F., McCarthy, M., Howse, M.L.P., and Williams, P.S. Factors affecting survival in advanced chronic kidney disease patients who choose not to receive dialysis. *Renal Failure* 2007; 29(6):653–659. DOI: 1080/08860220701459634

17. Carson, R.C., Juszczak, M., Davenport, A., and Burns, A. Is maximum conservative management an equivalent treatment option to dialysis for elderly patients with significant comorbid disease? *Clinical Journal of the American Society of Nephrology* 2009; 4(10): 1611–1619.

18. Lovell, N., Jones, C., Baynes, D., Dinning, S., Vinen, K., and Murtagh, F.E. Understanding patterns and factors associated with place of death in patients with end-stage kidney disease: a retrospective cohort study. *Palliative Medicine* 2017; 31(3): 283–288.

19. Murphy, E., Burns, A., Murtagh, F.E.M., Rooshenas, L., and Caskey, F.J. The Prepare for Kidney Care Study: prepare for renal dialysis versus responsive management in advanced chronic kidney disease. *Nephrology Dialysis Transplantation* 1st ed. 95: 2020; 1-8 DOI:10.1093/ndt/gffaa209.

20. Husbands, S., Caskey, F., Winton, H., Gibson, A., Donovan, J.L., and Rooshenas, L. Pre-trial qualitative work with health care professionals to refine the design and delivery of a randomised controlled trial on kidney care. *Trials* 2019; 20:224 1–13.

21. Young, J. Frailty – what it means and how to keep well over the winter months [Internet]. https://www.england.nhs.uk/blog/frailty/#:~:text=In%20medicine%2C%20frailty%20defines%20the,health%20and%20social%20care%20professionals. [Accessed 3 January 2021]

22. Clinical Frailty Scale. NHS Specialised Clinical Frailty Network https://www.scfn.org.uk/clinical-frailty-scale [Accessed 4 Sept 2022]

23. Chowdhury, R., Peel, N.M., Krosch, M., and Hubbard, R.E. Frailty and chronic kidney disease: a systematic review. *Archives of Gerontology and Geriatrics* ; 2016; 68: 135–142.

24. Hetherington, L., Prentice, J., Findlay, M., and Collidge, T. Clinical frailty scoring in patients with end stage renal disease: a predictor of mortality risk. *British Journal of Renal Medicine* 2020; 25 (2): 47–55.

25. Comprehensive geriatric assessment toolkit for Primary care practitioners. British Geriatric Society https://www.bgs.org.uk/sites/default/files/content/resources/files/2019-03-12/CGA%20Toolkit%20for%20Primary%20Care%20Practitioners_0.pdf [Accessed 4 Sept 2022]

26. McGrath, J., Almeida, P., and Law, R. The Whittington Frailty Pathway: improving access to comprehensive geriatric assessment: an interdisciplinary quality improvement project. *BMJ Open Qual* 2019; 8: e000798-7. DOI:10.1136/bmjoq-2019-000798

27. Ellis, G., Gardner, M., Tsiachristas, A., Langhorne, P., Burke, O., Harwood, R.H. et al. Comprehensive geriatric assessment for older adults admitted to hospital. *Cochrane Database of Systematic Reviews* 2017. Issue 9. Art. No:CD006211. DOI: 10.1002/14651858.CD006211.pub3

28. Santilli, V., Bernetti, A., Mangone, M., and Paoloni, M. Clinical definition of sarcopenia. *Clinical Cases in Mineral and Bone Metabolism* 2014; 11 (3): 177–180.

29. Kim, J.C., Kalantar-Zadeh, K., and Kopple, J.D. Frailty and protein-energy wasting in elderly patients with end stage kidney disease. *JASN. American Society of Nephrology* 2013; 24 (3): 337–351.

30. Goto, N.A., van Loon, I.N., Morpey, M.I., Verhaar, M.C., Willems, H.C., Emmelot-Vonk, M.H. et al. Geriatric assessment in elderly patients with end-stage kidney disease. *Nephron* 2019; 141 (1): 41–48.

31. Iyasere, O.U., Brown, E.A., Johansson, L., Huson, L., Smee, J., Maxwell, A.P. et al. Quality of life and physical function in

older patients on dialysis: a comparison of assisted peritoneal dialysis with hemodialysis. *CJASN* 2016; 11 (3): 423–430.

32. Roche, J.J.W., Wenn, R.T., Sahota, O., and Moran, C.G. Effect of comorbidities and postoperative complications on mortality after hip fracture in elderly people: prospective observational cohort study. *BMJ* 2005; 331 (7529): 1374–1375.

33. van Zwieten, A., Wong, G., Ruospo, M., Palmer, S.C., Teixeira-Pinto, A., Barulli, M.R. et al. Associations of cognitive function and education level with all-cause mortality in adults on hemodialysis: findings from the COGNITIVE-HD study. *American Journal of Kidney Diseases* Elsevier; 2019; 74 (4): 452–462.

34. Brown, E. and Farrington, K. Geriatric assessment in advanced kidney disease. *CJASN* 2019; 14: 1091–1093.

35. Nixon, A.C., Brown, J., Brotherton, A., Harrison, M., Todd, J., Brannigan, D. et al. Implementation of a frailty screening programme and Geriatric Assessment Service in a nephrology centre: a quality improvement project. *Journal of Nephrology* 2021; 34: 1215–1224.

36. Advanced kidney disease [Internet]. https://heeoe.hee.nhs. uk/sites/default/files/nhs_advanced_kidney_disease_ planning_for_end_of_life_care_booklet_dnacpr_info_ entry_pg_30.pdf [Accessed 4 Sept 2022]

37. O'Riordan, J., Noble, H., Kane, P.M., and Smyth, A. Advance care plan barriers in older patients with end-stage renal disease: a qualitative nephrologist interview study. *BMJ Support Palliat Care* 2020; 10 (4): e39.

38. Goff, S.L., Unruh, M.L., Klingensmith, J., Eneanya, N.D., Garvey, C., Germain, M.J. et al. Advance care planning with patients on hemodialysis: an implementation study. *BMC Palliative Care* 2019; 18 (64) DOI; 10.1186/s12904-019-0437-2

39. O'Halloran, P., Noble, H., Norwood, K., Maxwell, P., Shields, J., Fogarty, D. et al. Advance care planning with patients who have end-stage kidney disease: a systematic realist review. *Journal of Pain and Symptom Management* 2018; 56 (5): 795–807.E18.

40. Roberti, J., Cummings, A., Myall, M., Harvey, J., Lippiett, K., Hunt, K. et al. Work of being an adult patient with chronic kidney disease: a systematic review of qualitative studies. *BMJ Open.* 2018; 8 (9): e023507–29.

41. Karnik, J.A., Young, B.S., Lew, N.L., Herget, M., Dubinsky, C., Lazarus, J.M. et al. Cardiac arrest and sudden death in dialysis units. *Kidney International* 2001; 60 (1): 350–357.

42. Isles, C., Robertson, S., Almond, A., and Clark, D. The challenges of renal replacement therapy and renal palliative care in the elderly. *Journal of the Royal College of Physicians of Edinburgh* 2011; 41; 238–243.

43. Low, J., Smith, G., Burns, A., and Jones, L. The impact of end-stage kidney disease (ESKD) on close persons: a literature review. *Clinical Kidney Journal* 2008; 1 (2): 67–79.

44. Noble, H., Kelly, D., and Hudson, P. Experiences of carers supporting dying renal patients managed without dialysis. *Journal of Advanced Nursing* 2013; 69 (8): 1829–1839. doi: 10.1111/jan.12049.

45. Grubbs, V., Tuot, D.S., Powe, N.R., O'Donoghue, D., and Chesla, C.A. Family involvement in decisions to forego or withdraw dialysis: a qualitative study of nephrologists in the United States and England. *Kidney Medicine* 2019; 1 (2): 57–64.

46. Noble, H., Meyer, J., Bridges, J., Kelly, D., and Johnson, B. Patient experience of dialysis refusal or withdrawal—a review of the literature. *Journal of Renal Care* ; 2008; 34 (2): 94–100.

47. Shrestha, A. and Burns, A. End-stage kidney disease on dialysis: an observational study of modality change from maximum conservative management. *BMJ Supportive & Palliative Care* 2021: Published Online First: 15 March 2021. DOI: 10.1136/bmjspcare-2020-002839

48. Detering, K.M., Hancock, A.D., Reade, M.C., and Silvester, W. The impact of advance care planning on end of life care in elderly patients: randomised controlled trial. *BMJ* 2010; 340:c1345. doi: 10.1136/bmj.c1345.

49. Abadir, P.M., Finucane, T.E., and McNabney, M.K. When doctors and daughters disagree: twenty-two days and two blinks of an eye. *Journal of the American Geriatrics Society* 2011; 59: 2337–2340. doi: 10.1111/j.1532-5415.2011.03700.x.

50. Wade, D.T. and Kitzinger, C. Making healthcare decisions in a person's best interests when they lack capacity: clinical guidance based on a review of evidence. *Clinical Rehabilitation* 2019; 33 (10): 1571–1585.

51. Highet, G., Crawford, D., Murray, S.A., and Boyd, K. Development and evaluation of the Supportive and Palliative Care Indicators Tool (SPICT): a mixed-methods study. *BMJ Support Palliat Care2014*; 4 (3): 285.

52. Couchard, C., Labeeuw, M., Moranne, O., Allot, V., Esnault, V., Frimat, L. et al. A clinical score to predict 6-month prognosis in elderly patients starting dialysis for end-stage renal disease. *Nephrology Dialysis Transplantation* 2008; 24 (5): 1553–1561.

53. Cohen, L.M., Ruthazer, R., Moss, A.H., and Germain, M.J. Predicting six-month mortality for patients who are on maintenance hemodialysis. *CJASN* 2010; 5 (1): 72–79.

54. Wilson, J. A mixed method, psychosocial analysis of how senior health care professionals recognise dying and engage patients and families in the negotiation of key decisions. [Internet]. Smith P, Lucey H, editors. https://purehost.bath. ac.uk/ws/portalfiles/portal/187948864/WILSON_Joanne_ PhD_Thesis_FINAL28.09.2017.pdf [Accessed 4 Sept 2022]

55. Ryan, L. and Brown, E. Supporting and maintaining the frail patient on long-term renal replacement therapy. *Clinical Medicine.* 2020; 20 (2): 139–141.

56. Burns, A., Wilson, J., and Jones, H. Weekly "priorities MDT" meeting – an initiative to guide a holistic approach to care in frail, struggling renal patients. How do staff perceive this intervention three years on? *British Journal of Renal Medicine* 2019; 24: 88–92.

57. Dorman, S. and Brogan, A. Personalised care: what matters to you? *BMJ: British Medical Journal* [Internet]: https://blogs. bmj.com/bmj/2020/03/06/personalised-care-what-matters-to-you [Accessed 4 Sept 2022]

58. British Medical Association. *Mental Capacity Act Tool Kit.* British Medical Association 2008.

59. Mannix, K. *With the End in Mind: Dying, Death and Wisdom in an Age of Denial.* William Collins. 2019. *ISBN: 9780008210915*

60. Sekkarie, M.A. and Abdel-Rahman, E.M. Cultural challenges in the care of refugees with end-stage renal disease: what western nephrologists should know. *Nephron* 2017; 137 (2): 85–90.

61. Krawczyk, M. and Gallagher, R. Communicating prognostic uncertainty in potential end-of-life contexts: experiences of family members. *BMC Palliat Care.* 2016; 15 (1): 59.

62. National Institute for Health and Care Excellence (NICE). Planning and managing end of life care for a child or young person with a life-limiting condition. 2020

63. Wilcock, A., Howard, P., and Charlesworth, S. *Palliative Care Formulary,* 7e. Pharmaceutical Press. 2020

64. Secora, A., Alexander, G.C., Ballew, S.H., Coresh, J., and Grams, M.E.. Kidney function, polypharmacy, and potentially inappropriate medication use in a community-based cohort of older adults. *Drugs Aging* 2018; 35 (8): 735–750.

65. Low, J.K., Crawford, K., Manias, E., and Williams, A. Stressors and coping resources of Australian kidney transplant recipients related to medication taking: a qualitative study. *Journal of Clinical Nursing* 3rd ed. 2017; 26 (11–12): 1495–1507.

66. Ashley, C. and Dunleavey, A. The renal drug handbook. CRC Press .2018. ISBN:978-1-138-62479-5

67. Shirazian, S., Grant, C.D., Aina, O., Mattana, J., Khorassani, F., and Ricardo, A.C. Depression in chronic kidney disease and end-stage renal disease: similarities and differences in diagnosis, epidemiology, and management. *Kidney International Reports* 2017; 2 (1): 94–107.

68. Joint Formulary Committee. British National Formulary (online) [Internet]. London: BMJ Group and Pharmaceutical Press. http://www.medicinescomplete.com (accessed 28 March 2021).

69. Booth, S. and Johnson, M.J. Improving the quality of life of people with advanced respiratory disease and severe breathlessness. *Breathe* 2019; 15 (3): 198–215 p 215.

70. Marshall, K. Breathlessness: causes, assessment and non-pharmacological management. *Nursing Times* 2020; 116 (9): 24–26.

71. Johnson, M.J. and Currow, D.C. Opioids for breathlessness: a narrative review. *BMJ Supportive & Palliative Care* British Medical Journal Publishing Group; 2020; 10 (3): 287–295.

72. O'Connor, N.R., Dougherty, M., Harris, P.S., and Casarett, D.J. Survival after dialysis discontinuation and hospice enrollment for ESRD. *Clinical Journal of the American Society of Nephrology* 2013; 8 (12): 2117–2122. doi: 10.2215/cjn.04110413.

73. Murtagh, F.E.M., Addington-Hall, J.M., and Higginson, I.J. End-stage renal disease: a new trajectory of functional decline in the last year of life. *Journal of the American Geriatrics Society* 2011; 59 (2): 304–308.

74. Douglas, C., Murtagh, F., Chambers, E.J., Howse, M., and Ellershaw, J. Symptom management for the adult patient dying with advanced chronic kidney disease: a review of the literature and development of evidence-based guidelines by a United Kingdom Expert Consensus Group. *Palliative Medicine* 2009; 23 (2): 103–110.

75. Wilson, J., Laverty, D., Mann, T., Hayes, A., and Hart, D. *Third Edition: Care after Death.* Hospice UK. 2020 47.

19 Palliative Care for People Living with Mental Illness and People with Intellectual Disabilities

Jed Jerwood and Gemma Allen

Introduction

The only way death is not meaningless is to see yourself as part of something greater: a family, a community, a society.
[1, p. 127]

Palliative care in the United Kingdom is thought to be some of the best in the world, yet we know this only benefits a minority of the population [2]. Despite a focus on improving accessibility to palliative care, some groups of people face significant barriers, remaining marginalised, and underrepresented in services. Within this chapter, we explore some of the issues associated with the provision of palliative care for people with mental ill health and intellectual disability.

In 2015 [refreshed in 2021], the National Palliative and end-of-life Care Partnership published the Ambitions for Palliative and end-of-life Care [PEOLC] [3]. The framework proposes six ambitions to improve access and quality of PEOLC, including "each person gets fair access to care" highlighting the inequalities which exist for some people and communities.

I live in a society where I get good end-of-life care regardless of who I am, where I live or the circumstances of my life.
[3, p. 3]

For people living with mental illnesses and people with intellectual disabilities, many barriers to accessing high quality palliative care exist. On an interpersonal level these include negative attitudes, stigma, fear, and prejudice among health-care professionals [HCP's]. Structurally, barriers include the separation between mental health, physical health, and intellectual disability services, silo working between specialisms and commissioning arrangements. Both groups experience prejudice which leads to poor health outcomes, compounded by negative past experiences in health and social care services, issues relating to communication differences and accessibility issues.

Undoubtedly, people living with mental illnesses and people with intellectual disabilities share some common experiences and are clearly disadvantaged when accessing palliative and end-of-life care services. It is important to consider the specific needs of each group separately, with unique wishes, life experiences, and abilities.

Many people with intellectual disabilities have mental health needs and may also be mental health service users. Similarly, there are many mental health service users who also have intellectual disabilities and differences. People living with mental illnesses and intellectual disabilities often encounter other disadvantages which compound their experience of marginalisation such as living in poverty, a lack of family or social support, experience of loneliness and isolation, substance use, as well as less access to employment, leisure, and social activities.

These experiences and the chances of falling through the gaps in service provision often means people with mental ill health and people with intellectual disability do not receive palliative care until the very last days of life, or indeed at all.

This chapter is concerned with approaches and attitudes. For most of the people it concerns, the components of treatments and management of symptoms require many of the same interventions as the general population. However, the *way* that care is delivered, the *timing* of

Handbook of Palliative Care, Fourth Edition. Edited by Richard Kitchen, Christina Faull, Sarah Russell and Jo Wilson.
© 2024 John Wiley & Sons Ltd. Published 2024 by John Wiley & Sons Ltd.

interventions and the *approaches* to engagement and communication may differ.

The chapter includes the views and experiences of people living with mental illness and people with intellectual disability on their care needs and experiences of accessing care. It provides guidance on how to improve palliative care experiences and accessibility to make sure that when vulnerable people most need care and support, at the end of their lives, they are able to receive it.

Language and Terminology

There is a wide variety of terminology used to describe mental ill health including specific conditions such as schizophrenia, bipolar disorder, depression, anxiety, personality disorders, phobias, and many more. Umbrella terms such as severe mental illness [SMI] or common mental disorders [CMD] are also used to define severity. Language is emotive and many different views are held about the terminology used.

For this chapter, the term "people living with mental illness" has been used, to be more inclusive and to reflect the fact that it is not the specific diagnosis of an individual psychiatric disorder which leads to marginalisation in palliative care, but more the stigma surrounding mental illness as a whole.

In the United Kingdom, the term "learning disability" is understood and accepted and it should be noted that "learning difficulty" is different to "learning disability." However, internationally the term "intellectual disability" is widely used and gradually becoming the more recognised term. Within this chapter, we have used the term intellectual disability.

Across the world, health services are structured differently, and the extent of mental health and intellectual disability care systems differs in different countries. However, the stigma surrounding mental illness and intellectual disability, like the stigma surrounding death and dying, is universal and the barriers experienced by both defined populations are common across health systems.

Stigma around Death and Dying

The fear of death and dying is deep seated. The emotions which arise when we think about our own mortality can be difficult and lead to an avoidance of discussion about death. Beliefs about death and dying are often religiously and culturally anchored and in the UK, the health-care system has evolved in society where attitudes to death and dying are quiet, still, and sombre, and largely not discussed [4, 5].

Health-care professionals are often motivated by a desire to help people recover and, particularly in mental health services, death is seen to be a failure or something to be avoided. More broadly, advances in health care have led to higher expectation about curability and life expectancy.

Despite recent attention and an increase in discussion and initiatives to encourage conversations about death, dying, and grief [such as Death Cafés, Dying Matters Awareness Week, Hospice Care Week, and Good Grief Festival], the dying person can often experience feelings of withdrawal and an avoidance of conversations about dying and end-of-life care. Likewise, HCPs outside of the palliative care sector often do not feel confident speaking with patients about death and dying. For the dying person living with mental illness or intellectual disabilities this can mean that they are doubly disadvantaged, with staff lacking confidence in either speaking about death and dying or addressing their care needs. This leads to raised anxiety in HCP's about their role and feelings of abandonment in the dying person.

Palliative Care for People with Mental Ill Health

The first part of the chapter aims to explore some of the barriers experienced by people living with mental illnesses when accessing palliative care, the issues which arise for HCP's in thinking about providing care for a dying person with a mental illness and an incurable condition, and to present some examples of strategies for improving care experiences and breaking down barriers. The chapter draws on recent research by the author [6, 7], which includes the views of patients and carers, as well as HCPs from a range of backgrounds, to better understand the palliative and end-of-life care needs of people living with mental illnesses and incurable conditions.

Mental Health in the UK

Around 1 in 4 people will experience a period of mental ill health in their lifetime [8]. For many people, this is a brief event in response to a stressful or difficult period in their lives. In the UK, around 1 in 6 people report symptoms of a common mental disorder such as depression, anxiety, panic disorder, phobias, and obsessive compulsive disorders [9]. However, around 1 in 20 people live with a severe or persistent mental illness or condition such as schizophrenia, bipolar disorder, or personality disorder which has a significant impact on their day to day lives and functioning [10, 11].

In the UK, and in many other health-care systems, mental health and physical health services have traditionally been commissioned and provided separately. Within the health-care system, people who have more severe and persistent mental illnesses are cared for in secondary mental health services. The mental health system is structured around community mental health teams: e.g. multidisciplinary teams of psychiatrists, psychological therapists, community psychiatric nurses, occupational therapists, and social workers as well as other recovery and employment support services. People are referred via their General Practitioner [GP] when their mental health needs cannot be supported in primary care or following an acute admission to hospital or crisis presentation. During their journey through the mental health system, people may receive support in the community as an inpatient, and access a range of psychological therapies, occupational therapies, and recovery orientated support services. Many people spend many years within the mental health system, and currently, many service users have co-existant physical health problems, exacerbated by their mental illness and some of the medications they have been prescribed. In recent years there has been a national focus on improving the physical health of people within the mental health system to address this but has not included a focus on improving access to palliative care [12–16].

Health Inequalities and Mental Health

Adults living with long-term mental illnesses still die up to twenty years younger than the general population, which is one of the biggest health inequalities in the UK [14, 17, 18]. Early mortality in people living with long-term mental illness is mostly due to preventable causes associated with other socio-economic disadvantages such as living in poverty, poor quality housing, poor diet, lower levels of physical exercise, poorer diet, and higher rates of tobacco, drug, and alcohol use [15, 19]. Sometimes people living with mental illness present later with symptoms and may not feel able to attend routine screening and this can lead to later diagnosis, and then poorer prognosis, of life-threatening conditions. In addition, when accessing health services, people living with mental illness are often subject to "diagnostic overshadowing," where physical symptoms are attributed to mental illness [20]. People with mental illness report feeling dismissed, ignored, and fobbed off by health services, not having physical symptoms treated seriously, not finding health services accessible or joined up, and consequently continue to have poorer health outcomes [21].

For far too long, people of all ages with mental health problems have been stigmatised and marginalised, all too often experiencing an NHS that treats their minds and bodies separately. Mental health services have been underfunded for decades, and too many people have received no help at all, leading to hundreds and thousands of lives put on hold or ruined, and thousands of tragic and unnecessary deaths.
[21, p. 3]

Stigma and Mental Illness

Stigma towards people with mental illness dates back to the earliest of records. References to negative stereotypes of people with mental illnesses are evident in ancient Greek writings [22]. The separation of the mentally ill, which is arguably still evident in the commissioning and provision of mental health services, has long been a feature in all societies. People with mental illness have been taken away, locked up and ostracised, with the aim of "protecting society," throughout history [23, 24]. Fear of people with mental illness comes from two places – fear of attack, which comes from the unusual or distressing beliefs and behaviours people may experience when acutely mentally unwell; and the fear of contamination that somehow the mental illness can be caught, spread, or passed on [25].

Although legislation and clinical practice now focuses on detaining those who may be a risk to themselves, and for the minimum period possible, the perceived risk to others is still a key consideration in the assessment of mental health. While a small minority of people may pose a risk to others, and some may pose a risk to themselves at times, the vast majority of people with mental ill health pose no risk at all [26–28].

Even though contemporary understanding of mental ill health in clinical practice has evolved a long way from these early misconceptions, the stigma which surrounds mental illness continues to be very powerful in health-care settings and in wider society. This is compounded by portrayals of mental illness in the media, news, on television and in film. People with mental illness are portrayed as killers, psychopaths, dangerous, and violent. In addition, portrayals also present people with mental ill health as unable to make decisions, understand and as vulnerable members of society who need to have decision-making removed from them.

Experiences in Healthcare

In health-care settings, people who don't fit into perceived norms can be difficult for health-care professionals to work with, especially in busy, pressurised services [28–30]. People living with mental illness sometimes present differently to other people, they may show their distress more, feel more anxious, or seem suspicious of service providers. When unwell, sometimes people with mental illness may hold unusual beliefs, especially about death and dying, medications and medical treatments, and may present with unusual or different behaviours to other patients. People may find it hard to organise themselves, attend appointments and communicate with services. This leads services and HCP's to withdraw [7]. HCP's are subject to the same media and societal stereotypes and despite receiving anti-discriminatory practice and mental health awareness training, may still feel some of the same fears and anxieties about working with people who may feel very different to themselves [23, 28, 31]. The stigma and fear about mental illness continues to be pervasive and persistent.

Many people living with mental illness have had negative experiences in health care. Sometimes people will have experienced being detained against their will under the Mental Health Act 2007 [32]. Some people have had experiences of their health-care needs going unmet, ignored, or have felt fobbed off by services. It is common for physical ill health to be neglected and symptoms to be missed. For many people, they have felt misunderstood, not had access to the right kind of support at the right time with regard to their mental health needs, and experienced conflict with their care teams.

The symptoms of some mental health conditions that can cause people to feel paranoid, suspicious, or mistrustful of health-care services have often been exacerbated or reinforced by actual experiences. So when a person with mental ill health becomes unwell with an incurable physical condition, it can trigger negative past experiences which make that person less likely to seek or accept help and support. It might feel difficult to talk

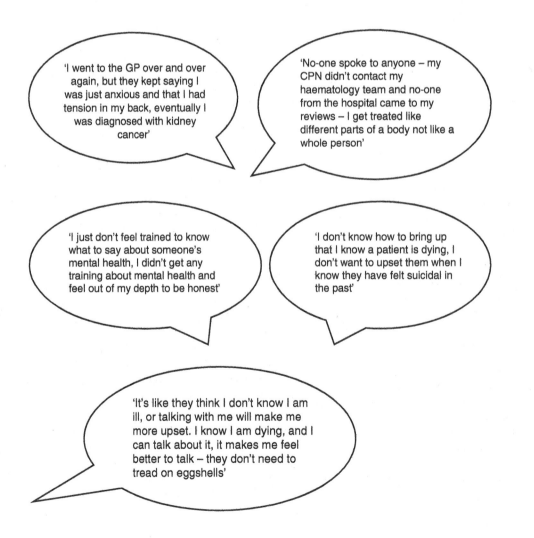

about the end-of-life with someone who has experienced suicidal feelings or who experiences very low mood. HCP's may be fearful of "getting it wrong" or causing distress and consequently, avoid difficult conversations but this can leave the person who is ill feeling abandoned or avoided.

A Note on Risk

An excessive focus on risk stems from stigma surrounding mental illness. The perceptions of people with mental ill health as dangerous or risky to others, or vulnerable and a risk to themselves, can lead to an avoidance of discussions between HCP's and their patients.

Discussions about palliative and end-of-life care, death and dying, and people with mental ill health often focus on risk. HCP's across mental health and palliative care often feel worried about having conversations about the end-of-life with people with mental ill health for fear of upsetting or de-stabilising the person [6, 33–35]. Conversations between HCPs regarding advance care planning [ACP] or involving the person in their own care can become risk-focused and issues of mental capacity and ability to be involved are often pre-occupying for professionals. In contrast, patients and carers often feel left out of care planning discussions or experience a feeling of being treated differently to other people when decisions about care are being made.

Most people with experience of mental illness have mental capacity to enable them to take part in care planning discussions and want to be involved. People living with mental illness can often feel anxious and being left out of discussions or not being told information about their health, prognosis, or treatment and care options can exacerbate these feelings.

Barriers to Accessing Palliative Care

There are barriers at all levels for people with mental ill health needing palliative care, both in terms of access and experience within services. Specialist palliative care providers, hospital, mental health, primary care, and other community services all have a role in the provision of palliative care. Barriers exist at three levels as highlighted in Table 1: (1) at system level, (2) within clinical practice and (3) with the patient themselves. The barriers are highlighted below with quotes from HCP, patient, and carer research participants.

Table 1 Barriers to palliative care.

Barriers to Palliative Care
SYSTEM
Structural Barriers
Silo working
Separation between mental health and physical health services—gaps between services
Unclear referral pathways
Lack of co-ordination of care
PRACTICE
Stigma and Prejudice
Lack of confidence
Avoidance of the patient
Fear of mental illness
Fear of talking about death and dying
Diagnostic overshadowing
Paternalism and risk averse practice
Lack of understanding of available services and care pathways [mental health and palliative care]
Lack of clarity of roles and responsibilities
PATIENT
Unusual beliefs or behaviours
Challenging or unusual presentations
Fear of services or negative past experiences in health care
Anxiety about meeting new people
Fear of dying
Isolation and lack of social and family support
Fear of discrimination
Lack of understanding of breadth of palliative care and services available
Loss of support due to physical health

How Can We Improve Care and Break down Barriers?

At both an individual or service level, as well as at a system level, there are ways that everyone involved in the care of people living with mental illness and an incurable condition can help reduce these barriers and improve the experience of accessing a receiving care.

Individual Level – What Can I Do?

Leaning In – Getting Alongside

It is important for health-care professionals [HCPs] in all settings to be able to see the person before them, rather than a series of labels and diagnoses. Consider your own fears and anxieties which arise when meeting a patient who has a mental illness. What are you worried about? Talk to other HCP's about your concerns and share knowledge and expertise.

Use your skills from having other difficult conversations to have these conversations. Ask the person what they know about their illness; do they understand the treatment options available to them? Do they understand what palliative care is in its widest definition? Do they know what is available locally in the palliative care system?

Ask how their mental illness affects them. What helps? What makes it worse? How can symptoms be alleviated? What might you need to know or look out for? How might you know if they were to become unwell? Are there other professionals or services involved in the person's care that you need to be in contact with?

If you notice yourself retreating or avoiding ask why? What is going on and getting in the way of you being alongside the person and how can you address this? What support might you need?

Care Co-ordination and Multi-agency Working/Communication between Services

There may be multiple organisations involved in a person's care or they may be very unsupported. People may not have good relationships with health-care professionals or family and may have support from other service users or community organisations. For good palliative and end-of-life care to be provided, multiple agencies need to be involved. Care needs to be co-ordinated and agencies will need to communicate. It may not be obvious who is co-ordinating care – for some people, their GP might be the best person, for others their care co-ordinator from their mental health team might be or for others a community nurse or other professional from a hospice might take the lead. However, it is important that all agencies stay involved with the person's care as their illness progresses. Hospice teams may need support from mental health teams and vice versa. Supporting the person to maintain contact with other services and specialisms is important.

Often patient care IT systems do not allow information sharing across agencies. It is important that agencies and professionals communicate with each other directly. Multi-agency meetings, involving the patient, are also essential to support the delivery of holistic palliative care.

Involving the Person [and those important to them]

Recent research highlighted how often people living with mental illness are excluded from conversations about their care [7, 36]. In contrast, patients and carers were very clear about wanting to be involved, feeling able to cope with being involved and that being excluded exacerbated their anxiety and feeling of isolation rather than feeling protective.

When working with people with mental illness it is important to establish early on, who they would like involved in their care, and as importantly, who they would not like involved in their care. Many people have very limited social and family support networks, and may have professionals or informal care networks who provide day to day support. Some people may have complex family relationships and it is important not to make assumptions about who is and is not involved. A person may have carers who also have mental health needs of their own and so having open conversations early on about who the preferred and most appropriate people to be involved in different aspects of care is essential.

For example, someone may want their family to be informed about their changing health status if they are not able to inform them themselves but may want a support worker to be the person attending health appointments and helping with advance care planning discussions.

Early Conversations and Referrals/Advance Care Planning

The benefits of early referral to palliative care are well documented [37]. For people with mental ill health this is all the more important because of the multiple disadvantages many face. They may need more time to build relationships with new services, but also may benefit even more than the general population from some of the interventions within palliative care, before end-of-life such as respite, psychological support, day hospice, social work advice, and advance care planning. For the small minority of people with mental ill health who do receive palliative care, it is often in the last few days or weeks of life. The intensity of such conversations may mean that they have to take place in smaller sessions over a longer period of time. In addition, people may have multiple agencies involved in their care and it can take time to co-ordinate the roles and responsibilities of each element.

The key to early referral is helping people understand that palliative care is not about the very end-of-life and can be provided throughout an illness trajectory.

System Level—What Can We Do?

Each local health-care system is structured differently and different palliative care systems and services are available in different areas. For example, there may be greater involvement of the voluntary and community sector in some areas, hospice services differ depending on commissioning arrangements, there may be community palliative care teams, hospice at home services, and day hospice provision to differing degrees across the locality. Similarly mental health services can be structured in a range of ways and have different referral pathways. However, there are things which service providers can do to improve the care journey for the person living with a mental illness and requiring palliative and end-of-life care.

Strategic Commitment—Setting the Tone

System-wide acknowledgement of the need to make services more inclusive to people living with mental illness, and other excluded groups, is important. All too often, people living with mental illness are not even acknowledged as a marginalised or minority group in strategic or policy level discussions. At a local level, bringing stakeholders together to **set a commitment for improvement** is something that all localities can do.

Training and Education—Winning Hearts and Minds

Identifying **local champions** within services who are passionate about improving services can help to drive improvements forward. Many HCP's are not aware that people living with mental illness encounter barriers to accessing palliative care. In mental health services, there is a need to increase awareness of the mental health clinician's role in supporting access to and delivery of palliative care. In palliative care services there is a need for greater understanding and higher levels of confidence among HCPs working with people living with mental illnesses.

Care Pathways and Service Understanding—Who, How, and When?

Improving knowledge of the local health-care systems is critical to improving access to services. HCP's need quick and easy ways to identify appropriate services for people living with mental illnesses and incurable conditions. Knowing who, how, and when to refer is essential to improving the dying person's care journey. **A local system map** or service leaflet, highlighting what is available at each stage of a person's illness is helpful for the dying person, their family, and health-care professionals.

System-wide, patient held, care plans—Everyone Knows, Everyone Asks

Adoption of a system-wide, patient held care plan document which is used across services can support better integrated care. This can include advance care planning but is a broader document, which could be held electronically or in paper form, which includes all the care and services involved with the patient. If all services, including mental health services, are aware of the locally adopted document, it can be used in appointments to ensure that all areas of care have been considered and each service is aware of who is involved in that person's care, avoiding the gaps between services and improving communication and awareness between services and empowering the person receiving care.

Discussion Activity

Case Study—John's[1] *story*

John was a 48-year-old man with a history of schizophrenia. John had been a mental health service user for more than twenty years and had a CPN who visited him regularly at home and was aware of John's physical health problems but not involved in his physical health care.

John had presented several times to his GP with symptoms and queried a prostate problem, but his GP had told him he was too young to need further screening. After six months and multiple appointments, John was diagnosed with prostate cancer, learning that his cancer was incurable from the GP receptionist.

John had a history of moving around, he had lived overseas and had lived in and out of supported care services throughout adulthood. He was estranged from his family and lived alone with his rescue dog in supported housing.

As John's physical health deteriorated, he experienced an increase in pain and a reduction in mobility. His Housing Support Worker helped him to apply for a ground-floor flat, which was more suitable for his needs, but increased his isolation. As his health deteriorated, his mental health also became more difficult for John to cope with. He was unable to go fishing, in pain, and now living alone in his flat with his dog who he was struggling to care for. His CPN continued to monitor his mental health.

John's Housing Support Worker contacted a local Hospice and John was referred for an assessment that he was reluctant to attend. He met with a member of the well-being team who offered pain management and suggested he attend the day hospice where John became a regular member of the Wednesday Social Group. Staff were initially worried about his schizophrenia diagnosis but as they got to know John, found him to be a funny and wise member of the group. He

---

[1]Pseudonym used to protect confidentiality of patient.

would often tell stories of his adventures overseas and shared the stories behind his many tattoos.

As John's health deteriorated further, the Hospice staff helped John to plan his future care. He was admitted for respite to help with symptom control, and during his stay planned for his dog to be rehomed. No mental health support was available to John in his final weeks of life and with his health deteriorating he died in the hospice six weeks later. His funeral took place, led by the Hospice Chaplain and attended by many of his day hospice friends and members of staff.

During John's admission, the Hospice did not contact his mental health team, his CPN did not visit and was not informed of his death for over a month.

Questions

- How effective was communication in John's story? Consider communication with John and between HCP's and services.
- How did John benefit from referral to palliative care?
- How could John's care have been improved? Think about his care journey from diagnosis to his death.

Palliative Care and People with Intellectual Disabilities

Intellectual Disability

The World Health Organisation definition of an intellectual disability is when the following three criteria are present: (1) a significantly reduced intellectual ability to understand new or complex information, (2) to learn and apply new skills [impaired intelligence] resulting in a reduced ability to cope independently [impaired social functioning] and (3) beginning before adulthood, with a lasting effect on development [38].

The level of daily living support an individual with intellectual disabilities will require is dependent on the degree of their intellectual disability. There is often a difference in individual communication skills, concept, and understanding of language with variations on the degree of care and support that a person will need.

There are different types of intellectual disability, and this can be distinguished by:

- **Mild to moderate intellectual disability**—The person may require some level of support with everyday tasks, learn to develop independence, be employed, live independently, and maintain relationships.
- **Severe and profound disability**—The person is likely to have severe limitations in capacity, conceptual skills, understanding, communication skills, and personal care. They are likely to require a high level of support to meet their care needs.

Health Concerns for People with Intellectual Disabilities, Disadvantaged in Life—and Death?

In the UK, there are more than 1.5 million people with an intellectual disability [39]. However, with increasing childhood survival rates, advances in care and an ageing population it is predicted that the number of people with an intellectual disability over the age of 60 years will increase, thus more people living longer with multiple and complex conditions and an increased need for palliative and end-of-life care.

Study findings suggest that people with intellectual disabilities are at an increased social disadvantage with poor access to health care, unmet care needs and delayed diagnosis of long-term conditions and progressive disease. People with an intellectual disability often experience indifferences in equality, poorer health outcomes and increased rates of significant health issues with a lower life expectancy than the general population and often dying preventable deaths [40].

The 2007 *Death by Indifference* report [41] shared several distressing accounts of people with intellectual disabilities who were alleged to be disproportionately affected and died from unnecessary, premature, and avoidable deaths. Since then, several independent inquiries and studies have followed highlighting further investigations into how and why people with an intellectual disability are dying younger than the general population, with poor health-care outcomes and failings in the health-care system for people with intellectual disabilities.

The *Confidential Inquiry into the Premature Deaths of People with Learning Disabilities* [CIPOLD] report [42] investigated the deaths of people with intellectual disabilities and described distinctive findings regarding avoidable deaths and failings within the health-care system. Furthermore, it identified that people with an intellectual disability were less likely to access specialist palliative care and the end-of-life care people received was un-coordinated with improvements required for the support that the dying person and their families receive. Many more reports have followed including The Care Quality Commission [2016] thematic review *A Different Ending: Addressing Inequalities in End-of-Life Care* [43]. The review identified and recognised that certain groups of people, including those with intellectual disabilities, experience inequitable care at the end-of-life with providers not understanding or considering their needs.

The learning from deaths of people with a learning disability [LeDeR] programme was established in 2015 as a service improvement programme in response to the CIPOLD recommendations. The programme aimed to learn from and

Table 2 Intellectual disability impairment level and median age of death [45].

Impairment Level	Median Age of Death
Mild intellectual disability	62
Moderate intellectual disability	63
Severe intellectual disability	57
Profound and multiple intellectual disability	40

Table 3 Barriers accessing palliative and end-of-life care for people with intellectual disabilities.

Late Diagnoses or Uncertain Prognostic Indicators
Institutional discrimination
Individual needs not considered or understood by health-care professionals
Lack of confidence—health-care professionals
Inadequate training and awareness of the needs of people with intellectual disabilities
Structural barriers and "gatekeepers" of services
Difficulty expressing pain and other symptoms
Poor communication between services and with the individual
Uncoordinated care
Difficulty navigating appointment booking systems.
Lack of understanding about Accessible Information Standard
Misconception of palliative care services
Lack of involvement in future care conversations
Silo-working
Assumptions made by health-care professionals
Lack of reasonable adjustments

prevent future avoidable premature deaths, supporting local steering groups to review deaths and identify significant issues, to improve health outcomes of people with an intellectual disability and reduce discrimination and inequity people with an intellectual disability experience. The publication of the 2018 LeDeR annual report [44] reviewed the findings from 1311 deaths of people with an intellectual disability who had died between June 2016 and November 2017. It presented the significant indifference in mortality for someone with an intellectual disability with the findings once again reporting poor coordination and care for people with intellectual disabilities, lack of understanding and awareness of individual needs and delays in care.

The LeDeR review [45] reported the median age of death for a man with an intellectual disability is just 60 years of age and 59 years for a woman. In comparison to the general population, the difference in median age of death between men with an intellectual disability is 23 years and for women 27 years. Table 2 presents the disparities in mortality age dependant on the level of impairment the individual has, with people with a profound or severe intellectual disability having a much lower life expectancy in comparison to a person with a mild to moderate intellectual disability.

Barriers Accessing Palliative Care for People with Intellectual Disabilities

There are a comprehensive range of challenges in delivering good palliative and end-of-life care for people with intellectual disabilities. When considering barriers that people with intellectual disabilities experience accessing wider health-care services [Table 3] it is essential to understand the gaps in knowledge and inequalities that lead to multiple disadvantages at the end-of-life. There may be access barriers if people are unaware of services, lack of reasonable adjustments made by the provider, poor previous experiences within health and social care services, structural or institutional barriers, and indirect biases that often exist within systems. Communication barriers between the individual, caregivers and services can result in lack of advance care planning opportunities and late referrals to palliative care.

Reasonable Adjustments

Under the Equality Act 2010 [46] health and social care services have a legal responsibility to create reasonable adjustments for people with an intellectual disability. Reasonable adjustments help to address and reduce health inequalities people with intellectual disabilities experience, access health screening programmes, and health services.

Take a moment to consider your organisation

- How do you communicate with people with an intellectual disability?
- Is information available in accessible formats?
- Are reasonable adjustments in place for appointments?
- Does your service give priority appointments or allow extra time for someone with an intellectual disability?

There are several ways that we can reduce barriers people with intellectual disabilities experience, enabling better access to palliative care services and improving end-of-life care for people with an intellectual disability and their caregivers.

Training and Education

Improved awareness of intellectual disabilities for health care professionals. How does the disease/condition present? How does the individual person with an intellectual disability report or describe discomfort, pain, distress, or other symptoms? What tools can be used to measure pain or distress?

Accessible Information and Reasonable Adjustments

Consider how people with an intellectual disability access screening programmes and health care appointments. What steps can be put in place to improve experiences? How do we identify how we can adapt services? What resources are available to support individuals with limited or non-verbal communication?

> **Case study 1: Applying reasonable adjustments within a Hospice**
>
> In 2017, The Mary Stevens Hospice in the Midlands, UK, was aware that their services were not accessible for people with an intellectual disability. The hospice commenced a programme whereby they invited people with intellectual disabilities to the hospice to conduct peer reviews and put recommendations into practice. They ensured staff were aware of reasonable adjustments for people with intellectual disabilities and ways in which they could do this. The hospice published easy read material, including an advance care plan, created a library of pictorial resources around death, dying and bereavement, installed accessible signage, created sensory spaces, and developed education for health-care professionals that is co-delivered with people with intellectual disabilities. In addition, the Hospice facilitates regular focus groups and workshops with people with intellectual disabilities to better understand the needs and concerns of this group.

Advance Care Planning with People with Intellectual Disabilities

Recognising when people with intellectual disabilities are approaching end-of-life can be challenging. For people with unidentified health needs it can often result in overlooked opportunities to discuss personal values and preferences planning for end-of-life care.

Advance care planning is an integral and important aspect to palliative care, with a series of ongoing discussions and opportunities for people to communicate choices and wishes, goals, and plans for future care so that personal preferences can be honoured at end-of-life with people better involved in their own decisions.

While advance care planning may not be beneficial to everyone, providing the opportunity to increase civic participation in these important conversations and communicate what is important can give individuals a sense of empowerment and control over their future care. Despite people with moderate to severe intellectual disabilities often having more complex communication skills or the inability to process or understand their prognosis it is still important to give them and their carers equal opportunities to communicate what matters most to them.

The case studies discussed shortly give examples of such introductory end-of-life conversations, outside the context of a medical environment and with people not within their final year of life. In all case studies, staff involved were skilled in these conversations but implemented new approaches to meet individual need, adapting their skills and using a range of resources to support the conversation.

> **Case study 2: Advance care planning conversations with people with a mild-moderate intellectual disability**
>
> Steven[2] is 54 years old and has a moderate intellectual disability and several physical disabilities. He lives with his wife who also has a mild intellectual disability and they both receive a daily care and support package. Steven is involved with several local advocacy groups and previously engaged in work focussed on equitable access to health care, reasonable adjustments and delivering awareness training to health and social care professionals.
>
> Steven joined a focus group for people with intellectual disabilities that met to discuss different issues about death and dying, including advance care planning. During the focus groups the facilitator used a variety of resources including easy read information and *Books Beyond Words* [47]. Steven was reluctant to participate in the session about advance care planning and stated that it was an "awful thing to think about" but wanted to stay and listen to the group discussions. Gradually, Steven became more engaged in the topic and participated in conversations, speaking openly about his own wishes for end-of-life and what matters most to him. By the end of the session, Steven had documented some of his choices to share with his wife, support worker, and GP. Following the focus group Steven has been involved in further advance care planning workshops, co-led by people with intellectual

---

[2] Pseudonyms used to protect confidentiality.

disabilities, using his story to engage and respond to other people's concerns.

> It is important that we speak about things that we are frightened of
> Steven—focus group member

Case Study 3: Involving and including people with profound multiple intellectual disabilities in conversations about future care

Tom[3] is a 24-year-old man with profound, multiple intellectual disabilities. He requires 24-hour care and support, and he lives with his brother who is his carer and Lasting Power of Attorney for both health/welfare and property/affairs. Tom attends a day care service twice a week and communicates non-verbally using limited Makaton signs and blinking. Tom attended a "What Matters to Me" day, whereby staff introduced conversations about priorities for end-of-life. Despite Tom's intellectual disability and limited communication Tom was supported to express several wishes that were important to him. These was documented within Tom's care plans and shared with his brother and wider multidisciplinary care team who were thankful that Tom had been included and involved in these discussions.

Bereavement Care—Why Is Bereavement Support Important?

Many people living with mental illness and intellectual disabilities have experienced bereavement. Unresolved losses can be a contributory factor to mental ill health and distress many people in mental health services and living with intellectual disability have experienced multiple losses.

This may make it even harder to think about their own care needs, should they become physically unwell. People in both groups are also often carers for people who may have incurable illnesses and will need access to bereavement support but can sometimes find their psychiatric diagnosis or intellectual disability is a barrier to accessing bereavement support.

There may be a role for the care teams involved with the person to provide bereavement support in this case or liaise with a bereavement service in some cases. Bereavement services may be concerned that they are not equipped to support a person's mental health needs or work with people with intellectual disabilities, but with support from other professionals who know the person well, can feel reassured that they are not solely responsible for a person's care and support and able to provide bereavement services.

> Going to the funeral is very important. Once a person has taken their final journey, you need to decide if you are going to the funeral or not. It's a question to think about! That's if you are even invited! Sometimes your family or carers decide that you shouldn't go to the funeral. That's wrong. From the family's perspective, they want to protect the person. The problem is, if the person wants to go to the funeral, but if the parents say no, it's very difficult. They don't have the right to make that decision. It's really, really important. Even if the person has severe and multiple disabilities, they still have feelings and emotions inside. They may know [that someone has died]. There is a way that they know. I don't know how, but they do know it inside.
> A person with intellectual disability from the GRASSroots group [48].

Public Health Approaches in palliative and end-of-life care for people with intellectual disabilities

> In the eighteenth century, to be born into a community was qualification enough to be part of that community, whatever a person's deviation from any sort of social norm. Communities adapted to people rather than people having to adapt to them. [49, p. 10]

When considering improvements to palliative care for marginalised groups, it is important to also look at a whole community approach, viewing the wider community as an equal partner to NHS and social care services and this is no less when working alongside people with intellectual disabilities. Various community development and engagement initiatives within the UK have enabled people to define their own needs, building not only the skills within the community to support people with death, dying, and bereavement but also community capacity. This approach helps to shift public attitudes and perceptions, developing a culture where people have open and honest conversations about their wishes and choices for end-of-life and supporting one another during times of ill health and grief. By "working with" rather than "doing to" a community's resilience can be strengthened, with inequalities tackled and challenged together, championing an equality led approach for palliative and end-of-life care.

The COVID-19 pandemic has highlighted the increased vulnerabilities, bias, and discrimination for people with intellectual disabilities. Inequalities have always existed for this group of people and they will continue to exist. It is up to everyone working in health and social care settings to recognise inequity, our role in perpetuating it, and the barriers that people with intellectual disabilities and other marginalised communities experience. Organisations

---

[3] Pseudonyms used to protect confidentiality.

Case Study—Using arts-approaches for advance care planning conversations

No Barriers Here [50] is a project co-developed by people with intellectual disabilities who wanted to explore creative ways for advance care planning conversations. Through arts-approached workshops the group worked with both chapter authors to initiate conversations with other people with intellectual disabilities.

Conversations during the workshops were facilitated using a creative approach such as collage, textiles, and weaving. The project ensured reasonable adjustments were in place and provided easy read information and support for people with intellectual disabilities to attend the workshops.

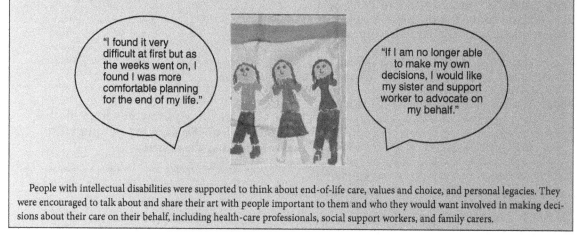

"I found it very difficult at first but as the weeks went on, I found I was more comfortable planning for the end of my life."

"If I am no longer able to make my own decisions, I would like my sister and support worker to advocate on my behalf."

People with intellectual disabilities were supported to think about end-of-life care, values and choice, and personal legacies. They were encouraged to talk about and share their art with people important to them and who they would want involved in making decisions about their care on their behalf, including health-care professionals, social support workers, and family carers.

must implement positive change to local and national policies, to be the difference and reduce disparities in how people with an intellectual disability live, die, and grieve.

It is vital that importance of excellent and co-ordinated care in the last hours, days, weeks, and years of life is recognised. People with intellectual disabilities often have little or no support, with a lack of communication between services and frequently do not experience a good death. Public health, community-led approaches have much to offer and HCP's and health-care organisations have a role to play as partners in these initiatives, advocating for excellence in palliative and bereavement care.

A horizon is where the known and the unknown meet. Where what can be seen meets with what is perhaps unknown, and it is individual and collective action that will enable expansion beyond the current patient population that traditionally access palliative and end-of-life care. If services and individuals listen and respond to people's needs, make reasonable adjustments, then care improves for the most vulnerable and for society as a whole.

Covid-19—Opportunities and Threats, Learning from the Pandemic

The impact of the Covid-19 pandemic has been felt across the world. In the UK, as in many other countries, the pandemic has illuminated wider health inequalities. As the pandemic progressed, data became available which highlighted the disproportionate impact the virus, and surrounding policy, was having on different groups of people. For people with mental ill health and intellectual disabilities, fears about the overuse of Do Not Attempt Cardio-Pulmonary Resuscitation [DNACPR] instructions emerged early on, delays in availability of vaccines for different vulnerable groups also impacted upon people with mental ill health and people with intellectual disability, in part due to the disproportionate levels of poor physical health experienced by both groups. In addition, lockdown measures and physical distancing resulted in increased isolation and loneliness for people already marginalised in our communities. For those with mental ill health or intellectual disabilities and living with long-term conditions, receiving palliative and end-of-life care or bereaved during the pandemic, the absence of social interaction and importance of human relationships has resulted in a marked change and increase in distress, behaviour, and understanding.

However, the developments in care during the pandemic also highlighted the role of palliative care, the importance of advance care planning, the importance of HCP's having the skills to provide and talk about palliative and end-of-life care and the importance of families and carers.

Conclusion

There continues to be persistent and increased health and socio-economic inequalities for people in the UK living with mental illness and with an intellectual disability, resulting in many people disadvantaged not only in life but in death and grief. However, small changes in practice have big impact. What makes a difference to people is a change in attitude and approach. The people and their carers and families who informed the research in this chapter were asking to be listened to, to be seen, to be included and to be empowered to participate in their own care decisions and care planning. Everyone in health care settings has a role to play in changing attitudes to people living with mental illness and with intellectual disabilities, to work together to make sure that the right support is in place the very end of their lives.

I just needed them to lean in, when I most needed them to lean in, they stepped back.
[51, p. 260] (John)

References

1. Gawande, A. (2014). *Being Mortal : Medicine and What Matters in the End.* New York: Metropolitan Books.
2. Dixon, J., King, D., Matosevic, T., Clark, M., and Knapp, M. (2015). *Equity in the provision of palliative care in the UK: review of evidence.* London: London School of Economics and Political Science, Political Social Services Research Unit.
3. National Palliative and End of Life Care Partnership. (2015). *Ambitions for palliative and end of life care: a national framework for local action 2015–2020.* London: NHS England.
4. Jalland, P. (2014). 'Bereavement and Mourning (Great Britain)', in *1914-1918-online. International Encyclopedia of the First World War* ed. by Ute Daniel, Peter Gatrell, Oliver Janz, Heather Jones, Jennifer Keene, Alan Kramer, and Bill Nasson, issued by Freie Universitat Berlin, Berlin 2014-10-08. DOI: 10.15463/ie1418.10178 Last modified: 2014-10-05. http://encyclopedia.1914-1918-online.net/article/Bereavement_and_Mourning_(Great_Britain).
5. Yalom, I. (2008). *Staring at the Sun: Overcoming the Terror of Death*, 2e. San Francisco: Jossey Bass.
6. Jerwood, J., Phimister, D., Ward, G., Holliday, N., and Coad, J. (2018). Barriers to palliative care for people with severe mental illness: exploring the views of clinical staff. *European Journal of Palliative Care* 25 (1): 20–25.
7. Jerwood, J., Ward, G., Phimister, D., Holliday, N., and Coad, J. 2021 Lean in, don't step back: the views and experiences of patients and carers with severe mental illness and incurable physical conditions on palliative and end of life care. *Progress in Palliative Care* (accessed 28 July 2021) 29 (5), 255-263.
8. NHS Digital. Adult psychiatric morbidity in England – 2007, results of a household survey. www.digital.nhs.uk/data-and-information/publications/statistical/adult-psychiatric-morbidity-survey/adult-psychiatric-morbidity-in-england-2007-results-of-a-household-survey (accessed 17 November 2021).
9. NHS Digital. Adult psychiatric morbidity survey: survey of mental health and wellbeing, England, 2014 – NHS Digital. www.webarchive.nationalarchives.gov.uk/ukgwa/20180328140249/http://digital.nhs.uk/catalogue/PUB21748 (accessed 17 November 2021).
10. Baker, C. (2018). *Mental health statistics for England: prevalence, services and funding.* Number 698. London: House of Commons Library.
11. NHS Digital. (2018). Mental health services monthly statistics. NHS Digital. www.digital.nhs.uk/data-and-information/publications/statistical/mental-health-services-monthly-statistics (accessed May 2021).
12. Royal College of Psychiatrists. (2013). *Whole-person Care: From Rhetoric to Reality – Achieving Parity between Mental and Physical Health.* London: Royal College of Psychiatrists.
13. Department of Health. (2016). Physical healthcare for people with mental health problems – GOV.UK. www.gov.uk/government/publications/physical-healthcare-for-people-with-mental-health-problems (accessed March 2021).
14. HM Government. Severe mental illness [SMI] and physical health inequalities: briefing – GOV.UK. www.gov.uk/government/publications/severe-mental-illness-smi-physical-health-inequalities/severe-mental-illness-and-physical-health-inequalities-briefing (accessed 5 January 2021).
15. ReThink Mental Illness. (2012). *20 years too soon: physical health – the experiences of people affected by mental illness.* London: ReThink Mental Illness.
16. Department of Health Midwifery and Allied Health Professions Policy Unit. (2016). *Improving the physical health of people with mental health problems: actions for mental health nurses.* London: HM Government.
17. Brown, S., Kim, M., Mitchell, C., and Inskip, H. (2010). Twenty-five year mortality of a community cohort with schizophrenia. *The British Journal of Psychiatry* 196 (2): 116–121. (accessed 23 March 2021).
18. National Institute for Health Research [NIHR] (2018). *Forward thinking: NIHR research on support for people with severe mental illness, a themed review of recent research.* London: National Institute for Health Research.
19. Wilson, R., Hepgul, N., Higginson, I.J., and Gao, W. (2020). End-of-life care and place of death in adults with serious mental illness: a systematic review and narrative synthesis. *Palliative Medicine* 34 (1): 49–68. (accessed 20 March 2021).
20. Noblett, J.E., Lawrence, R., and Smith, J.G. (2015). The attitudes of general hospital doctors toward patients with co-morbid mental illness. *The International Journal of Psychiatry in Medicine* 50 (4): 370–382. (accessed 23 March 2021).
21. Mental Health Taskforce. (2016). *The Five Year Forward View for Mental Health.* London: NHS England.

22. Arboleda-Flórez, J. (2003). Considerations on the stigma of mental illness. *The Canadian Journal of Psychiatry* 48 (10): 645–650. (accessed 23 March 2021).

23. Overton, S.L. and Medina, S.L. (2008). The stigma of mental illness. *Journal of Counselling & Development* 86 (2): 143–151.

24. Rössler, W. (2016). The stigma of mental disorders. *EMBO Reports* 17 (9): 1250–1253. (accessed 23 March 2021).

25. Stuart, H. and Arboleda-Flórez, J. (2001). Community attitudes toward people with schizophrenia. *The Canadian Journal of Psychiatry* 46 (3): 245–252. (accessed 23 March 2021).

26. Bates, L. and Stickley, T. (2013). Confronting Goffman: how can mental health nurses effectively challenge stigma? A critical review of the literature. *Journal of Psychiatric and Mental Health Nursing* 20 (7): 569–575. (accessed 28 July 2021).

27. Corrigan, P.W. and Rao, D. (2012). On the self-stigma of mental illness: stages, disclosure, and strategies for change. *The Canadian Journal of Psychiatry* 57(8):464–469. (accessed 2 August 2020).

28. Knaak, S., Mantler, E., and Szeto, A. (2017). Mental illness-related stigma in healthcare: barriers to access and care and evidence-based solutions. *Healthcare Management Forum* 30 (2): 111–116. (accessed 2 October 2021).

29. Conway, P. (2000). The unpopular patient revisited: characteristics or traits of patients which may result in their being considered as "difficult" by nurses. In: *Qualitative Evidence-based Practice Conference* (ed. P. Conway). Sheffield, United Kingdom: Education-line.

30. Feely, M.A., Havyer, R.D.A., Lapid, M.I., and Swetz, K.M. (2013). Management of end-of-life care and of difficult behaviours associated with borderline personality disorder. *Journal of Pain and Symptom Management* 45 (5): 934. (accessed 2 May 2021).

31. Ross, C.A. and Goldner, E.M. (2009). Stigma, negative attitudes and discrimination towards mental illness within the nursing profession: a review of the literature. *Journal of Psychiatric and Mental Health Nursing* 16 (6): 558–567. doi: 10.1111/j.1365-2850.2009.01399.x (accessed 2 April 2021).

32. Department of Health. (2007). *Mental Health Act*. London: HM Government.

33. Foti, M.E., Bartels, S.J., Van Citters, A.D., Merriman, M.P., and Fletcher, K.E. (2005). End-of-life treatment preferences of persons with serious mental illness. *Psychiatric Services* 56 (5): 585–591. doi: 10.1176/appi.ps.56.5.585 (accessed 2 February 2021).

34. Geppert, C.M.A., Rabjohn, P., and Vlaskovits, J. (2011). To treat or not to treat: psychosis, palliative care, and ethics at the end-of-life: a case analysis. *Psychosomatics* 52 (2): 178–184. doi: 10.1016/j.psym.2010.12.003 (accessed 2 June 2021).

35. Hill, R. (2005). End-of-life care for the patient with borderline personality disorder. *Journal of Hospice & Palliative Nursing* 7 (3): 150–161. (accessed 2 March 2021).

36. Knippenberg, I., Zaghouli, N., Engels, Y., Vissers, K.C.P., and Groot, M.M. (2020). Severe mental illness and palliative care: patient semi-structured interviews. *BMJ Supportive and Palliative Care* 1–7. (accessed 8 October 2021) doi: 10.1136/bmjspcare-2019-002122.

37. Haines, I.E. (2011). Managing patients with advanced cancer: the benefits of early referral for palliative care. *Medical Journal of Australia* 194 (3): 107–108. (accessed 8 October 2020).

38. World Health Organization. (2021). *Definition: intellectual disability*. New York: WHO.

39. MENCAP. How common is learning disability in the UK? How many people have a learning disability? | Mencap. https://www.mencap.org.uk/learning-disability-explained/research-and-statistics/how-common-learning-disability (accessed 17 June 2021).

40. Emerson, E., Baines, S., Allerton, L., and Welch, V. (2012). *Health Inequalities & People with Learning Disabilities in the UK: 2012 Health Inequalities & People with Learning Disabilities in the UK: 2012*. London: Department of Health.

41. MENCAP. (2007). *Death by Indifference*. London: MENCAP.

42. Heslop, P., Blair, P., Fleming, P., Hoghton, M., Marriott, A., and Russ, L. (2013). Confidential inquiry into premature deaths of people with learning disabilities [CIPOLD] final report. London (accessed 28 November 2021).

43. Care Quality Commission. (2016). *A Different Ending: Addressing Inequalities in End of Life Care*. London: Care Quality Commission.

44. University of Bristol. (2018). *Learning Disabilities Mortality Review [Leder] Programme Annual Report*. Bristol: University of Bristol.

45. University of Bristol. (2019). *Learning Disabilities Mortality Review [Leder] Programme Annual Report*. Bristol: University of Bristol.

46. HM Government. (2010). *Equality Act 2010*. London: HMSO.

47. www.booksbeyondwords.co.uk. Beyond words. https://booksbeyondwords.co.uk (accessed 17 November 2021).

48. PCPLD Network. (2017). *Delivering high quality end of life care for people who have a learning disability how to use this guide*. London: PCPLD.

49. Jarrett, S. (2020). *Those They Called Idiots*, 1e London: Reaktion.

50. Allen, G. No barriers here – ehospice. https://ehospice.com/uk_posts/no-barriers-here (accessed 17 November 2021).

51. Jerwood, J., Ward, G., Phimister, D., Holliday, N., and Coad, J. (2021). Lean in, don't step back: the views and experiences of patients and carers with severe mental illness and incurable physical conditions on palliative and end of life care. *Progress in Palliative Care* 29 (5): 255–263. (accessed 2 November 2021).

20 Care in the Last Days of Life and after Death

Nikhil Sanyal and Alistair Duncan

Special thanks to Jenny Booth RGN, Severn Hospice Shrewsbury for her support with pressure ulcer management.

Good quality end-of-life care is of the utmost importance and, if delivered well, is rewarding. There is no unified definition of palliative care however the tenets of what constitutes this area of practice are focused on the provision of holistic care for an individual, and those close to them, from diagnosis and especially during the last twelve months of life [1, 2].

The principles underlying the delivery of care in the last days of life remain constant despite an ever-changing clinical landscape that includes complicated treatments and an expanding understanding of diseases and their processes. Without the appropriate knowledge, approach and skills navigating end-of-life care can feel overwhelming to the professionals involved. However, failing to acknowledge deterioration in a person's condition and addressing the dying process does not prevent it from happening.

Palliative care as a specialty can be considered, at times, more of an art form than a science and you may find yourself adapting the advice within this chapter for the context in which you practice. If patients know that professionals are comfortable engaging in discussions on the topic of death, dying, and the end-of-life then they will be empowered to take an active role in planning and voicing their preferences. Achieving this will transform the patient's experience and hugely influence what those left behind recall of their loved one's last days.

Individualising end-of-life care was identified as a primary ambition by the National Palliative and End-of-Life Care Partnership in their national framework [3]. National guidance on the care in the last days of life have regularly been issued and reviewed over the last ten years. These have included a move away from the Liverpool Care Pathway which was abolished in 2014 following an independent review by Baroness Neuberger, and more

towards an individualised patient care plan. Individualised patient care plans for the last days of life are best exemplified by the One Chance to Get it Right report and Nice Guidance (NG31) [4, 5]. Services should strive to achieve equitable access to care for all, the maximisation of comfort and well-being, the improvement of community support and the delivery of coordinated care from a caring and competent workforce [3]. Furthermore, better recognition of palliative care outside of hospital has been estimated to improve care and reduce hospital costs by £180 million per year [6]. Therefore, not only does improving care of the dying patient improve outcomes for the individual involved and their family but financial savings can be passed on to others. NHS England's End-of-Life Care Programme aims to increase the percentage of people recognised as dying so that their needs can be individualised and care can be provided, where possible, in their preferred setting. The Gold Standards Framework system goes some way to helping professionals recognise those approaching the end-of-life and has also been shown to improve outcomes [7].

The topics covered within this chapter will include:
- how to recognise dying
- assessing the dying person
- supporting the dying person including symptom control measures at the end-of-life
- common concerns
- consideration of specific end-of-life scenarios
- care after death and bereavement support.

Many may feel that end-of-life care, once started, has an inevitability to it that renders our efforts futile however there is always something that can be done. The therapeutic power of listening – of sharing the heavy burden that comes with supporting someone to die peacefully – should never be underestimated.

Handbook of Palliative Care, Fourth Edition. Edited by Richard Kitchen, Christina Faull, Sarah Russell and Jo Wilson.
© 2024 John Wiley & Sons Ltd. Published 2024 by John Wiley & Sons Ltd.

Recognising Dying

Perhaps the most important step in providing good end-of-life care to patients and their families is the initial one – that of recognising that a dying process is imminent or is actually taking place [8]. Acknowledging and taking that first step is what allows all the other elements to unfold and follow on.

The recognition of dying allows healthcare professionals to tailor treatment plans to the patient's situation. Needless investigations and interventions can be avoided, and treatment can be honed. If patients, and those close to the patient in instances where the patient lacks capacity, are open to discussing preferences and priorities at the end-of-life then this can facilitate a personalised approach to advance care planning to prioritise what is important to the individual [9].

Identifying the dying process is fraught with difficulty and uncertainty [8, 10, 11]. Trying to distinguish between reversible deterioration and inevitable decline at the end-of-life is a skill which improves with experience and collaborative working with the wider multi-disciplinary team (MDT). To be certain about whether a patient is entering the dying phase of their illness or not is sometimes an impossibility and can pose one of the most significant barriers to recognising dying [12].

Barriers exist for patients and families as well as professionals. Some patients may simply not want to acknowledge their deteriorating health or their limited life expectancy. In extreme cases this denial may prevent engagement with professionals attempting discussions relating to any aspect of end-of-life care or future planning. Rarely is this impassable and facilitating the patient to speak with a trusted professional can often allow the initial steps to be taken.

Having an understanding of the traditional patterns of disease trajectory can sometimes help to shed some light on the matter although it is important to be mindful of the limitations to these models (see Figure 1) [13].

It is worth noting that these proposed trajectories do not take account of those patients who have more than one pathology or who may experience an acute event for example a severe infection or a stroke. Similarly, due to the less predictable nature of organ failure – such as heart failure or pulmonary fibrosis – opportunities to have advance care planning conversations are often missed, even when these diagnoses are understood to be life-limiting

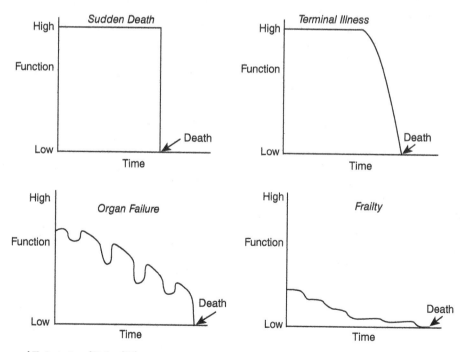

Proposed Trajectories of Dying

Figure 1 Proposed Trajectories of Dying [13].

and have limited treatment options. The dying process for these individuals often manifests as numerous clustered hospital admissions and many of these patients die in hospital, possibly because professionals have not recognised that repeat admissions and a decline despite our best treatment can be an indication of dying.

A number of tools exist to try and aid in the identification of people who are at risk of dying. Every tool is fallible, but most contain helpful information that can be taken into account when making a clinical judgement about prognosis and proximity to death [14]. Some examples of these tools include:

- GSF [7]
- SPICT [15]
- Karnofsky [16]
- AMBER care bundle [17]

No one tool can replace the value of assessing a patient and aligning the facts with the feeling. The tools are best used as prompts to begin conversations with patients and/or other professionals and are at their most effective if used over a number of sessions with a patient to chart a trajectory.

What Does Dying Look Like?

If we are to recognise dying when we see it then it is important to know what this process looks like [18]. Table 1 outlines some of the common features of the dying process and may, like the prognostication tools above, serve as a prompt to review the patient, their needs, and their current clinical plan.

Palliative care teams hold the recognition of dying in mind and often internally prognosticate (and validate with the MDT) in order to weigh up the active and palliative interventions that will promote that person's comfort – which is a term defined by the individual themselves – and stop any intervention that no longer contributes towards a patient's goals or comfort.

Previously, medical, nursing, and therapy undergraduate training in palliative care has historically been inadequate [19]. Other areas of education have often been prioritised despite death being a possible outcome in all avenues of medicine and healthcare. This approach is changing and education focussing on palliative care has increased. There is also a view that palliative care is focused on cancer and this is patently untrue. Patients who have treatment withdrawn, are too unwell for life-saving operations or who have progressive, degenerative pathology all deserve to receive high-quality palliative care. Thus,

Table 1 Common signs and symptoms of the dying phase.

Symptom/Sign	How This May Manifest
Increasing tiredness and fatigue	May spend increasing amounts of time sleeping/in bed
	Less interest in what is happening around them
	Less able to hold a conversation
Physically less able to do things	Deterioration in mobility and/or ability to transfer
	Spending increasing amounts of time in chair/bed
	More dependent on others for care needs
Changes in breathing	Breathing can become irregular and/or shallow
	Breathing can become noisy
Eating and drinking less	Reducing appetite/interest in food and/or drink
	Swallowing can become more difficult
	Likely to struggle with oral medications
Changes in appearance	Can look tired, pale, grey in colour
	Can appear increasingly cachectic
	Occasionally peripheries can take on a mottled appearance

healthcare professionals in all areas of practice should be equipped with the right skills and language to provide this.

The Government focus on avoidable deaths, while helpful, also instils a fear that death is avoidable, which is unhelpful when most deaths occur despite the best possible treatment [20]. Of course, we need to learn from our patients who die. However, by open conversation with patients and their families about dying we can start identifying important goals for that individual and ensure the death is an expected death rather than being seen as an avoidable death [21].

Assessing the Dying Person

Once dying is recognised the next steps involve assessing that individual and considering the needs that are unique to them. The dying process may have similarities from one individual to another but there will be important nuances to this that mark it out as particular to that person. The basics of palliative care help to address the processes common to all patients, but hopefully this section will also

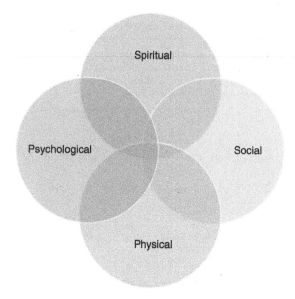

Figure 2 Components of a holistic assessment.

serve to help form a comprehensive assessment that leads to individualised and holistic care.

Holistic care can be broadly defined as care that incorporates the patient's physical, psychological, spiritual, and social care needs as seen in Figure 2 [22]. By taking into consideration all aspects of a person, allowing them to identify their own priorities and highlight the aspects of their experience that require attention from professionals is what allows us to call this process individualised [23]. This can be transformative for the patient and the people important to them.

There will be times where getting a sense of the individual is harder due to time pressures or emergencies but in the main there is often time to achieve this over many interactions rather than in one consultation. In addition to this, it is important to bear in mind that a person's priorities change over time. The needs identified during an initial assessment shortly after a palliative diagnosis has been made compared to the needs of the same person as they approach the end of their life could be very different emphasising the need for ongoing assessment. The assessment is best undertaken over a number of interactions using a multidisciplinary approach with a view to drawing on the expertise of different disciplines.

Most of us in healthcare have been trained to review individuals in a systematic way. As such this section aims to propose a possible approach to assessment (Table 2) but does not mean to imply there is only one way to do this. Similarly, as with all structured approaches, through

repeatedly trying new ways and adapting old ways of doing something you will formulate your own style of assessment of palliative patients that feels comfortable to you.

Building up a rapport where possible often encourages the patient to open up about certain things that they might otherwise have glossed over. As a "keeper of patient's secrets" we become privy to intimate knowledge of strangers in a very short space of time. This is a privilege but one that cannot be taken for granted.

Assessment of the dying person relies upon taking time to consider the individual, what is important to them and ensuring they have had the opportunity for all aspects of care to be discussed. As suggested by Figure 2, all of these different domains overlap and affect one another and assessing them allows us to provide individual, holistic, high-quality end-of-life care.

Finally, it is important to consider the needs of those close to the patient; for many this may be trusted people providing care, partners, friends, and/or family members. This may involve focusing on their psychological, emotional, and spiritual needs more so than physical needs however caring for someone at the end of their life is physically demanding. It may be that frailer patients have frail carers and it is important to be mindful of the pressure placed on them. Often, although not universally, those close to the patient may wish to take care of them and will attempt to do so unaided and ill equipped through lack of knowing what support is available. This is a big task which can be difficult for teams of professionals in specialist inpatient units, to undertake this as a small group of people caring for a loved one is no mean feat and can be overwhelming. With this in mind sometimes the assessments of the patient and their carer involve consideration as to how feasible continuing to care for them in their current residence is. This can be a hard discussion as many feel that moving from home to a hospice, for example, is a sign they have failed but the reality is that sometimes the needs of someone at the end of their life can become complex and challenging to manage at home even with maximal support.

Key summary points:
• Using a structured approach can help with holistic assessments while building experience/confidence
• Consider physical, psychological, and spiritual/religious needs
• Remember to focus on the person not the pathology
• Consider the needs of the patient but also their carers/families
• The holistic assessment also considers how feasible it is to continue caring for someone in their current locality as their needs change

Table 2 An example of an approach to holistic assessment.

Holistic Component	Points to Consider Covering
Physical issues Patients approaching the end-of-life often experience physical symptoms – trying to improve and/or control these where possible has the potential to enhance the quality of the time they have left to live.	• Symptoms – pain, nausea, vomiting, anxiety, breathlessness etc. • Mobility • Sleep disturbance • Appetite, nutrition & hydration • Excretion • Wounds and skin breakdown
Cultural, spiritual, and religious issues These can be distinct aspects of care or, for some individuals, exhibit a degree of overlap. Addressing this area of care helps to acknowledge the personhood of the individual, uncover additional support networks and can make all the difference in managing someone's pain, distress, or sense of isolation.	• Not being able to physically pray • Not being able to get to place of worship • Specific religious practices/customs that need to occur • Perhaps feeling disconnected from God/questioning faith • Sometimes strong religious beliefs can appear as barriers to treatments starting or stopping • Struggle to find a sense of meaning in life • Difficulty in achieving inner peace
Psychological issues Illness impacts upon how other people might perceive and relate to an individual and how the unwell individual perceives themselves. The implications are wide reaching and impact upon all domains of a person's life.	• Mood disturbance and emotional state • Existential distress • Fear of what is coming • Fear of what is being lost • Bereavement of the self – mourning the loss of who you feel you were • Sense of feeling like a burden
Social issues Social issues are varied and can include anything from family support to financial advice to discussions around how to meet a person's care needs.	• Relationships and the impact illness can have on this, including intimacy/sex • Concern for impact on family/children • Impact of ill-health on ability to provide and impact on finances • Provision of care • Place of care and place of death

Supporting the Dying Person

Having recognised the dying process and assessed the situation the focus moves onto how to support the dying person in their last days of life. By paying particular attention to physical needs (e.g. symptom control, reviewing medication and skin care), psychological needs (e.g. developing conversations around death/dying and advance care planning) and social needs (e.g. care packages, family support) the situation is approached in a holistic manner.

Physical

The management of physical symptoms is an important aspect of care. Many patients fear a painful or uncomfortable death making symptom control through the dying phase a shared goal between the patient and the HCPs delivering care. This concern is emphasised by studies which highlighted that over 50% of patients with a palliative diagnosis either malignant or non-malignant experienced pain [24, 25]. Physically the needs of patients will be unique to them however common themes to most patients involve us addressing current symptoms, appraising the effect of current medications and anticipating future problems.

A non-exhaustive list of symptoms commonly experienced in the last 48 hours of life, and the anticipatory medications frequently used to alleviate these symptoms, can be found in Table 3.

Given the prevalence of these symptoms in the last days of life good practice in palliative care often involves anticipatory prescribing. An example of the medicines used and

Table 3 Common symptoms at the end-of-life.

Symptom	Non-pharmacological Measures	Commonly Used Medications
Pain	Heat pads Repositioning	Non-opioids: Paracetamol (PO), NSAIDs (PO/SC) Weak Opioids: Codeine (PO), Dihydrocodeine (PO), Tramadol (PO) Strong Opioids: Morphine (PO/SC), Oxycodone (PO/SC), Diamorphine (SC)
Agitation/Anxiety	Open discussions regarding thoughts and fears (if well enough) Reassurance Ensure no reversible causes/contributors (e.g. urinary retention, hypoxia)	Midazolam (SC), Lorazepam (PO/SL) Levomepromazine (SC) Haloperidol (PO/SC)
Breathlessness	Oxygen if hypoxic Fan therapy (where appropriate) Cool cloth on face Breathing techniques (if well enough)	Strong Opioids: Morphine (PO/SC), Oxycodone (PO/SC), Diamorphine (SC)
Nausea/vomiting	Avoidance of triggers	Often a useful approach to tailor the antiemetic to the underlying cause however in the last days of life a broad spectrum agent e.g. Levomepromazine (PO/SC) is often best
Troublesome respiratory secretions	Repositioning Suction (if unconscious) Reassurance for people sitting alongside the patient	Hyoscine Butylbromide (SC) Glycopyrronium (SC) Hyoscine Hydrobromide (SC)

their appropriate initial doses can be seen in Table 4 (also note local guidelines in your area of practice).

Alongside these symptoms bowel management and urination may also require careful consideration during the dying process and if overlooked can become a source of anxiety and agitation. Constipation which was previously well controlled using oral laxatives may now need to be managed with suppositories if the person is unable to swallow oral medications. If the sensation to defecate is a source of anxiety or agitation for the individual then addressing this may bring considerable comfort.

Urinary retention can be another challenge for some individuals and can necessitate the use of a urinary catheter. Often, in the absence of retention, a catheter can be utilised as a person becomes increasingly fatigued and less able to mobilise out of bed to pass urine.

Table 4 An example of anticipatory prescribing at the end-of-life [26].

Symptom	Drug
Pain	Morphine sulfate 2.5 mg – 5 mg SC PRN (consider reducing if frail/elderly or renal impairment)
Nausea/vomiting	Levomepromazine 2.5 mg – 5 mg SC PRN
Agitation	Midazolam 2.5 mg – 5 mg SC PRN (consider reducing if frail/elderly or renal impairment)
Troublesome respiratory secretions	Hyoscine butylbromide 20 mg SC PRN

Oral care is another symptom control measure not to be overlooked. The vast majority of patients need some form of oral care as they approach the end-of-life. This part of a person's care is often viewed as a key nursing role however for those close to the patient who wish to take an active part in their care, they can often be supported to fulfil this role. The need for oral care may be as a result of a person's underlying illness (e.g. Oral cancer), therapeutic interventions (e.g. Antisecretory medications or oxygen therapy) or simply as a result of increased time spent breathing through the mouth and drying out the oral mucosa. In most cases the application of artificial saliva may be adequate however efforts should be made to ensure oral thrush, if present, is treated [27].

Pressure sores are common in patients at the end-of-life and this is often due to a combination of factors including, but not limited to, reduced skin integrity, poor circulation, reduced nutrition, side effects of medications, for example, steroids and increased time spent in one position. There is no excuse for someone developing pressure damage due to lack of adequate assessment or the provision of necessary equipment.

Commons areas for pressure damage include:

- Ears from nasal specs
- Bridge of nose if using face-masks or NIV
- Elbows
- Sacrum
- Hips
- Heels

Pressure sores can be graded from 1–4 and their treatment as detailed in Table 5 [28].

The possible impact of skin damage on patients who are dying can be physical (pain, malodour), social (embarrassment, impact on relationships) and psychological (lower self-esteem, distress if can see the wound) [29].

Employing pressure relieving practices and preventative measures is incredibly important if we are to help our patients avoid this added complication. Regular repositioning, barrier creams and dressings where appropriate alongside the use of a pressure relieving mattress are crucial in protecting the patient's skin. A heavy emphasis is placed on avoidance because once pressure damage has been sustained it can be difficult to reverse this process where the patient's general condition is deteriorating rapidly.

Suggested management of pressure ulcers is detailed in Table 6.

In situations where pressure damage has been sustained the appropriate use of dressings, barrier creams and/or treatment of infection are crucial in trying to reverse damage. In addition to this the involvement of tissue viability specialist nurses may be helpful for advice. No one should die from pressure damage but sadly this does still happen. For management of malignant wounds see Chapter 13 (Managing Complications of Cancer).

Often the rationalising of medications is prompted by a change in the patient's physical condition. This change in condition may be a deterioration in their ability to swallow

Table 5 Grading of pressure sores.

Depth	Grade	Description
Superficial	1	**Non-blanching erythema of intact skin. In darker skin may appear blue/purple.** May feel **warm, oedematous, or indurated.**
	2	**Partial thickness skin loss involving epidermis, dermis, or both.** May present as a **clear blister** often **without bruising.** Bruising suggests deeper injury.
Deep	3	**Full thickness skin loss.** May be able to see **subcutaneous fat, BUT bone or tendon cannot be.** Note that grade 3 ulcers **may be shallow in areas that have little subcutaneous fat naturally, e.g. bridge of nose.** NOTE: **Unclassified ulcers are now considered Grade 3.** These are full thickness ulcers where depth is obscured by slough or eschar. **Dry eschar** that is **intact and without fluctuance** is acting as a **natural barrier and should not be removed.**
	4	**Full thickness tissue loss with exposed bone or tendon.** Often has **tunnelling.**

Table 6 Management of pressure ulcers [30].

Category/Grade	Description	Dressing Choice
Category/Grade 1	Non blanching erythema of intact skin: persistent redness in light pigmented skin. Warmth, oedema, induration compared to surrounding skin. May include sensation and be painful.	Films for protection and observation: Hydrocolloid – e.g. Granuflex. Can be left up to 7 days.
Category/Grade 2	Partial thickness skin loss involving epidermis, dermis or both. Presents clinically as an abrasion or clear blister. Ulcer is superficial without bruising.	Hydrocolloid – e.g. Granuflex if low exudates. Combination Hydrocolloid/foam e.g. Aquafoam.
Category/Grade 3	Full thickness skin loss. Subcutaneous fat may be visible but bone, tendon not exposed. Often presents as a crater with or without undermining of adjacent tissue. Cavity may be filled with slough.	Alginate, flat/ribbon, or rope as primary dressing. Foam/Silver/Charcoal if odorous. Combination dressing if exudate's a problem. E.g. Carboflex – 5 layer. Ensure good protection of peri wound area to prevent excoriation from exudates.
Unclassified pressure ulcer – now Grade 3	Full thickness tissue loss in which actual depth is obscured by slough/necrotic tissue. Until slough/eschar is removed true depth cannot be determined but will either be grade 3/4.	Alginate Plus dressings as primary dressing. High absorbing foam as secondary dressings.
Category/Grade 4	Full thickness tissue loss with exposed tendon/bone. Often includes undermining and tunnelling. Can extend into muscle and or supporting structures e.g., fascia, tendon or joint capsule.	Consider Sharp/Surgical Mechanical/Enzymatic debridement. High absorbing Alginates as primary dressings. High absorbing Foam dressings as secondary dressings. Consider TNP (Topical Negative Pressure) on low suction if high exudate or odorous, and for patient comfort in palliative setting.
Suspected Deep Tissue Injury, Depth Unknown	Epidermis intact but affected area purple in colour or can be blood filled blister over dark wound bed. Over time skin will degrade and develop into deeper tissue loss. Wound may further evolve and become covered by thin eschar.	Hydrocolloid for protection. Observe site. Use pressure reducing strategies: elevation/dynamic mattress.
Moisture Lesions	Redness or partial thickness skin loss involving the epidermis, dermis, or both caused by excessive moisture from urine, faeces, or sweat. Not usually associated with a bony prominence but often seen alongside pressure ulcers of any grade.	Good skin hygiene. Barrier creams – E.g. Cavilon. No sting barrier sticks – Cavilon, Proshield.

or clear signs that they are moving towards the end of their life. In either case rationalising medications and reducing the medication burden to only those medications which are directed towards achieving symptom control and/or improving comfort is advisable. Additionally, it is important to ensure that medications not reliant on the oral route are available should they be required, and dose adjustment will be required when converting from the oral to subcutaneous route. For more information on deprescribing see Chapter 21 (Medicines Management in Palliative Care Including Syringe Pumps). For information on opioid conversion ratios see Chapter 10 (Pain and Its Management).

Psychological

Addressing psychological needs involves engaging with the patient and those people that are important to them to establish what they feel are the priorities. This may involve frequent or repeated conversations about how their symptoms are changing and the impact this is having on their life, for example, change in role in the family, dwindling independence, increasing reliance on others, perception of becoming a burden or discussions around their lived experience. It is common for the impact of a palliative illness to have significant impact on those people closest to the patient as well as the patient themselves [31].

There are no easy ways to "fix" these problems and often the therapeutic power comes from taking the time to listen, acknowledging and naming the problem(s) [32]. Although it is common for patients approaching the end of their lives to be low in mood and withdrawn if this tips over from being a normal human response to illness into a pathological response then medication may be effective in lifting mood.

Conversations around death and dying can be liberating for some patients and others might find these difficult topics to discuss. Exploring this at a pace the individual feels comfortable with, and potentially over multiple consultations may make this more accessible and hopefully result in a clearer idea around some of the things that might be important to that person in the future. This forms the basis of advance care planning (ACP). However, much like a birth plan sometimes the situation can change and dictate a different course of action.

As part of the ACP process ascertaining the presence of any prior decisions of the patient to appoint a power of attorney for finance or health is important as well as whether the patient has an advanced directive to refuse treatment (ADRT) and, if so, ensuring this is clearly communicated to all professionals involved.

Advance care planning should also include time spent discussing the escalation of care in the event of deterioration. It is key that patients and families are involved in these discussions and short of an emergency there is unlikely to be a valid reason not to do this. Discussing cardio-pulmonary resuscitation (CPR) is not always easy and may not be welcomed by all patients however offering them a discussion around this should not be shied away from simply because it can be hard. The way in which CPR is discussed will play a key role in how the patient understands the decision being made [33].

Reluctance to address advance care planning runs the risk of the patient losing capacity prior to the discussion taking place or trying to hold the conversation when the patient is almost too unwell to do so. This sometimes cannot be helped but sometimes prior opportunities have been missed or avoided. This can be due to many factors though there may be an assumption that it is "someone else's job." It is every clinician's responsibility. Failure to have these conversations can lead to unnecessary interventions, use of limited resources and worse outcomes for individual [34].

Preferences for who the patient would like with them around the time of death might be helpful to explore in advance (this is not always who we expect) as well as their after death preferences. This may delve deeper into thoughts/wishes on donating their body to science or tissue donation.

Social

When providing care at the end-of-life it is important to try and establish the patient's preferred place of care and death [35]. These two questions are different and may well provoke different answers. There are a multitude of factors which feed into the decision making process and where this can be identified ahead of time, laid out as part of an advance care plan, these wishes are far more likely to be honoured [36–38].

Important factors to consider when discussing this include not only the person's preference but the social support available in the community setting – this may take the form of lay carers and/or people close to the dying person, a formal funded package of care as well as essential services the patient is likely to need support from, for example, district nursing teams, GP services and community palliative care teams. Over time, as the patient deteriorates, they may need increased care to manage their continence, support with eating and drinking, and oral hygiene. At the very end-of-life, mouth care, eye care, and continence may require support from a team of trained professionals in order to maintain comfort and dignity. There may be situations where admission to an inpatient setting (e.g. Hospice) helps to meet a person's care needs or allows more timely symptom control and this will be different from one patient to the next.

For some patients who have a condition which has resulted in frequent hospital admissions (e.g. COPD, heart failure or cystic fibrosis) allowing them to get to know their hospital based medical and nursing teams well, the thought of admission to hospital may be one shrouded in safety and familiarity and an environment which has previously represented recovery. For these reasons, identifying a hospital setting as a preferred place of care, and perhaps even death, may be entirely logical, particularly if contact with other services and environments has been limited. However, no assumptions should be made [39].

Sensitive exploration of these issues ahead of time can be invaluable in trying to deliver patient centred end-of-life care, particularly if the patient is likely to lose capacity in the future. It is also key to review the social needs of those close to the patient if these have not already been addressed.

At any stage if you feel you have addressed, appraised, and anticipated what you can and things still feel uncontrolled then talk to colleagues and reach out for support from local services. This may be district nurses, occupational therapists, social workers, GP colleagues, hospice staff, and community palliative care teams. Supporting someone and their family/friends through the dying process is hard but you are not alone doing it.

Common Concerns

Providing excellent palliative care is no easy task. It requires being able to sit comfortably with uncertainty which may feel easier for some than others. This uncertainty resides in the fact that although there are commonalities between the dying process of individuals, everyone's experience of the dying process is unique. Therefore, even when comparing patients with the same condition the presentation and the management can vary greatly.

All of us recall looking after "Mrs. Smith." Mrs. Smith was the retired postmistress that was admitted with an aspiration pneumonia and a significant past medical history. Her family was concerned about her and you shared this with them and explained that antibiotics had been started but it seemed unlikely that she would recover from this, particularly in view of her frailty and co-morbidities. The expectation was that these antibiotics and her other treatments would be stopped within the next 24 hours, assuming no improvement was made, and that she would be "kept comfortable." The following day Mrs. Smith is sitting up in bed eating some porridge and speaking with the nurse, she smiles as you walk in and introduce yourself.

Sometimes the patients we think will die recover and the patients we think will recover die. We all get it wrong now and again and often these experiences, understandably, make us more wary about making predictions in the future [40]. Although prognostication is challenging what we can say with absolute certainty is that in these situations there is always a degree of uncertainty and we must coexist with this alongside our patients and those close to them.

Questions about prognosis are commonplace and rightly so. Any of us faced with the possibility of our own mortality might well want to know how long we have left. Whether explained as a time frame or measured by significant life events the question is the same and it is key not to miss this cue from patients or their loved ones.

One approach to answering this question is to:

- Find out **what the person already knows.**
- Ask if they **have asked this question to someone else** – if so, what did that person say? People often test healthcare professional's responses to see if what they have been told is accurate.
- Admit that prognostication is about providing your **"best guess."**
- **Avoid being too specific** – if told someone has four weeks then at that end of that time they may either live in fear that any day they may die or they may feel every day is a blessing.
- Explain that our best way of predicting this is based on **clinical condition** – that is, are they displaying any of the indicators of dying mentioned earlier? This also helps to broach the idea that *more tests* may not be appropriate.
- Explain that if we/they are **noticing changes in clinical condition week by week** then it is important we/they are **prepared to see changes on a weekly basis**. Likewise if there is change day by day then prognosis may be days.

Do not shy away from prognosis conversations as they may provide the opportunity to address not only important concerns for the patient and their loved ones but also key clinical decisions. These may include:

- Appropriateness of any ongoing treatments – e.g. IV fluids.
- The appropriate degree of escalation if this has not already been discussed that is, preferred place of care/death and resuscitation.
- Explaining that the normal dying process involves people eating and drinking less as the natural requirements of

the body change. This is an emotive topic, understandably, but often, if explained clearly and sensitively, relatives understand.

- It is appropriate to be observant for signs of dehydration but not interpreting this from a dry mouth, which is very common at the end-of-life.
- Be aware that supplemental fluids or feeding can actually contribute to symptoms during the dying phase such as chest secretions, nausea, vomiting or breathlessness.

Fluids and Feeding – an emotive topic often raised by relatives or people close to the patient rather than the patient themselves. Eating and drinking less is a natural part of the dying process and sometimes, for those that are aware the patient is dying, simply explaining this can be reassuring in itself [41]. However, looking only at this simple fact might fail to encompass the wider connotations that lots of us associate with food and drink. In many cultures, within families, in groups of friends, cooking for one another can be more than the simple provision of food. It is an act that shows caring, that demonstrates concern for another person's well-being and can be an expression of love for some. Finding yourself in a situation where you can no longer effectively express this can be an added blow to the realisation that the person you care about is dying. Practical conversations around how to modify meals can be helpful for both the patient and those caring for them. Sometimes emphasising the importance of small portions, "little and often," and abandoning meals that the patient no longer finds appetising and trying to accommodate the food that they do find enticing may help. Listening to these concerns is important and acknowledging them can hold therapeutic value for all parties involved.

Conversations about clinically assisted fluid and nutrition can be challenging and equally as emotive as those held in relation to natural eating and drinking. Often these conversations take time and careful exploration of what people believe is being provided by clinically assisted nutrition and/or hydration is a helpful place to start. Talking through the clinical indications for commencing these treatments can sometimes help to focus the conversation. For more guidance see NICE guidance NG31 (Care of dying adults in the last days of life) [5] and GMC guidance (Treatment and care towards the end-of-life: good practice in decision making) [42].

Returning to our earlier example, Mrs. Smith was started on her IV fluids because she was septic secondary to her aspiration pneumonia. Fluid was given to increase her circulating volume to give her the best chance of recovering from this illness. Despite the administration of these fluids, and her antibiotics, she has continued to deteriorate

and is unlikely to recover. We now need to weigh up the burdens and benefits she is experiencing in relation to these treatments. Gently moving through this conversation in as sensitive a manner as possible should hopefully help establish mutual understanding and highlight the importance of prioritising the patient's comfort as they approach the end of their life.

Hope – many professionals fear that holding conversations relating to a person's uncertain recovery or the fact that a person might be approaching the end of their life they will automatically stifle their hope. Discussing significant clinical events is never an easy task and by its very nature the news we are delivering is often "bad," or undesirable at the least, but unfortunately this does not mean it is a task that can be avoided unless the patient themselves refuses to have that conversation. In sharing significant news, where we have permission to do so, this allows a person, over time, to process what is happening to them. As a natural part of this we can reframe our experiences and in doing so we can reframe what we hope for and desire. Returning to Mrs. Smith, after discussions with her about the recent deterioration in her condition and why she isn't improving her thoughts might turn from hoping for recovery to hoping for a more comfortable period of time, easier breathing or perhaps a pain free death. Trying to broach these subjects where possible help to avoid the instillation of false hope which has the potential to be damaging and to distract a person from what is truly important to them at a point in their life where time might be precious.

So, what if you recognise all of the above and discuss this with your colleagues only to find they disagree? They may even be shocked by your suggestion that you think the patient "is palliative." Do not be alarmed. Difference of opinion is common but someone thinking differently to you does not mean you are wrong. There may be many factors at play in the clinical workings of a team be they conscious or subconscious. Some of the hardest discussions we have are with our colleagues. We would suggest being open to their views but if you reach an impasse consider a second opinion or involvement of your palliative care team for guidance and support.

Specific Scenarios

This section will provide guidance around certain situations which can arise at the end-of-life and often pose concern for healthcare professionals and sometimes patients. As always, if faced with a scenario that you are unsure how to tackle then referring to your local palliative care team is likely to yield useful advice specific to the situation you and your patient are in. Furthermore, we advocate professionals only working within the scope of their own practice and competence.

Prescribing opioids in naïve patients – it is very common that someone approaches the end of their life having never had an opiate before. The opposite can also be true and for advice in managing pain it is best to refer to Chapter 10, Pain and its management.

As a person approaches the terminal stages of their life the oral route is often compromised and frequently a result of fatigue and weakness which are common symptoms. As such subcutaneous administration is often used and drug choice can therefore be limited by this. A common approach is to **start low** and **titrate to need** (Appendix A). There is a common concern that opioids may hasten death by inducing respiratory depression; this is not the case if prescribed at appropriate doses and used for appropriate indications.

Breathlessness – this is a common symptom at the end-of-life even in the absence of respiratory pathology. This may be due to acute changes such as aspiration pneumonia, chronic conditions such as COPD or the build-up of respiratory secretions as part of the natural dying process. This symptom is often under-treated. Breathlessness can be a challenging symptom and is often coupled with anxiety. Non-pharmacological measures (open windows, handheld fans, reassurance) can be considered, however, in the terminal phase of illness it is unlikely that a patient will be well enough to engage fully with these and the reliance upon pharmacological management increases. Opioids are useful in reducing the sensation of breathlessness and benzodiazepines can help to alleviate the anxiety that often accompanies this symptom (Appendix B).

Open conversations about Cheyne-Stokes respirations is also advised. Reassure the relatives that this is a reflex action, that their loved one will not be aware of this change and it is **not a sign that they are distressed**. Explain that the pauses between breaths will gradually increase in length until eventually a pause is not followed by another breath. Relatives usually find this discussion supportive, and it can help to reduce their distress and anxiety.

Troublesome Respiratory Secretions

Excess respiratory secretions are commonplace at the end-of-life. Not always, but often, by this point in a person's illness they are likely to be spending the vast majority of their time asleep or they may well be completely unconscious.

Explanation and reassurance for people sitting with the patient is often the most important measure in managing the situation. Medications, for which there is mixed/little evidence can be used (Appendix C). Hyoscine butylbromide and glycopyrronium bromide, are anti-muscarinic drugs that help reduce the production of secretions but have limited impact on what is already there. Sometimes gentle repositioning helps move the fluid and alleviate any noise.

Nausea and Vomiting

This is a common symptom among palliative patients. It is always important to consider what the triggers and causes are as medical management can then be targeted to likely receptors. Appendix D outlines a protocol of managing nausea and vomiting in someone who is in the last days of life.

Terminal Agitation

In assessing any patient experiencing agitation as part of the dying process it is important to consider reversible or contributory causes for this symptom, for example, urinary retention, hypoxia, pain. In some situations no modifiable factors will be found and agitation may be as a result of the person's deterioration. Alleviating this with the appropriate medications is important (Appendix E).

Bleeding – This is a relatively rare event even in patients with an identified risk factor. These may include:
- Fungating wounds – particularly head and neck, axillary, and groin tumours
- Use of anticoagulation
- Liver failure – causing deranged clotting factors
- Presence of varices

Where this situation can be anticipated often measures can be put in place ahead of time and consideration can be given to preventative treatments where appropriate as well as a treatment escalation plan. Common points to consider include:
- Preventative treatments can be considered where appropriate, for example, Radiotherapy.
- Anticoagulation/antiplatelet treatment should be reviewed with particular attention paid to benefits versus risks.
- Treatment escalation plan including preferences around place of care/death and resuscitation status.
- Ensuring appropriate medications and dark towels are available in current place of care.

Appendix F shows management of bleeds in palliative patients and applies to community and hospital settings.

Seizures

Seizures can be a concern, perhaps owing to a previous diagnosis of epilepsy, or, as a result of the disease process the person is dying from, for example, a metastatic cancer which has spread to the brain. In the terminal stages of life this symptom is often managed using benzodiazepines. In the dying phase of illness Midazolam is the medication of choice (Appendix G). Where a patient has been established on an antiepileptic regime which has controlled their symptoms well it may be possible to continue this medication but for some this may not be possible and an alternative option may need to be considered.

Managing pain at end-of-life in those already on analgesic patches – In patients who have had stable pain controlled with buprenorphine or fentanyl patches it is good practice to continue with these. If the patient then develops breakthrough pain then a syringe driver may be warranted as opposed to increasing the strength of the patch, the titration of which needs to be undertaken slowly making them unsuitable for unstable pain at the end-of-life. **NB:** if using a syringe driver with a patch, ensure the PRN dose remains a **1/6th of the total daily dose of opioid (this would include the patch and the syringe driver)**. For more information on analgesic patches see Chapter 10 (Pain and Its Management).

Diabetes at the end-of-life – there is very clear guidance from diabetes.org.uk [43] on how to manage diabetes at the end-of-life. This includes guidance on what to do if someone is type 1 or type 2 diabetic. Uncontrolled blood sugars can add to patient's symptom burden and should be managed. The management plan may be influenced by the location of the patient, for example, community or inpatient.

Care after Death

The next steps for someone after they have died are likely to vary depending on the place of death and local protocols, however, national guidance helps to standardise this [44]. It is good practice to familiarise yourself with local processes as this will enable you to provide clear information for the recently bereaved at a time when they may be emotional and struggle to take on information.

Confirming Death

When a person has died their death must be verified by listening for breath sounds, heart sounds, checking for a central pulse, examining their pupils and checking there is no response to pain. This process can be completed by anybody who has been trained to do so and is underpinned by guidance for healthcare professionals [45, 46]. Following this a death certificate can subsequently be completed along with any other paperwork required to facilitate funeral plans unless there is reason to discuss the person's death with a coroner or procurator fiscal.

Personal Care after Death and Next Steps

Care after death will vary from one individual to the next and is likely to be influenced by cultural and religious practices that the person and/or the people close to them may wish to observe. Where possible try to establish ahead of time what the person's preferences might be. Be mindful that in certain religions, such as Islam, it is important to observe funeral rites within 24 hours after death. If this is likely to be relevant to your patient it is important to consider how this can be supported over a weekend or bank holiday, especially the writing of the Medical Certificate of the Cause of Death (MCCD).

After death many individuals value spending some time with the deceased person. This may simply be time spent sitting with the person or it may be important for them to be involved in the process of "laying out" the body, washing the person and completing last offices. A useful online resource is "Opening the Spiritual Gate" which outlines common religious practices and requirements around death and dying [47].

If someone dies at home then the family should have been made aware prior to this of who to call. This may be the district nursing team who will come and provide personal care after death as well as remove any medical devices present, that is, syringe drivers or catheters. They will also support those present through the next steps.

Care after death will be determined in part by the setting in which a person dies alongside their personal wishes and religious beliefs. Certain aspects of this care may need to be arranged swiftly but it is also acceptable if those close to the patient wish to wait for other people to arrive and pay their respects. Once they feel ready the person's loved ones can contact a funeral home of their choosing to notify them of the death. Individual funeral homes will have their own ways of working and this may impact on the option of viewing the body in the funeral home.

It is often clear prior to a patient's death if their case is going to require a discussion with the coroner or a formal referral before a death certificate is issued. It is important that loved ones are made aware of this and the rationale for the referral. Otherwise, upon receipt of the MCCD from the doctor involved there is a requirement for the death to be formally registered with a registrar within the appropriate number of days (5 days for a death within the UK, excluding Scotland where the death is registered within 8 days). Anyone can register a person's death and this may be a health professional if an individual has no next of kin.

See Chapter 8 (Integrating new perspectives: Working with loss and grief in palliative care) for information on bereavement.

Conclusion

Providing end-of-life care is everybody's responsibility. There is almost no area of healthcare which does not meet people nearing the end of their lives. This makes it imperative that all of us have a basic understanding of how to approach care in the last days of life.

Being able to have a conversation with a patient and those important to them about "what matters to them" and about approaching the topic of death with kindness and honesty means that patients can have conversations, and as a professional you can role model this for colleagues.

In reading this chapter it is possible you might be a person with a natural interest in this area of healthcare and hopefully you will feel able to not only provide good quality palliative and end-of-life care but also help educate those around you and challenge poor practice when/ if you see it.

References

1. NHS. (2018). *What end of life care involves*. Available from: https://www.nhs.uk/conditions/end-of-life-care/what-it-involves-and-when-it-starts (4 April 2021).

2. Marie Curie (2018). *What are palliative and end of life care?* Available from: https://www.mariecurie.org.uk/help/support/diagnosed/recent-diagnosis/palliative-care-end-of-life-care (4 April 2021).

3. National Palliative and End of Life Care Partnership. (2015). *Ambitions for palliative and end of life care: A national framework for local action 2015-2020*. Available from: https://endoflifecareambitions.org.uk/wp-content/uploads/2015/09/Ambitions-for-Palliative-and-End-of-Life-Care.pdf (4 April 2021).

4. Leadership Alliance for the Care of Dying People. (2014). *One chance to get it right: Improving people's experience of care in the last few days and hours of life*. Available from http://www.professionalpalliativehub.com/resource-centre/one-chance-get-it-right (11 November 2021).

5. National institute for clinical excellence. (16 December 2015). *Care of Dying adults in the last days of life* (NICE guideline NG31). NICE. Available from: https://www.nice.org.uk/guidance/ng31/resources/care-of-dying-adults-in-the-last-days-of-life-pdf-1837387324357 (11 November 2021).

6. NHSEngland. *About end of life care*. Available from: https://www.england.nhs.uk/eolc/introduction (4 April 2021).

7. Clifford, C., Thomas, K., and Armstrong-Wilson, J. (16 January 2017. Going for Gold: The Gold Standards Framework programme and accreditation in primary care. *End of Life Journal, BMJ*, 6:1–10. Available from: https://goldstandardsframework.org.uk/cd-content/uploads/files/End%20Life%20J-2016-Clifford-.pdf (21 September 2022).

8. Taylor, P., Dowding, D., and Johnson, M. (25 January 2017. Clinical decision making in the recognition of dying: A qualitative interview study. *BMC Palliative Care*. 16(11): 1–11. Available from: https://link.springer.com/content/pdf/10.1186/s12904-016-0179-3.pdf (11 November 2021).

9. Wright, A., Zang, B., Ray, A. et al. 8 October 2008. Associations between end of life discussions, patient mental health, medical care near death and caregiver bereavement adjustment. *JAMA*. 300(14): 1665–1673. Available from: https://www.ncbi.nlm.nih.gov/pmc/articles/PMC2853806 (11 November 2021).

10. Qureshi, S.P., Jones, D., Skinner, J., and Wood, M. (1 March 2008. Challenges to recognising the dying patient in acute care – perceptions of senior and newly graduated Scottish doctors. *BMJ Supportive & Palliative Care*. 8 (Supplement 1): A1–79. Available from: https://spcare.bmj.com/content/bmjspcare/8/Suppl_1/A7.3.full.pdf (11 November 2021).

11. McKinstry, Z. P104- Recognising dying in adults: Identifying patients in the last 12 months of life, *BMJ Supportive and Palliative Care*, 2017. Available from: https://spcare.bmj.com/content/7/Suppl_1/A38.3 (11 November 2021).

12. Murray, S., Boyd, K., and Sheikh, A. (17 March 2005. Palliative care in chronic illness. *BMJ*. 330: 611. Available from: https://www.bmj.com/content/330/7492/611.full (11 November 2021).

13. Lunney, J.R., Lynn, J., and Hogan, C. (2002). Profiles of Older Medicare Decedents. *Journal of the American Geriatrics Society* 50: 1108–1112. Available from: https://agsjournals.onlinelibrary.wiley.com/doi/full/10.1046/j.1532-5415.2002.50268.x?sid=nlm%3Apubmed (21 September 2022).

14. Simmons, C., McMillan, D., McWilliams, K. et al. (2017 May. Prognostic tools in patients with advanced cancer: A systematic review. *Journal of Pain and Symptom Management*, 53:5, 962–970. Available from: https://www.sciencedirect.com/science/article/pii/S0885392416312313?via%3Dihub (21 September 2022).

15. Highet, G., Crawford, D., Murray, S., and Boyd, K. (2014). Development and evaluation of the supportive and palliative care indicators tool (SPICT): A methods-study. *BMJ Supportive & Palliative Care* 4 (3): 285–290. Available from: https://pubmed.ncbi.nlm.nih.gov/24644193 (11 November 2021).

16. Yates, J., Chalmer, B., and McKegney, P. (1980). Evaluation of patients with advanced cancer using the Karnofsky performance status. *American Cancer Society* 45: 2220–2224. Available from: https://pubmed.ncbi.nlm.nih.gov/7370963 (11 November 2021).

17. Carey, I., Shouls, S., Bristowe, K. et al. (2015). Improving care for patients whose recovery is uncertain. The AMBER care bundle design and implementation. *BMJ Supportive & Palliative Care* 5: 405–411. Available from: https://spcare.bmj.com/content/5/4/405.info (11 November 2021).

18. Van Der Werff, G., Paans, W., and Nieweg, R. (2012). Hospital nurses' views of the signs and symptoms that herald the onset of the dying phase in oncology patients. *International Journal of Palliative Nursing* 18 (3): 143–149. Available from: https://www.magonlinelibrary.com/doi/full/10.12968/ijpn.2012.18.3.143?rfr_dat=cr_pub++0pubmed&url_ver=Z39.88-2003&rfr_id=ori%3Arid%3Acrossref.org (21 September 2022).

19. McMahon, D. and Wee, B. (171717 July 2019. Medical undergraduate palliative care education (UPCE). *BMJ Supportive & Palliative Care*. 0:1–3. Available from: https://ora.ox.ac.uk/objects/uuid:fbcf409b-168f-4651-83f1-4c14b31c3dba/download_file?safe_filename=bmjspcare-2019-001965.pdf&file_format=application%2Fpdf&type_of_work=Journal+article (11 November 2021).

20. National Quality Board. (2017). *National Guidance on Learning from Deaths*. Available from: https://www.england.nhs.uk/wp-content/uploads/2017/03/nqb-national-guidance-learning-from-deaths.pdf (11 November 2021).

21. Kastbom, L., Milnerg, A., and Karlsson, M. (2017). A good death from the perspective of palliative cancer patients. *Supportive Care in Cancer* 25: 933–939. Available from: https://pubmed.ncbi.nlm.nih.gov/27837324 (11 November 2021).

22. International association for hospice and palliative care. *6 Principles of palliative care [internet]*. Available from: https://hospicecare.com/what-we-do/publications/getting-started/6-principles-of-palliative-care (6 April 2021).

23. Ahmed, N., Ahmedzai, S., Collins, K., and Noble, B. (2014). Holistic assessment of supportive and palliative care needs: The evidence for routine systematic questioning. *BMJ Supportive & Palliative Care* 4: 3. Available from: https://pubmed.ncbi.nlm.nih.gov/24644199 (11 November 2021).

24. Murtagh, F., Addington-Hall, J., Edmonds, P. et al. (1 September 2010). Symptoms in the month before death for Stage 5 Chronic Kidney Disease patients managed without dialysis. *Journal of Pain and Symptom Management*. 40(3), 342–352. Available from: https://doi.org/10.1016/j.jpainsymman.2010.01.021 (11 November 2021).

25. International Association for the Study of Pain. (2008). *Global Year against Cancer Pain, Epidemiology of Cancer Pain. International Association for the Study of Pain*. Available from: Cancer Pain - International Association for the Study of Pain (IASP) (iasp-pain.org) (30 June 2021).

26. Lock, A. et al. (2019). *West Midlands Palliative Care Physicians Palliative Care Guidelines for the Use of Drugs in Symptom Control*. Birmingham: West Midlands Palliative Care Physicians Society.

27. Marie Curie. *Mouth Care*. Available from: https://www.mariecurie.org.uk/professionals/palliative-care-knowledge-zone/symptom-control/mouth-care (8 June 2021).

28. *Scottish Adaptation of the European Pressure Ulcer Advisory Panel (EPUAP) Pressure Ulcer Classification Tool*. (2020 December). Available from: https://www.healthcareimprovementscotland.org/programmes/patient_safety/tissue_viability_resources/pressure_ulcer_grading_tool.aspx (11 November 2021).

29. Gibson, S. and Green, J. (2013 May). Review of patients' experiences with fungating wounds and associated quality of life. *Journal of Wound Care* 22 (5): 265–275.

30. European Pressure Ulcer Advisory Panel. (2019). *Prevention and treatment of pressure ulcers/injuries*. Available from: https://www.epuap.org/wp-content/uploads/2016/10/quick-reference-guide-digital-npuap-epuap-pppia-jan2016.pdf (13 November 2021).

31. Ullrich, A., Ascherfeld, L., Marx, G. et al. (2017). Quality of life, psychological burden, needs and satisfaction during specialized inpatient palliative care in family caregivers of advanced cancer patients. *BMC Palliative Care* 16 (31). Available from: https://bmcpalliatcare.biomedcentral.com/articles/10.1186/s12904-017-0206-z (11 November 2021).

32. Maguire, P. (14 December 1985. 291: 1711–1713. Available from). Barriers to psychological care of the dying. *BMJ* https://www.bmj.com/content/bmj/291/6510/1711.full.pdf (11 November 2021).

33. Sterie, A.C., Jones, L., Jox, R., and Truchard, E. (2021 Available from). "It's not magic": A qualitative analysis of geriatric physicians' explanations of cardio-pulmonary resuscitation in hospital admissions. *Health Expectations*. https://pubmed.ncbi.nlm.nih.gov/33682993 (11 November 2021).

34. Redwood, S., Simmonds, B., Fox, F. et al. (2020 October). Consequences of "conversations not had": Insights into failures in communication affecting delays in hospital discharge for older people living with frailty. *Journal of Health Services Research & Policy* 25 (4): 213–219.

35. Skorstengaard, M., Neergaard, M., Andreassen, P., Brogaard, T. et al. (2017 November). Preferred place of care and death in terminally ill patients with lung and heart disease compared to cancer. *Journal of Palliative Medicine* 20: 11.

36. Bannon, F., Cairnduff, V., Fitzpatrick, D. et al. (2018). Insights into the factors associated with achieving the preference of home death in terminal cancer: A national population-based study. *Palliative & Supportive Care* 16 (6): 749–755.

37. Cohen, J., Houttekier, D., Onwuteaka-Philipsen, B. et al. (2010). Which patients with cancer die at home? A study of six European countries using death certificate data. *Journal of Clinical Oncology* 28: 2267–2273.

38. Gomes, B., Calanzani, N., Koffman, J., and Higginson, I.J. (2015). Is dying in hospital better than home in incurable cancer and what factors influence this? A population-based study. *BMC Medicine* 13 (1): 1.

39. Cross, S., Wesley, E., Kavalieratos, D., Tulsky, J., and Warraich, H. (2020 August). Place of death for individuals with chronic lung disease: Trends and associated factors from 2003–2017 in the United States. *Chest* 158 (2): 670–680.

40. Krawczyk, M. and Gallagher, R. (2016). Communicating prognostic uncertainty in potential end-of-life contexts: Experiences of family members. *BMC Palliative Care* 15 (1): 59. Available from: https://bmcpalliatcare.biomedcentral.com/articles/10.1186/s12904-016-0133-4 (11 November 2021).

41. Marcolini, E., Putnam, A., and History, A.A. (2018 June). Perspectives on Nutrition and Hydration at the end of life. *Yale Journal of Biology and Medicine* 91 (2): 173–176.

42. GMC. (2010). *Treatment and care towards the end of life: good practice in decision making*. GMC. Available from: Treatment and care towards the end of life - ethical guidance summary - GMC (gmc-uk.org) (11 November 2021).

43. Diabetes UK. (2021 Available from). *End of Life Guidance for Diabetes Care*. Diabetes UK. EoL_TREND_FINAL2_0.pdf (amazonaws.com) (25 October 2022).

44. Wilson, J., Laverty, D., Mann, T. et al. (2020 Available from). *Care after Death, Guidance for Staff Responsible for Care after Death*, 3e. Hospice UK. https://www.hospiceuk.org/what-we-offer/clinical-and-care-support/clinical-resources?utm_campaign=1544209_IPC+newsletter+-+COVID-19+update+October+2020+-+PDL-CCON-121054-1809&utm_medium=email&utm_source=dotdigital&dm_i=4JL6%2cX3IP%2c2XH24Z%2c43NKX%2c1 (11 November 2021).

45. Hospice UK and National Nurse Consultant Group (Palliative Care). (2020 Available from). *Special Edition of Care after Death: Registered Nurse Verification of Expected Adult Death (Rnvoead) Guidance*. Hospice UK. https://www.hospiceuk.org/what-we-offer/clinical-and-care-support/clinical-resources?utm_campaign=1544209_IPC+newsletter+-+COVID-19+update+October+2020+-+PDL-CCON-121054-1809&utm_medium=email&utm_source=dotdigital&dm_i=4JL6%2cX3IP%2c2XH24Z%2c43NKX%2c1 (11 November 2021).

46. Academy of Medical Royal Colleges. (2008). *A Code of Practice for the Diagnosis and Confirmation of Death*. PPG Design and Print Ltd. Available from: https://www.aomrc.org.uk/wp-content/uploads/2016/04/Code_Practice_Confirmation_Diagnosis_Death_1008-4.pdf (11 November 2021).

47. Cheshire and Merseyside Palliative Care Network. Opening the spiritual gate. Available from: www.openingthespriritualgate.net/all-faiths (28 June 2021).

48. NHS Scotland. *Scottish Palliative Care Guidelines*. Available from: https://www.palliativecareguidelines.scot.nhs.uk (22 October 2021).

Appendix A – Managing Pain in the Last Days of Life for Opioid Naïve Patients

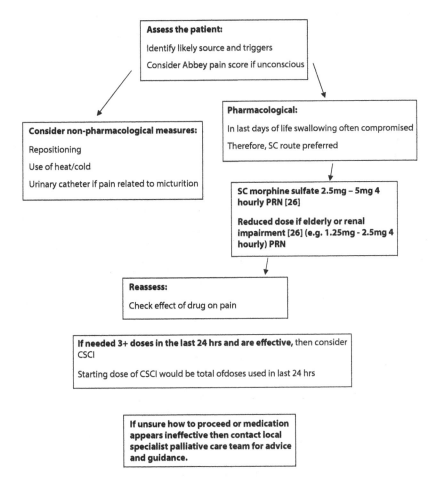

Assess the patient:

Identify likely source and triggers

Consider Abbey pain score if unconscious

Consider non-pharmacological measures:

Repositioning

Use of heat/cold

Urinary catheter if pain related to micturition

Pharmacological:

In last days of life swallowing often compromised

Therefore, SC route preferred

SC morphine sulfate 2.5mg – 5mg 4 hourly PRN [26]

Reduced dose if elderly or renal impairment [26] (e.g. 1.25mg - 2.5mg 4 hourly) PRN

Reassess:

Check effect of drug on pain

If needed 3+ doses in the last 24 hrs and are effective, then consider CSCI

Starting dose of CSCI would be total ofdoses used in last 24 hrs

If unsure how to proceed or medication appears ineffective then contact local specialist palliative care team for advice and guidance.

Handbook of Palliative Care, Fourth Edition. Edited by Richard Kitchen, Christina Faull, Sarah Russell and Jo Wilson.
© 2024 John Wiley & Sons Ltd. Published 2024 by John Wiley & Sons Ltd.

Appendix B – Managing Breathlessness in the Last Days of Life

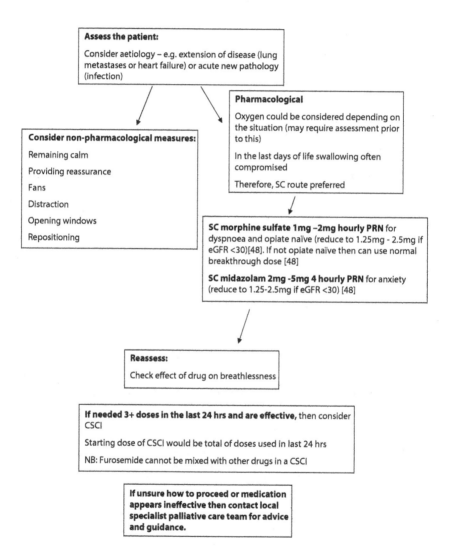

Assess the patient:

Consider aetiology – e.g. extension of disease (lung metastases or heart failure) or acute new pathology (infection)

Consider non-pharmacological measures:

Remaining calm

Providing reassurance

Fans

Distraction

Opening windows

Repositioning

Pharmacological

Oxygen could be considered depending on the situation (may require assessment prior to this)

In the last days of life swallowing often compromised

Therefore, SC route preferred

SC morphine sulfate 1mg –2mg hourly PRN for dyspnoea and opiate naïve (reduce to 1.25mg - 2.5mg if eGFR <30)[48]. If not opiate naïve then can use normal breakthrough dose [48]

SC midazolam 2mg -5mg 4 hourly PRN for anxiety (reduce to 1.25-2.5mg if eGFR <30) [48]

Reassess:

Check effect of drug on breathlessness

If needed 3+ doses in the last 24 hrs and are effective, then consider CSCI

Starting dose of CSCI would be total of doses used in last 24 hrs

NB: Furosemide cannot be mixed with other drugs in a CSCI

If unsure how to proceed or medication appears ineffective then contact local specialist palliative care team for advice and guidance.

Handbook of Palliative Care, Fourth Edition. Edited by Richard Kitchen, Christina Faull, Sarah Russell and Jo Wilson.
© 2024 John Wiley & Sons Ltd. Published 2024 by John Wiley & Sons Ltd.

Appendix C – Management of Respiratory Secretions in the Last Days of Life

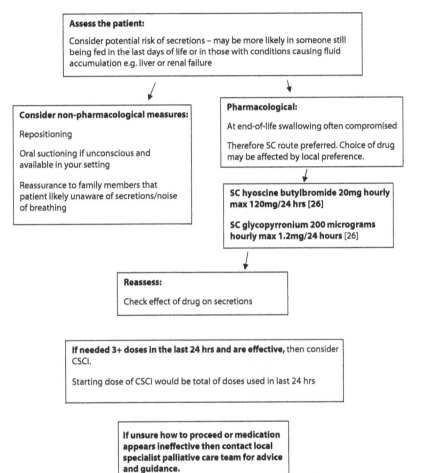

Assess the patient:

Consider potential risk of secretions – may be more likely in someone still being fed in the last days of life or in those with conditions causing fluid accumulation e.g. liver or renal failure

Consider non-pharmacological measures:

Repositioning

Oral suctioning if unconscious and available in your setting

Reassurance to family members that patient likely unaware of secretions/noise of breathing

Pharmacological:

At end-of-life swallowing often compromised

Therefore SC route preferred. Choice of drug may be affected by local preference.

SC hyoscine butylbromide 20mg hourly max 120mg/24 hrs [26]

SC glycopyrronium 200 micrograms hourly max 1.2mg/24 hours [26]

Reassess:

Check effect of drug on secretions

If needed 3+ doses in the last 24 hrs and are effective, then consider CSCI.

Starting dose of CSCI would be total of doses used in last 24 hrs

If unsure how to proceed or medication appears ineffective then contact local specialist palliative care team for advice and guidance.

Handbook of Palliative Care, Fourth Edition. Edited by Richard Kitchen, Christina Faull, Sarah Russell and Jo Wilson.
© 2024 John Wiley & Sons Ltd. Published 2024 by John Wiley & Sons Ltd.

Appendix D – Management of Nausea and Vomiting in Last Days of Life

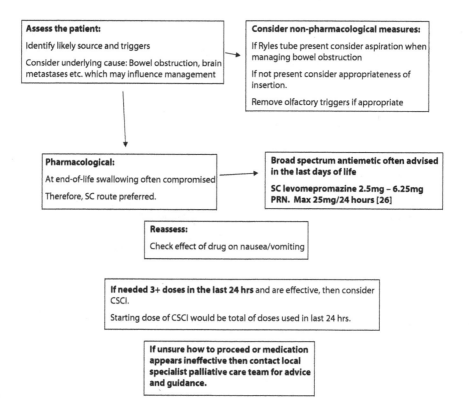

Assess the patient:

Identify likely source and triggers

Consider underlying cause: Bowel obstruction, brain metastases etc. which may influence management

Consider non-pharmacological measures:

If Ryles tube present consider aspiration when managing bowel obstruction

If not present consider appropriateness of insertion.

Remove olfactory triggers if appropriate

Pharmacological:

At end-of-life swallowing often compromised

Therefore, SC route preferred.

Broad spectrum antiemetic often advised in the last days of life

SC levomepromazine 2.5mg – 6.25mg PRN. Max 25mg/24 hours [26]

Reassess:

Check effect of drug on nausea/vomiting

If needed 3+ doses in the last 24 hrs and are effective, then consider CSCI.

Starting dose of CSCI would be total of doses used in last 24 hrs.

If unsure how to proceed or medication appears ineffective then contact local specialist palliative care team for advice and guidance.

Handbook of Palliative Care, Fourth Edition. Edited by Richard Kitchen, Christina Faull, Sarah Russell and Jo Wilson.
© 2024 John Wiley & Sons Ltd. Published 2024 by John Wiley & Sons Ltd.

Appendix E – Management of Terminal Agitation in the Last Days of Life

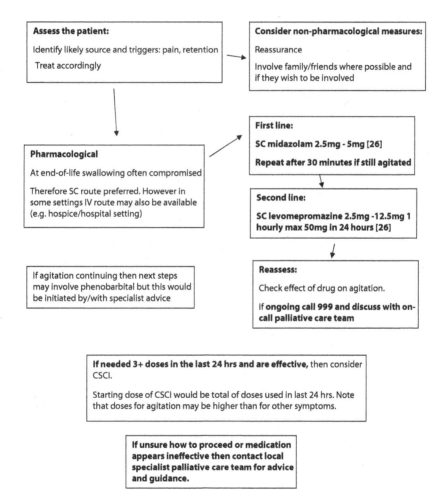

Assess the patient:

Identify likely source and triggers: pain, retention

Treat accordingly

Consider non-pharmacological measures:

Reassurance

Involve family/friends where possible and if they wish to be involved

Pharmacological

At end-of-life swallowing often compromised

Therefore SC route preferred. However in some settings IV route may also be available (e.g. hospice/hospital setting)

First line:

SC midazolam 2.5mg - 5mg [26]

Repeat after 30 minutes if still agitated

Second line:

SC levomepromazine 2.5mg -12.5mg 1 hourly max 50mg in 24 hours [26]

If agitation continuing then next steps may involve phenobarbital but this would be initiated by/with specialist advice

Reassess:

Check effect of drug on agitation.

If **ongoing call 999 and discuss with on-call palliative care team**

If needed 3+ doses in the last 24 hrs and are effective, then consider CSCI.

Starting dose of CSCI would be total of doses used in last 24 hrs. Note that doses for agitation may be higher than for other symptoms.

If unsure how to proceed or medication appears ineffective then contact local specialist palliative care team for advice and guidance.

Handbook of Palliative Care, Fourth Edition. Edited by Richard Kitchen, Christina Faull, Sarah Russell and Jo Wilson.
© 2024 John Wiley & Sons Ltd. Published 2024 by John Wiley & Sons Ltd.

Appendix F – Management of Bleeding in Last Days of Life

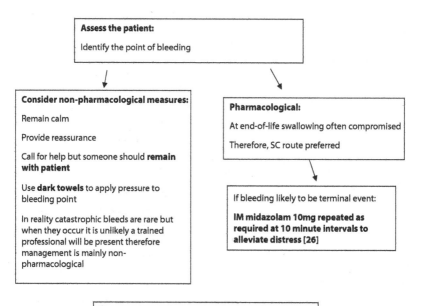

Assess the patient:

Identify the point of bleeding

Consider non-pharmacological measures:

Remain calm

Provide reassurance

Call for help but someone should **remain with patient**

Use **dark towels** to apply pressure to bleeding point

In reality catastrophic bleeds are rare but when they occur it is unlikely a trained professional will be present therefore management is mainly non-pharmacological

Pharmacological:

At end-of-life swallowing often compromised

Therefore, SC route preferred

If bleeding likely to be terminal event:

IM midazolam 10mg repeated as required at 10 minute intervals to alleviate distress [26]

Reassess:

If survives bleed then review any medication that may be contributing to bleed i.e. anticoagulation

If unsure how to proceed or medication appears ineffective then contact local specialist palliative care team for advice and guidance.

Handbook of Palliative Care, Fourth Edition. Edited by Richard Kitchen, Christina Faull, Sarah Russell and Jo Wilson.
© 2024 John Wiley & Sons Ltd. Published 2024 by John Wiley & Sons Ltd.

Appendix G – Management of Seizures in Last Days of Life

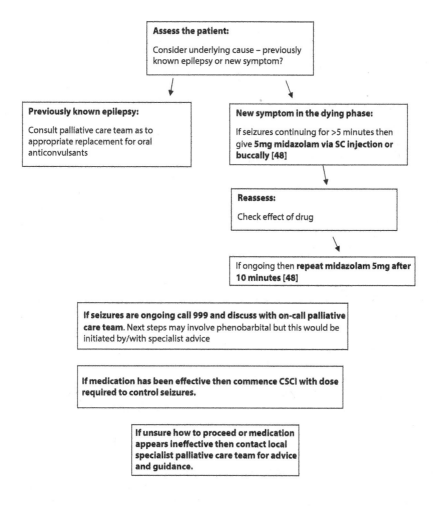

Assess the patient:

Consider underlying cause – previously known epilepsy or new symptom?

Previously known epilepsy:

Consult palliative care team as to appropriate replacement for oral anticonvulsants

New symptom in the dying phase:

If seizures continuing for >5 minutes then give **5mg midazolam via SC injection or buccally [48]**

Reassess:

Check effect of drug

If ongoing then **repeat midazolam 5mg after 10 minutes [48]**

If seizures are ongoing call 999 and discuss with on-call palliative care team. Next steps may involve phenobarbital but this would be initiated by/with specialist advice

If medication has been effective then commence CSCI with dose required to control seizures.

If unsure how to proceed or medication appears ineffective then contact local specialist palliative care team for advice and guidance.

Handbook of Palliative Care, Fourth Edition. Edited by Richard Kitchen, Christina Faull, Sarah Russell and Jo Wilson.
© 2024 John Wiley & Sons Ltd. Published 2024 by John Wiley & Sons Ltd.

21 Medicines Management in Palliative Care Including Syringe Pumps

Kerry Parker and Michelle Aslett

Introduction

A large proportion of patients requiring palliative care have symptom control needs and will require medicines to manage them, often alongside any regular medicines they are already prescribed. With palliative care encompassing non-malignant conditions, the complexity of medicines management is just as challenging as those with a cancer diagnosis undergoing advanced treatments or living longer with their disease.

Medicines management concerns all those involved in the prescribing, supply, administration, and guidance of drugs, and healthcare professionals within palliative care will vary with the differing responsibilities they have to contribute to the safe and effective use of medicines.

Definition of Medicines Management and How This Applies to Palliative Care

Medicines management and medicines optimisation has been defined as "the clinical, cost-effective and safe use of medicines to ensure patients get the maximum benefit from the medicines they need, while at the same time minimising potential harm" [1] and as a "system of processes and behaviours that determine how medicines are used by the NHS and patients" [2].

Medicines Management incorporates the clinical and legal approaches of the pharmacy team and learning from medicines related incidents, specifically related to medicines usage, which could have, or did, lead to patient harm. Examples of medicines-related incidents include:

- Prescribing errors
- Administration errors
- Unintentional omissions
- Near misses (preventable medicines-related patient safety incidents which could have led to patient harm)

This may involve local-level working with teams to address practice and processes or may be national and involving the Medicines Health Regulatory Agency (MHRA) via the yellow card scheme.

Medicines optimisation is ensuring that the right patients get the right choice of medicine, at the right time [3]. The goal is to help patients to:

- improve outcomes/experience with their medicines;
- take medicines correctly for maximum benefit without impacting their quality of life, for example, having to reconfigure mealtimes;
- avoid taking unnecessary medicines and reduce wastage;
- improve medicines safety.

Ultimately medicines optimisation can help encourage patients to take ownership of their treatment [4]. This ethos matches that of palliative care where the patient is at the centre and supported to make informed decisions.

Pharmacy Teams in Palliative Care: A Key Member

Palliative care requires a multidisciplinary approach – National Institute for Health and Care Excellence (NICE) guidance specifically recommends that an effective specialist palliative care team incorporates the range of expertise provided by pharmacy teams. Palliative care is delivered in a variety of healthcare settings so patients and

Handbook of Palliative Care, Fourth Edition. Edited by Richard Kitchen, Christina Faull, Sarah Russell and Jo Wilson.
© 2024 John Wiley & Sons Ltd. Published 2024 by John Wiley & Sons Ltd.

healthcare professionals may interact with different members of the pharmacy team.

Pharmacists are registered with the General Pharmaceutical Council (GPhC) to work in the UK. Their main role and responsibilities ensure:

- the quality of medicines supplied to patients
- supplies of medicines are within the law
- medicines prescribed to patients are suitable
- advising patients about medicines including how to take them, what reactions may occur, and answering patients' questions
- advising other healthcare professionals about safe and effective medicines use, and safe and secure supply of medicines.

Pharmacy technicians work under the supervision of a pharmacist and are registered professionals (GPhC). Their roles span all areas of pharmacy practice, from the purchasing, manufacture, preparation, supply, and final check of medicines to assisting medicines use reviews and administration of medicines.

Traditionally roles were within hospital, community, industry, and academia but now wider reaching and cross-interface pharmacy teams work within GP practices, care homes, Clinical Commissioning Groups (CCGs)/Integrated Care Boards (ICBs), Primary Care Networks (PCNs), and hospices.

The role of a palliative care pharmacy team comprises "clinical, educational, administrative and supportive" responsibilities. Many pharmacists are independent/non-medical prescribers, whose skills are best placed to support patients particularly where specialist medicines are required including managing their own patient caseloads.

On average, palliative care patients take 8 (range 0–17) different medications [5]. Changing formulations, reducing medicines burden, education, and support helps patients as well as their family/carers. Where compliance or lack of usual administration routes become an issue, the pharmacist can advise on alternative options for symptom control.

Pharmacists working in the palliative care MDT can help to address psychological and social circumstances that influence a patient's approach to medicines. This may be anxiety over the use of opioids and fear it is hastening death, patients trying to maintain their independence for as long as possible but being told medicines may affect their driving, or it may be family members with addiction issues which affect availability of medicines in the home. A partnership between the pharmacy team and patient as well as the wider MDT is essential.

The pharmacy team can help their healthcare settings with education, guideline development, audit, incident reviews, and reflections. They support the controlled drug accountable officers (CDAOs) who will feed into the controlled drug local intelligence network (CDLIN). There are regional and national pharmacist specialist interest groups that provide education catered for the team working at a higher level as well as sharing of practice, research, and networking.

Use of Drugs beyond Their Licence

In palliative care, medications are often prescribed outside the terms of their marketing authorisation (previously called a product license). A marketing authorisation is granted by a regulatory body to a pharmaceutical company for a specific medicinal product. It stipulates the terms of use, including indications, doses, routes, and patient populations for which it can be marketed [6].

"Off-label" is a term commonly used to describe the use of a medicinal product beyond the specifications of its marketing authorization, that is, using a licensed medicine for a purpose not covered by its marketing authorisation [6]; examples include antidepressants for neuropathic pain, subcutaneous administration of some medicines, and administration of medication via feeding tubes. Surveys suggest that up to one quarter of prescriptions in palliative care come into this category [7, 8].

An **unauthorised** (unlicensed) medicinal product is a product that does not have a marketing authorization granted for medicinal use in humans. These include:

- "specials" – special order products made in the UK by a manufacturer
- trial drugs
- "manipulated products" where two or more medicinal products have been mixed for administration, for example, syringe pump.

In the UK, doctors and independent prescribers may legally prescribe off-label and unlicensed products where it is accepted clinical practice and within their clinical competence. This will be backed up by local organisation governance and policies which will also determine any requirements around administration, dispensing and documentation [9–11]. The prescriber must be fully informed about the actions and uses of the medicinal product, be assured of the quality of the particular product, and in the light of published evidence, balance both the potential good and the potential harm which might ensue [9–11].

It is recommended that the patient (or their advocate if no capacity) are made aware why a medicine is being used "differently" to what the patient information leaflet tells them and for them to give informed consent and documented in the patient notes. In palliative care this can be a challenge as off-label use is so widespread and the burden of these discussions for most drugs use would not be manageable, so the decision remains with the prescriber regarding how to proceed with these discussions. A joint position statement has also been produced by the British Pain Society and the Association for Palliative Medicine, together with a patient information booklet [12].

Administration via feeding tubes is an unlicensed activity for most drugs but may be necessary for patients who are unable to swallow. Prescribers should refer to evidence-based resources and liaising with the pharmacy team on formulation options, timings or interaction concerns with feeds or other medicines and ensuring the tube is not at risk of the patency being affected by the drugs being administered.

Medication Compliance Aids

Patients taking multiple medicines may have difficulty in adhering to the regimen prescribed. Supporting patients struggling with compliance to medication regimens is a complex issue that should be approached in a way tailored to each individual [13, 14].

Certain patients find compliance aids helpful that contain tablets for the day indicating the time to be taken like "Redidose" boxes and blister packs. Some

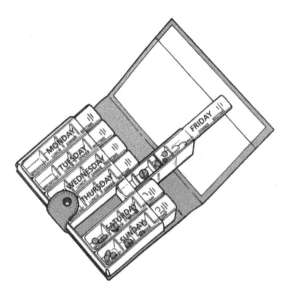

Figure 1 The Redidose 7 day pill dispenser.

devices include alarms and electronic dispensers to aid patients in remembering to take medications when due. Other aids available include downloadable apps which alarm when medications are due or send text reminders to patients.

There is little evidence to suggest whether these devices improve compliance, safety, satisfaction, or convenience with taking medications [15]. Patients interviewed about their use of compliance aids reported that most had purchased the systems because taking multiple medicines did not fit well in their lives and some found them helpful in giving them more control over their medicines. Rather than reminding them "to take" medication, the devices allowed patients to check whether "they had taken" medication and thus relieved the anxiety. Often, other measures were employed in addition to the compliance aid itself [16].

Many commonly prescribed medicines may not be suitable for use in compliance aids as storage outside of the original manufacturer packaging may negatively affect stability. Drugs for when required use or those subject to frequent dose changes are not appropriate for use in compliance aids.

No system is optimal for all patients and their ability to cope at home with a particular device should always be assessed before recommending [17]. The pharmacist may be able to offer alternative solutions such as the use of large print labels, diaries, and charts. Preparation of Pharmacy issued blister packs is time-consuming and expensive process; therefore, they should only be initiated for patients following review by a suitably trained healthcare professional.

Deprescribing

Deprescribing is "the process of tapering, stopping, discontinuing, or withdrawing drugs, with the goal of managing polypharmacy and improving outcomes. Clinicians typically attempt to taper or stop agents based on clinical experience, rather than using an evidence-based approach" [18].

• St. Anne's Hospice in Manchester reported patients who had one-week prognosis still took on average 11 regular tablets [19].

• This reveals a large drug burden on elderly patients and those with limited life remaining. Therefore, deprescribing is an important consideration.

• A Dutch study investigated patient, relative and HCP perceptions towards end-of-life medication management.

They identified multiple factors that can influence deprescribing decisions including lack of time, burdens for patients, lack of guidelines, uncertainty about life expectancy, and unknown consequences of withdrawing medication [20].

Deprescribing is an intentional planned process supervised by healthcare professionals, and with the patient and their carer. The aims of this process are to:
• Improve quality of life by reducing medications which may be contributing to symptoms, for example, increased falls, dry mouth affecting nutritional intake.
• Reduce medication burden – As life expectancy increases, so does the risk of multi-morbidities and subsequently the risk of polypharmacy [21].
• Avoid worsening of disease or causing withdrawal.

In the presence of life-limiting illness, the need to continue preventative medicines becomes less certain as they are unlikely to improve health or offer continued long-term health benefits [22]. Statins are one of the most common medications that are discontinued by specialist palliative care professionals; not only do they have multiple side-effects and interactions, but in patients with short prognosis they are more likely to cause harm than benefit.

Barriers to deprescribing medicines include:
• Patient and/or family reluctance – it may be viewed that the healthcare professional is "giving up" on them.
• Prognostication particularly in non-malignant conditions being unclear.
• Fear of predisposing a clinical event.
• Fear of the patient upsetting their other doctor or consultant – "I've always been told to take bisoprolol by my cardiologist."
• Differing opinions between specialists and/or generalists.
• Fear by the healthcare professional of where the discussion may lead – "does this mean I'm dying?"

Deprescribing requires good communication skills to start discussions and have honest conversations with patients and their families/carers. Most patients are happy to not take medication, but for some patients their medicines are the only element of control left in their life – to give this up means they perceive they have lost all control.

At the time of writing, there are no specific guidelines around stopping medicines for patients with a short prognosis. Guidance tends to focus on reducing medicines in relation to risk of side-effects in the elderly (STOPP/START) but research is ongoing to help support healthcare professionals in making these decisions alongside clinical judgements. More recently the OncPal deprescribing guideline has been published to support clinicians with discontinuation of medications which have limited benefit in palliative cancer patients [23].

Considerations:
• It is sometimes better not to start a medicine than to tackle deprescribing in the future, particularly in certain therapeutic areas.
• Older people, those who are approaching the end-of-life and those with increasing frailty are frequently prescribed unnecessary or higher risk medicines and should have more frequent medication reviews.
• Initiating discussions around deprescribing can be opportunistic with a changing patient, for example, loss of swallow but can ideally be approached during other advanced decision-making.
• Don't forget the inhalers – if the patient does not have the lung capacity and/or dexterity to use their devices then they are going to only be more prone to oral thrush than benefit from the inhaled medicine.

Complementary and Alternative Medicines

Complementary and alternative medicines (CAMs) are treatments that fall outside mainstream healthcare. These range from acupuncture and homeopathy, to aromatherapy, and colonic irrigation. The availability of CAMs on the NHS is limited and varies by region.

Herbal medicines contain active ingredients made from plant parts, such as leaves, roots, or flowers. Not all herbal products are medicines, some can be classified as food supplements or cosmetics. In the UK this is regulated by the "Traditional Herbal Medicine Scheme" [24].

Homeopathy is a system of medicine which is regulated by the Homeopathic National Rules Scheme in the UK. Homeopathic products should not be confused with herbal remedies. Some homeopathic products are derived from herbal active ingredients, but the important distinction is that homeopathic products are extremely diluted and administered according to specific principles. No legal regulation of homeopathic practitioners currently exists in the UK.

Many cancer patients (around 36% in one European study) use CAMs during or after therapy [25, 26]. Usage may depend on previous approaches to conventional medicines, lifestyle, and healthcare choices but also on the stage of disease, treatment decisions, and often at the point in time where patients/families are willing to try anything. Stories on social media of "cancer cures" bring hope to affected people. Patients are more likely to source information on alternative treatments from online and neighbours/friends than they are healthcare professionals [26]. This cohort of people are vulnerable and can become a target for fraudulent business [27].

It is important to address patient's queries and concerns around CAMs – failure to do so may mean the patient does not disclose important information on products they are using which may contribute to their symptoms, or feels they are not being listened to by their healthcare professionals and that their questions are being dismissed. To help patients make informed decisions, we need to listen to their queries and find the information out to discuss with them. Using reliable sources of information such as accessing medicines information services can help gain information to discuss with patients and guide discussions around risk and benefits of using such treatments.

Counselling points:
• There is a risk of adverse effects with herbal medicines and the potential for interaction with conventional medicines.
• Some herbal medicines may not be suitable for younger or older patients.
• If a patient has an adverse effect to the herbal medicine they are taking, they should stop taking the herbal medicine and inform a healthcare professional such as a pharmacist or a doctor.
• Patients should be advised to continue taking their prescribed medication if they are taking a herbal medicine; any changes to a prescribed medication should only be done following consultation with the prescriber.

As with standard medicines, reporting of adverse effects from herbal medicines is essential to understand more about these products and their interactions. Patients and professionals can report these online at the yellow card scheme.

Cannabis Oil (CBD)

CBD oil is available to buy legally as a food supplement from health stores, however there is no guarantee of product quality or robust evidence of health benefits [28]. The claims made in the press for CBD use are:
• Anxiety
• Pain
• Insomnia
• Treat/cure cancer

The main pharmacologically active compounds of *Cannabis sativa* are cannabidiol (CBD) and tetrahydrocannabinol (THC). Unlike THC, pure CBD is not psychoactive

and is not a controlled substance. The CBD oils that are on sale at time of publication contain low concentrations of CBD; however, it is difficult to purify CBD from plants to the point that no trace of THC remains [28]. The MHRA states that if a CBD product "contains any controlled cannabinoids, unintentionally or otherwise then it is highly likely that the product would be controlled" under the Misuse of Drugs regulations.

Some cannabis-based products are available to buy over the internet without a prescription. It's likely most of these products will be illegal to possess or supply as they will likely contain THC and may not be safe to use. CBD and THC can affect how other medicines work and interfere with liver function.

At the time of writing, there is ongoing research into medicinal cannabis and currently there are only three licensed forms for specific indications in the UK:
• Sativex (MS spasticity)
• Epidyolex (rare forms of childhood epilepsy)
• Nabilone (nausea and vomiting post chemotherapy when other treatments have not worked)

Claims of CBD "curing cancer" are not evidence based and so it is important to guide patients to respected sources of information so they can make informed decisions. The Macmillan and Cancer Research websites are useful resources to help guide those discussions.

Anticipatory Prescribing and Accessing Medicines

Deficiencies in communication, forward planning, pain management, and co-ordination of care can lead to avoidable suffering for patients with terminal illness. The Dying Without Dignity report (2015) highlighted that end-of-life care could be improved for 350,000 people a year in England alone [29]. One of the main themes highlighted was the importance of achieving good round-the-clock symptom control for all patients.

Certain symptoms including pain, nausea, vomiting, agitation, breathlessness, and terminal secretions are very common at the end-of-life, regardless of the cause of terminal illness. Due to the predictability of these symptoms occurring, the practice of anticipatory prescribing or "planning ahead" is common within palliative care and should be considered alongside making decisions about resuscitation and other advanced care plans. Not all patients will develop all symptoms listed above, however, it is considered best practice to prescribe and supply anticipatory medications in advance of need.

The purpose of anticipatory prescribing is to ensure:
- a supply of drug is available in a patient's home for immediate use needed (including diluent)
- all appropriate equipment including needles and syringes are available to administer the drugs
- appropriate medications can be administered in a timely fashion by a clinician without delays
- reduced distress to patients and families/carers
- avoid unnecessary hospital admissions

All healthcare professionals involved with end-of-life care should familiarise themselves with their local guidance and drug formularies. Guidelines are often prescriptive in terms of doses and medications to be used for management of symptoms in terminal illness, however it is important that practitioners always apply these in a patient-centred way, for example, patients with reduced renal function may require alternate opioids or dose reductions to those outlined in guidelines. Ensuring individualisation of care and treatments to meet the patient's clinical and social situation is essential to providing good quality symptom control. Unfamiliarity with the drugs is a risk and so liaising with specialist palliative care teams is necessary to ensure appropriate prescribing.

Common medications prescribed in anticipation of patient need include:
- an opioid – for pain and dyspnoea
- a benzodiazepine (usually midazolam) – for restlessness and agitation
- an anti-emetic – for nausea and vomiting
- an anti-cholinergic medication – for terminal secretions

Planning ahead for end-of-life symptom management in complex patients is critical, not only in terms of medication supply, but also addressing issues that may contribute to symptoms, for example, stopping smoking suddenly therefore needing nicotine patches to prevent agitation, or patients becoming unable to take oral anti-epileptics and a plan needed for prevention of seizures. Anticipatory prescribing for management of terminal haemorrhage is also encouraged if patients are at risk of developing these symptoms.

Some areas of the UK use Just in Case (JIC) box initiatives to support the practice of anticipatory planning. The JIC is an approved, readily identifiable container which contains all appropriate medications, equipment, and necessary documentations to facilitate prompt medication administration once symptoms develop. As these JIC boxes commonly contain controlled drugs it is essential that the security of the box, while in the patient's home, is maintained to minimise the risk of medications being unlawfully diverted.

Several regions have implemented commissioned schemes working with community pharmacies to hold a stock of essential end-of-life care medicines to ensure timely access to common medications used in palliative care [30]. These schemes are not fool proof and with issues around wholesaler deliveries, supply disruptions and manufacturing delays, a back-up system with hospital pharmacies may be required.

Overall, the best practice is to plan and access medicines not too soon before needed but before a distressing situation arises. Regular review of the symptom control needs of these patients over time is essential.

Use of the "Syringe Pump" for Continuous Subcutaneous Infusion of Medications in Palliative Care

Oral administration of medications may become inappropriate for several reasons during a patient's illness and drug administration by continuous infusion can be an alternative way to achieve symptom control. In the UK the subcutaneous (SC) route is primarily used for continuous infusion in palliative care, as it is well tolerated by patients and easily achievable in community settings. Administration of medications via continuous infusion provides steady-state plasma concentrations thus providing constant therapeutic benefit and reduced need for repeated bolus injections.

Continuous subcutaneous infusions (CSCI) are delivered using a portable, battery-operated device called a syringe pump. These devices deliver precise doses of medications over a set period of time, most commonly over 24 hours. An example is the T34 syringe pump. Use of CSCI is as effective as continuous IV infusion and intermittent bolus injections. In settings where it may be difficult to guarantee that regular intermittent injections will be administered on time, a CSCI is likely to provide better round-the-clock symptom management. Within palliative care the use of the syringe pump is firmly established to administer drugs for symptom control, either alone or in combinations according to the recognised compatibilities of different drugs [31–37].

The use of these devices is not without risk – between January 1, 2005 and June 30, 2010, the NPSA received reports of 8 deaths and 167 non-fatal incidents involving ambulatory syringe pumps [38]. Following concerns, a harmonised European Standard was drawn up identifying features of syringe pumps that would reduce the risk of incidents in practice – the recommendations include:

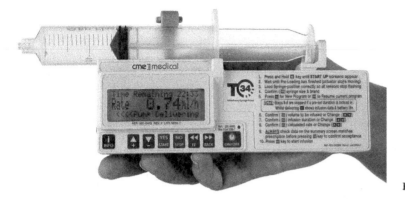

Figure 2 The T34 syringe pump.

- all syringe pumps to be calibrated in millilitres per hour
- mechanisms to stop the infusion if connections and fittings are incorrect
- alarms to indicate if the syringe becomes disconnected from the pump
- locks to prevent tampering with the syringe/device
- internal log memory to record pump events

Indications for Using the CSCI

For patients able to take and absorb oral drugs, administration of medications via CSCI is unlikely to improve symptom control and may be burdensome, with increased reliance on healthcare professionals to set up and manage the infusion device. However, continuous subcutaneous infusion can be useful route of medication administration when used appropriately. Common indications include:

- Persistent nausea and/or vomiting
- Swallowing difficulties
- Intestinal obstruction
- Oral/pharyngeal lesions
- Profound weakness/cachexia
- Patient preference
- Comatose or moribund patient

Prescribing of continuous infusions involves anticipating and responding to a patient's medication requirements over the next 24 hours. Any changes in symptoms experienced may necessitate additional injections to supplement the infusion therefore, medication should also be prescribed and be available, for immediate administration in case of breakthrough symptoms. This is sometimes referred to as "rescue medication."

Alternative routes of drug administration such as sublingual, buccal, rectal, or transdermal should be considered where appropriate. Long-term delivery of medications via subcutaneous infusion is rarely indicated but may be necessary for some patients. For many patients once symptoms are controlled, it is often possible to reconvert to oral formulations.

Explanation to the Patient and Carers

Before initiating a CSCI, explanation should be provided to the patient and their carers on the nature and intention of the procedure. It is important to explain to the patient and family:

- the reason for administering medication via this route
- how the device works (including the need for a battery change every 24 hours)
- the advantages and possible disadvantages of using a syringe pump
- how to seek assistance when the CSCI alarms
- The process for returning them after the patient has died.

Some patients may find the syringe pump obtrusive and disconcerting, many may have reservations and some fear that the implementation of a syringe pump equates with impending death. Questions should be invited, anxieties acknowledged, and appropriate reassurance given.

Medications Used in Syringe Pump

The administration of medications via CSCI is off-label for the majority of drugs administered this way. However, there is extensive clinical experience and reputable reference sources to support prescribing and administration of drugs via this route [6, 39–42]. Advice should be sought from local palliative care specialists on unusual drugs or combinations before prescribing. Many of the medications used are found in Table 1. Note that while the heading "sedative" is used for some medications, as they cause

Table 1 Drugs used in syringe pump.

Medication	Ampoule Size	Indication	Dose Range Per 24 Hours	Comments
Opioids				
Morphine Sulfate	10 mg/ml, 15 mg/ml, 20 mg/ml, 30 mg/ml (1 and 2 ml amps)	Pain, dyspnoea	Start: For opioid naive patients – refer to regional guidelines* for initial dose. For patients already on oral Morphine start at 50% of current total daily dose. Increase as necessary by 30–50% increments. No maximum dose.	• Is first-line choice of opioid in most areas. • Regular administration should be avoided in patients with GFR < 30 ml/min
Diamorphine	Crystalline powder 5 mg, 10 mg, 30 mg, 100 mg, 500 mg amps. Must be reconstituted with water prior to administration.	Pain, dyspnoea	Start: For opioid naive patients – refer to regional guidelines* for initial dose. For patients already on oral Morphine start at one-third of current total daily dose of oral morphine. Increase as necessary by 30–50% increments. No maximum dose.	• Alternative opioid to Morphine if high doses are required in a syringe pump. • Highly soluble • Final concentration should not exceed 250 mg/ml in syringe for administration via CSCI
Oxycodone	10 mg/ml (1 and 2 ml amps) 50 mg/ml (1 ml amps)	Pain, Morphine intolerance	Start: For opioid naive patients – refer to regional guidelines* for initial dose. For patients already on oral Oxycodone start at 50% of current total daily dose of oral Oxycodone. Increase as necessary by 30–50% increments. No maximum dose.	• If mixing with Cyclizine do not exceed 3 mg/ml Cyclizine
Alfentanil	1 mg/2 ml, 5 mg/10 ml and 5 mg/1 ml amps	Alternative to Morphine on advice of palliative care specialist, particularly in renal failure.	For opioid naive patients – refer to regional guidelines* or local palliative care team for initial dose. If converting from other opioids seek specialist palliative care advice	• Incompatibility may occur with Cyclizine
Hydromorphone	10 mg/ml, 20 mg/ml, 50 mg/ml amps (unlicensed special order)	Alternative to Morphine in cases of intolerance – on advice of palliative care specialist.	Start: At 50% of current total daily dose of oral Hydromorphone. If converting from other opioids seek specialist palliative care advice	• Unlicensed product is available as a special order from Martindale Pharma • Expensive

(Continued)

Table 1 *(Continued)*

Medication	Ampoule Size	Indication	Dose Range Per 24 Hours	Comments
Fentanyl	100 micrograms/2 ml and 500 micrograms/10 ml amps	Alternative to Morphine on advice of palliative care specialist, particularly in renal failure.	For opioid naive patients – refer to regional guidelines* or local palliative care team for initial dose. If converting from other opioids seek specialist palliative care advice	• Volume issues may restrict administration at high doses
Methadone	10 mg/ml and 50 mg/ml amps	Only on advice of palliative care specialist.	Seek advice from a palliative care specialist	• Can cause adverse reaction at site of infusion • Wide variation in individual plasma concentration • Long half-life leads to tendency to accumulate
NSAIDs				
Ketorolac	30 mg/ml amps	Bone pain on recommendation of palliative care specialist	30–60 mg	• Well tolerated • Use with caution in renal failure • Can be nephrotoxic • Short-term use only • High incident of GI bleeding; co-prescribe gastro-protective drug • Irritant therefore dilute with the largest possible volume of sodium chloride 0.9% • Very alkaline – high risk of precipitation in combination
Parecoxib	20 mg/ml (2 ml amps). Need reconstituting prior to administration.	Bone pain on recommendation of palliative care specialist	Start: 20–40 mg daily. Increase up to maximum of 80 mg/24 hours if beneficial for pain control.	• Limited compatibility data currently available • Use with caution in renal failure • May be suitable to administer as SC bolus once or twice daily
Anti-Emetics				
Haloperidol	5 mg/ml amps	Drug induced nausea; metabolic causes; anti-psychotic	1–5 mg reduce starting dose in renal impairment and elderly.	• Central dopamine receptor antagonist – avoid in parkinsonism • Mildly sedating • Settles agitation and psychosis

(Continued)

Table 1 (*Continued*)

Medication	Ampoule Size	Indication	Dose Range Per 24 Hours	Comments
Metoclopramide	5 mg/ml (2 ml amps)	Impaired gastric emptying	30–100 mg	• Dopamine receptor antagonist – avoid in parkinsonism • Non-sedating • Possibility of extra-pyramidal/dystonic side effects or tardive dyskinesia with prolonged use in younger women
Cyclizine	50 mg/ml amps	Intestinal obstruction; movement induced nausea, raised intra-cranial pressure	50–100 mg	• Anti-histamine (H_1) and anti-cholinergic • May cause drowsiness • Must not dilute with sodium chloride • Known compatibility problems in some combinations
Ondansetron	2 mg/ml (2 ml and 4 ml amps)	Chemotherapy or radiotherapy induced nausea and vomiting	8–24 mg	• $5HT_3$ antagonist – of not effective within 72 hours discontinue
Sedative and Anti-Emetic				
Levomepromazine	25 mg/ml amps	Nausea; restlessness and agitation; psychosis	Nausea – 5–25 mg (doses in excess of 35 mg cause sedation and are rarely necessary for nausea) Restlessness/Agitation – 25–75 mg; titration according to response. Very rarely doses as high as 200 mg/24 hours may be needed for severe terminal agitation, this should be managed under the supervision of a specialist in palliative care	• Effective anti-emetic • Useful for terminal agitation • Could be administered as SC bolus injection due to long half-life • May cause skin reactions at infusion site
Sedatives				
Midazolam	10 mg/2 ml preferred in palliative care. Other ampoules sizes are available.	Anxiety; terminal agitation and restlessness; dyspnoea; anti-convulsant, myoclonus	10–30 mg (common range), doses of up to 100 mg can be used	• Water soluble benzodiazepine • Large inter-individual variability in steady-state plasma levels

(Continued)

Table 1 (*Continued*)

Medication	Ampoule Size	Indication	Dose Range Per 24 Hours	Comments
Clonazepam	1 mg/ml amps (unlicensed in the UK, available as a parallel import)	Anxiety; terminal agitation and restlessness; anti-convulsant, neuropathic pain	500 micrograms–8 mg	• Less water soluble than midazolam • May be irritant • May cause confusion • Expensive
Anti-Cholinergics				
Glycopyrronium	200 microgram/ml (1 ml and 3 ml amps)	Terminal secretions	600 micrograms–1.2 mg	• Slower onset of action than Hyoscine Butylbromide • Less likely to cause confusion than Hyoscine Hydrobromide
Hyoscine Butylbromide	20 mg/ml (1 ml amps)	Severe Colic; Terminal Secretions; Intestinal Obstruction	20–120 mg (doses of up to 240 mg may be used)	• Less likely to cause sedation than Hyoscine Hydrobromide
Hyoscine Hydrobromide	400 micrograms/ml amps 600 micrograms /ml amps	Terminal Secretions, Sedation	600 micrograms–2.4 mg	• Rarely used in practice due to undesirable side effects and high cost • Dry mouth – extra attention to good oral hygiene
Anti-Convulsants				
Midazolam	See above			
Clonazepam	See above			
Levetiracetam	100 mg/ml (5 ml amps)	Seizures	500 mg–3 grams (Doses >2g will need to be split into 2 syringe pumps)	• May cause infusion site reactions – monitor site closely upon initiation • Volume restrictions mean doses above 2 grams may require splitting between multiple T34 pumps
Sedative and Anti-Convulsant				
Phenobarbital	30 mg/ml amps 60 mg/ml amps 200 mg/ml amps	Seizures, status epilepticus, terminal agitation	Management of Seizures: Up to 400 mg/24 hours Terminal Agitation: Typical dose is 800–1,200 mg/24 hours but can range 200–3,800 mg/24 hours.	• Stat bolus doses of IV/IM Phenobarbital should be trialled before initiation of CSCI – see PCF for full dosing information • Phenobarbital should be administered via a separate syringe pump. Due to its alkaline pH, it is likely to be *incompatible* with most drugs

(Continued)

Table 1 (*Continued*)

Medication	Ampoule Size	Indication	Dose Range Per 24 Hours	Comments
Miscellaneous				
Octreotide	50 micrograms/ml amps 100 micrograms/ml amps 200 micrograms/ml 5 ml amps 500 micrograms/ml amps	Reduces GI secretions; volume of vomit in intestinal obstruction; volume of enterocolic fistula	500 micrograms initially – if ineffective stop after 48 hours. If effective titrate to lowest effective dose (usual range 50–600 micrograms/24 hours)	• Expensive
Tranexamic Acid	100 mg/ml (5 ml amps)	Haemostatic – for prevention or treatment of bleeding	1000–2000 mg/24 hours	• Limited compatibility data – infuse in separate syringe pump • Case report data only
Ketamine	10 mg/ml (20 ml vial) 50 mg/ml (10 ml vial) 100 mg/ml (10 ml vial)	Difficult to control cancer pain; especially of neuropathic origin on recommendation of palliative care specialist	Seek advice from specialist palliative care	• Inhibits NMDA receptor • Psychomimetic side effects (may need Midazolam/Haloperidol to cover) • Contra-indication in raised intra-cranial pressure and seizures • Caution in hypertension/cardiac problems • Irritant therefore dilute with sodium chloride 0.9% to largest possible volume

This list is not exhaustive; it covers many of the drugs used in palliative care. See other chapters for specific indications and usage.
SC = subcutaneous; GI = gastrointestinal; CSCI – continuous subcutaneous infusion
*Dosing in opioid naive patients should be based on regional and national guidance – physicians should always consider patient factors including renal function and frailty when deciding on dose to prescribe and implement appropriate dose reductions.

drowsiness, in this context these medications are used to help manage agitation and distress towards the end-of-life when non-pharmacological methods have not been successful.

> **Information Resources: Drug Compatibility in Palliative Care**
>
> - Wilcock A, Howard P, and Charlesworth S. *The Palliative Care Formulary (7th Ed.)* London: Pharmaceutical Press, 2020.
> - Dickman A and Schneider J. *The Syringe Pump: Continuous Subcutaneous Infusions in Palliative Care (4th Ed.)* Oxford: Oxford University Press, 2016.
> - www.palliativedrugs.com
> - www.pallmed.info
> - www.sign.ac.uk
> - www.medicinescomplete.com (access to electronic version of the PCF – subscription required).

For certain drugs, with long half-lives, for example, levomepromazine, dexamethasone, it may be more practical to administer via bolus injection once or twice daily. Certain characteristics can also make drugs less suitable for continuous infusion, for example, dexamethasone has the potential to cause psychological stimulation, meaning that infusion overnight may disturb sleep.

If following the commencement of an infusion the drug dosages need to be altered, a new syringe should be set up rather than altering the rate of the current infusion. Alteration of the rate will deliver all the drugs at an increased or decreased speed risking poor symptom management for the patient. Alteration of infusion rate will also affect the time of next refilling of the syringe, risking a period with no infused medication if the supply runs out before the next district or community nursing visit.

Compatibility and Stability of Medications used in Syringe Pumps

Combination of drugs in a single syringe for infusion is common practice within palliative care as it allows for multiple symptoms to be treated while reducing the need for multiple infusion devices and cannula sites, promoting patient acceptance and comfort.

Under the UK Medicines Act (1968) mixing of drugs in this way, whereby one drug is not a vehicle of administration for the other, as detailed in the summary of product characteristics, creates an unlicensed medicine. This legislation was amended following public consultation (MLX356)

when the MHRA along with the Commission on Human Medicines recommended that changes should be made to the original legislation. These changes apply to palliative care and other clinical areas where mixing of medications is accepted as standard practice; the changes allow prescribers to mix medicines and prescribe medications for mixing by other registered healthcare professionals [43]. When prescribing medicines intended to be mixed, the prescriber should:
- provide written instructions on how to do so
- must satisfy themselves that the person mixing and administering the medications is competent to undertake the task safely and effectively
- exercise due diligence to ensure compatibility information is checked using reputable information sources when recommending combinations of medications for subcutaneous infusion
- select a suitable diluent for the infusion

The responsibility for the potential consequences of prescribing medications beyond their marketing authorisation remains with the prescriber.

Consideration of the compatibility of drugs is vital to ensure efficacy of therapy. Interactions between drugs can be difficult to predict and may produce different effects, including a reduction in stability resulting in precipitation or crystallisation of the drug solution. This may cause the infusion cannula to become blocked, the injection site to become inflamed, and the treatment to be ineffective.

Many drug and dosage combinations have been used in syringe pumps. Access to compatibility databases such as on palliativedrugs.com has allowed for nationwide information sharing on drug combinations that may be successfully implemented for symptom management in palliative patients.

In the UK, drugs are usually diluted with water for injection unless there is a specific requirement to use sodium chloride. In particular, 0.9% saline should not be used to dilute cyclizine or higher concentrations of diamorphine (≥ 40 mg/ml) as there is a high risk of precipitation. The number of drugs combined in a single syringe should be kept to a minimum; advice should be sought from specialist palliative care professionals or medicines information pharmacists when using unusual drugs or combinations via syringe pump.

Most drugs used in syringe pumps are water soluble and can therefore be mixed. However, some drugs, for example, phenobarbital (made up in propylene glycol), are immiscible with aqueous solutions and should not be used in the same syringe as other drugs. Where situations arise that drug compatibility issues or volume restrictions limit the ability to mix several drugs in a single syringe; it is possible to use multiple infusion devices.

The major factor leading to incompatibility is the relative concentration of each drug. Other factors include pH, storage conditions, temperature, and ionic strength. Many salts in aqueous solution undergo degradation. Higher concentrations may lead to lower efficacy due to instability or precipitation of drugs. Correct storage temperatures should be observed for all drugs during the administration of the infusion. Where high concentrations of drugs are being infused, change in temperature (particularly cold) can reduce solubility and therefore induce precipitation of the drugs within the syringe. Exposure to high temperatures may also cause incompatibility reactions to occur. The syringe contents should also be protected from direct sunlight by placing in an opaque pouch, holster, or pocket to prevent photodegradation of the contents of the syringe. Physical examination of the contents, although a guide to compatibility, does not guarantee absence of chemical reaction [44–56].

If the contents of the syringe become cloudy or discoloured before or during infusion, the syringe should be discarded immediately. Should incompatibility problems persist, and alternative drugs or routes are not available, then a second syringe pump may be required to infuse drugs separately. Alternatively, the use of bolus injections may be considered if the drug has a longer duration of action, provided that the patient's skin condition will make bolus injections tolerable.

Site of the Infusion

An appropriate choice of infusion site will help to minimise site problems. Changing the infusion site may be necessary if it is painful or appears to be inflamed or swollen. The frequency of this will vary between patients and depend on the combination of drugs used. The extension set and needle should be changed at each resiting [57]. Should there be persistent problems with irritation at the injection site, consider the following options:
- Reducing the concentration of drugs (i.e. larger volume).
- Changing the drug or considering an alternative route.
- Mixing drugs with 0.9% saline (if compatible).
- Using a plastic (Teflon or Vialon) cannula.
- Applying hydrocortisone 1% cream to the skin around the needle entry site and covering it with an occlusive dressing.
- Adding dexamethasone 0.5–1 mg to the infusion (if compatible). Dexamethasone should not be routinely added to infusion solutions unless there is a specific problem with infusion sites [58] and palliative care teams should be involved with the decision-making.

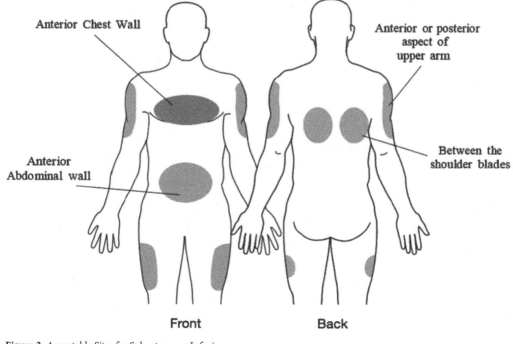

Figure 3 Acceptable Sites for Subcutaneous Infusion.

Choice of Site for the Infusion Cannula

Suitable sites for placement of the butterfly needle include:
- upper chest
- outer upper arm
- anterior abdomen
- thighs
- area over the scapula may be used in confused or disorientated patients

Avoid:
- deltoid area in bedbound patients who require regular turning
- sites over bony prominences in cachectic patients
- broken skin
- areas of inflammation
- recently irradiated areas
- tumour sites
- oedematous/lymphaedematous areas.

The exact placement may be influenced by the patient's preference, by the disease process and by common sense.

Management of Subcutaneous Infusions

Dedicated syringe pump monitoring charts should be used to ensure that the drug mixture is monitored throughout the infusion. It is essential that the following checks are made regularly:
- Drug and doses correct.
- Signs of irritation or inflammation at the injection site.
- Any evidence of leakage at the various connections.
- The pump is working (light flashing/intermittent motor noise).
- The set rate is correct and the corresponding amount of fluid infused.
- Any signs of crystallisation or precipitation (cloudiness).
- The tubing is not kinked.

The Gosport Report and Its Implications for Palliative Care

In 2018 the Gosport Independent Panel published a report following an investigation into the failings of care at Gosport War Memorial Hospital between 1988 and 2000. The implications of this report have far-reaching consequences for modern-day palliative care and highlight the importance of ensuring appropriate governance and safety practices are implemented by all healthcare professionals working with high risk medications including opioids.

The panel reported the following outcomes and practices of concern following their review [59, 60]:
- at least 450 patients are likely to have died after administration of inappropriate doses of opioid medications;
- opioids appear to have been initiated without appropriate clinical indication and documentation as to the rationale behind treatment;
- large dose ranges for medications were prescribed, allowing nursing staff with little training or knowledge in palliative care to initiate doses of opioids and sedatives with limited support from medical staff;
- patients were often administered combinations of medications via syringe pump at exceptionally high doses; the administration of these drugs, doses and combinations was directly linked to patient fatalities;
- once patients were started on a syringe pump, they were not reviewed clinically by a medical professional and doses were escalated regardless of patient response;
- the routine practice of prescribing excessively high doses of opioids without justifiable medical cause went unchallenged by pharmacists and consultants;
- none of this practice was patient-centred; the approach was consistent across all patients admitted regardless of clinical condition(s) and symptom need; because it suited the service that was available;
- concerns were raised by families and by some nursing staff at the hospital, but these went unaddressed by the hospital management, local police force, and the crown prosecution service, despite multiple investigations into the practices at the hospital.

The report highlighted that the indiscriminate use of medications via syringe pump was directly contributable to patient fatalities at the hospital; this prompted review within specialist palliative care to ensure the safety of local prescribing practices when administering drugs via continuous subcutaneous infusion.

The media reports of the events also raised concerns in patients and their families who were receiving specialist palliative care interventions at the time of the reports. Extra reassurances and communication skills were required during this period.

Since the events at Gosport War Memorial Hospital, and prior to the release of the report, person-centred pharmacy practice in hospital, hospice, and primary-care settings has significantly changed. Pharmacists have become key members of multi-disciplinary teams and are better placed to challenge inappropriate prescribing practice. Medication governance and assurance processes for the safe use of opioid medications have also strengthened since the events that occurred at Gosport [59–61].

Following the Shipman Inquiry in 2007 all organisations are now legally required to appoint a Controlled Drugs Accountable Officer (CDAO), whose role it is to manage the safe and secure handling of controlled drugs within the organisation. Controlled Drugs Local Intelligence Network (CDLIN)s have also been established to support sharing of information and areas of good practice. Implementation of electronic prescribing systems also supports with data collection and can analyse unusual patterns and trends in prescribing in ways which were not available during the time of the events at Gosport.

The practice of anticipatory prescribing of syringe pumps is now discouraged by the Association of Supportive and Palliative Care Pharmacists as the risks of this practice are thought to outweigh the benefits. The practice of range prescribing of medications for administration via syringe pump in generalist settings is also challenged.

It is important to constantly review and audit practices, whether as a healthcare professional or as an organisation, to ensure processes and management of patients with palliative care needs is appropriate, patient-centred, and safe.

Steroids in Palliative Care

Corticosteroids have been shown to be effective for a variety of uses in the palliative care setting. The most commonly used systemic corticosteroid in palliative care is dexamethasone. Research has shown that as many as 50% of patients with advanced disease may be prescribed systemic corticosteroids during their illness [62]. Common indications for steroid treatment in palliative care include:

- Raised intracranial pressure
- Anorexia
- Nausea and vomiting
- GI obstruction
- Liver capsular pain
- Raised SVCO
- Spinal cord compression

All patients prescribed corticosteroids should be given treatment for the shortest time using the lowest effective dose to limit the risk of inducing adrenal insufficiency [63]. Ongoing need for corticosteroids should be reviewed on a regular basis. When administering corticosteroids regularly they should be given once daily in the morning, or twice daily with the last dose before 2 p.m. as this reduces suppression of the hypopituitary-adrenal axis and may prevent corticosteroid-induced insomnia.

Dexamethasone has a higher glucocorticoid activity and insignificant mineralocorticoid effect compared to other corticosteroids [6] and is the best choice for clinical scenarios where high-dose anti-inflammatory treatment is required. Note that 2 mg oral dexamethasone is approximately equivalent to 15 mg oral prednisolone. It also has a longer duration of action which means doses are no more than once or twice a day. Alongside the potency which can mean fewer tablets, it helps aid medication compliance with administration.

A proton pump inhibitor (or H2-antagonist if available) should be co-prescribed with corticosteroids for all patients taking NSAIDS or those with two or more of the following risk factors [64]:

- Advanced malignancy
- Previous history of peptic ulcer disease.
- Starting dose of corticosteroids is equivalent to or greater than 8 mg dexamethasone.

Gastro-protection should also be considered for patients taking other drugs which increase the risk GI irritation and bleeding including: SSRIs, aspirin, anticoagulants, and bisphosphonates.

Side effects of corticosteroids include candida infection, weight gain, bruising, thinning of the skin, diabetes mellitus, proximal myopathy, and cushingoid features. Hyperglycaemia is a recognised side effect of corticosteroid therapy, in both diabetic and nondiabetic patients. It is therefore important to monitor glucose levels in all patients receiving regular corticosteroid therapy.

Corticosteroids should be discontinued once symptoms have resolved, or reduced to the lowest effective dose required. The Committee on Safety of Medicines (CSM) has recommended that systemic corticosteroids should be gradually withdrawn in patients who have received treatment for longer than three weeks.

For patients struggling to take tablets there are two options – licensed oral liquids are available (N.B.: different strengths are available therefore check carefully the strength a patient tells you due to risk of errors) or the tablets can be dissolved in water (unlicensed use).

For patients unable to take oral dexamethasone, doses of less than 8 mg may be administered via a bolus subcutaneous injection. If a greater dose is required, dexamethasone can be given twice daily subcutaneously (morning and lunchtime).

Dexamethasone injection is available as 3.3 mg/ml (1 and 2 ml amps) and 3.8 mg/ml (1 ml amps). To convert between PO and SC routes, both 3.3 mg and 3.8 mg dexamethasone *base* of the injectable formulations can be considered approximately equivalent to dexamethasone *base* 4 mg PO. This is to avoid wastage of volumes and complexity of drug calculations in preparing the dose [6].

For patients in the dying phase of their illness where they may be moribund and no longer able to take medication, it is generally acceptable to discontinue corticosteroids abruptly [6, 65, 66], maintenance doses may be required to prevent withdrawal syndrome and/or where their clinical condition/symptom control indicates steroids to continue, for example, brain tumour and brain metastases which may be causing seizures and headaches.

Monitoring Required with Corticosteroids

- For courses over seven days, monitor blood glucose regularly during treatment (e.g. every 1–2 weeks), particularly in patients at risk of diabetes [6].
- Monitor for symptoms which might indicate hyperglycaemia, for example, increased thirst, increased frequency of micturition.
- Steroid-induced diabetes will require medication management alongside the continued use of the steroids, remembering that as the steroids are weaned down/withdrawn, so too will the diabetes medication need to be adjusted. Diabetes UK have produced guidance to support [67].

Controlled Drugs

Controlled drugs (CDs) in the UK are subject to the requirements of the Misuse of Drugs Regulations 2001. The legislation categorises these drugs into five schedules [24, 68].

Prescriptions written by non-medical prescribers can be prescribed on the green FP10SS or purple FP10PN/FP10SP prescriptions forms [69].

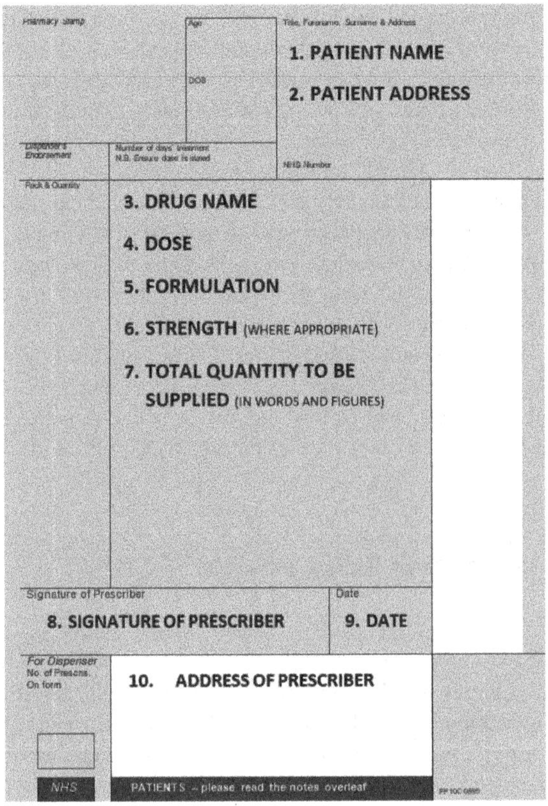

Figure 4 CD Requirements.

The legal requirements for prescriptions for controlled drugs in schedules 2 and 3 to be valid are outlined in Figure 4. It is an offence for a prescriber to issue an incomplete prescription and it is illegal for a pharmacist to dispense a CD unless all the information required by law is given on the prescription.

Table 2 Categories of Controlled drugs list - GOV.UK (www.gov.uk)

Schedule 1	LSD and ecstasy-type substances – have virtually no therapeutic use	
Schedule 2	Principal opioids and major stimulants	Medical and dental prescribers are allowed prescribe all CDs in schedules 2–5 for the purpose of treating organic disease.
Schedule 3	Most barbiturates plus buprenorphine, midazolam, tramadol, and temazepam. Gabapentin and pregabalin since 2019 due to concerns around increasing abuse of these medications	Nurse and pharmacist independent prescribers can prescribe, administer, and give directions for the administration of Schedule 2–5 CDs for the purpose of treating organic disease or injury since 2012.
Schedule 4	Mainly benzodiazepines	
Schedule 5	Low dose and dilute preparations of some of the schedule 2 drugs e.g. morphine sulfate oral solution 10 mg/5 ml	

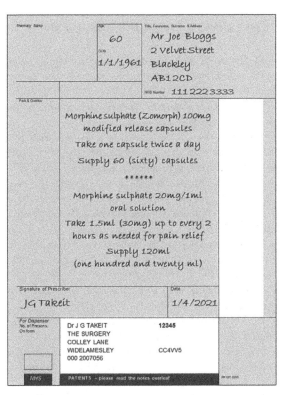

Figure 5 Example of completed FP10 for oral controlled drugs.

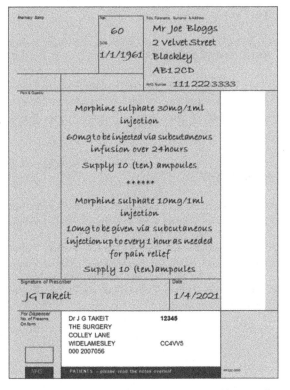

Figure 6 Example of completed FP10 for injectable controlled drugs.

For CDs in schedules 2 and 3 prescribers must specify the quantity of medication they want dispensed in both words and figures, the RPS advises that it is best practice to prescribe in terms of dosage units [24]. Failure to comply with the regulations will result in inconvenience to the patient and delay in supplying the necessary medicines.

Prescriptions written for CDs in schedules 2–4 are valid for 28 day after the date on the prescription, it is considered good practice to supply only an appropriate amount for the needs of the patient and if more than 30 days' supply is given, then a note to justify the reason should be included in the patient records [24].

Examples of completed CD prescriptions are shown in Figures 5 and 6.

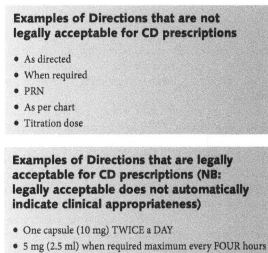

Examples of Directions that are not legally acceptable for CD prescriptions

- As directed
- When required
- PRN
- As per chart
- Titration dose

Examples of Directions that are legally acceptable for CD prescriptions (NB: legally acceptable does not automatically indicate clinical appropriateness)

- One capsule (10 mg) TWICE a DAY
- 5 mg (2.5 ml) when required maximum every FOUR hours
- 10 mg subcut prn for pain every TWO hours

Taking CDs Abroad

If a patient travelling abroad requires more than three calendar months' supply of CD, the licencing law requires the patient to seek a licence from the Home Office. The licence however has no legal status outside the United Kingdom and does not ensure safe passage through the customs of the country of destination. The patient must contact the Embassy or High Commission in the United Kingdom to clarify the requirements for taking CDs through the customs of the destination country or countries [24].

Unwanted Medicines or Disposal of CDs after a Death at Home

A patient or their representative may return unwanted medicines, to a community pharmacist for destruction. Because CDs are the property of the patient they should, where possible, be returned for destruction by the patient or the patient's representative, unless there are concerns that leaving these medications in the patients' home after their death creates a risk of misappropriation of these medications for example known history of substance abuse [24, 70].

The Role of Pharmacy in Future Palliative Care

The pharmacy team are essential to palliative care teams in hospital, hospice, and community services. Their role has advanced from that of medicines management to include clinical advice and treatment management alongside information provision to empower patients.

Supporting patients at their preferred place of care, often home, means that services must adapt to this need, demonstrated with the recent COVID-19 pandemic. The role of the pharmacist is not only in the strategic side of co-ordinating services to help access medicines or providing support to generalist teams with complex specialist medicines, but has now advanced into consultant roles with pharmacists managing their own caseloads of patients either as in-patients, outpatient clinics, or home visits.

Research in palliative care has also developed over the years and now with interest not only in assessing the impact of services but also in new therapies, there is an opportunity for pharmacists to be involved from a quantitative and qualitative perspective.

Initiatives to support access to medicines at home especially around carer administration of symptom control medicines (e.g. CARiAD study [71]) provides opportunities for pharmacists and pharmacy technicians to support and educate those involved.

Strategic input into process mapping of patient journeys, commissioning services and national projects is key to keeping the pharmacist at the frontline of innovation alongside their healthcare colleagues.

Key Learnings from the Chapter

- Medicines Management and Medicines Optimisation involve healthcare professionals and patients/carers/families.
- The pharmacy team play a key role in specialist palliative care service delivery.
- Anticipatory planning is essential and appropriate prescribing and availability of symptom control medicines can reduce distress or inappropriate admissions.
- Controlled Drugs have multiple legal requirements and their risk of diversion is high – consideration needs to be given to this while not denying patients access to essential medicines.
- Staff involved need to be competent and trained in the medicines they are using within their practice – unfamiliarity can lead to errors and patient harm. Local guidance and key resources need to be available. "Off-label" prescribing and evidence base needs to be clear.
- Syringe pumps/CSCIs remain the mainstay of delivering consistent symptom control.
- It is imperative to keep communication channels open when patients are considering using CBD/CAMs and to ask them to keep HCPs informed if they are using it.
- Wherever possible, deprescribing should be performed as a partnership between the patient (and carer) and the prescriber.

Acknowledgements

This chapter has been updated from the previous edition written by Dr Christine Hirsch and Dr Maria McKenna. Some content of the original chapter remains with permission.

References

1. Royal College of Nursing. *Medicines Management*. Available from: https://www.rcn.org.uk/clinical-topics/medicines-management (accessed 11 April 2021).
2. National Institute for Health and Clinical Excellence. (2015). *Medicines optimisation: the safe and effective use of medicines to enable the best possible outcomes.* (NICE Guideline – NG5). Available from: https://www.nice.org.uk/guidance/ng5/chapter/Introduction (accessed 11 April 2021).

3. National Institute for Health and Clinical Excellence. (2016) *Medicines optimisation.* (NICE Quality Standard). Available from: https://www.nice.org.uk/guidance/qs120/resources/medicines-optimisation-pdf-75545351857861 (accessed 11 April 2021).

4. Royal Pharmaceutical Society. (2013) *Medicines optimisation: helping patients to make the most of medicines.* Available from: https://www.rpharms.com/Portals/0/RPS%20document%20library/Open%20access/Policy/helping-patients-make-the-most-of-their-medicines.pdf (Accessed 11 April 2021).

5. Thompson, J. (2019). Deprescribing in palliative care. *Clinical Medicine* 19 (4): 311–314.

6. Wilcock, A., Howard, P., and Charlesworth, S. (2020). *Palliative Care Formulary*, 7e. London: Pharmaceutical Press.

7. Atkinson, C. and Kirkham, S. (1999). Unlicensed uses for medication in a palliative care unit. *Palliative Medicine* 13: 145–152.

8. Todd, J. and Davies, A. (1999). Use of unlicensed medication in palliative medicine. *Palliative Medicine* 13: 466.

9. General Medical Council. (2013). Good practice in prescribing and managing medicines and devices. www.gmc-uk.org (accessed 11 April 2021).

10. Royal Pharmaceutical Society (2016). A competency framework for all prescribers. www.rpharms.com (accessed 11 April 2021).

11. Royal Pharmaceutical Society (2016). Prescribing specials. Guidance for the prescribers of specials. www.rpharms.com (accessed 11 April 2021).

12. The British Pain Society (2012). *Use of medicines outside of their UK marketing authorisation in pain management and palliative medicine.* Available from: https://www.britishpainsociety.org/static/uploads/resources/files/useofmeds_professional_final.pdf (accessed 11 April 2021).

13. Aronson, J. (2007). Compliance, concordance, adherence. *British Journal of Clinical Phamacology* 63 (4): 383–384.

14. Bergman-Evans, B. (2006). AIDES to improving medication adherence in older adults. *Geriatric Nursing* 27: 174–182.

15. Furmedge, D. (2018). Evidence and tips on the use of medication compliance aids. *BMJ* 362.

16. Lecouturier. (2011). Medication compliance aids: a qualitative study of users' views. *British Journal of General Practice* 61 (583): 93–100.

17. Cramer, J. (1998). Enhancing patient compliance aids in the elderly: role of packaging aids and monitoring. *Drugs Aging* 12 (1): 7–15.

18. Thompson, W. and Farrell, B. (2013). Deprescribing: what is it and what does the evidence tell us? *Canadian Journal of Hospital Pharmacy* 66 (3): 201–202.

19. Phippen, A., Pickard, J., Steinke, D. et al. Identifying, highlighting, and reducing polypharmacy in a UK hospice inpatient unit using improvement Science methods. *BMJ Open Quality 2017* 6. doi: 10.1136/bmjquality.u211783.w5035. published Online First 10 March 2017.

20. Dees, M.K., Geijetman, E.C.T., Dekkers, W.J.M. et al. (2018). Perspectives of patients, close relatives, nurses, and physicians on end-of-life medication management. *Palliative and Supportive Care* 16: 580–589.

21. Gao, L., Maidment, I., Mathews, F.E. et al. (2018). Medication usage change in older people (65+) in England over 20 years: findings from CFAS I and CFAS II. *Age and Ageing* 47: 220–225.

22. Todd et al. (2012). I don't think I'd be frightened if the statins went. *BMC Palliative Care* 15: 13.

23. Lindsay, J. et al. (2014). The development and evaluation of an oncological palliative care deprescribing guideline: the "OncPal deprescribing guideline". *Support Cancer Care* doi: 10.1007/s00520-014-2322-0.

24. Royal Pharmaceutical Society. (2019). *Medicines, Ethics and Practice*, 43e. London: Pharmaceutical Press.

25. Molassiotis, A., Fernadez-Ortega, P., Pud, D. et al. (2005). Use of complementary and alternative medicine in cancer patients: a European survey. *Annals of Oncology* 16: 655–663.

26. Muecke, R., Paul, M., Conrad, C. et al. (2016). Complementary and alternative medicine in palliative care. a comparison of data from surveys among patients and professionals. *Integrative Cancer Therapies* 15 (1): 10–16.

27. Delgado-Lopez, P. and Corrales-Garcia, E. (2018). Influence of internet and social media in the promotion of alternative oncology, cancer quackery, and the predatory publishing phenomenon. *Cureus* 10 (5).

28. Millar, S.A., Stone, N.L., Bellman, Z.D., Yates, A.S., England, T.J., and O'Sullivan, S.E. (2019). A systematic review of cannabidiol dosing in clinical populations. *British Journal of Clinical Pharmacology* 85 (9): 1888–1900.

29. Parliamentary and Health Service Ombudsman. *Dying without dignity Investigations by the Parliamentary and Health Service Ombudsman into complaints about end of life care.* Available from: https://www.ombudsman.org.uk/sites/default/files/Dying_without_dignity.pdf (accessed 11 April 2021).

30. Specialist Pharmacy Service. Practice examples for using alternative supply routes for end of life medicines. Available from: https://www.sps.nhs.uk/articles/practice-examples-for-using-alternative-supply-routes-for-end-of-life-medicines (accessed 11 April 2021).

31. Russell, P.S.B. (1979). Analgesia in terminal malignant disease. *BMJ* 1: 1561.

32. Dickinson, R.J., Howard, B., and Campbell, J. (1984). The relief of pain by subcutaneous infusion of diamorphine. In: *Advances in Morphine Therapy The 1983 International Symposium on Pain Control. Royal Society of Medicine International Symposium Series*, 64 (ed. E. Wilkes and J. Lenz), 105–110. London: Royal Society of Medicine.

33. Oliver, D.J. (1985). The use of the syringe driver in terminal care. *British Journal of Clinical Pharmacology* 20: 515–516.

34. Coyle, N., Mauskop, A., Maggard, J. et al. (1986). Continuous subcutaneous infusions of opiates in cancer patients with pain. *Oncology Nursing Forum* 13: 53–57.

35. Beswick, D.T. (1987). Use of syringe driver in terminal care. *Pharmacology Journal* 239: 656–658.

36. Bruera, E., Brenneis, C., Michaud, M. et al. (1987). Continuous subcutaneous infusion of narcotics using a portable disposable device in patients with advanced cancer. *Cancer Treatment Rep* June 1987; 71: 635–637.

37. Bottomley, D.M. and Hanks, G.W. (1990). Subcutaneous midazolam infusion in palliative care. *Journal Pain Symptom Manage* 5 (4): 259–261.

38. National Patients Safety Agency. (2010). Available at: http://www.nrls.npsa.nhs.uk/alerts/?entryid45=92908 (accessed 11 April 2021).

39. Dickman, A. and Schneider, J. (2016). *The Syringe Driver: Continuous Subcutaneous Infusions in Palliative Care*, 4e. Oxford: Oxford University Press.

40. SIGN Guideline 106. (2008). Control of pain in adults with cancer: Scottish Intercollegiate Guidelines Network, Scottish Cancer Therapy Network. Available at: www.sign.ac.uk (2008).

41. Back, I. (2011). www.pallmed.netDrugcompatibilitydatabase.

42. PalliativeDrugs.Com. *Syringe driver survey database*. Available at: https://www.palliativedrugs.com/syringe-driver-database-introduction.html. (accessed 11 April 2021).

43. MHRA. Public consultation (MLX356). (2009). *Proposal for amendments to medicines legislation to allow mixing of medicines in palliative care*. Available at: Medical and non-medical prescribing: mixing medicines in clinical practice - GOV.UK (www.gov.uk) (accessed 11 April 2021).

44. Allwood, M.C. (1984). Diamorphine mixed with antiemetic drugs in plastic syringes. *British Journal of Pharmacology Practical* 6: 88–90.

45. Collins, A.J., Abethell, J.A., Holmes, S.G. et al. (1986). Stability of diamorphine hydrochloride with haloperidol in prefilled syringes for subcutaneous infusion. *Journal of Pharmacology* 38 (Suppl.): 51.

46. Regnard, C., Pashley, S., and Westrope, E. (1986). Anti-emetic/diamorphine compatibility in infusion pumps. *British of Journal Pharmacology Practical* 8: 218–220.

47. Allwood, M.C. (1991). The compatibility of high dose diamorphine with cyclizine or haloperidol in plastic syringes. *International Journal of Pharmacology Practical* 5: 120.

48. Allwood, M.C. (1991). The stability of diamorphine alone and in combination with antiemetics in plastic syringes. *Palliative Medicine* 5: 330–333.

49. Allwood, M.C., Brown, P.C., and Lee, M. (1994). Stability of injections containing diamorphine and midazolam in plastic syringes. *International Journal of Pharmacology Practical* 3: 57–59.

50. Fielding, H., Kyaterekera, N., Skellern, G. et al. (2000). The compatibility and stability of octreotide acetate in the presence of diamorphine hydrochloride in polypropylene syringes. *Palliative Medicine* 14: 205–207.

51. Smith, J., Hirsch, C., Marriott, J. et al. (2000). The stability of diamorphine and glycopyrrolate in PCA syringes. *Pharmacology Journal* 265: R69.

52. Negro, S., Reyes, R., Azuara, M. et al. (2006). Morphine, haloperidol, hyoscine N-butylbromide combined in s.c. infusion solutions: Compatibility and stability. *International Journal of Pharmacology* 307: 278–284.

53. Grassby, P.F. and Hutchings, L. (1997). Drug combinations in syringe drivers: the compatibility and stability of diamorphine with cyclizine and haloperidol. *Palliative Medicine* 11: 217–224.

54. Fawcett, J.P., Woods, D.J., Munasiri, B. et al. (1994). Compatibility of cyclizine lactate and haloperidol lactate. *American Jouranl of Hospital of Pharmacy* 51: 2292.

55. Grassby, P.F. (1996). Personal communication.

56. Gardiner, P.R. (2003). Compatibility of an injectable oxycodone formulation with typical diluents, syringes, tubings, infusion bags and drugs for potential co-administration. *Hospital Pharmacy* 10: 354–361.

57. Mitten, T. (2001). Subcutaneous infusions: A review of problems and solutions. *International Jouranl of Palliative Nursing* 7 (2): 75–85.

58. Reymond, L., Charles, M.A., Bowman, J. et al. (2003). The effect of dexamethasone on the longevity of syringe driver subcutaneous sites in palliative care patients. *Medical Jouranl of Australia* 178: 486–489.

59. Panel, G.I. (2018). *Gosport Independent Panel Report*. London: s.n. Available at: https://www.gosportpanel.independent.gov.uk (accessed 11 April 2021).

60. Royal Pharmaceutical Society. *Gosport Report*. Available at: https://www.rpharms.com/about-us/who-we-are/expert-advisors/hospital-expert-advisory-group/gosport-report (accessed 11 April 2021).

61. Godlee, F. (2018). Lessons from Gosport. *BMJ* 362: K2923.

62. Hanks, G.W., Trueman, T., and Twycross, R.G. (1983). Corticosteroids in terminal cancer – a prospective analysis of current practice. *Postgraduate Medical Journal* 59: 702–706.

63. Committee on Safety of Medicines and Medicines Control Agency. (1998). Withdrawal of systemic corticosteroids. *Current Problems in Pharmacovigilance* 24: 5–7.

64. Ellershaw, J.E. and Kelly, M.J. (1994). Corticosteroids and peptic ulceration. *Palliative Medical* 8 (4): 313–319.

65. (2009). Merseyside and Cheshire palliative care network audit group. *Corticosteroids in Palliative Care*. Expert Consensus.

66. Rousseau, P. (2004). Sudden withdrawal of corticosteroids: A commentary. *American Journal of Hospice and Palliative Care* 21: 169–171.

67. Diabetes UK. (2018). End of life diabetes care: clinical care recommendations. Available at: UKhttps://www.diabetes.org.uk/professionals/position-statements-reports/diagnosisongoing-management-monitoring/end-of-life-care (accessed November 2021).

68. National Prescribing Centre. (2009). *A Guide to Good Practice in the Management of Controlled Drugs in Primary Care*, 3e. England: National Prescribing Centre. (accessed 11 April 2021).

69. Pharmaceutical Services Negotiating Committee. *Is this prescription form valid?* Available at: https://psnc.org.uk/dispensing-supply/receiving-a-prescription/is-this-prescription-form-valid (accessed 11 April 2021).

70. Care Quality Commission. *Disposing of medicines.* Available at: https://www.cqc.org.uk/guidance-providers/adult-social-care/disposing-medicines (accessed 11 April 2021).

71. Poolman, M. et al. (2019). CARer-ADministration of as-needed subcutaneous medication for breakthrough symptoms in homebased dying patients (CARiAD): study protocol for a UK-based open randomised pilot trial. *Trials* 20 (1): 105.

Further Reading

1. Ashley, C. and Dunleavy, A. (2018). *The Renal Drug Handbook: The Ultimate Prescribing Guide for Renal Practitioners*, 5e. CRC Press.

2. Bernard, S.A. and Bruera, E. (2000). Drug interactions in palliative care. *Journal of Clinical Oncology* 18 (8): 1780–1799.

3. *British National Formulary.* Guidance on prescribing in terminal care (in the first section of the book).

4. Centre for Palliative Care Research and Education. (2010). Queensland health. In: *Guidelines for Subcutaneous Device Management in Palliative Care*, 2e. Australian Government Department of Health and Ageing. Available at: www.health.qld.gov.au/cpcre (accessed 11 April 2021).

5. NHS Scotland. (2010). Palliative care guidelines – Subcutaneous infusion of medication via a McKinley pump or syringe driver. Available at: Syringe Driver Pump – West Midlands Palliative Care (westmidspallcare.co.uk) (accessed 11 April 2021).

6. Smyth, J. (2015). *The NEWT Guidelines for administration of medication to patients with enteral feeding tubes or swallowing difficulties.* 3e.

7. Trissel, L.A. (2011). *Handbook on Injectable Drugs*, 16e. Houston, TX: American Society of Health System Pharmacists Inc.

8. Urie, J., Feilding, H., McArthur, D., et al. (2000). Palliative care. *Pharmacology Journal* 256: 603–614.

9. Watson, M., Lucas, C., Hoy, A., et al. (2011). palliative care guidelines plus. Available at: http://book.pallcare.info/index.php (accessed 11 April 2021).

22 Spirituality in Palliative Care

Margaret Holloway

Introduction

Spiritual care has been embedded in palliative care from the outset. In Cicely Saunders' vision for hospice she talked about "total care for total pain," delivered by a multidisciplinary team which included a chaplain alongside clinicians and others. Spiritual care is included in definitions of palliative care [1–4], including for children, which the WHO defines as, "active total care of the child's body, mind and spirit" [1 p. 13].

A chaplain is identified as one of the core professions in today's multidisciplinary palliative care team [5] while at the same time competency in spiritual care is included in standards for other disciplines [6, 7]. Service delivery programmes specify its inclusion, including the recording of spiritual needs and preferences [8, 9]. Indeed, it is argued that suffering and distress at the end-of-life cannot be alleviated without a "deep knowledge of the nature of suffering," integrating spiritual perspectives alongside psychological and socio-cultural [10 p. 799].

In its origins, Saunders' vision was simple. Both nursing and social work trace their beginnings in charitable religious foundations and ministering to the dying and bereaved has always been a significant element in the religious pastoral role, across all religions. However, in contemporary palliative care, the progressive secularisation of western societies alongside greater awareness within palliative care of the complexities of working in contexts of religious and cultural pluralism, combined with crossing of boundaries between health and care professions, have led to a more complex scenario [11, 12]. Questions are raised for the clinical team which have very real import in practice.

- What do we *actually mean* by spiritual care?
- How do we recognise spiritual need?

- How do we distinguish spiritual pain and distress from emotional or psychological needs?

In fact, *what is the evidence* that spiritual care should remain an embedded part of palliative care and how do the research findings of academics translate into the daily realities of diverse palliative care settings across the globe?

Assuming that we can find answers to those dilemmas,
- Who is best placed to address those needs, especially if the patient or family does not identify as religious?

Yet who except a dedicated religious or spiritual advisor has the skills or capacity to offer spiritual care in the daily round of palliative care? This chapter will seek to unpack these questions before returning to the holistic vision which remains at the heart of modern palliative care across the globe.

Understanding Spirituality

Despite the fact that much spirituality research continues to be concerned with definitions and concepts, finding one definition of spirituality which is universally acceptable has been "notoriously difficult" [13] and practitioners commonly find the notion of spirituality too vague [14–16]. However, there *is* consensus over elements within different definitions [17, 18] which provide clues to usefully understand spirituality in the clinical or practice setting.

First, something as "basic" [14] as spirituality, which relates to the essence of our being [19], which is experienced in community *and* resonates with personal cultural scripts [20, 21], cannot be reduced to a "one size fits all" concept. Nevertheless, shared "psycho-spiritual" elements [22] can be found within each of the world's religions and "humanistic spirituality" "allows for both secular and religious orientations to find common ground in the notion of what it is to be human" [13, 23, 24]. Explorations of

Handbook of Palliative Care, Fourth Edition. Edited by Richard Kitchen, Christina Faull, Sarah Russell and Jo Wilson.
© 2024 John Wiley & Sons Ltd. Published 2024 by John Wiley & Sons Ltd.

spiritual practice in contemporary society suggest that death is one of the key factors in understanding this phenomenon [25]. Our task as practitioners, is, first, to understand our own spirituality in the face of death, from which foundation we can reach out to connect with the spirituality of the other person [21].

Fundamentally, this is about finding meaning within what may be chaotic, contradictory, or at first sight senseless. There is plentiful evidence that the process of seeking and finding meaning is a constant and enduring feature of human existence [26] which, in contemporary secularised societies, manifests as the creation of personalised meanings out of the spiritual traditions and resources which are available [27].

Other approaches to conceptualising spirituality focus on its attributes, for example, love, joy, peace, hope. Discussions of spirituality and spiritual care at the end-of-life emphasise meaning and connectedness but draw these attributes into the process. For example, the US National Consensus Project on Palliative Care defined spirituality as:

> "…the aspect of humanity that refers to the way individuals seek and express meaning and purpose and the way they experience their connectedness to the moment, to self, to others, to nature, and to the significant or sacred." [28 p. 887]

Cicely Saunders has been credited with promoting this concept of spirituality as meaning-making [29], representing the despair of the dying person as spiritual pain. This brings us to another aspect of spirituality – that it is intrinsically bound up with the darkness of life, including the suffering of those with terminal disease. Those definitions of spirituality which emphasise its positive force may, at first reading, jar with the realities of dying in circumstances (such as pandemic) when all that counts for best practice appears to be undermined. Some writers deal with this by "embracing the paradox" of death [30] and seeking to understand the relationship between negative and positive feelings and experienced spirituality [31].

From my own practice and research into spirituality in death, dying, and bereavement, I have reached the conclusion that it is useful to understand spirituality as a coming-together of three dimensions [32]:

• Spirituality is concerned with meaning and purpose, in particular, the *search* for meaning.
• Spirituality is experienced through relationships, and those relationships may be with an external or "higher" source, or sources of spiritual strength may be found in families, friends, or communities.
• Spirituality promotes certain behaviours and practices, within oneself and also towards the other person.

The European Association for Palliative Care takes a similar approach, describing spiritual care as multi-factorial and embracing [33]:

• Existential challenges (e.g. questions concerning identity, meaning, suffering and death, guilt and shame, reconciliation and forgiveness, freedom and responsibility, hope and despair, love and joy).
• Value-based considerations and attitudes (what is most important for each person, such as relationships with oneself, family, friends, work, nature, art and culture, ethics and morals, and life itself).
• Religious considerations and foundations (faith, beliefs, and practices, the relationship with God or the ultimate).

We shall explore these dimensions further in this chapter to seek out how, as health and care practitioners, friends and family, we can offer spiritual care which may transform the negativity of dying and bereavement by illuminating its darkness.

Assessment of Spiritual Need

A literature review of spiritual care at the end-of-life [14] found that tools which help identify spiritual need are popular with practitioners. Both language and emphasis have shifted from Cicely Saunders' identification of spiritual *pain* to an approach which looks at spirituality as both resource and potential root problem. (Table 1).

Narrative and Biographical Approaches

In keeping with the hospice and palliative care philosophy of helping a person to live until they die, of focusing on those things which are important to this individual and their family, tools which derive from narrative and biographical

Table 1 Assessing spirituality as both resource and problem.

Purpose of assessment	Outcome of assessment
Facilitate connection with spiritual resources within self, family, and community	*Strength and support*
Identify unmet spiritual needs and what might meet those needs	*Holistic care*
Identifying where deep spiritual distress is source of agitation	*Spiritual care the priority in restoring well-being*

approaches have been widely used. For example, broad, general questions might be used to elicit sources of meaning or comfort in the person's life. The FICA [34] and HOPE [35] tools both use a mnemonic as a shorthand device.

The FICA Assessment Tool

This suggests four sets of questions stemming from the domains of:

 i) Faith, belief, and meaning
 ii) Importance (of faith) and influence
 iii) Community
 iv) Addressing these issues/actioning a care plan.

In each area, the practitioner or clinician begins with trying to ascertain the importance of faith or a faith community in the person's life. Where the person does not identify any formal religious background, the questioning moves to trying to establish what are alternative sources of meaning or broader spiritual support in their life.

The HOPE Assessment Tool

By contrast, the HOPE tool starts from broader sources of hope and meaning (under the heading "sources of hope, meaning, comfort, strength, peace, love and connection") and in so doing establishes whether religious faith is one of these and if so, how important it is. For example, the practitioner/clinician may ask what helps to sustain the person in difficult times and may specifically ask whether organised religion is one of their sources of support. If the answer is "yes," under the heading "Organised religion," questions are used to delve into *how* it is that their faith helps, whether they derive significant support from a faith community, for example, or, indeed, whether some aspects (such as attending religious services) are not important. If, however, the person points to the prime importance of friends and family, for example, the assessment moves into looking at "Personal spirituality or practices," independent of organised religion. It is important to remember (although the tool does not make this clear) that these personal practices may co-exist with participation in formal religion or they may serve as an alternative spirituality. For this reason, the first section of the assessment, which looks broadly at sources of meaning and sustenance, is extremely important, and, skilfully conducted, should lead gently into the deepest hopes and fears of the person facing death. The fourth section, "Effects on medical care and end-of-life issues," allows the clinician/practitioner to explore the implications of the spiritual or faith position which the person has shared, for their treatment.

Both these tools take the same approach of seeking out the spiritual resources which this person has to draw upon and facilitating or strengthening their access to them, taking account of beliefs which the person holds which have important implications for their treatment, especially end-of-life care decisions.

Spiritual Pain or Distress

Narrative and biographical approaches are also useful in illuminating the pain of deep spiritual distress. Spiritual pain has been described as,

> "pain operating at a deeper level of consciousness … manifest in a wide variety of symptoms such as constant and chronic pain; withdrawal or isolation from spiritual support systems; conflict with family members and friends; anxiety, fear or mistrust; anger; self-loathing; hopelessness; feelings of failure … unforgiveness; despair; and fear or dread" [36 p. 4].

The key to determining that what is being manifested is *spiritual* distress, as well as the emotional and psychological affects, is that gentle probing will uncover a religious or spiritual issue at its root or core.

Certain factors commonly promote spiritual distress and may, when combined, promote crisis:
- Loss of a faith which was once important in the person's life;
- A sense of alienation, dissonance, or deep conflict in the inner self;
- A need to find answers leading to wrestling with unresolved questions, sometimes referred to as the "groanings" of the soul;
- A model of an external deity or force which is punishing, unforgiving, disappointed, manipulative, and controlling [37]. However, it is important to balance appropriate psychiatric care for depression at end-of-life with separate recognition of existential despair, in which complete desolation, profound meaninglessness, hopelessness, helplessness, and powerlessness may be experienced [38]. The following story (Box 1) illustrates how a psychiatrist and art therapist worked together to address the deep pain manifested in depression and existential despair.

Holding to a model of a negative external deity or force is commonly associated with a history of abuse or very strict religious upbringing and has been described as "negative religious coping" [39]. Box 2 illustrates how the spiritual care advisor was able to help the patient find peace by connecting her with other elements of her faith.

Box 1: A journey out of despair

Tim developed a brain tumour at the age of 30. He became withdrawn when diagnosed, including with his wife. Following psychiatric in-patient treatment for severe depression, Tim was referred to Ella, an art therapist working in palliative care. The psychiatric episode appeared to have been triggered by existential despair – Tim had been brought up to believe that if he worked hard, the rewards would follow, and now he felt both cheated and a failure. When he started to draw after about a month, he became very anxious and at times angry and frustrated. Ella sees her role as being available to the patient, as a resource or companion on their therapeutic journey. With Tim, she tried to create a calm accepting environment in which his drawings could be lodged, although he then discarded them. Two days before he died, Tim did one final drawing which he presented to Ella for her to keep. Ella believes that Tim had finally found a new way of valuing his life. He appeared to be reconciled with himself as well as with his wife.

Models of Spiritual Care

In addition to models for assessing spiritual need, there are numerous models designed to guide practitioners in addressing those needs and providing spiritual support. Sometimes this will be as part of a comprehensive

Box 2: Finding forgiveness and peace

Sandra was a woman in her 50s suffering from an inoperable brain tumour. She had already lost her sight when admitted to the hospice. Maureen, the spiritual care advisor, was called in by the nurses because of Sandra's extreme agitation, screaming pronouncements of a religious nature – "I'm going to burn in hell." Sandra and her husband, David, belonged to a Christian evangelical church. She appeared to be in spiritual anguish. Maureen did not attempt to engage in spiritual ministry through conversation but by gently holding and stroking Sandra's face, repeatedly assuring her that she was "safe and secure." This was the only thing which calmed Sandra, and the nurses, who had felt there was little they could do for Sandra, began to do the same. When Sandra died, a fortnight after her admission, she was peaceful. The funeral reflected her spiritual life as a singer and song-writer and Maureen found it uplifting.

assessment and holistic model of care and sometimes the spiritual needs may be the starting point. People have a diversity of spiritual need and thus require support from a range of practitioners (see a model for interdisciplinary

working [40]) with differing levels of skill, as in the Marie Curie Religious and Spiritual Competencies model [41]. This identifies four levels of interaction that take place in the hospice and the different competencies which are required at each level. This starts with a basic awareness of spiritual need and the listening and communication skills to engage with patients about these, which, it argues, are required of all staff or volunteers in their casual contacts with patients, their families, and carers; Box 3 provides an example of this level of interaction. The complexity progresses from there through the ability to recognise and refer "difficult needs" and develop a spiritual care plan to address those needs (see Box 1 for a case example) to the fourth level, appropriate only for those staff or volunteers whose primary responsibility is spiritual and religious care, whether of patients, visitors, or other staff. At this level, the worker may expect to be engaging with complex spiritual and existential needs; Box 2 and the Fellow Traveller *Interpreting* stage provide case examples of this level.

Popular among practitioners is the notion of spiritual companioning. The fellow traveller model of spiritual companioning (Figure 1) illustrates how different practitioners with their varying skillsets may, together, carry out spiritual care in practice.

By asking the question "What can I do for you?" and in careful listening to the answer, all practitioners can identify if and when another person on the team might be better able to meet this person's needs [42]; however, as emphasised in the Fellow Traveller model, this does not have to mean that the original team member withdraws, but that they work together with a colleague to best support the different aspects of care.

So how do these models help in the everyday realities of practice? Commonly, practitioners report that they do not feel equipped to address spiritual issues [43–45]. It is important to find a model or approach which is both do-able and inclusive. That means, one with which the individual worker feels comfortable and which can be delivered within their particular work environment [46, 47] and, most importantly, can be adapted so as to be appropriate for the individual person in their family, community, and cultural context. The "models" presented in this chapter in fact do just that, and their different approaches can be combined.

What they do not offer is step-by-step guidance as to what the worker might do or say at any given moment or in any particular circumstance. However, the following three principles, all of which are embedded within the tools and models presented in this chapter, offer a framework:

JOINING

Spiritual awareness. Start where the person is.

Appropriate for every worker

Robert is a palliative care consultant physician. He is treating Luke, a young man with an aggressive osteo-sarcoma. Robert feels helpless in the face of Luke's pain, which seems to consume his whole being. He asks Luke if there is anything else he can do for him. Luke asks to see the chaplain, although he had not indicated any religion on admission.

LISTENING

Spiritual sensitivity. Assessment of significance of spiritual issues.

Every worker up to a point

Elsie and her family are referred to Mike, the hospital social worker, because of family conflict. Elsie has been a spasmodic church-goer throughout her life but she used to attend the Communion service when she was a day hospice patient and she has expressed regret that she doesn't feel "up to" participating now. Her daughter, Susan, has told nursing staff that her mother's "return to religion" was purely to do with loneliness after her husband's death and they are all better off without a God who allows such suffering. Susan's daughters, Louise and Samantha, are both very close to their grandma and cannot bear the thought that she might die soon. Both girls attend Church parade as Girl Guides and have asked for prayers to be said for their gran. Susan is angry and dismissive of this. Mike begins to see Susan separately, gently untangling with her, feelings of anger and loss. Simultaneously, he arranges for the chaplain to offer communion to Elsie at her bedside and for the church youth worker to talk to Louise and Nicky.

UNDERSTANDING

Spiritual empathy. *Only workers with understanding of own spirituality*

Cathy is a palliative care nurse who works with a young couple, Nicky (who has breast cancer) and Sean and their three-year old son, Liam. Cathy feels that by shouldering some of the practical and physical burden and struggle for the family, the palliative care team gave Sean and Nicky the space to complete emotional and psychological tasks. She describes Nicky as having embarked on her last journey when she entered the hospice, investing ordinary events with new meaning which seemed "almost spiritual," although Cathy says she herself is not religious.

INTERPRETING

Spiritual exploration

Only workers with specialist training or in conjunction with religious professional/spiritual care advisor

Laura is a social worker in a children's hospital who had supported Vicky, a lone mother whose child (Maddie) had a life-limiting condition. After Maddie dies, Laura feels at a loss to deal with Vicky's questions, such as where Maddie is now, and suggests she speak to the chaplain, Phil. When Vicky angrily dismisses this idea, Laura talks to him herself. Phil suggests that she focus with Vicky on those things which help her feel connected to Maddie. This helps to some extent but Vicky returns to questions about the After Life which leave Laura out of her depth. She tells Vicky that that she had found the chaplain friendly and open when she had shared with him her own struggles over Maddy's death. Vicky is struck by this and says she would like to talk to Phil.

Figure 1 The fellow traveller model. (adapted from [20]).

1. Our starting point must be the needs of the person and those around them, to be open to the clues they give about their sources of meaning and spiritual support.

2. We must understand enough about our own spirituality and journey, to be comfortable with that of the other person [47–50].

3. We should neither under-estimate nor over-estimate what we can offer, at any point and for however fleeting a moment.

Research has identified what it is that those healthcare workers who are comfortable engaging in spiritual care say that they do in practice [14, 51]:

- "Being there"
- Helping to find sources of meaning
- Supportive care – "holding a safe nurturing space"
- Empathy and compassion – entering into "weak places"
- Attentive listening
- Sharing the journey
- Sustaining

From this we might conclude that spiritual care is as much about *being* as *doing*. The notion, familiar to palliative care workers, of "sharing the pain" is one such example.

With those principles in mind, there are certain "hooks" or anchors in spiritual care practice.

Box 3:   Sharing the pain

Neil has motor neurone disease and attends the day-care unit in his local hospice. His daughter also has motor neurone disease and is currently an in-patient in the hospice. Gillian is a healthcare assistant on the day-care unit. She and Neil form a special connection built partly around shared memories of having grown up in the same area at the same time, but, most especially, Gillian's daughter, who was the same age as Neil's daughter, had died about a year ago. Neil talks about his fear of dying and shares his deep sorrow, grief, and guilt about his daughter's impending death and frustration that he cannot even hug his wife when she needs comfort, nor articulate his love for his family. Sometimes Gillian just sits with him while he cries, where other people seem to avoid his pain. Just before he dies, he is able to tell his wife that he loves her; she tells Gillian that this was healing for them both.

Transcendence, Transformation, Wholeness, and Hope

Listening to the other person's story of their life, including their spiritual journey (although they may not couch it in traditional religious terms), allows us to reach behind the patient receiving palliative care to the person facing their own death. They may find fresh understanding of who they really are and what is important to them [52]. In recognising this, the carer, "knows that the person lying apparently helpless in the bed, whose medical progress is now termed deterioration, has important inner steps still to take, steps which may sometimes become strides" [30 p. 28].

For me, four concepts underpin the task of supporting the person in their spiritual journey at the end-of-life (Figure 2) (see [20] for a fuller exploration of these).

The notion of *transcendence* carries with it a whiff of "other worldliness," which has led some to bring it down to the mundane and everyday by suggesting that it is about "making the best of things" [53]. Yet spiritual care must be about supporting the person in more than that.

• It may not be possible to change a situation or circumstance, but the problem is *transcended* when it no longer has the painful, negative, or oppressive impact which it did.

• In this process, change or growth takes place within, which is in itself *transformational*.

Suppose, however, that the source of the spiritual pain this person is experiencing lies in a relationship which has broken down, and it may not be possible to repair that relationship – perhaps because the person has died, perhaps because they are not able or willing to forgive. Or it might be a traumatic event of long-lasting impact, which cannot itself be changed. This is where the twin concepts of wholeness and hope come into play.

• A helpful short-hand definition of *hope* comes from a group of mental health service users in an Australian study [54] that no matter how bad things seem, it is possible to hold on to the essential goodness of life.

• That means being able to experience *wholeness*: within myself and in relating to my immediate and wider environment. As one of my research respondents put it, "I've just had to make a whole of all the bits and pieces" [55 p. 304].

When the care-giver is able to facilitate the employment of hope, engender a sense of wholeness and transformational change which allows the dying person to transcend the darkness of their death, they are engaged in "co-creation of a new narrative" [56].

Spirituality and Spiritual Care in Multicultural Context

One of the criticisms of contemporary spiritual care is that it relies on definitions of spirituality derived from research in western, secularised societies; indeed, some have argued that "spiritual but not religious" has no meaning in other world views [58].

Spiritual Needs of Specific Cultural Groups

In addressing this deficit, one approach is to focus on the implications for palliative care of the beliefs and practices of particular groups. The Cicely Saunders Foundation has produced a set of recommendations for spiritual care with Black and Minority Ethnic Groups receiving palliative care [59]. Pointing out that for many of these patients their faith is strengthened during serious illness and that they wish to discuss the implications of their beliefs and spiritual needs with physicians, the report recommends that palliative care services should work in close partnership with local faith communities. There is a need to counter ignorance and discomfort on both sides.

The authors recommend a shared model of spiritual care between palliative care services and local faith groups, which addresses education and training, referral mechanisms, documentation of spiritual well-being in assessments, and provision of a range of spiritual resources

Spiritual Care – 4 concepts

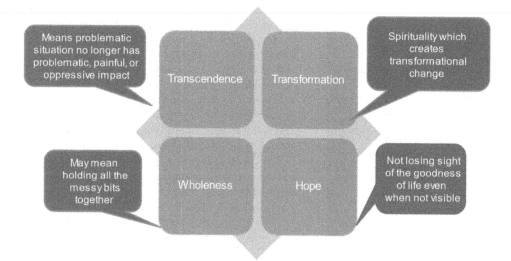

Means problematic situation no longer has problematic, painful, or oppressive impact

Transcendence

Transformation

Spirituality which creates transformational change

May mean holding all the messy bits together

Wholeness

Hope

Not losing sight of the goodness of life even when not visible

Figure 2 Conceptual building blocks of spiritual care [57].

and choice of spiritual care provider. These should be underpinned by culturally specific knowledge and awareness within the palliative care team, including the ability to recognise and explore spiritual beliefs and narratives which are potentially harmful, both to the patient's sense of wellbeing, but also to their ability to make informed choices about treatment.

The relevance of these recommendations can be seen when looking at these examples of research into the needs of specific health groups.

- US Latinos living with cancer were found to have resorted to folk healing traditions for psycho-social-spiritual support because they experienced a lack of cultural fit with formal healthcare, preferring a holistic model which merges religious and health practices [62].
- In a longitudinal study of over 2000 HIV-infected Americans, women, non-whites and older people reported higher levels of religiosity and spirituality; importantly, 72% overall reported that their religious and spiritual identities informed their decision-making [63].

Box 4:   Research into spiritual needs of specific groups

- Among rural older Americans with serious diabetes and declining health, ethnicity was associated with private religious practice, with African Americans having higher levels of private practice than Native Americans, who in turn showed higher levels than white Americans. Public religious participation for all groups declined as their health declined, suggesting that this may result in unmet religious and spiritual needs at the end-of-life [59].
- Lack of understanding among healthcare professionals of the SE Asian practice of burning clothes to provide for the deceased can result in a psychiatric diagnosis [61].
- For devout Muslims, increased spiritual practice is a necessary part of their preparation for death and not simply for comfort [60].

A Transcultural Approach

A broader approach seeks to find points of connection between different faith and belief approaches, variously suggesting that there are universal elements in all religions [22] as well as common themes in how spirituality is understood and experienced [21, 65]. Using listening and empathic skills, the practitioner can thus engage with the unique experience of the other person at the end-of-life, "maintaining the spirit" by relating to the meanings sought and ascribed by them, where one's own traditions and practices may differ [21].

Reminding us that death is difficult across all cultures, an Australian study concluded that an important first step is to establish the "rules of engagement" around discussion of diagnosis and treatment [66]. This may be particularly important for chaplains, who come from a specific religious tradition, but may, in the "caring moment," find themselves ministering to people from a wide range of religious backgrounds and faith, or non-faith positions. For example, healthcare decisions are profoundly influenced by beliefs and values about death and what happens after death, and it is argued that chaplains should use their own experience of weighing the issues to offer comfort, support, and guidance, within the other person's framework of belief – religious or humanistic [30, 65–67]. Assumptions should not be made based on cultural identity alone; a study of Asian medical students from different cultural backgrounds found varying personal narratives despite strong identification with traditional beliefs and rituals [68].

Different emphases may emerge, such as a holistic appreciation of life and death embracing body-mind-spirit [65, 69] and death as transition from the material to the spiritual world [68] in Eastern spiritual approaches, where western perspectives tend towards a more dichotomous approach to life and death, particularly in highly secularised societies [67]. However, the question of "what makes us essentially human" [70] unites and connects across such divides. Perhaps challenging for modern palliative care, is the approach to suffering, which may be viewed as the gateway to a better life or ultimate fulfilment [71] and within which belief framework, it may be important for the person to pass from life to death in a calm and "mindful" state [72]. However, whilst arguing that traditional Buddhism has unique resources to support people who are dying – for example, evidence is put forward for the healing power of sutra chanting [73] – Japanese scholars continue to work on "closing the gap" between traditional Buddhist and modern healthcare as desired by many Buddhist followers today. In so doing they have identified significant accord with elements of the "good death" in western culture, such as achieving reconciliation in relationships, saying goodbye and relinquishing of unnecessary concerns [72]. Likewise, the Federation of Islamic Medical Associations has benchmarked their palliative care services against the mapping undertaken by the World Health Organisation, including of good spiritual care [74].

Conclusion

This chapter has discussed spiritual care at the end-of-life in its multi-faceted complexity and rich diversity. At the same time, the message is simple:

- Spiritual care is not an add-on but an essential part of providing holistic care for the person and their family at the end-of-life;

- It follows, therefore, that all members of the palliative or healthcare team must be able to first, recognise spiritual need and spiritual distress or pain, and second, engage with this aspect of care as far as they are able; in some cases, this will mean referral at a particular point to a more appropriate person to meet these needs;

- Not everyone (patients or staff) comes from a confirmed belief position or adheres to a particular religious faith so we need to understand a broader spirituality and make connections between this within ourselves and within the other person.

There are multiple tools available to assess spiritual need and offer spiritual care and this chapter has presented a range. Despite this, we know that health and social care practitioners can feel confused, inhibited or simply overwhelmed by the challenges of supporting people and their families at the end-of-life, such that spiritual care can seem one thing too much and best left to the spiritual or religious professional. They, in turn, can feel that their own identity may be off-putting for the person from a totally different background and perhaps that their training has not equipped them to bridge this divide. Yet we have looked at how much unites us in our common humanity as we face death. What is most important is that you, the reader, can find in these resources those which resonate with your own understandings and experiences of spirituality and with which you can engage as you travel with the dying person and those close to them. Holistic care is essentially about engaging our whole selves with the whole person in need. It is this, however it is achieved, which lies at the heart of palliative care.

References

1. Connor, S. (ed) (2020). *Global Atlas of Palliative Care*. 2e. Worldwide Hospice Palliative Care Alliance. London, UK. https://urldefense.com/v3/_https://www.thewhpca.org/resources/global-atlas-on-end-of-life-care__.

2. Open Society Foundation. (1998). *Project on Death in America. Report of Activities July 1994 – December 1997*. New York: OPI/PDIA.

3. Chapple, H.S., Bouton, B.L., Chow, A.Y.M. et al. (2017). The body of knowledge in thanatology: an outline. *Death Studies* 41 (2): 118–125.

4. Westminster Health Forum Keynote Seminar. (9 December 2008). *Palliative and End of Life Care*. London: Westminster Health Forum.

5. Kobayashi, R. and McAllister, C.A. (2013). Similarities and differences in perspectives on interdisciplinary collaboration among hospice team members. *American Journal of Hospice & Palliative Care* 31 (8): 1–8.

6. National Association of Social Workers. (2004). *NASW Standards for Palliative and End of Life Care*. Washington: NASW.

7. NHS Education for Scotland. (2009). *Spiritual care matters*. Edinburgh.https://www.nes.scot.nhs.uk/media/23nphas3/spiritualcaremattersfinal.pdf. Accessed 17 Feb 2023.

8. Enguidanos, S.M., Cherin, D., and Brumley, R. (2005). Home-based palliative care study: site of death, and costs of medical care for patients with congestive heart failure, chronic obstructive pulmonary disease, and cancer. *Journal of Social Work in End-of-Life & Palliative Care* 1 (3): 37–55.

9. National End of life Care Programme. (2012). *End of life care coordination: record-keeping guidance*. https://www.bl.uk/collection-items/end-of-life-care-coordination-record-keeping-guidance. Accessed 17 Feb 2023.

10. Krikorian, A., Limonero, J.T., and Maté, J. (2012). Suffering and distress at the end of life. *Psycho-Oncology* 21: 799–808.

11. Scheurich, N. (2003). Reconsidering spirituality and medicine. *Academic Medicine* 78 (4): 356–360.

12. National Council for Palliative Care. (2010). *The Missing Piece: Meeting People's Spiritual Needs in End of Life Care*. London: NCPC.

13. Nolan, S. and Holloway, M. (2013). *A-Z of Spirituality*. Basingstoke: Palgrave Macmillan.

14. Holloway, M., Adamson, S., McSherry, W., and Swinton, J. (2011 online February). *Spiritual care at the end of life: a systematic review of the literature*. https://www.gov.uk/government/publications/spiritual-care-at-the-end-of-life-a-systematic-review-of-the-literature.Accessed 17 Feb 2023.

15. Ross, L. (2006). Spiritual care in nursing: an overview of the research to date. *Journal of Clinical Nursing* 15 (7): 852–862.

16. Taylor, E.J. (2003). Spiritual needs of patients with cancer and family caregivers. *Cancer Nursing* 26: 260–266.

17. Burke, G. (2007). *Spirituality: Roots & Routes. A Secular Reflection on the Practice of Spiritual Care*. London: Age Concern Reports.

18. Stephenson, P.S. and Berry, D.B. (2015). Describing spirituality at the end of life. *Western Journal of Nursing Research* 37 (9): 1229–1247.

19. Gilbert, P. (2011). The spiritual foundation: awareness and context for people's lives today. In: (2007) *Spirituality, Values and Mental Health: Jewels for the Journey* (ed. M.E. Coyte, P. Gilbert, and V. Nicholls). London: Jessica Kingsley.

20. Holloway, M. and Moss, B. (2010). *Spirituality and Social Work*. London: Palgrave Macmillan.

21. Holloway, M. (2006). Death the great leveller? towards a transcultural spirituality of dying and bereavement. *Journal of Clinical Nursing* 15 (7): 833–839.

22. Sutherland, M. (2005). Spirituality and pastoral care in the rapidly changing culture of health care. *Contact* 145: 42–46.

23. Lines, D. (2002). Counseling within a new spiritual paradigm. *Journal of Humanistic Psychology* 42: 102.

24. Muramoto, S. and Hoffman, E. (2005). Humanistic psychology in Japan. *Journal of Humanistic Psychology* 45: 465.

25. Rowson, J. (2014). *Spiritualise: Revitalising Spirituality to Address 21st Century Challenges*. London: Royal Society of Arts.

26. Inall, Y. and Lillie, M. (2020). Meaning and mnemonic in archaeological studies of death. *Mortality* 25 (1): 7–24.

27. Holloway, M., Hukelova, M., and Bailey, L. (2018). *Displaying self: memorialisation in contemporary society*. University of Hull. https://remembermeproject.wordpress.com/ Accessed 17 Feb 2023.

28. Puchalski, C., Ferell, B., Virani, R. et al. (2009). Improving the quality of spiritual care as a dimension of palliative care: the report of the Consensus Conference. *Journal of Palliative Medicine* 12 (10): 885–903.

29. Walter, T. (1997). The ideology and organization of spiritual care: three approaches. *Palliative Medicine* 11 (1): 21–30.

30 Lloyd [Holloway], M. (1995). *Embracing the paradox: pastoral care with dying and bereaved people*. Contact Pastoral Monographs No 5, Contact Pastoral Limited Trust: Edinburgh.

31. Culliford, L. (2011). *The Psychology of Spirituality: An Introduction*. London: Jessica Kingsley.

32. Holloway, M. (2012). Social work. In: *The Textbook of Spirituality in Healthcare* (ed. M. Cobb, C. Puchalski, and B. Rumbold). Oxford: Oxford University Press.

33. European Association for Palliative Care, Spiritual Care Reference Group. *What is spiritual care?* https://www.eapcnet.eu/eapc-groups/reference/spiritual-care (accessed 23 November 2021). 2017.

34. Puchalski, C.M. and Romer, A.L. (2000). Taking a spiritual history allows clinicians to understand patients more fully. *Journal of Palliative Medicine* 3: 129–137.

35. Anandarajah, G. and Hight, E. (2001). Spirituality and medical practice: using the HOPE questions as a practical tool for spiritual assessment. *American Family Physician* 63: 81–89.

36. Burton, R. (2004). Spiritual pain: origins, nature and management. *Contact* 143: 3–13.

37. Holloway, M. (2007). *Negotiating Death in Contemporary Health and Social Care*. Bristol: Policy Press.

38. Parker, M. (2004). Medicalizing meaning: demoralization syndrome and the desire to die. *Australian and New Zealand Journal of Psychiatry* 38: 765–773.

39. Phelps, A., Maciejewski, P., Nilsson, M. et al. (2009). Religious coping and use of intensive life-prolonging care near death in patients with advanced cancer. *Journal of American Medical Association* 301 (11): 1140–1147.

40. Puchalski, C.M., Lunsford, B., and Miller, T. (2006). Interdisciplinary spiritual care for seriously ill and dying patients: a collaborative model. *The Cancer Journal* 12 (5): 398–413.

41. Marie Curie Cancer Care. (2003). *Spiritual & religious care competencies for specialist palliative care*. http://ahpcc.co.uk/wp-content/uploads/2014/07/spiritcomp.pdf Accessed 17 Feb 2023.

42. Hegarty, M. (2007). Care of the spirit that transcends religious, ideological and philosophical boundaries. *Indian Journal of Palliative Care* 13 (2): 42–47.

43. Arnold, E.M., Artin, K.A., Griffith, D. et al. (2007). Unmet needs at the end of life: perceptions of hospice social workers. *Journal of Social Work in End-of-Life & Palliative Care* 2 (4): 61–83.

44. Dane, B. and Moore, R. (2005). Social workers' use of spiritual practices in palliative care. *Journal of Social Work in End-of-Life & Palliative Care* 1 (4): 63–81.

45. Ross, L., McSherry, W., Gisked, T. et al. (2018). Nursing and midwifery students' perceptions of spirituality, spiritual care and spiritual care competency: a prospective, longitudinal, correlational European study. *Nurse Education Today* 67: 64–71.

46. Luckhaupt, S.E., Yi, M.S., Mueller, C.V. et al. (2005). Beliefs of primary care residents regarding spirituality and religion in clinical encounters with patients: a study at a midwestern U.S. teaching institution. *Academic Medicine* 80 (6): 560–570.

47. National End of Life Care Programme. (2011). *Talking about End of Life Care: Right Conversations, Right People, Right Time.* London: Crown Publications.

48. Messikomer, C.M. and De Craemer, W. (2002). The spirituality of academic physicians: an ethnography of a Scripture-based group in an academic medical center. *Academic Medicine* 77 (6): 562–573.

49. Héliot, Y. (2020). *Religious Identity and Working in the NHS.* NHS Employers/University of Surrey.

50. van Otterloo, A., Aupers, S., and Houtman, D. (2012). Trajectories to the New Age. The spiritual turn of the first generation of Dutch New Age teachers. *Social Compass* 59: 239–256.

51. Gilbert, P. (2013). *Spirituality and End of Life Care.* Hove: Pavilion.

52. Stanworth, R. (2004). *Recognizing Spiritual Needs in People Who are Dying.* Oxford: Oxford University Press.

53. Kellehear, A. (2000). Spirituality and palliative care: a model of needs. *Palliative Medicine* 14: 149–155.

54. Jevne, R. (2005). Hope. The simplicity and complexity. In: *Interdisciplinary Perspectives on Hope* (ed. J. Elliott), 259–289. New York: Nova Science.

55. Lloyd [Holloway], M. (1996). Philosophy and religion in the face of death and bereavement. *Journal of Religion and Health* 35 (4): 295–310.

56. Hodge, D. (2000). Spiritual ecomaps: a new diagrammatic tool for assessing marital and family spirituality. *Journal of Marital and Family Therapy* 26 (2): 211–216.

57. Holloway, M. (2015). Spirituality at the sharp end; the challenging world of social work and social care. *Journal for the Study of Spirituality* 4 (2): 121–135.

58. Yip, K. (2005). A dynamic Asian response to globalization in cross-cultural social work. *International Social Work* 48 (5): 593–607.

59. Selman, L., Harding, R., Speck, P. et al. (2010). *Spiritual Care Recommendations for People from Black and Minority Ethnic (BME) Groups Receiving Palliative Care in the UK, with Special Reference to the sub-Saharan African Population.* London: King's College London/Cicely Saunders Foundation.

60. Arcury, T.A., Stafford, J.M., Bell, R.A. et al. (2007). The association of health and functional status with private and public religious practice among rural, ethnically diverse, older adults with diabetes. *The Journal of Rural Health* 23 (3): 246–253.

61. Ow, R. and Saparin, N.H.B. (2014). Malay Muslim Worldviews: some thoughts for social work practice in Singapore. *Journal of Religion & Spirituality in Social Work* 33 (1): 73–94.

62. Bhagwan, R. and Chan, C.L.W. (2014). Indigenous spirituality: an introduction. *Journal of Religion & Spirituality in Social Work* 33 (1): 1–3.

63. Rosario, A.M. and De La Rosa, M. (2014). Santería as informal mental health support among U.S. Latinos with cancer. *Journal of Religion & Spirituality in Social Work* 33 (1): 4–18.

64. Lorenz, K.A., Hays, R.D., Shapiro, M.F. et al. (2005). Religiousness and spirituality among HIV-infected Americans. *Journal of Palliative Medicine* 8 (4): 774–781.

65. Ahmad, W. (2018). Spiritual care at the end of life: western views and Islamic perspectives. *International Journal of Human and Health Sciences* 2 (2): 65–70.

66. Carey, L.B. and Cohen, J. (2008). Religion, spirituality and health care treatment decisions: the role of chaplains in the Australian clinical context. *Journal of Health Care Chaplaincy* 15: 25–39.

67. Ai, A.L. and McCormick, T.R. (2010). Increasing diversity of Americans' faiths alongside baby boomers' aging: implications for chaplain intervention in health settings. *Journal of Health Care Chaplaincy* 16: 24–41.

68. Bharathy, A., Malayapillay, M., and Russell, V. (2013). Crosscultural narratives on death and bereavement among medical students: implications for undergraduate curricula. *International Journal of Medical Education* 4: 68–74.

69. Chan, C.L.W., Ng, S.M., Ho, R.T.H., and Chow, A.Y.M. (2006). East meets West: applying Eastern spirituality in clinical practice. *Journal of Clinical Nursing* 15 (7): 822–832.

70. Kirkland, R. (2008). "Enhancing life?" Perspectives from traditional Chinese value systems. *Journal of Law, Medicine & Ethics*, Spring, 26–40.

71. Department of Health. (2009). *Religion or Belief. A Practical Guide for the NHS.* London: Crown publications.

72. Watts, J.S. and Tomatsu, Y. (eds.) (2012). *Buddhist Care for the Dying and Bereaved.* Boston: Wisdom publications/The Jodu Shu Research Institute.

73. Taniyama, Y. and Becker, C.B. (2014). Religious care by Zen Buddhist monks: a response to criticism of "funeral Buddhism." *Journal of Religion & Spirituality in Social Work* 33 (1): 49–60.

74. Ebrahim, A., Fadel, H. & Mishal, A.(eds).Federation of Islamic Medical Associations. (2016). Medical care at end of life. In: *Encyclopedia of Islamic Medical Ethics – Part III.* Amman-Jordan: Jordan Society for Islamic Medical Sciences.

23 Creating Space, Clarity and Containment in order to Sustain Staff: Managing the Emotional Impact of Palliative Care Work

Barbara Wren

Introduction

Palliative care is concerned with improving the quality of life of patients and their families facing the problems associated with life-limiting illness, through the prevention and relief of suffering. It integrates the psychological, physical, social, cultural, and spiritual aspects of a patient's care, acknowledging and respecting the uniqueness of each patient and their family. While a specialist area, all medicine requires an understanding of the application of palliative care to the relief of suffering in serious illness, and at end-of-life. It can be an immensely rewarding and enriching area within which to work while also posing predictable emotional challenges for the practitioner. Learning to meet these challenges provides a subtle opportunity for healthcare staff to make sense of their own personal relationship to vulnerability, suffering, death and dying, and integrate this understanding into their roles in ways that can increase self-awareness, effectiveness, and impact. The aim of this chapter is to describe how the well-being of palliative care providers can be enhanced by helping both individuals and systems to attend to themselves, and to the contexts and complexity of their work in order to realistically manage its psychological challenges. Psychologically informed interventions will be described along with a consideration of the importance of good role and team design and containing[1] management, to maximise the potential for working in palliative care to be fulfilling and rewarding, while managing its predictable emotional risks and reducing the likelihood of burnout.

The Context of Palliative Care Practice

Working in palliative care involves supporting people at a time when their relationship to themselves, their bodies, their families, and their future is changing in unwanted ways. Fear of pain, disfigurement, decay, loss of control, independence, and dignity, and ultimately loss of life are profound fears we all carry. Being confronted with these experiences will evoke primitive feelings (including the fear of abandonment and annihilation) that practitioners will need to manage in order to carry out their work. Most will have developed defences[2] to protect themselves, however, these can become threatened (at a time of personal

---

[1]Containment is a crucial function of both managers and organisations. It refers to the skill of enabling individual staff and the team to manage their work in a way that connects them effectively to their task while ensuring effective management of emotions at work that enables clinicians to work within role boundaries.

[2]Defenses are strategies people use to separate themselves from unpleasant events, actions, or thoughts to manage psychological threats and unwanted feelings, such as guilt, shame, fear, and helplessness.

Handbook of Palliative Care, Fourth Edition. Edited by Richard Kitchen, Christina Faull, Sarah Russell and Jo Wilson.
© 2024 John Wiley & Sons Ltd. Published 2024 by John Wiley & Sons Ltd.

loss for example, or of overwhelming exposure to death and dying which has been a feature of working in health care during the COVID-19 pandemic). It is in the context of these powerful emotional experiences that palliative care is provided. In addition, the necessary imperative it requires of moving from a curative stance to that of palliation may, for many clinicians, evoke uncomfortable and challenging feelings of vulnerability, helplessness, and impotence. Of course, working in palliative care also provides profound opportunities for experiences of intimacy, and expressions of creativity, tenderness, and love, which are immensely rewarding but pose other challenges. For example, how to work within boundaries, and across multiple contexts, to set limits for oneself and others, and to sensitively navigate the many transitions from intimacy to objectivity and back again, that must occur throughout the progression of an illness, to ensure that its trajectory is managed appropriately over time in the interests of the patient, their family, and the health-care system. Pre-qualification training for doctors, nurses, and allied health professionals' focusses of necessity on content and clinical skills and there is little time to train these relational skills which are key both to the quality of the work and the resilience of staff. Psychological interventions can facilitate the development and deepening of these skills and of practitioner self-awareness and psychological flexibility both of which are the cornerstones of self-care.

The Emotional Complexity in Palliative Care Work

Working in palliative care poses several predictable challenges all of which make psychological demands on practitioners:

• Communicating effectively to be able to sensitively address the complex ethical, psychological, and social issues that arise and ensure that care evolves to meet changing needs of patients and their families as illnesses progress.

• Keeping two contexts in view at the same time: working to maximise well-being, reduce suffering and prolong life while keeping in mind and addressing the realistic possibility of deterioration and death. Helping patients and families to navigate various transitions between these two realities over time.

• Managing uncertainty and supporting patients and family systems to manage uncertainty often indefinitely.

• Providing effective support for those living with advanced illness who are suffering from a complex mix of effects such as fatigue and disability, while navigating painful changes in roles and identities within work and family systems.

• Containing[3] anxiety in patients and families and other health-care professionals while managing complex and sometimes high-risk clinical scenarios.

• Withstanding and addressing anger, aggression, denial, grief, and profound sorrow as individuals and family systems come to terms with the reality of suffering and dying, death, and loss.

• Bearing witness to suffering and making decisions about what level to address and alleviate it as illnesses progress e.g. physical, emotional, cognitive, relational, and/or spiritual.

• Coming to terms with their own vulnerability and making sense of their own relationship to feelings of helplessness, impotence, and fears of "failure" to avoid over-intervention (e.g. surgery with poor chances of significant change for patients, extending chemotherapy to avoid confronting dying, repeated onward referral), unnecessary prolonging of suffering or unhelpful management of hope in patients, family, and health-care systems.

• Managing their own occasional feelings of fear, revulsion, and disgust in response to patient physical deterioration, in order to facilitate patients' acceptance of bodily changes, and help them manage associated feelings of shame, and fears of abandonment.

• Managing natural feelings of tenderness, longing, desire for intimacy, and attachment, evoked by the work in a way that ensures that health professionals stay in role and on task (even though being close to these feelings may fulfil deep needs in the health professionals, both known and unknown, seen and unseen).

• Managing their relationship to their own personal experiences of loss in order to maintain well-being and promote an effective relationship to their role that is underpinned by an awareness of their motivations and their limits, and the limits of the system they are working in. These loss experiences may have drawn them towards this work in ways that they are aware or unaware of and can over time cause difficulties (for themselves and others)

---

[3]Containment: refers to the skill of enabling individual patients and families to safely feel, express and manage the range of emotions evoked by serious illness and dying, in a way that connects them to reality and to their own resources, hopes, and needs, while managing each stage of illness.

without opportunities to acknowledge and understand them. They can also create opportunities for growth if processed in a way that will allow the individual to recalibrate their relationship to work and to their palliative care role.

• Working with complex systems both family, and health and social care systems.

• Working creatively to respond over time to a range of needs, preferences, spiritual belief systems, and cultures.

• Attending sensitively to the uniqueness and newness of each patient's illness experience despite one's own knowledge of an illness' trajectory. Balancing hope and reality by pacing and tailoring information to patients' and families' process of adaptation to progression of an illness and the reality of their predicament.

Navigating this emotional complexity and attending to its relational[4] nature will optimise the potential for positive staff experience. This has benefits for staff but also for patients. Staff experience creates the emotional climate within which patients are cared for and will mediate key aspects of the patient experience including the extent to which patients feel safe, held, and understood, able to manage their anxiety, and to adapt to change over time. A productive relationship with palliative care staff and teams helps patients to relate to their bodies and their ill-health with dignity, control, and realism, and to trust that health-care providers can help them manage hope over time without becoming overwhelmed by fear. This experience has huge potential to realign their relationship to themselves and their illnesses and to cope with the acceptance of realities that will change their futures, their relationships to their bodies, and their families.

Considering the Options

How can we optimise the experience of staff doing palliative care work? This chapter will outline the range of options available from each of the following positions:

Looking inwards: *Individual well-being*
Providing opportunities to develop and maintain a productive relationship to oneself, one's role, job content, and the work system through the development of self-awareness, self-compassion, and psychological flexibility.

Looking outward: *Work design*
Attending to the job, role, and team and how they are managed. Ensuring that the work is well structured, and

that staff feel psychologically safe by building in role clarity, good work design, effective teamwork, and containing management.

The view from above: *Thinking systemically*
Managing the impact of palliative care work in the context of the hospital or community system.

Putting it all together: *Reciprocity and meaning*

Designing psychological interventions in order to connect all three levels above and attend to the importance of working both from the inside out (that is how individuals relate to their role and job content) and the outside in (how the system impacts on individuals and teams). Attending to this meaning and reciprocity when crafting responsive, creative psychological interventions.

Looking Inwards: *Individual Well-being*

Well-being at work is:

> The ability to reach the highest potential possible for the individual, the role, and the organisation. Staff will feel engaged, stretched, and challenged in their work and enjoy growing and learning. They will feel a sense of pride in themselves, their work, and their team. It includes short term emotional outcomes such as levels of happiness and conversely of distress (which will have cognitive and performance consequences), and longer term psychological and physical functioning. It is demonstrated behaviourally by productivity, satisfaction, commitment, and engagement.

A general sense of well-being provides an overall sense of purpose that gives direction and meaning to people's actions at work. People with higher levels of well-being are more likely to interpret events at work positively, deal with other people more constructively, perform better at tasks, react to positive and negative feedback more constructively and learn and solve problems more effectively [1].

Cognitive style (the relationship to oneself)
This is the way in which individuals make sense of what happens to them, their patients, and their work, i.e. how they attribute outcomes, whether they are they optimistic or pessimistic? Do they generalise? Do they catastrophise? What attributions do they make for the reasons why events occur the way they do? How do they relate to themselves? Do they tend to be self-critical, or are they able to be supportive to themselves when they are distressed or under

---

[4]The fact that the quality of the work is dependent on the relationship to oneself, one's colleagues, the patient and their family, and the health-care system.

strain? The concepts of psychological flexibility and self-compassion, two elements of cognitive style, have been used to develop individual and group interventions to improve well-being at work.

Psychological Flexibility

Psychological flexibility is the ability to stay in contact with the present moment regardless of unpleasant thoughts, feelings, and bodily sensations, while choosing one's behaviours based on the situation, personal values, and the palliative care role requirement. It describes the ability to recognize and adapt to various situations; adapt mind sets or behavioural repertoires when necessary, maintain balance among important life domains; and be aware, open, and committed to behaviours that are congruent with deeply held values. In many forms of dysfunction, these flexibility processes are absent [2]. Individuals with greater psychological flexibility are less likely to struggle with unwanted thoughts and feelings, more in touch with present moment experience, and more likely to base actions on values and goals (rather than current internal states). Psychological flexibility has been found to be powerful predictor of absenteeism, and workplace performance [3,4].

Healthy Responses to Negative Events

Health-care work is demanding and difficult. Healthcare contexts are complex, competitive, and under high strain. Negative events at work are inevitable. How do individuals make sense of their negative experiences e.g. tensions with other teams, anxieties about quality of care in different parts of the system, disruptions, and interruptions, disappointment in the outcome of a good referral they have made, worry about the quality of a service they are dependent on, loss, aggression, families in denial, and frightened patients? Can they persevere despite the pain these experiences are causing them? Are they able to understand and make sense of these experiences aside from their own emotional reactions to them in order to reposition their relationship to an individual or part of the health-care system that is causing difficulty in order to do their work effectively? Can they maintain their equilibrium and their ability to work within the limits these difficulties may have revealed? Can they experience sadness, loss, anger, aggression, and frustration without being unduly overwhelmed and at the same time manage to stay in role

and on task?[5] What resources will they need to achieve this? The following is an overview of emotional resources they can draw on.

Self-compassion

Self-compassion entails being warm and understanding towards oneself rather than ignoring pain or attacking oneself with self-criticism at times of suffering, feelings of failure, or being inadequate. Being self-compassionate involves recognizing that being imperfect, failing, and experiencing life difficulties is inevitable, and learning to cultivate ways to be gentle with oneself when confronted with painful experiences [5]. Mindfulness based cognitive therapy (MBCT), developed from Jon Kabat-Zinn's [6] mindfulness-based stress reduction programme, aims to increase self-awareness and thus can positively influence levels of self-compassion. The goal of this approach to become able to see oneself separately from the negative thoughts and moods one is experiencing. Compassion-focused therapy (CFT), developed by Paul Gilbert [7], focuses on the use of compassionate mind training to facilitate the development of self-compassion through connecting to experiences that instil feelings of safety and contentment. All these interventions help healthcare providers develop their self-care resources, enabling them to maintain compassion for themselves while fielding high levels of emotional demands [8].

By creating space to think and to **choose** a response to emotionally difficult experience these interventions may also help palliative care providers avoid the pitfall of internalising system difficulties. That is attributing difficulties solely to themselves and how "good" or "bad" a practitioner they think they are rather than remaining aware of the contributions of system problems e.g. when there are resource limitations, poor communication, or organisational incoherence. Self-compassion creates more space for a realistic appraisal of the reality of what can and cannot be achieved in a work role and work system. This can manage any tendency to reject oneself instead of accepting that painful, unwanted emotions may be being produced by the work and the work system (rather than being a symptom of failure, incompetence, weakness, or innate "badness").

Relationship building abilities

Positive and productive relationships are the second cornerstone of well-being at work. How do individuals connect with others? Are they able to make connections in

---

[5]On task: focused on the palliative care role and what is required of it.

which all parties in a relationship feel heard, understood, and listened to? Do they have a sense of their own impact? Can they establish and manage boundaries in a work relationship that are appropriate for their context and purpose? Can they create a sense of trust in their relationships? Are they able to be sensitive to spoken and unspoken communication and tailor their behaviours accordingly? Are they able to negotiate intimacy and distance, that is to come close enough to palliative care patients to comfort and treat them, and bear witness to their pain and suffering but also to then reposition themselves sensitively (so that a patient or their family do not feel abandoned or criticised) in order to be objective (to revise a treatment plan for example, or make on onward referral or challenge unrealistic hope)?

Emotional Intelligence

Emotional intelligence is the ability to "monitor one's own and others' feelings, to discriminate among them, and to use this information to guide one's thinking and action" [9]. Skills in understanding and managing one's own emotions, as well as noticing emotions in others and responding appropriately and sensitively allow caregivers to manage the relational aspects of providing palliative care. Those higher in emotional intelligence will have greater skills in attending to the meaning of patient and colleague behaviour and responding in a way which is congruent with that meaning and more likely to promote good communication and understanding and ultimately a more positive patient experience.

Sense of Coherence

A sense of coherence describes to the ability to maintain equilibrium at times of difficulty. A sense of coherence helps people to stay well and even able to improve their health despite stressful experiences and situations. Antonovsky [10] described three key components of an individual's sense of coherence. These are:

• Comprehensibility—the cognitive component, that is the ability to understand one's experiences of life and work, and to be understood by others.

• Manageability—the perception that one can manage the situations in which one finds oneself (and to access appropriate help to achieve this if needed)

• Meaningfulness—the sense that in times of adversity life is meaningful enough to find the motivation to continue.

In many ways palliative care is concerned with providing patients and their families with a sense of coherence throughout their illness experience by ensuring that they can relate to it as comprehensible, manageable, and

meaningful, and are able to persevere without despair. In order to provide this sense of containment to distressed patients, health-care providers themselves need a sense of coherence. It can be achieved through a reconnection with fundamental values and beliefs [11–13], through good management, and teamwork. It is enhanced by organisational coherence, and interventions which allow staff to regularly connect to meaning and values and to make sense of their experience of work from several different perspectives.

Problem solving skills

Working in palliative care requires solving problems at several different levels: clinical, relational (patients and colleagues and the wider system), operational, strategic, and at the level of the family system. Problem solving abilities enable health-care staff to assess problems, consider a range of solutions and chose the next step while anticipating consequences both intended and unintended. Systems thinking [14] can be an invaluable addition to problem solving skills allowing clinicians to engage with the complexity of palliative care contexts in order to achieve realistic, joined up solutions for patients and their families. Team meeting, case discussions and presentations, role consultation and coaching can all develop individual and team problem solving skills.

Looking Outward: Work Design

The impact of work stress is determined by the interaction between the person exposed, the skills and resources described above, and the system they work in. We know how to design work roles to minimise negative system impacts and promote healthy working. The six dimensions of work that will impact on well-being are: the relative balance of demands, control and support, the design of the role, relationships with colleagues, and the way in which change is managed [15]. Jobs with high levels of demands but low levels of control and support create the most work strain. High demand jobs with high control and support produce productive challenge, learning, growth, and staff engagement. Managers are often limited in their ability to reduce the level of demands that their staff are exposed to in modern health care and therefore focusing on increasing control and support is important in protecting well-being.

Role clarity

Role clarity is protective of well-being. To be effective an individual at work needs to be clear about their role and their task i.e. what does the role need to achieve for palliative care patients and their families? They need support for the role e.g. ensuring it is well resourced, provided with clarity and well positioned so that all those interacting with a role know its purpose, what it needs, and what it will provide. Both factors increase the likelihood that a role will be taken up with maximum effectiveness and minimum strain. Role clarity also includes knowing where one role ends and other begins, that is clarity about interfaces and interdependencies.

Teamwork

Multi-disciplinary teamwork underpins both good staff and patient experience and is a protection against stress, error, and risk [16]. The cornerstone of good teamwork is clear roles, clear team processes i.e. meetings, opportunities for reflection, and learning. Good management of team and group processes ensure the team remains on task and that the organisation gets what it needs from the team and the team gets what it needs from the organisation. Poor staff experience can be a result of poorly structured and led teamwork, a team with little time to reflect on experience, or to learn and change through this reflection. Team development and team supervision all provide opportunities for teams to process work experiences and have the potential to reduce work strain. Well led and well managed teams can protect staff from toxins in the system.

Management

Managers have a significant impact on the work experience of health-care staff both positive and negative. Various studies have linked poor management style to emotional exhaustion in staff [17]; low job satisfaction and intention to leave [18]. A line manager's behaviour and the culture they create in their team is the biggest influence on an employee's work experience. By improving their management capabilities managers can improve their own well-being as well as that of their team, achieving better results, and benefitting the organisation. The UK CIPD (Chartered Institute of Personnel and Development) have produced a management competency framework which identifies the skills and behaviours of managers that promote good teamwork and protect staff well-being [19]. Good management is containing.

The View from Above: Thinking Systemically

Finally, the well-being of the palliative care provider will be impacted by the network of systems within which the work takes place, the way in which interdependencies and interfaces are managed, and the extent to which the system supports the task of palliative care. Effective working requires the ability to work across contexts and systems with self-awareness and the ability to make sense of and adapt to different system contexts in order to maximise the impact of palliative care work.

Most health-care organisations are primarily focused on patient treatment and recovery. They are fast paced systems under high strain constantly striving to meet patient demands, to survive in a turbulent world and to innovate in response to rapid growth in medical and scientific knowledge (all of which have achieved immeasurably improved outcomes for patients). Medicine has extended the limits of what can be achieved, and hoped-for, in patient outcomes. Patient expectations are high and in Western societies exposure to death, dying, and their rituals is more limited than in previous generations.[6] Acknowledging endings and limits in this context is painful. Denial of limits may profoundly impact the culture of some medical systems with visible and invisible impacts on palliative care providers which need to be attended to in the interests of their well-being, skills development, and the quality of their services. In his book Being Mortal, Atul Gawande writes about how "our ideas about how to deal with our finitude have got the reality wrong."

You don't have to spend much time with the elderly or those with terminal illness to see how often medicine fails the people it is supposed to help. The waning days of our lives are given over to treatments that addle our brains and sap our bodies for a slivers chance of benefit. They are spent in institutions – nursing homes and intensive care units – where regimented, anonymous routines cut us off from all the things that matter to us in life. Our reluctance to honestly examine the experience of ageing and dying has increased the harm we inflict on people and denied them the basic comforts they most need. Lacking a coherent view of how people might live successfully all the way to their very end we have allowed our fates to be controlled by the imperatives of medicine, technology, and strangers. [20, p. 9]

Confronting the limits of treatment is challenging for organisations and their clinicians and may lead to palliative care work being side-lined and devalued in overt or covert ways while the reality of limits and of death are being denied. The potential for organisational splitting (that is working with suffering, dying and death being disconnected and seen as other from the main "business" of a hospital), and for palliative care to be related to, not as an

---

[6]The Covid pandemic has changed some of this and highlighted the need for more and better palliative care provision.

integral part of medicine but a "go to" service when clinicians have run out of options poses immense challenges for palliative care providers in their ability to provide quality care in a timely way. Maintaining the well-being of palliative care providers requires attending to this aspect of the context and creating opportunities for its impact on individuals and teams to be named and explored. As well as addressing the impact of this splitting on the quality and resourcing of palliative care provision, the high burden on practitioners needs to be regularly attended to in the interests of staff well-being.

Putting It All Together: Reciprocity and Meaning

Maintaining the well-being of palliative care providers requires attending to the impact of providing care in these complex contexts. Designing palliative care work to create the conditions for productive, satisfying working is the first step. Then creating psychologically facilitated interventions that support individuals and teams to attend to seen and unseen layers of the work (as described in the section below), and of the system that enables it, will allow them to sustain themselves over time. Making sense of organisational cultures allows for a consideration of how the system is relating to the suffering, dying, and death of all its patients and will enable those providing palliative care to position their roles and their work wisely and with reference to system and individual limits. This increases the likelihood that clinicians can maintain their well-being over time while attending to their patients and to themselves with authenticity. These approaches will all be described in more detail in the following sections.

The work of palliative care is provided in a complex system with many layers of context. The innermost layer is the relationship between the clinician and the patient. What occurs in this relationship will influence a patient's relationship to their illness, their body, and their predicament. The relationship is reciprocal and will also impact on the clinician who will be exposed to profound emotions e.g. anxiety, fear, hope, desperation, sadness, anger, resignation, longing, and rage. The system's ability to support the clinician to withstand strong emotions while translating their experience of this relationship into the design of meaningful palliative care interventions is key to the quality of the work. If the work is well designed and they are well held by the system, then the clinicians' ability to listen to and attend to their patients is sustaining and meaningful not just for patients but for themselves.

Authenticity and Meaning: Maybe Patients and Practitioners Have Similar Needs

One of the challenges of palliative care work is the shift that clinicians must make from "saving lives" to slowing down to attend to patient's needs and bear witness to their suffering. For many, shifting gears can feel threatening, but it is essential. How do palliative care practitioners make sense of what their patients need from them while retaining their equilibrium? Listening closely to patients allows for palliative care to be provided with reference to the meaning and context of an illness and the hoped-for quality of remaining time. Helping clinicians honour and develop their creativity and deepen their ability to pay attention to meaning develops their courage to simply listen [21, 22]. The profound impact on patients of feeling contained and heard by clinicians is immensely rewarding to the clinician and this experience can over time help them manage their fears of impotence and helplessness. *If we can stop and listen, patients tell us what they need.* This allows the task of medicine to be refocused and the work of palliative care to deepen.

In recent years some powerful writing has shared stories of death and dying providing insights into the palliative care patient experience. By describing the realities of their experience patients tell us what they need:

> Yes, I am scared but not all the time. When I was first diagnosed, I was terrified. I had no idea that the body could turn against itself and incubate its own enemy. I had never been seriously ill in my life before: now suddenly here I was face to face with my own mortality. There was a moment when I saw my body in the mirror for the first time. Overnight my own flesh had become alien to me, the saboteur of my hopes and dreams. It was incomprehensible and so frightening. I cried "I can't die," I sobbed "not me. Not now." But I'm used to dying now. It's become ordinary and unremarkable, something everyone does at one time or another. If I am afraid of anything its of dying badly, of getting caught up in some process that prolongs my life unnecessarily. No, there is nothing good about dying. It is sad beyond belief. But it is part of life and there is no escaping it. Once you grasp that fact good things can result. [23, p. 34]

In *When Breath Becomes Air* [24], Dr Paul Kalanathi describes his own attempt to work alongside his oncologist to treat his lung cancer and his hope that she would share his data, give him a prognosis, and treat him like a medical colleague. She did not collude and so he wrote:

> It occurred to me that my relationship to statistics changed as soon as I became one. What patients seek is not scientific

knowledge but existential authenticity. My doctor hadn't given me back my identity. She'd protected my ability to forge a new one. And finally, I knew I would have to. [24, p. 36]

And later in a paragraph that captures the creativity and sensitivity required of those working in palliative care:

The tricky thing about terminal illness is that as you go through it your values are constantly changing. You try to figure out what matters to you and then you keep figuring it out. It felt like someone had taken away my credit card and I was having to learn how to budget. Death may be a one-time event but living with terminal illness is a process. [24, p. 54]

Intervening to Manage the Impact of Palliative Care Work

If we can stop and listen, patients tell us what they need. Interventions to protect staff well-being must model this process and allow palliative care practitioners to stop and listen to themselves and each other. Providing opportunities for staff to move away from their task focus is key. Creating confidence that this is possible without causing them harm or undue anxiety and that they will be able to return to their tasks, intact and able to resume their role, is central to the creation of the safety needed to explore the complex emotional experiences at the heart of palliative care work. Slowing them down and paying close attention to what they say, allows staff to listen to themselves and to begin to risk moving, even temporarily, away from busyness. When we create regular opportunities to pause and listen to staff, stories of their work experience, and its contexts eventually emerge and begin to take shape. Though this takes time, as health-care staff find it easier to listen to and tell their patients' story rather than their own.

Interventions need to be designed to give permission to shift the focus to themselves, to help them find ways to listen and attend to their own experience and to develop their confidence that they can manage the transition out of, and back to, role and task. And then when they have shared the story of their work – or the story of themselves that their relationship to the work reveals – these interventions can help them to make sense of their experiences by considering the levels of context in their stories. For example, their inner worlds and the ways in which they relate to themselves, their relationship to their palliative care role and what drives it, their reciprocal relationship to

their work system and their colleagues, and finally their understanding of how their organisation is relating to the task of palliative care and as a result positioning and impacting on them.

Psychologically informed interventions can be provided at the following levels:

Individual

Clinical supervision, role consultation, and coaching all allow palliative care clinicians to have a space within which to process the impact of their work. Regular facilitated one to one meetings provide an opportunity to explore the meaning of, and relationship to, this work, and over time deepen understanding of self and how to make sense of and manage difficulty. Space can be used to discuss ongoing clinical cases, deepen understanding of a clinician's own impact, address blind spots and make sense of heaviness, tiredness, and stuckness. This happens through understanding the impact of serious illness, group dynamics, and the family system, and exploring why a clinician may find certain cases, patients, and families more difficult and others more rewarding. Complex issues such as caring for a colleague or continuing to work while managing the impact of one's own illness can all be covered in these spaces. Clinical supervision also creates opportunities for a detoxification of aspects of the work and the work system and an externalising of difficulty that can deepen understanding over time of the reciprocal nature of the work and how to understand and manage oneself in relation to its emotional intensity. Processing emotion creates space to think more clearly and return to role refreshed.

Team

Team supervision allows palliative care teams to come together regularly to reflect on the impact of the work both individually and collectively. This has several benefits. Group members have an opportunity to connect to colleagues as a community and develop a sense of how colleagues are feeling and how their experience compares to others. There is a development of a shared understanding of the impact of the work and its contexts and of similarities and differences between team members. Having a clear structure for these sessions and holding them at regular intervals creates a sense of containment, coherence, and connection. Facilitators can explore concepts such as self-compassion and psychological flexibility and relate these to ongoing cases whose impact may be discussed in the group thus deepening participant's understanding of their relationship to themselves, their role, and their work content. The impact of the organisational context and its pressures can be named and noticed and managed and there can be huge relief for participants in having problems externalised. Coping strategies can be explored and shared and the difficulty and meaningfulness of the work can be regularly attended to both normalise difficult feelings as well as to highlight and celebrate the profound contribution palliative care makes to patients and their families. Having a repetitive group structure, for example the same opening and closing exercise, models ways of entering and leaving this non-task space, provides time to settle, and beds down a way of paying attention outside the group: "what has been the most meaningful part of your work this week?" "What was the smallest moment of reward in your day yesterday?" "What has been most challenging since we last met?" are all useful questions for the opening section. Over time if team supervision becomes part of a palliative care service it is hoped that even when immersed in the chaotic, fragmented busyness of a hospital or community service or knee deep in the sorrow or aggression of a patient and their family, the palliative care practitioner has a sense of a space they can safely return to where they will have an opportunity to release the feelings these experiences have evoked without self-censure, judgement, or pressure to "perform," and simply be listened to.

Organisational

Organisational level reflective space creates opportunities for staff in a hospital or community setting to come together at regular intervals to reflect on how they are relating to the suffering, dying, and deaths of their patients. There are several methods that can be used including the use of prepared stories from staff such as in Schwartz Rounds [25], the use of patient stories (for example a patient talking of their experience of terminal illness) and psycho educational sessions where psychologists reflect on common dilemmas and issues in relation to working in this area and there are opportunities for staff to ask questions and share some of their own experiences. Once again, the value is in shifting away from task and towards meaning and creating safety to explore the humanity that makes this difficult work possible. Organisational level space allows a hospital community to observe itself at regular intervals and consider how it is meeting the needs of palliative care patients and this enables individual palliative care staff who attend these sessions to deepen their understanding of how their organisational context may be impacting on their work.

Conclusions

The emotional challenges of working in palliative care are predictable and can be managed. Once the basics are in place (role clarity, good work design, effective multi-disciplinary teamwork, and good management), interventions to protect staff health can help by allowing for the release of deeper emotions that may be evoked by the work but need to be denied to successfully take up the clinical role. The psychological challenge of palliative care work is to stay in touch with meaning, without being overwhelmed by it, while staying in role and on task. Embedding regular psychologically informed interventions that support staff to engage with emotional complexity will allow a slow repetitive process to take hold in which it is hoped that staff will deepen their capacity to attend to meaning and to become more comfortable with witnessing without solving and listening without rescuing. Creating team and organisational spaces that deepen the ability to do this (for colleagues and for oneself), will enhance the ability to do this for patients and increase the likelihood that staff can stay well, do meaningful work, and continue to authentically relate to themselves and their task.

References

1. Robertson, I. and Cooper, C. (2017). *Wellbeing, Productivity and Happiness at Work*, 2e. London: Palgrave Macmillan.
2. Kashdan, T. and Rottenberg, J. (2010). Psychological flexibility as a fundamental aspect of health. *Clinical Psychology Review* 30 (7): 865–878.
3. Bond, F. and Bunce, D. (2003). *Reducing Stress and Improving Performance through Work Reorganization*. BOHRF.
4. Bond, F.W., Flaxman, P.E., and Bunce, D. (2008). The influence of psychological flexibility on work redesign: mediated moderation of a work reorganization intervention. *Journal of Applied Psychology* 93: 645–654.
5. Neff, K. (2003). Self- compassion: an alternative conceptualization of a healthy attitude towards oneself. *Self and Identity* 2.
6. Kabat-Zinn, J. (2018). *The Healing Power of Mindfulness*. London: Piatkus.
7. Gilbert, P. (2010). *The Compassionate Mind*. London: Constable Press.
8. Ballat, J. and Campling, P. (2011). *Intelligent Kindness: Reforming the Culture of Healthcare*. London: The Royal College of Psychiatrists.
9. Goleman, D. (2020). *Emotional Intelligence*. London: Bloomsbury.

10. Antonovsky, A. (1987). *Unraveling the Mystery of Health – How People Manage Stress and Stay Well*. San Francisco: Jossey-Bass Publishers.
11. Fredrickson, B. (1998 September). What good are positive emotions? *Review of General Psychology* 2 (3): 300–3019.
12. Fredrickson, B. and Joiner, J. (2002 March). Positive emotions trigger upward spirals toward emotional wellbeing. *Psychol. Sci.* 13 (2): 172–175.
13. Seligman, H. (2005). Empirical validation of positive psychology interventions. *American Psychologist* 60 (5): 410–421.
14. McCaughan, N. and Palmer, P. (2006). *Systems Thinking for Harassed Managers*. Oxford: Routledge.
15. HSE. (2004). *The stress management standards*. HSE website.
16. Firth Cozens, J. and Harrison, J. (2010). *How to Survive in Medicine*. London: Wiley BMJ books.
17. Michie, S. et al. (1999). *Reducing Work Related Ill-health and Sickness Absence in NHS Staff*. London: Nuffield books.
18. Buttigrecy, S. et al. (2011 November). *Well-structured Teams and the Buffering of Hospital Employees from Stress*. Health Services Management Research.
19. Chartered Institute of Personnel and Development. (1999). Line management behaviour and stress at work. London: CIPD.
20. Gawande, A. (2014). *Being Mortal: Medicine and What Matters in the End*. London: Profile Books.
21. Clarke, R. (2019). *Dear Life*. Great Britain: Little Brown.
22. Mannix, K. (2019 and 2021). *With the End in Mind and Listen*. London: William Collins.
23. Taylor, C. (2017). *Dying: A Memoir*. Edinburgh: Cannongate Books.
24. Kalanathi, P. (2017). *When Breath Becomes Air*. London: Vintage Books.
25. Wren, B. (2016). *True Tales of Organisational Life*. London: Karnac Press.

24 Patient/Individual and Carer Wellbeing

Tes Smith

Introduction

This chapter will focus on the well-being of the individual "patient" and their carers. In order to do that we will firstly, explore the terms "patient" and "carer". For the purpose of consistency, the individual "patient" will be referred to as the "cared for" and carer as "the carer". Implicit in the discussions is that the patient / cared for must always be seen as an individual with a unique set of needs. The impact and complexity of the role of the carer will be explored to enable understanding of their potential needs. There is also a question at times, as to whether someone is a formal or informal carer. It is not as simple as whether someone is paid or not, although that is sometimes a useful way to differentiate. Paid care and thus the carers (from an agency or by way of a personal assistant agreement) are usually accessed through local authority or NHS assessment, care package and allocation of benefit (this is a complex aspect to care and more information can be found on personal health budgets and personal budget information in the helpful sources section). There is a group referred to as "young carers". These are people under the age of 18, who are to be considered for the importance of their caring role and the impact of this on their lives.

It should be recognised that it is hard to be "struggling" or "unwell" in daily life without assistance wherever and however one lives. In the UK, the most people in need can have access to four times a day care provision if they meet the criteria, sometimes 24hr care at home can be funded through continuing health care, though much more rare than it is common place. Unless they privately fund care it is during the "in between times" that it is helpful, and expected, for family and friends step in. For those that live alone, or for those who have no family/friends, this can mean a sudden change to coping, and retaining independence, presenting people with less life choices and indeed at times the need to enter residential/care home settings. In the UK, the care settings available to people at end-of-life usually start with them in their own homes and accessing acute hospital services during diagnosis and treatment phases. As their prognosis changes people then access supportive/palliative care via hospices, care agencies and community services. Hospices provide ongoing care and or access to other services that cannot be accessed via traditional NHS or social care provision, and this can be said of the hospice provision in the United States of America (USA) too. In the UK, some care can be accessed via a perceived seamless NHS service, though in reality people need to pursue care services and or access privately paid support in a robust manner. In the USA this can be insurance led, which also predetermines levels of care accessible. In Europe there are significant variances from country to country and in India and Asia there is a mixed yet developing economy of support outside the hospital process that is apparent in some areas. This is often led by charitable organisations.

There is a well-being approach discussion in the context of palliative and end-of-life care (PEOLC) [1–6] in the UK. Similar approaches worldwide are developed or still being developed in line with the model of care in that area/country. This chapter is UK focused with the supposition that much of the discussion can be adopted in other countries and adapted to the model of care within.

The approach in the UK is that care is offered from referral until the death of the cared for and then moves into bereavement care for the carer. A framework for discussion is provided to form a rapid assessment tool to aid professionals when working with those that come to their service. This framework supports any professional's

Handbook of Palliative Care, Fourth Edition. Edited by Richard Kitchen, Christina Faull, Sarah Russell and Jo Wilson.
© 2024 John Wiley & Sons Ltd. Published 2024 by John Wiley & Sons Ltd.

requirement to identify and assess those that are in need, whether they are the cared for or the carer, at point of entry to any services. There is also a guide for the receiving organisations/professionals to consider.

This chapter considers professions/roles/interventions that can support the cared for and carers. These roles can be within multidisciplinary teams (MDT) or accessed by MDT members by way of referral to teams and organisations. These roles include palliative care social work (PCSW) accessed via hospices; occupational therapy (OT); physiotherapy; complementary therapy (CT) and other therapies; and allied health professionals (AHP) encompassed within the banner of health and well-being support. These professionals can offer strategies, support and advice within the arena of PEOLC, particularly with a focus on supporting carers. This chapter does not have the capacity to address all forms of therapy whether they be mainstream, conventional or alternative; it will, however, highlight a few that are commonly used within the area of PEOLC, in the UK and the USA, with varying availability in other parts of the world. Additionally, case studies from current practice will illustrate the different roles and interventions, concluding with the need to consider carer support after the death of the cared for (all names/identifiable information have been changed). There will also be other sources for help and support available and links to professional associations and national bodies for carers. A discussion about care for the professionals is also outlined as the chapter concludes.

What is a Patient?

The use of the term patient itself is subject to much debate, in that traditionally a medical approach has been to describe people as patients linked to their medical condition. This can manifest in negative ways e.g. '…the MND in bed 13'

This debate began in the 1950's with a book entitled *Patients are people too* and it invited the medical profession to view people as people and *not as a patient with a diagnosis. They also* recognised that "People are not only sick persons … they are single; they are married; they have children as well as hope, aims, and aspirations for the future … for relief from long term illness, but, more important, for independence and personal dignity" [1 p.8].

The debate continues to the present day. Baroness Julia Neuberger asked, "Do we need a new word for patients?" "The word 'patient' conjures up a vision of quiet suffering, of someone lying patiently in a bed waiting for the doctor

to come by and give of his or her skill, and of an unequal relationship between the user of healthcare services and the provider. The user is described simply as suffering, while the healthcare professional has a title, be it nurse or doctor, physiotherapist or phlebotomist." [2 p.1756].

Another view is that of Smith who highlights: "People are often described or labelled as 'patients, clients or service users', this can run the risk of dehumanising the person and potentially lose the essence of person-centered approaches." Smith further suggests complexity of situations must be explored and not assumed in order to understand [3 p.66]. The term "family and carer" will be used interchangeably to describe those who are important to the individual. In these times of complex family structures, it is imperative that workers recognise different "families", lifestyles and choices. It is not appropriate to assume it is the family who will be the carers or who is most important to the individual and this is something that must be checked early on in interactions with the individual [3 p.66–68].

Current experience is that to become the cared for changes so much for an individual, and key to any intervention is the recognition that this position regardless of the term used, be that patient, client, service user, dependent or cared for, is a significant change for that individual and will require time and understanding in order to support their new needs. When someone is facing a life limiting illness, they are essentially facing the fact that their lives will end prematurely and can indicate some need for support. These needs are unique and different for each individual, and this was identified by Kubler-Ross: "the terminally ill patient has very special needs which can be fulfilled if we sit and take time to sit and listen and find out what they are" [4 p.10].

What is a Carer?

In the UK it is recognised that there is a legal requirement to identify and assess the needs of the cared for and of carers [5]. In the USA, many Government programmes allow family members to get paid for caring, and in Europe there are programmes and ways of supporting carers, though often more using formal carers as opposed to support for the family. In Asia, carer support has less recognition, though Carers Worldwide as a charity is starting to make inroads into recognition of this [6]. There is still much work to do to have carers recognised in the same way as the UK and USA. In the UK, many iterations of health and social care legislation (up to the Care Act 2014, updated 2020) articulate that need [7–9]. Additionally,

The National Institute for Health and Care Excellence (NICE) identify the breadth of the legislative requirements: "Healthcare practitioners should be aware of the requirement to offer a carer's needs assessment in line with the Care Act 2014, and a young carer's needs assessment in line with the Children and Families Act 2014." Also, that: "People managing and delivering services should think about what practical and emotional support can be provided to carers of adults approaching the end of their life and review this when needed." Noting that: "When carer's needs are identified, consider that the support needs of a young carer are likely to be different to those of an older carer" [10]. Young carers are those under 18 years of age and the Carers Organisation in the UK estimate 1 in 5 school children are carers [11]. The Health Affairs publication blog in 2017 estimated the number in the USA was over 1 million aged 8–18 years [12]. Carers Worldwide estimated that in India and Nepal 9% of carers were under 17 but believed the number to be much higher in reality [6]. For younger carers particularly, much should be considered as to how their role sits with education, friendships and fun, as the carer role can be at times all consuming.

There is a history of debate as to who and what constitutes being a carer. In the UK now, "A carer is anyone, including children and adults, who look after a family member, partner or friend who needs help because of their illness, frailty, disability, a mental health problem or an addiction and cannot cope without their support. The care they give is unpaid" [13].

For many though it is through an informal route that they became a carer and often through their relationship with the cared for, be it through partner, family, friend or, at times, by default i.e. there is no one else to provide for the individual. It is important to recognise that entering into a carer relationship means that the carer's and cared for becomes a different relationship often with little chance to negotiate or challenge that new aspect to the relationship. "It can be difficult for carers to see their caring role as separate from the relationship they have with the person for whom they care whether that relationship is as a parent, child, sibling, partner, or a friend" [14].

In practice, it is important to recognise what the previous role/relationship was, and how it has now changed for both. The impact can include changes to the dynamics of relationships; position in families and relationship break down; children and young adults becoming the carer as opposed to the usual natural event of being cared for and enabled to develop and grow into adulthood. Children can be identified as "practical" care givers, though not always

seen as carers from a psychological perspective. For example, they can be told they are the reason a person continues to live, or they brighten their day, or the cared for wants to live long enough to see them graduate, marry etc. This role that's given will impact a child further when the person dies and must be acknowledged and worked with. It can also be recognised that this may need revisiting as an issue as the "child" grows older.

The term next of kin (NOK) is used frequently in health and care situations within conversations between families and professionals to "name" a key person, yet in the UK has no legal status. One must also be mindful that carer and NOK are different terms, albeit they may at times be one and the same person, at other times they are not; this distinction is important not least within complex "family dynamics" and caring situations. This distinction is true for all and it is often a mistake by professionals who ask: "Who is your next of kin?", when the questions they should actually ask are for example: "Who is your carer? Who will care for you? Who else should we discuss arrangements with?" Under the Mental Capacity Act it is essential that we identify if there is a Lasting Power of Attorney for Health and Welfare as they represent the individual/patient voice, once the individual has lost mental capacity. This may or may not be the main carer [15].

In groups or families, and especially, where relationships and communications may either tense and/or complicated, it is important to establish who the unpaid carer is as they have legal right to assessment and support. Carers can sometimes feel they are the ones with the right to access patient information, though the individual with mental capacity may wish for another to have a view and represent them. The term NOK, should also not be confused with the role of "nearest relative" under the Mental Health Act, 2007 [16]. This is a legal term, which has responsibilities under this Act. It enables a nominated family member to act on behalf of the individual, when mentally unwell (not incapacitated as per the Mental Capacity Act) and ensure they are being safeguarded under the Mental Health Act https://www.mind.org.uk/ information-support/legal-rights/nearest-relative/about-the-nearest-relative/ [17–20]. The NOK versus carer issue is even more distinct for certain cultures and groups within our communities, in that in some cultures who follow the patriarchal model, for example the eldest son may be the NOK, yet it's the daughter-in-law that may be the carer.

Ultimately becoming, being, and being "classed" as a carer, whether it be formally or informally, is a complex, hard and for some rewarding place to be. Carers UK explain there are currently estimated 6.5 million carers looking after people/the cared for, be this voluntarily or due to the circumstance they find themselves in [11]. Moving from informal to formal carer status is a complex process. Informal carers are often hidden, though formalisation in the UK, i.e. if self-identified and or by a professional, usually mean that one can become recognised through an assessment and payment via the benefit system. The impact on people caring can be a few hours a week or 24 hours a day, and during extreme times such as the recent COVID-19 pandemic, the sense of responsibility can be intense. The mix of isolation, restricted access to usual forms of support and access to the information and advice needed to keep caring is challenging: "Being a carer can be very stressful. Many carers say they experience negative emotions including guilt, resentment, anger, loneliness and depression" [11].

Caring and Being the "Cared For"

The situation of becoming a carer is often unexpected and can be gradual or sudden. The relationship of a care situation can be complex and should always be seen and assessed within its unique set of circumstances. The cared for is already in a compromised unplanned place, in that they need someone to help them whether it be mentally, physically or practically and that can take some adjustment. Also, the question of where they want to be cared for needs understanding. Often it is their wish to remain in their home. This is supported by public policy [21]. That accepted, we also know that the ideas and needs of the individual and those close to them can also at times be at odds and this must be recognised and navigated by those looking to support them.

How to Begin with Wellbeing Support

Wellbeing is essentially achieving a positive outcome that is meaningful for an individual person within their set of circumstances. In wider society it is an often an indicator that encourages a holistic approach to disease prevention, rather than concentrating just on the treatment of disease. The first professional to assess the individual and their carer should be cognisant of the need to take a holistic approach and to establish what is the very specific need of this cared for / carer relationship. Careful and considered conversations need to take place and be repeated/reviewed

as the situation may/will change. Good communication is key to engage and assist those being assessed. However, the ability to get communication right is not easy. We all need to be able to reflect and recognise where we have not connected with the cared for / carer and make further effort to establish rapport.

Experience tells us that initially people will only be able to focus on the now, and then as things progress, they will move to a position of "what if?" or "why?" and ultimately "did I do enough?" after the event. It is important that professionals feel able to have open conversations with the carer and cared for to enable the initiation of support. Some people believe these conversations can take away hope, but it is a rare situation that non-verbal cues do not reveal the actual reality of the situation and future direction for the cared for. Thus the frame for any assessment and intervention should begin by considering the communication approach and articulation of the reality of the situation for both the cared for and the carer. From that starting point this enables an honest commencement as to the needs and shape of the offer of support and ideas as to how the individual and carer may approach the future and management of it. This is the requirement of the first contact the carer and cared for have with professionals, whether it be via the general practitioner (GP), hospital clinic, primary or social care and or sometimes through advice lines. At times people will not know what help they want or need, and it is for the professionals to "spot and guide".

Therefore, the very first questions for any worker approaching an individual with a view to completing a plan of intervention and or assessment should be:

- Who is this person in front of me?
- What are their needs in relation to their condition?
- Who is important to them? [22]
- Do they have mental capacity for the decisions being made?
- How is the person in respect to the Mental Capacity Act – do they have an LPA for health and wellbeing and / or an LPA for finance?

This starting point enables the professional frame their ideas and questions. From that start it is possible to move to a fuller discussion with either the carer, cared for or both depending on who has presented initially for help, and or appears to be struggling. The framework devised in Box 1 is a guide/prompt for professionals at first contact e.g. GPs, hospital clinics, district nurses.

Box 1: A framework for discussion with the individual

Recognise that a carer and cared for situation is present
- Identify who is the carer and cared for (sometimes those that become carers already have their own challenges to manage)
- What was the relationship before?
- Acknowledge what has changed for them both and as individuals
- Identify the timeframe they believe they wish to look at in terms of strategies to cope
- Agree whether they wish to be seen individually or separately
- What currently do they feel they need support with?
- Explore the preferred mechanisms for support
- Do they have any knowledge of practice or interventions that may help? Agree whom the individual would like involved – together or individually
- Agree what level of information should be shared. What language and terminology is going to make most sense to those involved?
- Agree how the next steps in terms of treatment or symptom management or intervention will be accessed
- Identify where they may access this support; hospices are often the place to start as well as other local voluntary sectors
- If a formal care package support is needed refer to the local authority/council for a needs assessment (social care)
- Gain agreement from the carer and cared for to refer to other organisations
- Acknowledge they are important, and it is indeed a very relevant and important outcome for them both that further support be obtained

Box 2: Advice for organisations that receive referrals identifying the need for help and support

- Review the information received with the cared for and carer, separately and together where possible
- Remember that the situation may have changed since referral and/or they may have more questions to ask
- Ascertain what it is that is the biggest area of need for support
- Offer ideas, as sometimes people are not able to identify one issue, as they can be overwhelmed by many
- Look for "physical" cues from the carer (often easier to articulate than saying one is stressed):
  - "I am so tired"
  - "I don't relax"
  - "I've not got much appetite"
  - "I haven't time to …"
  - "I feel lost"
- From the cared for cues could be:
  - "I'm a burden"
  - "I worry about X"
  - "I don't like to ask"
- Ensure time is given to both to explore next steps and what interventions may help them e.g. talking things through and practical steps, to therapeutic interventions via complementary therapy, art, music and others.
- Agree to share the ideas for support, now and for the future. This should include the carer and cared for's preferences for care and who would be the provider of this.
- Ascertain where the carer feels their threshold for care is and are there any barriers, worries or training needs.
- Agree onward referrals to other systems of support for the family and friends if required.
- Agree when the above will be reviewed and discuss the realistic tweaks that can be made as changes to need occur.

For organisations receiving referrals, it can be challenging to identify the priority of needs, as at times carer needs are not identified, just those of the cared for. Box 2 offers further prompts/guidance. Carer needs will require exploration and understanding; at times needs are not always obvious nor are the solutions. In the complex health, social care and voluntary care landscape, another issue may be where to obtain accessible help for individuals. This does require a level of local knowledge and at times trusting that referring to one organisation will result in effective signposting to another if appropriate to meet an identified need.

NICE published the quality standard for EOLC [23], clearly outlining the complexity for those approaching end-of-life and the need to access a range of support and interventions. Further, the start of an assessment can be at whatever point the individual and/or their carer meet services and at times people will need access to different professionals and interventions [10].

The following are brief examples of some of the professionals (other than doctors and nurses) that have a role in supporting the cared for and their carers. This is not a definitive group, rather a focus on a few professionals. These and other relevant UK organisations and links are provided at the end of the chapter.

Physiotherapist

The skill and profession of physiotherapy as part of the MDT also takes a holistic approach that involves the individual patient directly in their own care. They work with the carer to help explain, and at times train them how to work with the cared for and use equipment needed to care safely. Physiotherapists can be accessed within hospital teams and community primary care teams. They are also often included within hospice teams. They too are key to providing a range of interventions to help both the cared for and the carer. Physiotherapy can be helpful for people of all ages with a wide range of health conditions; often other professionals may query how can a physiotherapist work with someone nearing end-of-life or who will not "recover" from their illness.

Case study A: A physiotherapist's perspective

In palliative and end-of-life care practice, a physiotherapist brings both practical and functional help and strategies to the individual. While working with the person and their family/carer, daily functional challenges can be overcome to make life easier and more enjoyable. This is achieved by assessing what they can do and want to do and help them achieve this with advice. Therefore, the physiotherapist can concentrate on what is important to them as they face life limiting illness and end-of-life.

In practice I concentrate on:

- Non-pharmaceutical pain management: passive, assisted or active exercise if the individual can manage this and not fatigue, and use of TENS (transcutaneous electrical nerve stimulation) machine.
- Comfortable positioning in bed/chair (if person can be supported to sit out of bed). This will include positioning and support with cushions and pillows or with sleep system (where the individual has been assessed for this and if available).
- Maintaining good airway and chest management for chest infection and breathlessness management.
- Use of manual therapies techniques where appropriate.

Physiotherapy professionals support people to live within their new optimum/way of living and have many ways to assist with symptom control and showing new ways to do everyday tasks, as well as keeping the body in the best shape it can be as it deals with the illness within. Manual therapy is one of the techniques utilised in PEOLC, rarely available in mainstream NHS services, and hospices are a real source of expertise in this technique (Figure 1).

Social Worker

Social workers are multi-skilled registered professionals who can access support following an assessment via the local (social care) authority. They are located in many settings and have different roles according to the organisation within which they are employed. In the case of PEOLC, many hospices have palliative care social workers as key members of the Multi-Disciplinary Team (MDT). Many commentators have defined the role of the social worker [25–32]. In the UK the Association of Palliative Care Social workers articulate the role as: "Palliative care social workers are registered social workers that work predominantly or exclusively with people living with terminal illnesses. Social work is core to palliative care. With the other multi-disciplinary professional team surrounding the person and those important to them, the social worker ensures that services and interventions take account of the whole person as well as their family, whatever that means for them" [33]. PCSWs are further represented by European and International Associations.

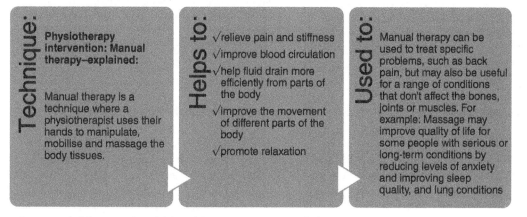

Figure 1 Manual therapy explained (adapted from NHS 2021 – Manual therapy [24]).

The social worker role is one that will support the carer and cared for. At times they will work individually and at times together. They are often proficient in counselling skills and enable acceptance pre and post bereavement, as well as enabling support with practical and psychosocial aspects faced by the carer and cared for. The case study below articulates a typical PCSW intervention and outcome for a carer and cared for:

Case study B: Carers' intervention – social worker:

I worked with M (69 yrs) for 18 months before her husband (P) died. She was referred for carers support as she was struggling in her caring role. P had a chronic health condition, so M had been caring for him for a long time. She was weary, worn out, frustrated and angry.

I supported her to get an increase in P's care package through liaising with Social Care, and to secure a sitting service so M could go out and socialise. I also referred her for complementary therapy to improve her well-being.

As we worked together, we explored her grief emotions around the loss of her husband's health, their future together and her change of role from wife to nurse, as she perceived it. I helped her to develop coping mechanisms as well as giving her permission to consider her needs. During the pandemic to weekly telephone support. Her feelings of isolation intensified. My calls were her only outlet for her feelings.

In the last month of life, P experienced a lot of pain. I enabled M to voice her helplessness and distress. Through liaising with my nursing colleagues at the hospice I empowered M to gain confidence in managing P's new symptoms at home.

At this point M needed to talk through her feelings for P, the negative feelings she had experienced towards him during the times he had been very demanding and unkind to her. My work was in helping M to become aware that as a carer she just needed to be good enough and not perfect.

On reflection, the value of my social work with M, lay in the fact that I was consistent through the whole process, created a safe place for her to explore her situation and was able to deal with the practical issues of caring which arose.

such things as being able to go outside, and have the room set up for maximal family engagement. Again, many hospices will employ and have access to OT support. Those in turn will have relationships with primary care and social care OTs to ensure seamless communications and access to services. The National End-Of-Life Care Programme 2011 was one of the first publications to articulate their role in relation to the role in achieving good quality EOLC, citing: "Occupational therapists' core skills and knowledge mean they are well placed to drive delivery of high-quality person-centred end-of-life care, … through: Effective communication and holistic assessment skills [34 p.14].

A case study illustrates the role and impact further:

Case study C: Occupational Therapy (OT) role and practice

I recently completed some breathlessness management intervention with a man who had a diagnosis of Motor Neurone Disease (MND). He was aware that MND presents differently in people and that the symptoms can vary in presentation and speed of how they affect people. The fear of breathlessness and not being able to get your breath is a real and all-consuming fear. He was very anxious about his breathlessness, resulting in even more reliance upon his wife for emotional and physical support. This was placing a strain on their marriage and increasing the carer "burden" felt by his wife. They both described this worry and increased pressure on them and that it was taking over their lives.

I completed a breathlessness management session. This was specifically designed to educate him regarding techniques to manage his breathlessness and reduce anxiety. I was able to also show and demonstrate the techniques with the wife so she could support and reassure effectively when they were alone.

Reflecting on my intervention, I believe that if we can empower people to become experts in their own condition and self-manage their symptoms, it reduces their reliance upon caregivers and restores their relationships to the usual status quo of husband and wife, as opposed to one spouse taking a caring role.

Occupational Therapist

The role of occupational therapy (OT) in PEOLC can at times be misunderstood. As OT is assumed to be for getting people well and concentrating on rehabilitation, the role of the OT at end-of-life can be a challenge. However, meaning and activity are vital to ensuring the well-being of the "cared for "as they die and occupational therapy is vital in achieving

Complementary Therapy (CT)

The title complementary suggests the belief that interventions that come under this umbrella are complementary to mainstream health interventions [13]. The list of interventions that this relates to is as well as, or instead of mainstream medical interventions and includes practitioners that may be professionally regulated or meet practice standards agreed by the professional standards authority [13]. It is often the case that those that practice within the role (paid staff, or more commonly volunteers in the hospice sector) within the PEOLC arena are trained in several interventions, which they can draw on when working with, cared for and their carers.

A personal reflection as a complementary therapist of working in palliative care: "Having worked in a variety of clinical settings, I can honestly say that in palliative care, true integrated care happens routinely. The attitude towards complementary therapy is refreshing – that of acceptance and openness to the role that it can play in the management of symptoms. Each role within the MDT brings a wealth of knowledge and ideas – when these disciplines communicate and collaborate like they do in the hospice setting, the patient benefits from true holistic care" [35].

connected to certain organs and body systems. Reflexologists believe that applying pressure to these parts offers a range of health benefits. There are not many studies on the medical benefits; a study in 2014 [36], cited no benefits at all to reflexology and medical conditions in the way of physiological and biochemical outcomes. Conversely a study conducted in 2011 did identify some benefit with pain management in woman with breast cancer [37].

As with any intervention be it words, hands on therapeutic intervention or experienced advice, if an individual/carer takes some comfort and indeed some positive impact from the intervention, it is worth its application. The following is a case study illustrating the benefits a carer can receive from reflexology.

Case study D: Complementary intervention – hand massage

I visited an elderly gentleman in the community with advanced Alzheimer's, being cared for, predominately, in bed by his wife. Every evening he would experience "sun downing" and became restless, agitated and confused. At this time of the day, his wife was also exhausted and becoming more disconnected from her husband. The complementary therapy intervention was a hand massage with a prescriptive cream made with essential oils of Lavender and Melissa. We also made this the last visit of the day to relax him close to the time he would become restless.

After the first visit, his wife reported that he settled quicker in the evening, with less frequent episodes of calling out and longer periods of sleep. However, these were short lived and by the following day, the agitation and restlessness were back. When we returned, we showed his wife how to perform the simple hand massage and provided regular blends of hand cream with Lavender and Melissa essential oils. The simple act of the massage combined with the therapeutic qualities of the essential oils was calming, even more so when done by his loved one. His wife felt useful, connected and empowered to manage these difficult episodes. They both enjoyed the simple act of gentle and comforting touch, improving the quality of time spent together.

Reflexology

Reflexology is a type of massage that involves applying different amounts of pressure to the feet, hands, and ears. It is based on a theory that these body parts are

Case study E: Complementary therapy intervention – Reflexology

This case study relates to a lady, in her fifties, caring for her husband with cancer and a short prognosis. She was experiencing anxiety and insomnia. She reluctantly accepted a visit, concerned she would be taking the appointment from someone who needed it more. Reassured that by supporting carers, we were supporting the patients, her husband had declined.

On my first visit, I explained therapies and let her choose – the rationale being that any therapy which enabled her to relax would be of benefit. She chose reflexology. During the first session, she found it hard to relax and just wanted to talk. Her husband would usually be upstairs and unwilling to engage. During that first therapy session she asked many questions about the hospice. She feared what the future held, and particularly whether she would be able to cope with her husband dying at home. They had two grown up daughters, one at university, the other in a nearby assisted living facility with learning disabilities. She was concerned the girls wouldn't cope with their dad's deterioration. Her husband refused help and she felt overwhelmed at the thought of what was to come.

I saw her weekly; each time concentrating on reflexes, helping balance her emotionally and physically. Whilst gently working her feet, we would discuss the things that were bothering her – this conversation was always led by her. I reassured her about the role of the hospice and the emphasis on symptom control and quality of life. I encouraged her to visit. We discussed the support that was available to her and her daughters and the services that they could access for advice and support. By session three, she gave me permission to refer & session four, we were still making progress with her sleep and mood.

Over time, the periods of silence during the sessions became longer and she relaxed. She reported that immediately after her reflexology sessions she slept better. She was felt calmer and more optimistic that she could cope. My last visit was emotional – she was very grateful for the reflexology. I reassured that she could contact us at any time for support. During a follow up call a few weeks after the last session, she confirmed they had visited the hospice and they were surprised at how lovely it was there. Her husband died a few months later at home, but the family had the full support of the hospice. The reflexology helped with her anxiety and improved her sleeping, but mainly, I think that the sessions helped her to be less fearful of the hospice.

Reiki

A hospice complementary therapist, explains below her understanding, and also the impact she has seen in practice:

"Reiki is a Japanese therapy used for the reduction of stress and relaxation. Based on the idea that we are all made of a universal energy and when energy is low, we are more likely to feel unwell, experiencing symptoms like pain or anxiety. During a session, the therapist uses their hands and channels more energy to the person, where it is utilised by the body wherever needed. It requires no special equipment and works alongside other therapies or conventional interventions to improve wellbeing. It supports the whole person physically emotionally, mentally and spiritually. Anecdotally, Reiki can be a comfort, relieving pain, decreasing anxiety and improving quality of life in a non-invasive way. Many people report feeling very calm, peaceful and may experience pleasant sensations of warmth and tingling. It is very common for people to report better sleep" (personal communication)[36].

The Reiki principles incorporate the mindset "just for today", which means being present. Reiki practitioners are often asked to provide Reiki when patients are nearing the end of their life. Reiki won't stop a person from dying, but it can help them to find peace and acceptance in the process. Agitation, restlessness and distress are not uncommon in someone who is actively dying. Being present with that person, sending positive, loving and compassionate intention (energy) can often help them to settle. Usually it's those individuals who have received Reiki whilst relatively well who request it when they are nearing death. If the person is too unwell to request it

themselves, their family may request it. They too get comfort from knowing that their loved one is receiving something in their final days that they have found so comforting in the past."

Through this time of the COVID-19 pandemic the team have also tried distance Reiki with some success which again will need more study and understanding.

Case study F: Reiki in practice

I worked with a cared for / carer couple in the community. Both of whom were retired nurses. The carer was a wife and was caring for her husband who had dementia and brain injury following several strokes. He was for the most part non-verbal and bedbound. We initially received a referral due to issues with the husband sleeping and settling at night, and provided a blend of oils to help. I offered reiki initially for support for the carer – she could receive it at home and since it's just a short 15-minute session, should not detract from her caring for her husband. She was keen but felt it should be her husband who received it, so I encouraged them both to try it. Recently, the husband's brother had died from COVID – they were a very close-knit loving family – his wife had tried to explain this to him, but he had not acknowledged it. She was very saddened by this and felt that she was grieving largely on her own for the loss of her brother-in-law. During the first reiki session, the husband was very peaceful – in fact they felt that he had mainly slept through it, but when he woke, he asked after his brother. His wife explained that he had died, and they both cried together. She is convinced that the reiki helped him to understand, to respond appropriately, release emotions and allowed them to be together in that moment of grief together.

Other Forms of Therapy

As people are complex, it would be expected that not one approach will fit all. There is a range of therapeutic approaches that have emerged and the application of many is sometimes less understood than the "conventional" roles of talking therapy and physical therapies. However, there is often access to several different therapies ether by way of volunteers and/or students (less so paid roles currently). Regulation is queried at times for the lesser-known therapies; anyone who refers to themselves for example as an art therapist, drama-therapist or music therapist in the UK must be registered with the Health and Care Professions Council (HCPC).

The range of therapeutic interventions are increasingly recognised as a form of communication and release for many emotions. For music therapy, we can often link a song or piece of music to a significant event. Most recently, many of us saw the moving video of the dancer living with dementia reacting to a familiar piece of music and still enacting the dance moves. It was Prima Ballerina: Marta C. González, first dancer of the New York Ballet in the 1960's, with Alzheimer's listening to Swan Lake and as the music plays, she starts to enact the dance moves still retained within her memory [38].

Music therapy can be useful: "(It) aligns to the holistic approach to palliative and end-of-life care (PEOLC), with an emergent evidence base reporting positive effect on a range of health-related outcomes for both patient and family carer alongside high client demand. However, the current service provision and the role of music therapists in supporting individuals receiving PEOLC in the UK is currently unknown" [39]. The provision in the UK is not consistent, yet more and more it is recognised as an effective therapeutic intervention/strategy and has many uses for both the carer and cared for in my experience, professionally and personally.

Art Therapy

Another lesser understood therapeutic intervention which is described by the British Association of Art Therapists, on line: "Art therapy is a form of psychotherapy that uses art media as its primary mode of expression and communication. Within this context, art is not used as diagnostic tool but as a medium to address emotional issues which may be confusing and distressing" [40]. They further explain its application is broad: "Art therapists work with children, young people, adults and the elderly. Clients may have a wide range of difficulties, disabilities or diagnoses. These include emotional, behavioural or mental health problems, learning or physical disabilities, life-limiting conditions, neurological conditions and physical illnesses" [41].

> ### Case Study G: Art therapy in practice
>
> I first met C (10), in August 2020 for an online assessment after receiving a referral from her mother who had contacted the Hospice. C's mother was concerned for her daughter's mental health after the death of her grand-

mother. Her grandmother died from cancer at their home in July under the care of the hospice. Her mother described how C had found it difficult to talk about how she was feeling: anxious, unhappy and withdrawn. We organised an online assessment session as coronavirus restrictions meant that face to face assessments and sessions could not take place.

The initial assessment with C to see how she was coping and to see if art therapy would be a beneficial and appropriate therapy for her. I also needed to determine if online sessions would be suitable for her.

She had a lot of unanswered questions, expressed a great deal of mixed and confused feelings. C voiced a love for art and was eager to ask about what art therapy entailed which I explained to her. It seemed that art therapy would benefit C in being able to think about her grandmother, share her memories, feelings and begin to process what had happened at her own pace.

In C's next few sessions, she decorated a memory box which she enjoyed doing, containing her feelings as well as her memories. Each image represented a memory, this supported her in talking about how she was feeling and began to help her process her loss. She symbolized her grandmother in the colours she used, and the flowers she painted. She illustrated their relationship, the loss she felt, her love for her grandmother, her family, culture, and faith, which is especially important to her and her family. This helped her feel validated and excepted. She filled the box with photos and treasures that her grandmother had given her which not only made her feel connected to her grandmother but assisted her in processing some raw emotions.

Working with Children

When we consider work with children this will be in many forms either as a care recipient, as a carer, or pre- or post-bereavement. All therapies have a contribution to make. There is much anecdotal evidence and discussion about addressing and supporting a child's experience showing is vital to enable them to have good mental health as adults. It is of course important to ensure close working with the GP, parents and the young person and that all consent and understand the boundaries associated with support and interventions.

Experience and stress will present in different forms and the skill of the practitioner will enable the right approach to be taken as the following case study demonstrates.

Case study H: Child therapy in practice

I initially met A, when her mother contacted the hospice. A had presented with severe anxiety two years after her grandmother had died at the hospice. Mum was worried by the severity of distress her daughter was experiencing, which she immediately connected to the loss of her beloved grandmother. A, who was then 16, was very anxious at the prospect of our appointments.

After several sessions, I was able to share my concerns with A – that she was presenting aspects of what is commonly called Obsessive-Compulsive Disorder (OCD). A described how she was experiencing increased anxiety and feelings of danger. These and other symptoms had troubled A since grandma's death.

I referred to theories about recovery from trauma to gain an insight into the impact and details of trauma and reading body language as a symptom of difficult experiences. A's behavioural patterns showed she found it difficult to concentrate at school and found little comfort in socialising with friends.

Emotions that may be seen in a child during this stage of grief:

Anger: I couldn't save my grandma! Why couldn't I help her? *Fear/Nerves*: I feel terrorised by what I saw! What if I get sick? Who will help me? *Therapeutic model*: A presented the symptoms of OCD common to those suffering post-traumatic stress disorder, therefore, my work with her is informed by Attachment Theory: A was very attached to her grandma.

With the restrictions of COVID, the lockdown has changed the nature of our work. We have continued our sessions online using video calling. This approach has been very successful, and A checks in with me on a weekly or on an ad hoc basis. I also maintained contact with her mother, whilst upholding the ethical framework of confidentiality. School closures during the COVID disruptions has offered us the opportunity to reflect on many aspects of A's life – many difficulties brought on by the lockdown period have been aired and shared.

A has also been offered uninterrupted counselling through the year. Online sessions outside of school hours and, therefore, have proved manageable and beneficial. A continues with her schoolwork and hopes to attend university.

Care after Death

This is an area that can be forgotten for carer's support; much focus and support is provided while they are active carers to enable them to continue to care. Once the cared for dies, that brings another dynamic of loss and grief for carers. This is again a complexity of emotion; for some they struggle with a mixture of grief and loss for the person who has died, relief at the end of the loved one's situation and the demands of being a carer, and for some the loss of the role of being a carer. They need to learn how to define themselves again whilst managing so many practical tasks at times and again the loss of the individual. Breen et al highlights this particular issue and suggests the need for: "…palliative care services to support family caregivers while caring and after the death, including those with normal grief. Palliative care services are moving towards harnessing a suite of strategies to meet the varied support needs of caregivers' pre-death. These strategies have benefits pre- and post-death, but we should not overlook the importance of post-death" [41 p.50].

Case Study I: A carers reflection: Before and after...

For two years: everyday had been focused on how mum was, wondering whether she would have a good or bad day, and would she end up in hospital again. Her condition was very unusual and required a lot of explanation and understanding though ultimately, she would die – we didn't know when. I worked and each day visited Mum and Dad at home – to help Dad keep caring and to support Mum. On the occasions she ended up in hospital I drove to the hospital each night and brought Dad home at the end of each day. Essentially every waking hour was managing the situation and as the final weeks barreled down on us – none of us were prepared. This was still incomprehensible – Mum the center, the essence of what we knew as us as a family was going to leave.

When she did die at home, nurses came as they said *they* wanted to have closure and say goodbye to her, collect equipment and sign off paperwork. No one thought to ask my Dad or I …"Were we ok? Would we cope? Did we need anything?" … was it that medically the job was done; the "patient" had died? For us in many ways it had just started … now we weren't carers anymore … we were adrift in a heart rendering place none of us wanted to be in nor sure how to do it – it was hard.

Many years on I reflected – what would have helped at that time? A kind word, a check in, an acknowledgement – even weeks later maybe… Perhaps this is why I have felt so passionately about carers support and ensure in practice we don't forget them after death…

And then: my father too came towards the end of his life, and the focus became all-consuming to be his carer and provide him with all he needed. He died 19 years later to the day of my mum's death, cared for at home by me, with the help of others. My experience this time was different – leading up to his death many of the professionals checked in with me to ask how I was doing and did I need anything.

After his death I received care and compassion and recognition of my loss as a daughter and a carer – a comfort and a welcome acknowledgement at a time of such pain, sadness and loss. I mattered – it mattered; I am grateful to those professionals who recognised that.

In practice, many hospices, hospitals and voluntary organisations offer bereavement support for carers in several forms: 1:1 counselling, group therapy and some offer a carer's lunch each year in which people are still acknowledged as a carer following the death of their cared for.

Caring for and Supervision of the Professionals Providing Care

In order to provide compassionate and meaningful care, staff and volunteers need to be looked after too in terms of supervision and development. Continuing professional development (CPD), lifelong learning, management supervision and appraisal process underpin the delivery of all the functions within an effective MDT and the delivery of high-quality services.

It is important that organisations provide a framework for all employees, inclusive of professional practitioners to explore discuss and examine their role, task completion and practice in a safe and supportive environment. Also to ensure that management and clinical supervision is accounted for in the support offered (Figures 2 and 3).

For many organisations in the UK there can now be a climate of what is described as management supervision as opposed to clinical supervision, or a combination of the two with some additional peer support mechanisms.

The message is look after practitioners and volunteers and ensure they have appropriate support mechanisms and the appropriate level of supervision for their role. They in turn can and will deliver great care and support for those in need.

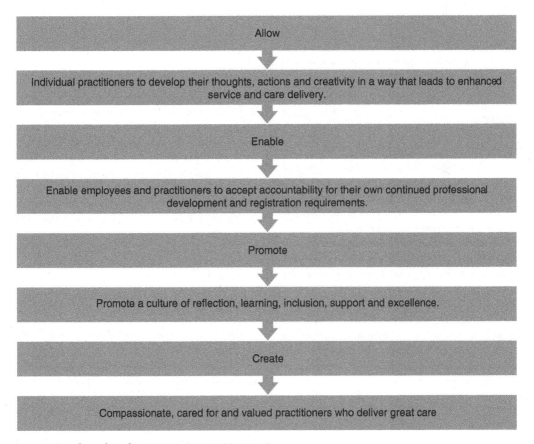

Figure 2 Regular and timely management supervision matrix.

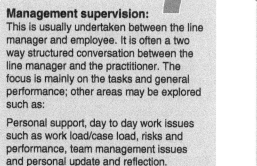

Management supervision:
This is usually undertaken between the line manager and employee. It is often a two way structured conversation between the line manager and the practitioner. The focus is mainly on the tasks and general performance; other areas may be explored such as:

Personal support, day to day work issues such as work load/case load, risks and performance, team management issues and personal update and reflection.

Issues such as priorities, balance of workload, levels of competence, and levels of training/CPD may also be incorporated in this form of management supervision.

'Clinical/professional' supervision:
Usually in the UK, professional registration required supervision. This is a formal process of support and learning in which individual practitioners are facilitated through self-reflection, either individually or in a group, with professional supervisors who can provide support, education and management functions, in meeting the needs of the supervisees in their continued professional development. This ensures compliance with regulatory bodies, professional standards and competencies are maintained and incorporated into the organisation

Figure 3 Management supervision vs clinical/professional supervision.

Summary

In summary, the complexity associated with being the carer or cared for is undeniably broad. Thus, the need for careful identification, listening, assessing and supporting in the right way is paramount. As each circumstance is unique to the carer and cared for, the access to a range of interventions to enable positive support is clear.

Early assessments and listening will help identify what the individual in the scenario will benefit from initially. It is important to remember the need to check and review and adapt approaches as circumstances change.

The use of the skills within the MDT and well-being therapists is essential to provide interventions that enable the carer to keep caring if that's their wish, and for the cared for to be assured their needs will still be met and their carer also looked after. It is vital this care continues after the "cared for" has died.

Personally and professionally one can perceive the carer role differently. For me, as articulated in Case Study I, it is through caring for my mum at end-of-life and more recently supporting my dad too, which showed me the

difference one can experience as a professional and a daughter. Most importantly the need to know someone is there to help you – that you matter, when you need it most as a carer is crucial.

The reasons a person becomes the cared for or the carer pale into insignificance for the carer, once trying to get through each day becomes the challenge. To adapt the idea in the "starfish story", we can't help all carers, but we can make a difference to one and/or those we can – our role is to help them do that when they cross our professional paths and organisations [42].

Acknowledgements

The author is currently Director of Services at Saint Francis Hospice, near Romford.

I am grateful for the support of the organisation to write this chapter and to have the space to develop the information contained within the boxes and images in the chapter based on my own professional and personal experiences. Also the case studies and personal reflections of some of the Therapies and Well-Being practitioners at

Saint Francis. They have provided insight and up to date case studies and applications of some of therapies mentioned here. My thanks go to them and colleagues for their hard work, commitment and passion, they all make such an impact on people and the work highlighted within really is a drop in the ocean of all they achieve. That is extended to all those working to improve peoples' journeys.

Finally, I am grateful for the gift my parents, Professor David and Margaret Smith, gave me by trusting me to be their carer as their lives came to an end, what we were to each other we are still. They were hard and emotional roller coasters, but ones I took on gladly and learnt so much from, and now I can share with others to help us all to be aware, compassionate and empathetic to the role of the carer.

With thanks to the following for their case studies:

Briony Townshend, palliative care social worker; Claire Smart, occupational therapist; Christine A Ezediuno, senior physiotherapist; Klaire Craven, complementary therapist; Emily Gray, child and family therapist, and art therapist; Stella Christou child and family therapist, counsellor

Referencing support: Brigid Hardy, business manager.

Sources of Further Information and Support:

- Bereavement Advice Centre – Information for Professionals https://www.bereavementadvice.org/topics/what-to-do-when-someone-dies/step-by-stepchecklist
- Dying Matters – Understanding death and dying https://www.dyingmatters.org/page/resources-understanding-death-and-dying
- Health Education England – Learning Hub (registration for access required) https://learninghub.nhs.uk
- Marie Curie – End-of-life care resource: providing care after death https://www.mariecurie.org.uk/professionals/palliative-care-knowledge-zone/finaldays/care-after-death
- NHS Education for Scotland – Support around death (SAD) https://www.sad.scot.nhs.uk

- Our Frontline – Mental Health at Work support by phone or text https://www.mentalhealthatwork.org.uk/ourfrontline
- Personal health budgets: https://www.nhs.uk/nhs-services/help-with-health-costs/what-is-a-personal-health-budget
- Personal budget(social care): https://www.nhs.uk/conditions/social-care-and-support-guide/money-work-and-benefits/personal-budgets
- RCN – conducting courageous conversations by telephone
- RCN – End-of-life care
- RCN – promoting wellbeing in the workforce https://www.rcn.org.uk/library/Subject-Guides/wellbeing-self-care-and-resilience
- Skills for Care – End-of-life care https://www.rcn.org.uk/library/Subject-Guides/wellbeing-self-care-and-resilience

National End-of-Life Programme route to success series:

- NEOLCP (2010a) *Holistic Common Assessment.* [on line] Available at: http://www.swscn.org.uk/wp/wp-content/uploads/2015/07/holistic-assessment.pdf
- NEOLCP (2010b) *Supporting people to live and die well a framework for social care at the end-of-life.* [on line] Available at: https://endoflifecareambitions.org.uk/wp-content/uploads/2016/09/supporting-people-to-live-and-die-well_summary.pdf, accessed January 2021
- NEOLCP (2011) *The route to success in end-of-life care –achieving quality for people with learning disabilities.* [online] Available at: https://www.england.nhs.uk/improvement-hub/wp-content/uploads/sites/44/2017/11/End-of-Life-Care-Route-to-Success-learning-disabilities.pdf, accessed December 2021
- NEOLCP The route to success in end-of-life care – Achieving quality for occupational therapy. Available on line: https://www.england.nhs.uk/improvement-hub/wp-content/uploads/sites/44/2017/11/End-of-Life-Care-Route-to-Success-Occupational-Therapy.pdf Accessed December 2021
- NEOLCP (2012) *The route to success in end-of-life care – achieving quality for lesbian, gay, bisexual and transgender people.* [on line] Available at: https://www.macmillan.org.uk/documents/aboutus/health_professionals/endoflifecarelgbtroutetosuccess.pdf, accessed December 2020
- NEOLCP (2012b) *The route to success in end-of-life care – achieving quality for social work.*

- [on line] Available at: https://www.england.nhs.uk/improvement-hub/wp-content/uploads/sites/44/2017/11/route-to-success-social-work.pdf. accessed January 2013. AND https://www.england.nhs.uk/improvement-hub/wp-content/uploads/sites/44/2017/11/route-to-success-social-work.pdf, accessed December 2020

Organisations providing information and support for carers, on line:

Carers Trust www.carers.org
Carers UK www.carersuk.org
Carers Direct www.nhs.uk/carersdirect

Therapy organisations and professional bodies

- Association for Dance Movement Psychotherapy UK https://admp.org.uk/
- Professional body for dance movement psychotherapists. Provides information about dance movement therapy and a register of accredited therapists.
- British Association of Art Therapists 020 7686 4216 https://baat.org
- Professional body for visual art therapists. Provides information about art therapy and a register of accredited therapists.
- British Association of Dramatherapists 01242 235 515 https://baat.org/art-therapy/what-is-art-therapy/ Professional body for dramatherapists (provides information about dramatherapy and a register of accredited therapists).
- British Association for Music Therapy 020 7837 6100 info@bamt.org bamt.org (Professional body for music therapists).
- Health and Care Professions Council (HCPC) 0300 500 6184 https://www.bamt.org/ Regulates some types of health professionals including art, drama and music therapists.
- The National Institute for Health and Care Excellence (NICE) https://www.hcpc-uk.org/ Information and clinical guidelines on recommended treatments for different conditions.

Worldwide resources (on line):

www.Usa.gov/disability-caregiver
https://www.usa.gov/disability-caregiver
www.Carersworldwide.org
www.carersuk.org

References

1. Field, M. (1958). *Patients are People*, 2e. New York: Columbia Press.
2. Neuberger, J. (1999). Do we need a new word for patients? lets do away with "patients". *BMJ* 318 (7200): 1756–1757.
3. Smith, T., Hayes, A. et al. (2013). *Pathways through Care at the End of Life: A Guide to Person-Centred Care*. Jessica Kingsley Publishers. (Chapters 2 & 3).
4. Kubler-Ross, E. (1970). *On Death and Dying*. London: Routledge.
5. Assessment Process for carers under the Care Act Available at: https://www.disabilityrightsuk.org/assessment-process-carers-under-care-act (accessed January 2022).
6. Carers Worldwide Available at: https://carersworldwide.org (accessed February 2022).
7. Department of Health (2008). *The End of Life Care Strategy*. London: DH.
8. Department of Health and Social Care (2010) Recognised, valued and supported: Next steps for the carers strategy. Available at: https://www.gov.uk/government/publications/recognised-valued-and-supported-next-steps-for-the-carers-strategy (accessed August 2020).
9. Department of Health and Social Care (2020). Care act 2014 – updated. Available at: https://www.gov.uk/government/publications/care-act-statutory-guidance/list-of-changes-made-to-the-care-act-guidance (accessed January 2021).
10. NICE (2019). End of life care for adults: service delivery. Available at: www.nice.org.uk/guidance/ng142 (accessed January 2022).
11. Carers UK Available at: https://www.carersuk.org (accessed January 2021).
12. Remler, D.K., Korenman, S.D., and Hyson, R.T. (2017). Estimating the effects of health insurance and other social programs on poverty under the affordable care act. *Health Affairs* 36 (10): 1828–1837.
13. NHS Commissioning (2020). Who is considered a carer? Available at: https://www.england.nhs.uk/commissioning/comm-carers/carers (accessed September 2020).
14. NHS (2021). Complementary and alternative medicine, guidance. Available at: https://www.nhs.uk/conditions/complementary-and-alternative-medicine (accessed January 2021).

15. MIND.org.uk. Available at: https://www.mind.org.uk/information-support/legal-rights/mental-capacity-act-2005/overview (accessed December 2021).

16. National End of Life Care Programme (2013). Available at: https://ehospice.com/uk_posts/supporting-people-to-live-and-die-well-social-care-at-the-end-of-life (accessed January 2022).

17. MIND.org.uk. Available at: https://www.mind.org.uk/information-support/legal-rights/nearest-relative/about-the-nearest-relative (accessed January 2022).

18. National End of Life Care Programme (2012). The route to success in end of life care – Achieving quality for occupational therapy. Available at: https://www.england.nhs.uk/improvement-hub/wp-content/uploads/sites/44/2017/11/End-of-Life-Care-Route-to-Success-Occupational-Therapy.pdf (accessed December 2020).

19. National End of Life Care Programme (2013). The route to success in end of life care – achieving quality for lesbian, gay, bisexual and transgender people. Available at: https://www.macmillan.org.uk/documents/aboutus/health_professionals/endoflifecare-lgbtroutetosuccess.pdf (accessed December 2020).

20. National End of Life Care Programme (2012). The route to success in end of life care – achieving quality for social work. Available at: https://www.england.nhs.uk/improvement-hub/wp-content/uploads/sites/44/2017/11/route-to-success-social-work.pdf (accessed December 2021).

21. NHS. Palliative and End of Life Care. Available at: https://www.england.nhs.uk/eolc (accessed January 2021).

22 Smith, T., Hayes, A. et al. (2013). *Pathways through Care at the End of Life: A Guide to Person-Centred Care*. Jessica Kingsley Publishers. (Page 67).

23. NICE (2011, updated 2017) Quality standard for end of life care. Available at: https://www.nice.org.uk/guidance/qs13 (accessed January 2021).

24. Manual therapy explained (adapted from NHS 2021 – Manual therapy) Available at: https://www.nhs.uk/conditions/physiotherapy/how-it-works (accessed January 2021).

25. Oliver, D. (ed.) (2012). *End of Life Care in Neurological Disease*. London: Springer. (Chapter 1, p 1-19).

26. Payne, M. (2007). Know your colleagues – role of social work in end of life care. *End of Life Care* 1 (1): 69–73.

27. Payne, M. (2012) Palliative care social work competencies: they need to show social work is social. [Blog] Available at: https://documento.mx/documents/palliative-social-work-competencies-5c1180b9afd3e (accessed January 2012).

28. Pierson, J. (2011). *Understanding Social Work – History and Context*. Berkshire: McGraw with Open University Press.

29. Reith, M. and Payne, M. (2009). *Social Work in End of Life and Palliative Care*. Bristol: Policy Press.

30. Rand, S., Vadean, F., and Forder, J. (2020). The impact of social care services on carers' quality of life. *International Journal of Care Caring* 4 (2): 235–259.

31. Sheldon, F. (1997). *Psychosocial Palliative Care*. Cheltenham: Stanley Thornes.

32. Sheldon, F. (2000). Dimensions of the role of the social worker in palliative care. *Palliative Medicine* 14: 491–498.

33. Association of Palliative Care Social Workers Available at: https://www.apcsw.org.uk (accessed January 2021).

34. Department of Health (2011). End of life care strategy – third annual report. Available at: https://assets.publishing.service.gov.uk/government/uploads/system/uploads/attachment_data/file/213730/dh_130570.pdf (accessed February 2022).

35. Craven, K. (2021). Personal communication.

36. McCullough, J., Liddle, S., Sinclair, M. et al. (2014). The physiological and biochemical outcomes associated with a reflexology treatment: a systematic review. *Evidence-Based Complementary and Alternative Medicine* 2014 Article ID 502123: 16. doi: 10.1155/2014/502123.

37. Sikorskii, A., Wyatt, G.K., Siddiqi, A.E., and Tamkus, D. (2011). Recruitment and early retention of women with advanced breast cancer in a complementary and alternative medicine trial. *Evidence-Based Complement and Alternative Medicine* 734517: doi: 10.1093/ecam/nep051.

38. YouTube (2020). Marta Gonzalez former Prima Ballerina with Alzheimer's. [Video]. Available from: https://www.youtube.com/watch?v=hsLLXY_wZYI (accessed 20 December 2020).

39. Cedar, S., White, M., and Atwal, A. (2018). The efficacy of complementary therapy for patients receiving palliative cancer care. *International Journal of Palliative Nursing* 24 (3): 146–151. doi: 10.12968/ijpn.2018.24.3.146.

40. BAAT British association of art therapists. what is art therapy? [On line] Available at: https://baat.org (accessed January 2022).

41. Breen, L., Aoun, S., O'Connor, M. et al. (2020). Effect of caregiving at end of life on grief, quality of life and general health: a prospective, longitudinal, comparative study. *Palliative Medicine* 34 (1): 145–154.

42. "The Star Thrower" (1996). from The Unexpected Universe by Loren Eiseley. Copyright © 1968 by Loren Eiseley and renewed 1996 by John A. Eichman, III.

Index

Note: Page numbers followed by *f* refer to figures and *t* refer to tables.